The Comparative Anatomy and Histology of the Cerebellum from Monotremes through Apes

The Comparative Anatomy and Histology of the CEREBELLUM *from Monotremes through Apes*

---

by

OLOF LARSELL, Ph.D.

edited by JAN JANSEN, M.D.

THE UNIVERSITY OF MINNESOTA PRESS, MINNEAPOLIS

Publication of this book was aided by a grant from the National Institute of Neurological Diseases and Blindness of the United States Public Health Service (grant NB 06794-01).

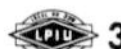 3

Library of Congress Catalog Card Number: 67-19421

ISBN 0-8166-0576-9

PUBLISHED IN GREAT BRITAIN, INDIA, AND PAKISTAN BY THE OXFORD UNIVERSITY PRESS, LONDON, BOMBAY, AND KARACHI, AND IN CANADA BY THE COPP CLARK PUBLISHING CO. LIMITED, TORONTO

PREFACE

THE first volume on myxinoids through birds of Olof Larsell's monograph, *The Comparative Anatomy and Histology of the Cerebellum*, was published in 1967. This second volume gives a comprehensive account of the morphogenesis and the morphology of the mammalian cerebellum from monotremes through apes. Originally Dr. Larsell planned to include the cerebellum of man in this volume and after his death, when I undertook to see the work through publication, I at first expected to follow his outline. But, so much material had been assembled that it appeared preferable to reserve the description of the human cerebellum for a third volume. Chapters on cerebellar connections and the cerebellar cortex, its histology and ultrastructure, will be included in the final volume.

In presenting the second volume of the monograph it appears appropriate to quote from Dr. Heinrich Klüver's Foreword to *The Vertebrate Visual System* by Stephan Polyak: "While it is true that we now live in an age abounding in 'functional' and 'dynamic' approaches, such approaches again and again appear to demand a return to 'form' and 'structure.' " In the text as well as in the illustrations of this monograph Dr. Larsell carries forward the best traditions of classical morphology. I am convinced that his work will meet the demand for a return to form and structure as a basis for future research in neuroanatomy and neurophysiology.

References to some recent contributions to the main topic of this volume have been added; otherwise I have made very few changes in Dr. Larsell's manuscript. Most of the illustrations that Dr. Larsell had planned (some finished, others half-finished or merely sketched) have been included.

The Bibliography bears testimony to Dr. Larsell's desire to acknowledge and do justice to the contributions of fellow scientists. Great efforts have been made to identify all references in Dr. Larsell's manuscript but unfortunately some remain unidentified. Even so I hope the Bibliography will prove a reliable guide to the literature on the development and morphology of the mammalian cerebellum.

It is a pleasure to acknowledge the helpful cooperation of a number of collaborators.

First I wish to express my sincerest appreciation to Dr. Robert S. Dow, whose initiative, constant efforts, and encouragement have made possible the publication of Dr. Larsell's monumental work.

My secretary, Mrs. Agnes Holter, rendered invaluable technical assistance in preparing the manuscript and considerably eased the burden of proofreading. Her help is acknowledged with deep gratitude. I also wish to thank Mrs. Maybelle Romig for her excellent secretarial assistance in the earlier stages of this work.

Mrs. Clarence Ashworth Francone, of the University of Oregon Medical School, prepared most of the illustrations. Some were made by Mrs. Inger Grøholt, of the Anatomical Institute, University of Oslo. I am greatly indebted to both these skilled artists.

Finally, I wish to express my appreciation to the entire staff of the University of Minnesota Press for their skillful handling of all technical and typographical matters.

JAN JANSEN
Anatomical Institute
University of Oslo, Norway

Oslo, November 1968

CONTENTS

The Comparative Anatomy and Histology of the Cerebellum from Monotremes through Apes

INTRODUCTION

AFTER descriptions of the human cerebellum by Malacarne (1776, 1780), Reil (1807–8), and other anatomists of the early nineteenth century, the attention of researchers was directed to the organ in subhuman mammals. Tiedemann (1821) published figures of the brain, including the cerebellum, of the lion, simians, and other mammals, and Rosenthal (1831) described the cerebellum of the seal. Huschke (1854) compared the cerebellum of man with that of mammals and, although he was writing in the pre-Darwinian period, he emphasized the comparative approach for an understanding of the organ. Bolk (1906, p. 26) commented that it was strange that Huschke's views attracted so little attention since they were the first to indicate the importance of the comparative approach which is the path that anatomical research has come to follow without allowing itself to be influenced by current schemes of cerebellar architecture based on the human cerebellum. Brief descriptions and beautiful illustrations of the cerebellum of the horse, ox, spider monkey, and other mammals were published by Leuret and Gratiolet (1839–57). Murie (1874) described the cerebellum of the sea lion and Ganser (1882) and Krause (1884) included this organ in their accounts of the brain of the mole and the rabbit, respectively. Other authors described the cerebellum of various mammals and man: Guldberg (1885) described the cerebellum in the whale and Loewe (1880) described it in man and various mammals. Stilling (1864–67, 1878) made a detailed study of the human cerebellum including a description of its nuclei to which Henle (1871, 1879) added important observations. Schwalbe (1881) and others divided the human cerebellum into various sections, and the lobules and fissures of the organ in man were analyzed in great detail by Ziehen (1903) who also described the cerebellum of a number of other mammals. Earlier this author (1897, 1901) had described it in the spiny anteater, *Echidna*,* and in *Ornithorhynchus*. Flatau and Jacobsohn (1899) attempted to homologize the lobules of the cerebellum in a series of mammals, including apes, in terms of the human cerebellum, and Ärnbäck–Christie–Linde (1900) called attention to the simple pattern of lobules and fissures in the cerebellum of shrews and small bats.

Fragmentary descriptions of the embryonic cerebellum were made by a number of early authors. Wenzel and Wenzel (1812) contributed observations on the organ in human and mammalian embryos, and Bollinger (1814) included the cerebellum in his description of the development of the human brain. Serres (1824–27) stated that the cerebellum appears during the seventh week in the human embryo and in the sixth day of incubation in the chick. According to the description, it is formed by the appearance of two laminae that come to rest against each other at the midline, which later gradually fuse and then fold so that transverse fissures appear in increasing numbers. According to Tiedemann (1816) a small thin plate arises from each side of the medulla oblongata at the beginning of the second month in the human embryo; these plates turn medially and rest against each other but do not fuse until later. Krishaber (1865) and Callender (1874) also dealt with the cerebellum in descriptions of the developing human brain. The cerebellum was divided by His (1874) into a middle part (vermis), formed in the median part of the brain tube, and two lateral parts, the hemispheres, that appear later. Mihalkovics (1877) described an expanded lamella which arches over the rhomboidal fossa and is separated by a constriction from the roof of the midbrain ventricle; it becomes thinner caudally and merges with

*The spiny anteater is referred to throughout this volume as *Echidna* or *Echidna aculeata*; however, the current preferred taxonomic classification is *Tachyglossus aculeatus*.

the tela of the rhomboidal fossa. He also recognized the paired cerebellar rudiments. About the same time, Alix (1877) and Koelliker (1879) described the developing cerebellum.

In a study of histogenesis of the cerebellum of rodents and reptiles Herrick (1891) observed a zone of cell proliferation at the lateral angle of the fourth ventricle which he regarded as having great significance in the development of the organ.

While the observations of many of the earlier authors cited above pointed to a bilateral origin of the cerebellum, others considered it unpaired at an early stage. Stroud (1895) studied the development of the organ in many stages of cat and human embryos and some stages of the pig and showed that it develops from bilateral alar plates that fuse across the midline, above the fourth ventricle, and by further growth form a median cerebellar mass.

Although the importance of comparative anatomy in the study of the cerebellum had been emphasized by many authors, no constant feature common to all mammalian cerebella had been made clear until Kuithan (1894, 1895), in sheep and human embryos, and Stroud (1895), in embryos of the cat and man, described a deep and universally present fissure which Kuithan called the sulcus primarius and Stroud named the sulcus furcalis. Both authors thought this fissure divides the cerebellum into anterior and posterior major divisions. Stroud carried his comparisons to a considerable number of adult cerebella of other species and relegated the deep sulcus horizontalis magnus of the adult human cerebellum to a subordinate position morphologically.

Stroud, in addition, made the important discovery that the laterorostral projection from the inferior posterior part of the cerebellum of the cat is divisible into two parts, separated by a fissure which he called the floccular sulcus. The ventral and smaller division, which Stroud called the flocculus, was considered to be homologous with the human flocculus; the dorsal and larger division was named paraflocculus and was subdivided into superior and medial or inferior parts. A fissure separating the paraflocculus from the main mass of the hemisphere was named the parafloccular sulcus. Although this sulcus was described as appearing before the floccular sulcus, some of Stroud's figures show the latter at earlier embryonic stages. Kuithan did not recognize the morphological importance of the paraflocculus, which he called the vermis lateralis in the sheep. The significance of Stroud's discovery of the paraflocculus for an understanding of the comparative anatomy of the cerebellum "can hardly be overstated" as Bradley commented in 1903. Stroud emphasized the importance of the embryonic approach for an understanding of cerebellar morphology. Subsequently he (1897) reported briefly on the adult cerebellum of a number of primates.

On the basis of studies of the brains of a large number of mammals, including representatives of virtually all orders, and embryonic stages of many species, G. E. Smith (1902, 1903a, 1903b, 1903c, 1903d) divided the cerebellum into lobus anticus, lobus medius, and lobus posticus. The anterior and medial lobes are separated by the fissura prima of this author, corresponding to the sulcus primarius of Kuithan and the sulcus furcalis of Stroud. The medial and posterior lobes are separated by a furrow appearing later which was called the fissura secunda by G. E. Smith. The posterior lobe is subdivided into the uvula and nodulus by the postnodular fissure which G. E. Smith (1903b, p. 370) recognized as the most precocious, although it is the shallowest, of the three early vermal fissures. It had been mentioned as the earliest furrow in some of his previous contributions. The paraflocculus was subdivided into dorsal and ventral limbs, corresponding to the superior and inferior or medial parts of Stroud. Part of the ventral limb (ventral paraflocculus) was described as forming a petrosal lobule which, in all primates except the anthropoid apes and man, was said to be lodged in a fossa of the petrous part of the temporal bone. Although G. E. Smith recognized that the paraflocculus and the much smaller flocculus are formed independently of each other, he nevertheless grouped them together as the "lobulus flocculi." In view of many of his clear illustrations of the lobules and fissures in the posterior part of the cerebellum, especially in some of the marsupials, it is strange that a greater distinction was not made between the nodulus and flocculus, on the one hand, and the paraflocculus and its vermal connections, on the other hand.

Bradley (1903, 1904, 1905) emphasized the need of extensive embryological studies in combination with comparative studies of the adult cerebellum in order to establish a sound basis for homologizing the cerebellar lobes and fissures. After extensive investigations on developmental stages of the rabbit, pig, sheep, ox, horse, and man, and on the adult cerebellum of a large number and variety of species, he divided the cerebellum into five transverse lobes, each including both median and lateral (hemispheral) parts. Some but not all of these lobes were subdivided by Bradley so that nine transverse segments are delimited by fissures of varying depth; the deepest of these, called fissure II, corresponds to the sulcus primarius of Kuithan, the sulcus furcalis of Stroud, and the fissura prima of G. E. Smith. Fissure IV of Bradley, which was the first fissure to appear in rabbit and pig embryos and is manifested early in the sheep, corresponds to the postnodular fissure of G. E. Smith. It is followed by the eventually much deeper fissure II; accordingly, the sequence is the same as that described by G. E. Smith. Lobe E of Bradley, corresponding to the nodulus, was shown to be continuous with the flocculus on either side; the entire transverse segment thus formed is delimited from lobule D by fissure IV and its lateral continuations. Bradley's (1904) generalized diagram of the mammalian cerebellum shows his lobule D subdivided into two transverse segments by his fissure *d*. This corresponds to the fissura secunda of G. E. Smith, although Bradley regarded it as a secondary furrow. The median (vermal) part of the lobe was divided into D_1 (pyramis) and D_2 (uvula); fissure *d* extends into the parafloccular part of lobe D, which results in a dorsal and a ventral paraflocculus. These are continuous with each other around the end of the fissure, as also illustrated by G. E. Smith (1903c). Fissure III of Bradley in the pig and other ungulates which have a complex pattern of vermal folia corresponds to the suprapyramidal fissure of G. E. Smith (prepyramidal fissure of more recent terminology). The fissure labeled III in Bradley's figures of the rabbit, rat, and some other species corresponds to the fissura secunda of G. E. Smith.

Bolk (1906) sought to establish a pattern of the cerebellar subdivisions which could be applied to all mammals. His studies were based entirely on adult cerebella except for a series on human embryos. The cerebellum of the primitive primate, *Lemur albifrons*, was selected as representing the typical subdivisions in simple form and the lobules were given descriptive names.

After comparing the relative development of the corresponding lobules in other species of various sizes and body forms with the muscular development of these species Bolk suggested a somatotopic functional localization in the cerebellum with reference to different parts of the body. His proposals led to experiments by van Rijnberk (1908) and others to determine the physiological effects of ablations of various parts of the cerebellum. These and other experimental studies on cerebellar localization have been reviewed by Dow and Moruzzi (1958).

The cerebellum was divided by Bolk into anterior and posterior lobes separated by the fissura primaria (fissura prima of G. E. Smith). The lobus medius and lobus posticus of G. E. Smith were not regarded as primary divisions because the fissura secunda does not extend onto the lateral surface of the organ but was described as confluent with various fissures in different species. On the basis of the primary medullary rays the anterior lobe was divided into lobuli 1–4; in many species lobulus 4 was subdivided into 4A and 4B. In the horse five distinct lobules were illustrated.

The four lobuli of Bolk were regarded as corresponding to the lingula, the lobulus centralis, and the culmen of the human cerebellum. Bolk (1906, p. 77) stated that he had been unable to decide whether the lobulus centralis or the lingula in man corresponds to his lobulus 1, but he favored the lingula. He did not name the fissures delimiting the lobules of the anterior lobe; in his illustrations, however, the furrow between his lobuli 3 and 4 corresponds to the preculminate fissure of the rat, cat, monkey, and human embryos. Lobuli 1, 2, and 3 of Bolk correspond, respectively, to lobules I, II, and III as I defined them in the rat (1952), cat and monkey (1953a), and pig (1954). Lobulus 4 of Bolk corresponds to the culmen which I subdivided into lobules IV and V.

Ariens Kappers, Huber and Crosby (1936), and Jansen (1954), using Roman numeral designations, identified the lingula with lobule I and the central lobule with lobule II, and assigned lobules III and IV to the culmen. Other authors appeared to regard both lobuli 1 and 2 of Bolk as included in the lingula.

The differences of interpretation are rooted in the identity of the preculminate fissure of man and mammals and the variability of the ventral part of the anterior lobe in man. These features of the cerebellum of mammals and man will be discussed in subsequent sections. At this point it is necessary to anticipate the detailed evidence pertaining to the human lingula and simply state that developmentally it is not a single morphological lobule but corresponds, in various degrees of atrophic development, to lobules I and II of the rat and other subanthropoids. Whether restricted to lobule I or also including lobule II, the lingula appears to be functionally related to the tail. In man the atrophy of these two lobules appears to be correlated with the loss of the tail and the modification of the basal tail muscles into elements of the pelvic diaphragm. In the following descriptions of the morphological development and adult pattern of the lobules and fissures in the rat and in other species, the functional factors will be taken into consideration.

The posterior lobe of Bolk is composed of an "unpaired" lobulus simplex, immediately behind the fissura prima; an unpaired lobulus medianus posterior; and paired hemispheral divisions called lobulus ansiformis, lobulus paramedianus, and formatio vermicularis. The lobulus simplex, as described by Bolk, extends from one side to the other of the posterior lobe. The lobulus medianus posterior comprises lobuli *a* (nodulus), *b* (uvula), and *c*. Lobulus *c* was divided in some species into c_1 (pyramis) and c_2, corresponding to the tuber vermis, folium cacuminis (folium vermis), and declive of man – the latter corresponds to the median part of the lobulus simplex.

The uvulonodular fissure, corresponding to the postnodular fissure of G. E. Smith, separates lobuli *a* and *b*; the fissura secunda separates lobuli *b* and c_1; and the prepyramidal fissure separates lobulus c_1 from c_2.

The hemispheral subdivisions of the posterior part of the cerebellum, according to Bolk, are independent of the vermal subdivisions and are separated from them by a deep paramedian fissure. The ansiform lobule is subdivided into crus I and crus II. There is no distinct boundary between the ansiform and paramedian lobules in many species and some authors have called the two lobules, together, the ansoparamedian lobule.

The formatio vermicularis of Bolk, separated from the principal mass of the hemisphere by the parafloccular fissure, includes a pars tonsillaris, pars circumcludens, lobulus petrosus, and pars floccularis. The ascending limb, or crus circumcludens of the formatio, was described as corresponding to the dorsal paraflocculus of Bradley and G. E. Smith, while the descending limb corresponds to the ventral paraflocculus. The flocculus is smaller and more laterally situated on the surface of the brachium pontis. Bolk misinterpreted the vermal relations of the subdivisions of his formatio vermicularis. The parafloccular lobe and flocculus of Riley (1929), which together correspond to Bolk's formatio vermicularis, were indicated by Riley as connected, respectively, with lobuli *b* and c_1 and lobulus *a* of Bolk.

Edinger (1910) and Comolli (1910) divided the mammalian cerebellum into the paleocerebellum and the neocerebellum. As described and diagrammatically illustrated by Edinger, the organ was divided into anterior, medial, and posterior transverse lobes. The anterior lobe, corresponding to the anterior lobe of G. E. Smith and other authors, is limited posteriorly by the sulcus primarius anterior of Edinger (fissura prima). The posterior lobe, which is composed of the nodulus and the two flocculi, is separated from the medial lobe by the sulcus primarius posterior which extends across the midline. The posterior sulcus and posterior lobe of Edinger correspond, respectively, to the posterolateral fissure and flocculonodular lobe of Larsell and Dow (1935) and Larsell (1935, 1936a, 1936b, 1937). The medial lobe is bilateral and was subdivided into lobule I (lateral part of lobulus simplex of Bolk), lobule II (lobulus ansoparamedianus), and lobule III corresponding to the human tonsilla, according to Edinger.

The paleocerebellum as defined by Edinger includes the flocculi, the nodulus, and the remainder of the vermis; as illustrated in his diagram the lateral part of the anterior lobe is part of the neocerebellum. The remaining and largest part of the neocerebellum is represented by the medial lobe on either side of the paleocerebellum. Thus a combination of the anteroposterior and transverse divisions of the organ is presented.

The concepts of Edinger and Comolli have exerted a wide influence in functional analysis of the cerebellum and many attempts have been made to refine them. On more precise anatomical grounds than those of gross morphology, such as fiber tract connections, a sharp distinction cannot be made between the paleo- and neo-cerebellum in Edinger's sense. The demonstration by Brodal, Kristiansen, and Jansen (1950) of a cerebellar hemisphere with pontine connections in birds has removed one of the principal foundations of the concept that the cerebellum of birds is vermis and, accordingly, paleocerebellum. The concept of longitudinal or anteroposterior divisions of the cerebellum, however, has been gaining increased anatomical and experimental support.

Ingvar (1918), on the basis of embryological, comparative anatomical, and experimental studies by the Marchi method, divided the mammalian cerebellum into anterior, medial, and posterior lobules, as he had divided the avian cerebellum. The anterior lobe of Ingvar, delimited posteriorly by the fissura prima, corresponds to the similarly named lobe of G. E. Smith and other authors. The middle lobe included the lobulus simplex, ansiform and paramedian lobes of Bolk, and a group of vermal segments collectively called the lobulus medius medianus, corresponding to the posterior part of Bolk's lobulus c_2. The posterior lobe of Ingvar included the nodulus, the uvula, a segment he regarded as the pyramis, and the flocculus and paraflocculus. The paramedian lobule of mammals, according to Ingvar, corresponds to the tonsilla of man. As will be seen later, this interpretation was in error.

After further studies, Ingvar (1928) presented a concept of cerebellar divisions based on the distribution of the afferent fiber connections. He compared the cerebellum to a three-story building. The basement or first level, including the nodulus, uvula, and lingula, receives vestibular root fibers; the next story, or spinal level, is composed of the anterior lobe, pyramis, and paraflocculus; and the remaining lobes mainly receive pontocerebellar fibers. Ingvar recognized that there must be overlapping of the afferent fibers systems in the cerebellar cortex. He believed that his scheme expressed not only the evolution of cerebellar functions but also the functional localization in the organ.

Jakob (1928) combined the schemes of cerebellar division proposed by Edinger and Ingvar. On the basis of studies of the differentiation of the cortex during development of the cerebellum in the human embryo by his collaborator Hayashi (1924), Jakob added a feature not previously described, namely, the pars intermedia. This forms a paravermal zone, on either side, which tapers caudalward from the rostral part of the hemispheres for an indeterminate distance. The intermediate zone of cortex becomes recognizable in the 5½-month-old fetus by its more advanced differentiation, as compared with the more lateral part of the hemisphere. It lies above the globose and emboliform nuclei, according to Jakob, whereas the greater part of the hemisphere covers the dentate nucleus; the fastigial nucleus lies beneath the vermal cortex.

While Jakob believed that the pars intermedia is limited to the rostral part of the hemispheres, Jansen and Brodal (1942), in experimental studies of corticonuclear connections, found indications that this zone continues into the caudal part of the cerebellum. These authors (1940, 1942) demonstrated that the lateral part of the hemispheres projects efferent fibers to the nucleus lateralis (dentatus), the intermediate part projects efferent fibers to the nucleus interpositus, and the vermis projects these fibers to the nucleus fastigii. Thus there are three longitudinal zones of cortex, but the pars intermedia, which is situated in the superficial medial part of the hemisphere, usually is not distinguishable from the adjacent cortex. Jansen (1954) found an inconspicuous paravermal ridge in the whale cerebellum which possibly indicates the presence of the pars intermedia. In some adult human cerebella I found suggestions of a similarly situated ridge. The longitudinal zones will be discussed further in another section.

Langelaan (1919) divided the cerebellum of human fetuses into ten transverse lobes, each including vermal and hemispheral parts. The first to the ninth, inclusive, correspond in general to the nine transverse divisions formed by the lobes and sublobes of Bradley. The tenth lobe of Langelaan, called the lobus nodiolovelaris by him and the gyrus choroideus posterior by Koelliker (1879), apparently corresponds to the germinal zone of the cerebellar margin since it is related to the choroid tela and the choroid plexus.

In a large series of adult mammals ranging from marsupials to man, Riley (1929) traced the individual folia from the vermal lobules into the hemispheral lobules. Employing the terminology of Bolk with some modifications and basing the vermal lobules on the primary branches (medullary rays) from the deep medullary mass, Riley divided the vermis into seven lobules in some species and into eight lobules in others; lobule 3 of Bolk was omitted in many because there was no primary ray between those leading to his lobuli 2 and 4. The latter lobule was subdivided into 4A and 4B in many species; these sublobules sometimes represented large segments separated by relatively deep fissures.

The entire cerebellum posterior of the fissura prima was called the posterior lobe. The intercrural fissure of the lobulus ansiformis was homologized with the horizontal fissure of man. The paramedian lobule, according to Riley, corresponds to the human lobulus biventer; it is related medially to lobulus c_1, the pyramis. The paraflocculus was said to be related to lobulus B by a separate peduncular attachment.

Studies of the morphology and fiber tract connections of the cerebellum of the mole, small bats, and the opossum (Larsell, 1934, 1935, 1936a, 1936b, 1937; Larsell and Dow, 1935), which are similar to those on amphibians and reptiles that have already been reviewed and supplemented, led to the morphological differentiation of the flocculonodular lobe and the corpus cerebelli as the primary divisions of the mammalian cerebellum. The posterolateral fissure, formed by confluence of the floccular sulcus of Stroud which appears early in differentiation, was recognized as the boundary between the primary cerebellar divisions. The floccular sulcus or lateral segment of the posterolateral fissure is the first cerebellar furrow to make its appearance in mammals as it does in birds. As the nodulus differentiates in the posteroventral margin of the cerebellar rudiment, it becomes delimited from the remainder of the vermal part of the organ by the vermal segment of the posterolateral fissure, with the two segments soon becoming confluent.

The flocculonodular lobe, as seen in silver- and myelin-stained preparations, is the principal terminus of primary and secondary vestibular fibers – some primary fibers also reach the lingula and the fastigial nucleus. This distribution was confirmed by experimental methods in the rat, cat, and monkey by Dow (1936, 1938). A vestibular commissure, corresponding to the vestibulolateral commissure of urodeles but lacking the lateral-line component, was recognized in the small mammals.

The corpus cerebelli is the terminus of spinal, trigeminal, bulbar, tectal, and pontine fibers related to the proprioceptive, exteroceptive, and cerebro-pontocerebellar systems. An anterior commissura cerebelli which is primarily composed of ventral spinocerebellar and trigeminocerebellar fibers corresponds to the cerebellar commissure of Herrick in urodeles. The corpus cerebelli is divided into anterior and posterior lobes by the fissura prima of G. E. Smith but the posterior lobe excludes the nodulus, flocculus, and their connecting fibers.

The cerebellar architecture of marsupials and insectivores was described in subsequent sections but it should be noted here that instead of the numerous lobules, already mentioned in larger mammals, the cerebellum of the mole, small bats, and soricine shrews is characterized by fewer divisions. In the opossum some of the lobules of the corpus cerebelli were so poorly defined as to be uncertain, but the flocculonodular lobe is well differentiated.

The ten folia of birds (Larsell, 1948, 1967) are separated by fissures that correspond to those of all but the smaller and more primitive mammals, in which there are fewer fissures. Those present can be homologized with individual furrows, from both birds and larger marsupial and placental mammals. Comparison of the developing and adult cerebellum of the white rat (Larsell, 1952) shows cortical folds similar to those of birds. These were called lobules I–X instead of folia because of their more prominent secondary foliation; the Roman numerals were adopted because of the confusion that resulted from earlier designations. Lobules I–V are included in the anterior lobe of the corpus cerebelli; lobules VI–IX are included in the posterior lobe; and lobule X is the nodulus of the flocculonodular lobe.

SENSE ORGANS AND PERIPHERAL NERVES

RECENT neurophysiological investigations have shown that the cerebellum is under the influence of a great variety – possibly all modalities – of sensory impulses. The following account is restricted to the proprioceptive organs in a narrow sense, since it only deals with the vestibular labyrinth, the muscle spindles, and the tendon spindles.

Acoustic Nerve and Labyrinth

ACOUSTIC NERVE

The acoustic nerve of mammals and man enters the medulla oblongata by a dorsal or lateral cochlear root and a ventral or medial vestibular root. The two roots unite distally to form the trunk of the acoustic nerve, which passes into the internal auditory meatus. The vestibular fibers enter the vestibular or Scarpa's ganglion situated at the bottom of this meatus, which is formed of the cell bodies that give rise to the fibers. The cochlear fibers separate from the vestibular part of the trunk and enter the cochlea; their cells constitute the cochlear or spiral ganglion, also called the ganglion of Corti, which is situated in the modiolus of the cochlea.

The peripheral processes of the vestibular ganglion cells form a posterior or superior utriculo-ampullary division and an anterior or inferior sacculo-ampullary division. The latter accompanies the cochlear nerve a short distance before dividing into two branches, one to the sacculus and one to the posterior ampulla of the semicircular canals. The superior division separates into a utricular branch and a smaller branch to the anterior or superior (in man) ampulla which accompanies the utricular branch for a short distance; a branch to the lateral ampulla also is given off by the superior division. The distribution of the subdivisions in various mammals and man has been described by Retzius (1881–84), Oort (1918), de Burlet (1929), Lorente de Nó (1926, 1931, 1933), Poljak (1927), Hardy (1934), Weston (1938, 1939), and others. Shute (1951a, 1951b) described the branches from serial sections of human embryos stained with silver.

According to Shute the superior ampullary branch joins the principal utricular nerve by a short stem shared by a small superior utricular nerve. The principal utricular nerve gives off a superior saccular nerve, first described by Voit (1907), to the upper part of the macula utriculi. This was usually considered a branch from the superior vestibular ganglion but Poljak (1927) traced the nerve of Voit, in the cat, to the inferior vestibular ganglion through an anastomosis with the main utricular nerve. Shute found a similar anastomotic fascicle in the human embryo and believed that the nerve of Voit is partly continuous with it, with most of the cells of origin being situated in the inferior vestibular ganglion.

The main branch to the saccule comes from the inferior vestibular ganglion and is distributed to the basal part of the macula sacculi. A small bundle of fibers extending from the inferior vestibular ganglion to the entrance of the cochlear nerve into the cochlea was described by Oort (1918) as a vestibulocochlear anastomosis. Kolmer (1924), Lorente de Nó (1926), and Berggren (1932) believed, as did Oort, that this branch represents an aberrant cochlear bundle. Poljak (1927) regarded it as an aberrant vestibular bundle which possibly includes sympathetic fibers. G. L. Rasmussen (1946, 1953), however, found that it does not rejoin the cochlear nerve and continue with it centralward, as Oort and others believed, but rather is composed in part of efferent fibers that arise in the region of the contralateral superior olivary complex. These fibers cross the midline and emerge from the medulla oblongata between the two divisions of the vestibular nerve at a point unrelated to the entrance of the cochlear nerve and dorsal to the rootlets of the intermediate nerve. Their contralateral origin and efferent nature were demonstrated by degeneration of the fibers following lesions in the floor of the fourth ventricle between the facial colliculi. These efferent fibers, called the olivocochlear fascicle by G. L. Rasmussen, join the cochlear nerve between its basal and second turns and become part of a spiral formation at the external margin of the cochlear ganglion. They could be followed into a delicate spiral lamina in all the turns of the cochlea, but not into the organ of Corti. Terminals on the hair cells, described by Portmann and Portmann (1952) and others, could not be confirmed by G. L. Rasmussen (1953, 1960), but electron microscopic and histochemical studies by C. A. Smith and G. L. Rasmussen (1963) have demonstrated efferent fibers in the spiral nerves of the organ of Corti beneath the internal hair cells and in the tunnel. Some fibers of Oort's bundle, the spiral bundle of the cochlear ganglion, and other spirals within the osseous spiral lamina were said to be unrelated to the olivocochlear fascicle but instead were regarded, for the most part, as primary cochlear afferents (G. L. Rasmussen, 1953). According to Shute (1951a) cochlear fibers of Oort's bundle are processes of the last cells of the cochlear ganglion that enter the developing cochlea. Efferent fibers to the vestibular labyrinth, which will be discussed again later, have been described in Oort's nerve by G. L. Rasmussen and Gacek (1958) and by Gacek (1960).

An inconstant small bundle extending from the beginning of the cochlear ganglion to the inferior part of the macula sacculi was described in man by Hardy (1934). He believed that this bundle to the sacculus is a true branch of the cochlear nerve and suggested the term cochleosaccular nerve. According to Shute the cochlear ganglion makes no contribution to the innervation of the macula sacculi.

Lorente de Nó (1926) described a faciocochlear anastomosis in mice which he thought was composed of sympathetic fibers from the internal carotid plexus to the cochlea by way of the petrosal nerves and the tympanic plexus. He also found vasomotor fibers on the blood vessels of the labyrinth. A slender strand of fibers between the geniculate ganglion and the cochlear nerve was described by Shute (1951b) as a faciocochlear anastomosis, probably including sympathetic fibers.

According to Powell and Cowan (1962), who studied the projection of the cochlea upon the nuclei of the brainstem of the cat and rabbit by the methods of Nauta, Glees, and Bodian, the primary auditory nerve fibers terminate in the anteroventral, posteroventral, and dorsal cochlear nuclei. No fibers were seen ending in the superior olivary or medial trapezoid nuclei. The cochlear nuclei project to the two pre-olivary nuclei of the same side, to the contralateral medial trapezoid and lateral lemniscal nuclei, and to the proximal halves of the medial superior olive of both sides.

Involvement of vestibular divisions of VIII nerve in one cat, in addition to almost complete destruction of cochlea, produced degeneration which was clearly traceable dorsomedially around spinal V tract to the four vestibular nuclei. The interstitial nucleus of VIII nerve shows very heavy preterminal and terminal degeneration in the form of solid boutons and pericellular fragmentation. The distribution of the terminal degeneration in the vestibular nuclei is limited to the central part of the superior nucleus, to the rostral and ventral parts of the lateral nucleus, and to the lateral part of the medial nucleus. In the inferior nucleus degeneration was found throughout its entire mediolateral extent. As Walberg *et al.* (1958) have pointed out, the majority of large cells of the lateral vestibular nucleus do not appear to be in direct contact with primary vestibular afferents since their perikarya and dendritic processes are singularly free of terminal degeneration.

VESTIBULAR LABYRINTH

The subdivisions of the membranous labyrinth of mammals differ in some respects from those of lower vertebrates. The papilla neglecta, papilla lagena, and the ramulus lagenae of the vestibular nerve were found in monotremes by Alexander (1904) but they do not exist in most mammals. According to de Burlet (1929) part of the papilla lagenae of *Echidna* is surrounded by a perilymphatic space lacking trabeculae, as in the cochlea. The ganglion cells of the nerve fibers that end in this part of the lagena, which presumably is auditory, are situated in close relation to the modiolus of the osseous spiral lamina, that is, intraotically, whereas those whose fibers end in the trabeculated part of the lagena were found in the internal auditory meatus and hence are intracranial (Weston, 1938, 1939).

The size range of vestibular fibers is not so great in mammals as in lower vertebrates but Lorente de Nó (1926, 1928, 1931), in Golgi and Cajal preparations of young mice and kittens, and Poljak (1927), in mouse and man, subdivided the individual units of the vestibular labyrinth on the basis of the characteristic fiber sizes represented.

The macula utriculi was divided by Lorente de Nó (1931) into an anterior and marginal region in which fine fibers terminate, an adjacent crescent-shaped region in which large fibers end, a medial and posterior region characterized by large fibers, and a posterolateral region in which medium-sized and small fibers terminate. The macula sacculi was divided into an anterior region of large fibers, a medial region of large fibers, and a superior and posterior marginal region of fine fibers. These regions of the macula sacculi are less distinctly defined than in the macula utriculi. The cristae ampullares have a central region characterized by large fibers, an intermediate region of medium-sized fibers, and a marginal region of fine fibers. These fibers of various sizes become arranged into five groups which Lorente de Nó followed into cell groups of the vestibular ganglion and from them to the subdivisions of the vestibular nuclear complex.

As has been long known, the sensory epithelium of all divisions of the vestibular labyrinth includes hair cells and supporting cells. Wersäll (1956) differentiated two types of hair cells in light and electron microscopic studies of the cristae ampullares of the guinea pig. Two types of cells also were found in the maculae of the sacculus and the utriculus by Engström (1958). Those called type I by Wersäll are flask-shaped, with short, small necks; their bodies are surrounded by terminal calyces of large fibers. The type II cells are cylindrical in form but vary somewhat in both shape and length. They are innervated by small nerve fibers. The small nerve-fiber endings are of two types: granulated and nongranulated. Granulated endings also occur on the external surface of the calyces that surround the type I cells. Engström (1958) suggested that the granulated endings are efferent. Certain differences in the internal organization of the two types of cells appeared in electron microscopic studies. Both types are distributed throughout the ampullary cristae but type I cells are localized chiefly at the summits and type II cells are chiefly at the peripheries (Wersäll, 1956). In the maculae type I cells mainly exist in the central regions and type II cells are more abundant at the peripheries. The proportion of type II cells appears to be greater in the maculae than in the cristae (Wersäll, 1960).

The electron microscopic studies of the hair cells and their innervation by Wersäll (1954, 1956, 1960), Wersäll, Engström, and Hjorth (1954), Smith (1956), Engström (1958), and Engström and Wersäll (1958) have so recently been reviewed by Brodal *et al.* (1962) that reference is made to these latter authors. It should be noted here that according to Wersäll (1960) the ray, an elasmobranch, has only one type of hair cell – type II. The nerve fibers, which vary considerably in diameter, were said to end at the bases of the hair cells as granulated and nongranulated terminals. Some are large but no calyces occur; type I cells accordingly are lacking. On the basis of comparisons of the hair cells of rays and mammals, Wersäll concluded that the type I cells represent a phylogenically more highly developed variety which is more sensitive than type II but not essential to the basic function of the vestibular labyrinth. They represent a mechanism of response within a limited area of the neuroepithelium. The type II cells were believed to respond to stronger, more widely spread stimuli.

Physiological studies reviewed by Dow and Moruzzi (1958) indicated that the ampullary cristae are stimulated by movements of the endolymph of the semicircular ducts, produced by angular acceleration (Camis, 1928; Fischer, 1956; Gernandt, 1959; and others). Kinetic reflexes result from this. The macula of the utricle is stimulated by the forces of gravity, linear acceleration, and centrifugal forces, according to McNally and Tait (1934), Adrian (1943), Löwenstein and Roberts (1949, 1951), and others. Stimulation of the utricle results in static reflexes. The sacculus has been subjected to bilateral destruction without effect on labyrinthine reflexes (Versteegh, 1927; Löwenstein, 1936; and others). Ashcroft and Hallpike (1934), Löwenstein and Roberts (1951), and others believed that the macula sacculi is associated with the cochlea as a receptor of slow vibrational stimuli.

There is no evidence that the cochlea or the cochlear nuclei of mammals have connections with the cerebellum except through the midbrain auditory centers, with which the cochlear nuclei are connected by the lateral lemniscus. Therefore, except for occasional references, the cochlea and cochlear nuclei will be omitted from consideration.

Vestibular Nuclei

The vestibular nuclear complex of mammals classically was divided into four principal nuclei: the lateral nucleus of Deiters, the superior nucleus of Bechterew, the medial nucleus of Schwalbe, and the descending (inferior) nucleus of Ramon y Cajal. After the earlier studies of Deiters, Bechterew, Schwalbe, and others, Ramon y Cajal (1909–11) described the nuclei in young mice and kittens; Stokes (1912) and Voris and Hoerr (1932) described them in the opossum; Winkler and Potter (1911), Meessen and Olszewski (1949), and others described them in the rabbit; Winkler and Potter (1914) described them in the cat; and Sabin (1897), Jacobsohn (1909), Marburg (1924), Ziehen (1934a), Olszewski and Baxter (1954), and others described them in man.

Confusion in terminology about the delimitation of the individual nuclei led Brodal and Pompeiano (1957) to a restudy of the nuclear complex in kittens. These authors based the subdivisions on the cytoarchitectonic features of the component groups of cells, as shown in Nissl preparations, supplemented by the connections of these groups as demonstrated in experimental-anatomical studies by Brodal and his associates. Brodal and Pompeiano refined the definitions of the principal nuclei and added several distinct groups of cells that either are included in the larger masses or are topographically related to them. Some of these groups had been described by earlier authors, but the topographically related groups had not been clearly differentiated from the principal nuclei.

The embryonic origin of the vestibular nuclei, according to Harkmark (1954) who made experimental studies of cell migrations in chick embryos, is not from the rhombic lip but from the neuroepithelium medial of it. According to Hugosson (1957) the vestibular nuclei of mouse, human, and other embryos develop from the dorsolateral cell column of the medulla oblongata and the cochlear nuclei from the dorsal column. Vraa-Jensen (1956) found that the majority of the cells in Deiters' nucleus in chick embryos and adult hens correspond to somatic sensory cells, but the mature giant or Deiters' cells, characteristic of this nucleus in lower vertebrates as well as in mammals, resemble motor elements in size, distribution of Nissl granules, and staining properties. Hamberger and Hydén (1949) and Jacobsohn (1910) also regarded them as being related to the motor cells. According to Vraa-Jensen, the giant cells are derived from the medial part of the matrix of the basal lamina in the chick embryo, where somatic and visceral motor cells also have their origin. Vraa-Jensen also believed that Deiters' cells form a link in the motor pathway.

The vestibular nuclei and the cell groups included within them, or related topographically, in the cat have recently been summarized by Brodal (1960) and Brodal, Pompeiano, and Walberg (1962). For greater detail the reader is referred to the contribution of Brodal and Pompeiano (1957). In the following pages these accounts are relied on for brief descriptions of the vestibular nuclei and cell groups in the cat, rabbit, and man.

The lateral vestibular nucleus (nucleus of Deiters, giant-celled vestibular nucleus) in the kitten was defined by Brodal and Pompeiano as the part of the vestibular nuclear complex in which the characteristic cytoarchitectural element is represented by the giant cells of Deiters. The lateral part of the nucleus is entered by vestibular root fibers that spread within the nucleus in a way that separates its cells into minor groups. In addition to the giant cells, which vary considerably in size, the nucleus also includes smaller cells of various forms and sizes. These are intermingled throughout the nucleus except in a lateral projection called group *l* which consists of medium-sized cells only and was regarded as a special part of Deiters' nucleus.

Meessen and Olszewski (1949) divided Deiters' nucleus in the rabbit into four subnuclei all of which include giant cells, but only nucleus γ of these authors was said to consist exclusively of such cells. Some of the cell groups of Meessen and Olszewski, according to Brodal and Pompeiano (1957), correspond to part of the descending vestibular nucleus of the cat.

Deiters' nucleus in man, according to Olszewski and Baxter (1954), begins at the caudal pole of the motor trigeminal nucleus and extends a distance of 4 mm to a level caudal of the upper pole of the descending vestibular nucleus. Ziehen (1934a) gave the greatest length of Deiters' nucleus as 9 mm in man, which is an example of the difference in boundaries ascribed to this and the other nuclei by various authors. Deiters' nucleus is related dorsally to the lateral part of the floor of the fourth ventricle; laterally to the inferior cerebellar peduncle; medially to the medial vestibular nucleus; ventrally to the spinal trigeminal tract and nucleus and to the parvicellular nucleus of the reticular substance. Olszewski and Baxter divided the nuclear mass into a subnucleus lateralis and a subnucleus medialis, with the spinal root of the vestibular nerve which traverses the lateral part of Deiters' nucleus partly separating the two subnuclei.

Brodal and Pompeiano (1957) found that the giant cells of Deiters in the kitten are multipolar elements ranging from 30 μ to about 45 μ in the widest cross-sectional area of the perikaryon. They have coarse Nissl granules which are concentrically arranged around the cell nucleus. The smaller cells are of different types and sizes. The larger of these cells usually are multipolar, medium-sized elements, often oval or spindle-shaped; very small cells also occur. The caudal part of the nucleus was said to include relatively more and larger Deiters' cells and fewer smaller-sized cells than the rostral part, but the two regions gradually merge.

In the rabbit, Meessen and Olszewski (1949) found smaller cells of various sizes, and Deiters' cells in three subnuclei. A fourth subnucleus, called γ, includes Deiters' cells of larger size.

Olszewski and Baxter (1954) described the Deiters' cells in man as multipolar elements with coarse, deeply staining Nissl granules of varying size. Ziehen (1934a) recorded the greatest length of giant cells in the human lateral nucleus as 60 μ to 70 μ. Several other types of cells ranging from large to very small elements were included, as in the cat and rabbit. The characteristic cells of the subnucleus lateralis of Olszewski and Baxter were said to be large, rounded, or spindle-shaped multipolar elements with large, deeply staining Nissl granules. Occasional cells of the type characteristic of the mesencephalic trigeminal nucleus were found among them. The subnucleus medialis of Olszewski and Baxter was said to include a smaller number of large cells and many medium-sized cells. The latter are polymorphic and multipolar, with Nissl granules of medium size.

In Golgi preparations of newborn and very young mice and kittens Ramon y Cajal (1909–11) described the cells of Deiters' nucleus as being stellate and multipolar. These cells have long, spiny dendrites which are divided into numerous branches. Some of the dendrites were said to extend to the medial or the inferior nucleus and occasionally to the fascicle of the vestibular fibers. The axons of these neurons are thick fibers, lacking collaterals in their course through the nucleus. Sometimes the axons arise from dendrites. Fine collaterals of vestibular root fibers were said to form a rich plexus among the cells.

Hauglie-Hanssen (1968) found in Golgi preparations of the vestibular nuclei of newborn kittens that the nerve cells are rather well differentiated at this stage, with the dendrites showing definite spines.

The superior vestibular nucleus (nucleus angularis, nucleus of Bechterew) of the cat is covered dorsally by the brachium conjunctivum and the mesencephalic nucleus of the trigeminus lies dorsomedially of its rostral two-thirds. The caudal half of the nucleus borders ventrally on the lateral vestibular nucleus but cytoarchitectural differences between the two nuclei make the boundary fairly distinct.

Subdivisions of the superior nuclear mass have been made by various authors but much confusion about them has existed. Lewandowsky (1904) described an oval region in the dog which is situated dorsolaterally of Deiters' nucleus and extends forward beneath the brachium conjunctivum so that its dorsomedial end reaches the lateral wall of the fourth ventricle. He called this region the "nucleus supremus acustici." Onufrowicz (1885) described a similar region, possibly more ventrally situated, and Kohnstamm (1910) designated a cell mass between the sensory trigeminal nucleus and the main part of Bechterew's nucleus as the nucleus trigemino-angularis. Fuse (1912) was doubtful about the existence of Lewandowsky's nucleus but he referred to the nucleus of Onufrowicz and the nucleus of Kohnstamm.

In a comparative study of the nuclei of Deiters and of Bechterew in a large series of mammals, employing the Nissl and other techniques, Kaplan (1912–13) described dorsoangular, dorsolateral, central- or ventromedial, and ventrolateral groups of cells in Bechterew's nucleus. These groups are unequally differentiated in different mammalian orders. Kaplan regarded a ventral aggregation of cells in the dorsolateral group as possibly corresponding to the nucleus of Lewandowsky. Ariens Kappers (1947) believed that the nucleus of Lewandowsky corresponds to a cell mass called the vestibulocerebellar nucleus by Ramon y Cajal (1909–11) and Lorente de Nó (1933). Brodal and Pompeiano (1957), however, did not find sufficiently distinct cytoarchitectonic differences in the region of the superior vestibular nucleus of the kitten to justify subdivisions. These authors regarded the entire cell mass as the superior vestibular nucleus of Bechterew.

The cells of the superior nucleus, in Nissl preparations of the cat, are rather scattered and are of small or medium size. The small cells are stellate, spindle-shaped or rounded, and multipolar, with fine Nissl granules. Clusters of larger multipolar cells occur in the central part of the nucleus (Brodal and Pompeiano, 1957).

In the rabbit Meessen and Olszewski (1949) described the cells as being loosely arranged, having triangular to oval elements with abundant Nissl substance and short dendrites. Smaller spindle-shaped to oval cells also occur.

Most of the cells in man, according to Olszewski and Baxter (1954), are medium in size, rounded or oval in form, and have short dendrites. Intermingled with these are many smaller and a few larger but similar cells.

From Golgi preparations of young mice and other animals Ramon y Cajal (1909–11) described Bechterew's nucleus as being formed of numerous medium-sized multipolar cells separated by fascicles of lateroposteriorly directed fibers. The axons of the cells were said to emit some collaterals within the nucleus.

The medial vestibular nucleus (also known as the nucleus of Schwalbe, the nucleus triangularis, the nucleus dorsomedialis, or the nucleus principis) is situated beneath the floor of the lateral part of the fourth ventricle in the anterior region of the medulla oblongata and the posterior part of the pons. In the cat it extends rostrally approximately to the same level as the rostral end of the lateral nucleus; caudally it reaches the level of the anterior pole of the hypoglossal nucleus, and medially strands of cells connect it with the nucleus praepositus hypoglossi. The anterior part of the nucleus fuses to some extent with the nucleus of Bechterew, and the ventral part of its caudal region fuses laterally with the descending vestibular nucleus, but the dorsal part is separated from the latter by a zone free of cells (Brodal and Pompeiano, 1957). According to Winkler and Potter (1914) the medial nucleus of the cat comprises four groups of cells, but only the groups labeled *a* and *b* by these authors represent the medial nucleus proper as defined by Brodal and Pompeiano.

The literature includes various descriptions of the medial nucleus in the rabbit. Some divided it into an anterior nucleus medialis of Schwalbe and an elongated nucleus triangularis, extending caudalward. Meessen and Olszewski (1949) found no boundary that justified such a division; therefore they called the entire nucleus the triangularis and described it as forming the eminentia nuclei triangularis of the floor of the fourth ventricle.

In man Olszewski and Baxter (1954) found that the medial nucleus lies beneath the lateral part of the fourth ventricle and extends from the level of the caudal pole of the abducens nucleus to a level about 1 mm caudal of the upper pole of the hypoglossal nucleus.

The cells of the medial vestibular nucleus in the cat, according to Brodal and Pompeiano (1957), are closely arranged elements of medium size and of rounded, triangular, or polymorphic form. Nissl granules are small. Larger cells were said to occur at the middle levels of the nucleus.

In the rabbit Meessen and Olszewski (1949) described the cells as oval, triangular, and spindle-shaped elements of medium or small size that are irregularly arranged but interspersed with scattered larger cells. The smaller cells stain lightly in Nissl preparations, but the larger cells have big, dark-staining Nissl granules. The caudal part of the nucleus is very cellular; fewer and smaller cells occur at successive levels in a rostral direction but the transition is gradual.

The human medial vestibular nucleus, according to Olszewski and Baxter (1954), has irregularly arranged cells of oval, triangular, or spindlelike form. The spindle-shaped and round cells are small and stain lightly by the Nissl method. Scattered polymorphic cells of larger size have big, dark-staining Nissl granules.

In Golgi preparations of the mouse, Ramon y Cajal (1909–11) described the cells of the medial nucleus as small, triangular, spindle-shaped, or stellate elements surrounded, as in Deiters' nucleus, by a plexus of axonal branches. The dendrites of the neurons are small and divide repeatedly, with some extending considerable distances; they are studded with varicosities. The axons are small and nodulated.

Brodal and Pompeiano (1957) found that the inferior (spinal or descending) vestibular nucleus begins ventral of the caudal third of Deiters' nucleus, where the majority of vestibular root fibers enter the nuclear complex, and extends caudalward along the descending vestibular root. It is related medially to the nucleus medialis and ventrolaterally to the roots of the vestibular and glossopharyngeal nerves. Part of the nucleus as defined by these authors was included by Winkler and Potter (1914) in the medial nucleus. Some authors included the rostral part of the inferior vestibular nucleus in the nucleus of Deiters. As delimited on the basis of its cytoarchitectural pattern and the presence of the longitudinally directed fibers characteristic of it, the inferior vestibular nucleus forms a quantitatively large part of the vestibular nuclear complex (Brodal and Pompeiano, 1957).

The inferior vestibular nucleus of the rabbit is situated between the medial nucleus and nucleus cuneatus (Meessen and Olszewski, 1949).

Olszewski and Baxter (1954) found that the inferior nucleus in man extends from the upper pole of the lateral cuneate nucleus to the level of the caudal pole of the nucleus facialis. Its ventrolateral and medial relations are similar to those in the cat.

Brodal and Pompeiano (1957) found that the cytoarchitecture of the inferior vestibular nucleus is not entirely uniform. Small, medium-sized, and some large multipolar cells that approach the size of the giant cells of Deiters occur throughout. The large cells, regarded as displaced Deiters' cells, are especially abundant rostrally. Situated ventrolaterally in the caudal part of the nucleus, one or more densely packed aggregations of rather large cells were labeled group *f* by Brodal and Pompeiano. These cells differ from surrounding neurons by their larger size and their lack of primary vestibular fibers. They were regarded as a distinct division of the inferior nucleus and as similar to cell groups in the rabbit also called group *f* by Meessen and Olszewski (1949). Elsewhere the inferior nucleus of the cat consists of scattered cells situated close to the longitudinally directed vestibular root and other fibers.

In the rabbit the inferior nucleus is composed of dark-staining, slender cells of medium size; group *f* consists of larger, closely packed cells as in the cat.

Olszewski and Baxter (1954) described the cells of the inferior nucleus in man as less densely arranged than those of the medial nucleus. They are of medium size, oval or triangular in form, and multipolar, with long, slender dendritic processes. It has been said that the medial part of the nucleus is formed usually of smaller cells than those of the lateral part, but small elements similar to the larger cells are scattered among the latter throughout the nucleus.

Golgi preparations of young animals, according to Ramon y Cajal (1909–11), show small fusiform or triangular cells having long, varicosed dendrites. Larger cells in the lateral part of the nucleus have numerous richly branching dendrites that somewhat resemble those of Deiters' nucleus. The axons, some descending and others ascending, were said to accompany the descending vestibular root fibers.

The interstitial nucleus of the vestibular root as described from Golgi material of the mouse by Ramon y Cajal (1909–11) comprises two or three groups of cells situated among the intramedullary root fibers. The cells are polymorphic and have numerous dendrites that end within the limits of each cell group or extend to two or three groups. The axons pass either forward or posteriorly but they could not be followed to their destinations. Numerous collaterals, arising at right angles from the vestibular fibers that enclose the nuclear groups, divide to form an intricate plexus which envelops the cells.

Fuse (1912) and Poljak (1926) observed similarly situated cells and Klossowsky (1933) described a small nucleus among the vestibular root fibers of the cat, dog, rabbit, guinea pig, and man. In Nissl preparations the cells are polygonal in form and have deeply staining Nissl granules. Brodal and Pompeiano (1957) described the correspondingly situated cells in the kitten as being medium sized and usually elongated along the vestibular root fibers. Scattered giant cells were also seen occasionally. According to Powell and Cowan (1962) the interstitial nucleus of nerve VIII of the cat, following lesions of the vestibular nerve, shows preterminal and terminal degeneration.

Ramon y Cajal (1909, p. 770) regarded the interstitial nucleus of the vestibular root as possibly corresponding to the tangential nucleus of teleosts and birds, which he had described in 1908. Such a homology was favored by Ariens Kappers, Huber, and Crosby (1936), and Ariens Kappers (1947) stated that it is possible. Fuse (1912), however, regarded the interstitial nucleus of the vestibular root as an aberrant part of Deiters' nucleus, as did Brodal and Pompeiano (1957).

Comparison of the interstitial nucleus of the vestibular root of mammals with the tangential nucleus of lower vertebrates brings forth both similarities and dissimilarities. In birds and most reptiles the large fibers from the cristae ampullares end on cells of the tangential nucleus by spoonlike terminations (Larsell, 1967). Ariens Kappers (1947) found that elasmobranchii, amphibians, and some turtles have relatively small ampullary fibers that end as plexiform terminals among laterally situated polygonal cells. None of the ampullary fibers have spoonlike terminals in mammals but such terminals also are lacking in other mammalian nuclei, for example the oculomotor, in which they were found in various lower vertebrates. It has been demonstrated that the fibers from which collaterals reach the cells of the interstitial nucleus are connected peripherally with the ampullary cristae; thus their collaterals would correspond to those of the ampullary fibers in elasmobranchii, amphibians, and some reptiles. Other similarities appear when a comparison is made between the efferent connections of the tangential nucleus and the mammalian nucleus of the vestibular root, as described below.

The interstitial nucleus of the vestibular root in the cat contributes fibers to the ascending medial longitudinal fascicle as demonstrated by retrograde changes of some of its cells following section of this fascicle (Brodal and Pompeiano, 1958). Hemisection of the cord also affected cells of the ipsilateral interstitial nucleus (Pompeiano and Brodal, 1957a). As illustrated in figure 8 of these authors, complete hemisection of one side of the cord accompanied by injury to the ventral funiculus alone of the opposite side was followed by cell changes in the interstitial nuclei and also in cell group *l* of both sides. Only a few other cells of Deiters' nucleus were affected on the side with the limited lesion, in contrast to the numerous retrograde cells on the side completely hemisected. Although Pompeiano and Brodal made no such interpretation, it may be pointed out that since the descending medial longitudinal fascicle occupies the sulcomarginal fascicle of the ventral funiculus, the descending fibers from the interstitial nucleus of the vestibular root could be interpreted as being included in the descending medial longitudinal fascicle. If so, they would correspond to the descending fibers from the tangential nucleus of birds and reptiles.

The interstitial nucleus of the vestibular root appears to send no fibers to the cerebellum, as is also true of the tangential nucleus of birds and reptiles. As described below the interstitial nucleus differs from Deiters' nucleus in that it receives no fibers from the fastigial nucleus and none from the spinovestibular tract.

The primary vestibular fibers that give off collaterals to cells of the interstitial nucleus of the vestibular root traverse the nucleus and terminate elsewhere in the vestibular nuclear complex. As noted below ampullary fibers end in several of the vestibular nuclei. On the grounds of similarities to the tangential nucleus of birds and reptiles and differences from the lateral vestibular nucleus, as noted above, it appears justifiable to regard the interstitial nucleus of the vestibular root as corresponding to at least a part of the avian and reptilian tangential nucleus.

Comparison with the tangential nucleus of teleosts presents greater difficulties. This nucleus was divided by Tello (1909) and Beccari (1931) into dorsal and ventral parts (see Larsell, 1967). Differences in the apparent relations of these two divisions to the descending medial longitudinal fascicle and in the descriptions of the ampullary fibers that enter each one point to the need for renewed study of these nuclei in fishes in comparison with the tangential nucleus and its connections in other vertebrates.

Minor cell groups. Some of the minor cell groups differentiated by Brodal and Pompeiano (1957) are included within the larger nuclei; others are related to them only by juxtaposition.

Group *f* already has been mentioned in connection with the inferior vestibular nucleus. Many of its cells project fibers to the cerebellum (Brodal and Torvik,

1957) while others give rise to ascending fibers in the medial longitudinal fascicle. Brodal and Pompeiano (1957) considered this group to be a special part of the inferior vestibular nucleus.

Group *g* is situated below the caudal end of the medial nucleus, forming a dense collection of glia cells and a few nerve cells.

Group *l* has been mentioned as a special part of Deiters' nucleus.

Group *sv* is an aggregation of spindle-shaped cells between the caudal end of Deiters' nucleus and the rostral level of the external cuneate nucleus; it is situated immediately beneath the dorsal surface of the medulla oblongata. Brodal and Pompeiano regarded it as probably corresponding to a cell mass in man called the nucleus supravestibularis by Olszewski and Baxter (1954).

Group *x* is situated between the caudal half of the inferior nucleus and the rostral pole of the external cuneate nucleus. It receives no terminal vestibular fibers, which excludes it from the vestibular nuclei proper, but collaterals of the spinocerebellar tracts reach this cell group. Ipsilateral projections to the cerebellum were described by Brodal and Torvik (1957) and were said to contribute to the medial longitudinal fascicle (Brodal and Pompeiano, 1958).

Group *y*, situated lateral of the caudal part of Deiters' nucleus, probably is not part of the vestibular complex proper but may correspond to the nucleus cerebello-acusticus of Ramon y Cajal (1896), according to Brodal and Pompeiano.

Group *z*, situated immediately rostral of the nucleus gracilis and dorsolateral of the inferior vestibular nucleus, does not receive terminal vestibular fibers. It also differs in connections from the nucleus gracilis, with which there appears to be no relation.

A nucleus parasolitarius was described by Brodal, Pompeiano, and Walberg (1962) as probably corresponding to a nucleus so named by Allen (1923) in the guinea pig and to an area in man labeled nucleus parvocellularis compactus by Olszewski and Baxter (1954). It was difficult to see in Nissl preparations but it was evident in preparations with heavy preterminal fiber degeneration following lesions of the contralateral fastigial nucleus.

Considering the interstitial nucleus of the vestibular root as homologous with part of the tangential nucleus of lower vertebrates, five of the six vestibular nuclei of birds are represented in mammals. If the dorsolateral and ventrolateral vestibular nuclei of Sanders (1929) in birds are subdivisions of the nucleus of Deiters, as they were considered to be by Bartels (1925) and others, then the number of vestibular nuclei is the same in birds and mammals. Probably there is a correspondence of some of the subdivisions described in birds by Ramon y Cajal (1908), Craigie (1928), Sanders (1929), and others with subdivisions and cell groups in mammals. Attempts to relate individual cell masses of the vestibular complex and topographically adjacent cell groups of mammals to the vestibular nuclei and their subdivisions in birds only have led to confusion.

In Golgi preparations of kittens the neurons of the minor groups of the vestibular complex generally appear to be more multipolar than those of the major subdivisions. In particular this is true for the cells of groups *f* and *x*. The dendrites of these neurons are as a rule shorter and often more richly branched than those of the main vestibular nuclei (Hauglie-Hanssen, 1968).

AFFERENT CONNECTIONS OF VESTIBULAR NUCLEI

Vestibular root fibers. The primary vestibular fibers of mammals, as of lower vertebrates, bifurcate into ascending and descending branches after entering the medulla oblongata. This bifurcation and the branches were described from Golgi preparations by Koelliker (1891), Held (1892), and Ramon y Cajal (1896, 1909–11). The ascending branches give off numerous collaterals that spread into the anterior part of Deiters' nucleus and throughout the nucleus of Bechterew; according to Ramon y Cajal some of the fibers terminate in the latter nucleus and others continue into the cerebellum. The descending branches form the descending root of the vestibular nerve and extend as far as the inferior part of the inferior vestibular nucleus. The branches give rise to numerous collaterals directed medially into the medial vestibular nucleus and then branch and terminate in the inferior nucleus.

Lorente de Nó (1933) gave a more detailed description of distribution to individual vestibular nuclei, based on Golgi preparations of young mice and kittens, which will be discussed later. Partial descriptions of the distribution of vestibular root fibers, as seen in Marchi preparations, were contributed by Winkler (1907), Leidler (1914), Ingvar (1918), Dow (1936), and others. Walberg, Bowsher, and Brodal (1958), employing the silver techniques following lesions of the vestibular nerve in adult cats, analyzed the distribution of the root fibers to the vestibular nuclei. The distribution of degenerated vestibular root fibers following labyrinthectomy or surgical section of the vestibular nerve in the cat and monkey was described by Carpenter (1960b) on the basis of preparations by the Nauta-Gygax technique.

Studies using the preterminal and terminal fiber degeneration techniques demonstrated that primary vestibular fibers terminate in all four principal vestibular nuclei, but in restricted zones rather than distributed throughout each nucleus. According to the Oslo school, as summarized by Brodal *et al.* (1962), vestibular root fibers end in the rostroventral part of Deiters' nucleus, the central region of the superior or Bechterew's nucleus, the lateral parts of the medial nucleus, and all of the inferior nucleus except cell group *f*; degenerated fibers are few, however, in the ventrolateral part of the inferior nucleus and are nonexistent in the rostral ventrolateral part of this nucleus. Cell group *l* of Deiters' nucleus receives a small number of primary vestibular fibers and the interstitial nucleus of the vestibular root shows preterminal and terminal fiber degeneration, as well as degenerating fibers of passage.

Carpenter's (1960b) description differs in some respects. Heavy degeneration was described at the entrance of the vestibular root into the medulla oblongata, but no specific mention was made of the interstitial nucleus of the vestibular root or of cell group *l*. Fibers from the more medial part of the vestibular root were said to be distributed to the rostral parts of the inferior nucleus and the ventral half of Deiters' nucleus. Laterally situated vestibular root fibers were said to pass dorsally, as small fascicles, through the dorsal part of Deiters' nucleus toward the superior vestibular nucleus and the juxtarestiform body. Preterminal and terminal degeneration was described as heavy in all parts of the inferior nucleus, but most of the longitudinally arranged fibers that characterize this nucleus in preparations stained for normal fibers showed little degeneration, indicating that these are not vestibular root fibers. Degenerated fibers of various sizes, including many large ones, were found in the inferior nucleus. According to Carpenter, fine fiber degeneration is abundant in the lateral and ventral parts of the medial vestibular nucleus, with a few scattered fibers also appearing near the ependymal lining of the floor of the fourth ventricle. Coarse, degenerated preterminal fibers from the lateral part of the vestibular root were found in the superior vestibular nucleus and degeneration was said to have been especially abundant in the dorsal and lateral parts of this nucleus. Large degenerated fibers were found along the ventromedial border of the brachium conjunctivum, with some apparently passing into the cerebellum. Carpenter found no primary vestibular fiber degeneration in cell groups *x* and *z*, in accord with Brodal and Pompeiano (1958), who (1957) also added cell group *y* to the aggregations of cells lacking such fibers.

The vestibular fibers end on the soma and the dendritic processes of the cells of the principal nuclei end by terminal boutons. However, the giant cells of Deiters in the lateral nucleus and also the large cells in the rostral part of the inferior nucleus do not have such vestibular root terminals, unlike the small cells which have them in large numbers (Walberg *et al*, 1958).

Using Nauta, Glees, and Bodian methods on cats, Powell and Cowan (1962) found the terminal degeneration of vestibular root fibers limited to the central part of the superior vestibular nucleus, to the rostral and ventral parts of Deiters' nucleus, to the lateral part of the medial nucleus, and to the entire mediolateral extent of the inferior nucleus. The regions of the principal nuclei that are devoid of vestibular root fibers and also the cell groups that lack such fibers receive other afferents, which are described below.

Kaida (1929) and Camis (1930) believed that primary vestibular fibers enter the medial longitudinal fascicle, and it will be recalled that Ariens Kappers (1947) described ampullary fibers to the descending medial longitudinal fascicle in birds. Carpenter (1960b) found no root fiber degeneration in the medial longitudinal fascicle in the spinal cord, the midbrain, or the caudal part of the diencephalon.

Crossed vestibular root fibers were believed by Ramon y Cajal (1909–11) to occur in the region of the genu of the facial nerve but their termination was uncertain. Leidler (1914) and others believed that some root fibers may cross or that crossing is possible (Gray, 1926). A. T. Rasmussen (1932), however, found no evidence of contralateral root fibers. According to Addens (1934) the crossed fibers at the level of the facial genu are preganglionic fibers of the intermediate nerve. Ariens Kappers (1947) believed that all vestibular root fibers end ipsilaterally, a conclusion which was confirmed by the experimental studies of the Oslo school and of Carpenter and his associates.

According to Carpenter (1960b) a few primary vestibular fibers were followed in Nauta-Gygax preparations from the inferior vestibular nucleus into the region of the fasciculus solitarius and its nucleus and also into the region of the dorsal motor nucleus of the vagus and the dorsolateral reticular formation beneath the vestibular nuclei. Brodal *et al.* (1962), however, found no evidence of vestibular root fibers to the nucleus of the solitary tract or to the perihypoglossal nuclei.

Lorente de Nó (1926, 1931), employing a modification of the Cajal method on mouse and cat embryos, established that each subdivision of the labyrinth is connected by fibers to a particular part of the vestibular ganglion. The cells of the anterior and lateral ampullary cristae lie in the anterior and dorsal part of the ganglion but cells of the posterior cristae lie in the dorsocaudal region. Cells of the utricular macula lie in the intermediate region and those from the sacculus lie in the intermediate and ventrocaudal regions. The centrally directed fibers from the vestibular ganglion are gathered into five aggregations called groups I–V, each composed of fibers of several sizes.

The fibers of the three cristae come together, as they begin their course toward the medulla oblongata, and constitute a single fascicle which comprises group I and group II fibers. Group I includes only thin and medium-sized fibers from the peripheral parts of the cristae; the group II fibers are larger and come from the central parts of the cristae. The fibers from the utricular and saccular nerves enter the medulla oblongata a little farther caudally than those from the ampullary cristae. They undoubtedly are part of group IV, but whether group III is part of the utricular nerve, is from one of the regions of the macula utriculi, or represents large fibers from the centrum of the ampullary cristae could not be determined. Group V represents fibers from the posterior saccular nerve but some of the fibers of this nerve may be included in group IV, which also contains fibers from the anterior saccular nerve.

As seen in Golgi preparations of young mice and kittens these fibers bifurcate on entering the medulla oblongata into ascending and descending branches that are distributed to the subdivisions of the vestibular nuclear complex. Lorente de Nó's terminology of the vestibular nuclei differs in some respects from that of other authors. Brodal *et al.* (1962) interpreted this author's descriptions of the terminals of the five groups of fibers in terms of the vestibular nuclei as defined by Brodal and Pompeiano (1957). In accord with Lorente de Nó these authors concluded that no distinct selective distribution of afferents from the various subdivisions of the labyrinth to the individual vestibular nuclei is evident, although the fibers from the cristae and those from the maculae, in part, have different central distributions.

The superior vestibular nucleus apparently receives fibers only from the cristae, but such fibers were said to end also in the lateralmost part of the inferior nucleus and in the medial nucleus (Lorente de Nó's angular nucleus). Whether fibers to the lateral nucleus come entirely from the macula utriculi or in part from the ampullary cristae was uncertain. Some fibers of the group that ends in Deiters' nucleus possibly end in the medial nucleus. No reference to the interstitial nucleus of the vestibular root, cell group *l* of Deiters' nucleus, or other subdivisions or cell groups of the nuclei was made in relation to the distribution of the fiber groups of Lorente de Nó. It is not improbable that the collaterals to the interstitial nucleus described by Ramon y Cajal derive from ampullary fibers that terminate elsewhere and that some of the cell groups that receive vestibular root fibers may represent special areas within the larger nuclei in which ampullary fibers end.

Ascending vestibular root fibers to the cerebellum have been described by many authors. Ramon y Cajal (1909–11) found them in Golgi material, as already noted. Ingvar (1918), in Marchi preparations of the cat, followed root fibers to the flocculus, nodulus, uvula, lingula, and the cerebellar nuclei. In pyridine-silver series of the opossum and bat I followed fibers from the vestibular roots to the flocculus and nodulus, with some also apparently passing to the fastigial nucleus (1936a, 1936b). More recently in pyridine-silver and Golgi series of fetal and neonatal rats, I followed vestibular root fibers to the flocculus and nodulus but I found none leading to the fastigial nucleus. Fibers to this nucleus have been described by so many authors that there can be no doubt about their presence.

Lorente de Nó (1933) was uncertain of vestibular root fibers to the cerebellar cortex in his Golgi material of the mouse but Tello (1940) found vestibular root fibers to the cerebellum in Cajal preparations of mouse embryos. According to Dow (1936), who studied their distribution by the Marchi method in the rat and cat, root fibers pass to the ipsilateral flocculus, to the lateral half of the nodulus and adjacent parts of the uvula, and to the fastigial nucleus; subsequently Dow (1939) traced root fibers to the lingula also. Carpenter (1960b) used silver-degeneration methods to show that primary vestibular fibers are distributed medially to the cortex of the nodulus and uvula and around the fastigial nucleus, with some fibers entering this nucleus. Some appear to cross the midline but degeneration is somewhat more prominent on the same side as the labyrinthectomy. Preterminal degeneration was observed bilaterally to the lateral parts of the cortex of the lingula, but whether it was to lobule I or II, described in a subsequent section, or to both is not indicated. Degeneration to the flocculus is ipsilateral. The specific labyrinthine relations of the primary vestibular fibers to the cerebellum are not certain but they appear to be related to the macula utriculi and perhaps to the macula sacculi.

Spinovestibular connections. These were described from Marchi preparations by Thiele and Horsley (1901), Collier and Buzzard (1903), MacNalty and Horsley (1909), and others and from Golgi material by Lorente de Nó (1924). Some of the earlier authors described the fibers as ascending with the dorsal spinocerebellar tract and ending in the lateral or inferior vestibular nuclei. According to Lorente de Nó collaterals from the dorsal spinocerebellar tract primarily enter the ventrocaudal part of the inferior vestibular nucleus, but some enter the ventrolateral part of the medial nucleus. Johnson (1954) and Mehler, Feferman, and Nauta (1960), using the Nauta technique, described them in the cat and monkey, respectively. According to Johnson the fibers are ipsilateral and end in Deiters' nucleus. Mehler and co-workers found few degenerating fibers following lesions of the thoracic cord. Pompeiano and Brodal (1957b), using the Glees method, concluded that the spinovestibular fibers ascend with those of the dorsal spinocerebellar tract. The fibers may include collaterals but many of them are so coarse that they probably are not collaterals and a considerable number are derived from lumbosacral levels of the cord. The spinovestibular fibers end ipsilaterally in the dorsocaudal parts of Deiters' nucleus, in the caudalmost regions of the medial and inferior nuclei, and in cell groups *x* and *z*, that is, in the zones and cell groups that receive no primary vestibular fibers (Pompeiano and Brodal, 1957b; Brodal *et al.*, 1962). The distribution in Deiters' nucleus is in the zone which gives rise to vestibulospinal fibers to the lower levels of the spinal cord. Brodal *et al.* (1962) cited Bowsher as having found spinovestibular fibers in chordotomy cases in man which were restricted to the dorsal part of Deiters' nucleus and to a region corresponding to cell group *x* of the cat.

Connections from higher levels of the brain with vestibular nuclei. According to Pompeiano and Walberg (1957) fibers from the mesencephalic interstitial nucleus of Ramon y Cajal descend in the ipsilateral fasciculus longitudenalis medialis and are distributed throughout the medial vestibular nucleus, but are more abundant in its caudodorsal part. The total number of fibers was said to be small. No terminal degeneration in the vestibular nuclei was found by Pompeiano and Walberg after lesions of the nucleus of Darkschewitsch, the central gray substance, the reticular formation of the midbrain, the superior colliculus, the nucleus of the posterior commissure, the corpus striatum, or the cerebral cortex. The reticular formation of the pons and medulla oblongata, however, could not be excluded as sources of fibers to the vestibular nuclei.

Cerebellovestibular connections and fastigiovestibular fibers. Fibers from the fastigial nuclei to the vestibular complex have been described by many authors. Allen (1924) and A. T. Rasmussen (1933) concluded from Marchi preparations that fastigiovestibular fibers are bilaterally distributed. Those to the ipsilateral vestibular nuclei reach them through the juxtarestiform body, while those to the contralateral nuclei decussate in the cerebellum and reach the vestibular nuclei through the uncinate fascicle. Jansen and Jansen (1955), using the Brodal-Gudden method, concluded that the cells of the fastigial nucleus sending fibers into the ipsilateral restiform body are situated predominantly in the rostral half of the fastigial nucleus, while the decussating fibers, reaching the nuclei through the uncinate fascicle, are derived from cells in the caudal half of the nucleus.

Thomas, Kaufman, Sprague, and Chambers (1956), employing the Nauta-Gygax method after total unilateral destruction of the fastigial nucleus, found fiber degeneration in the vestibular nuclei of both sides. The contralateral path was said largely to avoid the superior vestibular nucleus and the dorsomedial part of Deiters' nucleus. The ipsilateral path avoids the ventrolateral part of Deiters' nucleus in which descending contralateral fibers predominate. Ipsilateral descending fibers to Deiters' nucleus were found chiefly dorsomedially. Degenerated fibers descend from these nuclei into the inferior vestibular nucleus, where some end. According to Cohen, Chambers, and Sprague (1958) the caudal part of the fastigial nucleus projects more predominantly contralaterally than does the nucleus as a whole. These authors believed that the nucleus interpositus and the nucleus lateralis (dentatus) also send fibers to the ipsilateral vestibular nuclei.

Carpenter, Brittin, and Pines (1958), who employed the Nauta-Gygax, Marchi, and Nissl techniques on cats following localized stereotaxic lesions of the fastigial nuclei, and Carpenter (1959), who employed the Marchi method after similar lesions in the monkey, described fibers from the caudal part of the fastigial nucleus as being predominantly crossed and entering the contralateral uncinate bundle of Russell. Descending fibers of the fascicle project to all the vestibular nuclei but the greatest number were said to pass to and through the lateral and inferior nuclei. Some fibers reach the paramedian reticular formation of the pons and medulla oblongata from the level of the abducens nucleus to that of the hypoglossal nuclei.

According to Walberg, Pompeiano, Brodal, and Jansen (1962) and Brodal *et al.* (1962), fastigial fibers that arise chiefly in the caudal part of the nucleus are distributed through the uncinate fascicle to circumscribed parts of all four principal contralateral vestibular nuclei and to cell groups *f* and *x*. Ipsilateral fastigial fibers were said to end in restricted parts of all four vestibular nuclei, with most of them coming from the rostral part of the fastigial nucleus.

The fastigiovestibular fibers end on all types of cells in the nuclei but the giant cells of the lateral and inferior nuclei have few contacts from fastigial fibers. The interstitial nucleus of the vestibular root and cell group *z* receive no fastigial fibers (Brodal *et al.*, 1962), but the medial longitudinal fascicle and the nucleus parasolitarius were said to receive them bilaterally. Fastigial fibers also reach the perihypoglossal nuclei, but Carpenter (1960b) found none entering the medial longitudinal fascicle.

Corticovestibular fibers. Allen (1924), Hohman (1929), Bender (1932), A. T. Rasmussen (1933), Dow (1936, 1938), and others have described fibers from the cerebellar vermis and/ or flocculus to vestibular nuclei. According to Dow, fibers from the nodulus pass to all the vestibular nuclei and to the dorsal part of the reticular formation. Walberg and Jansen (1961) described fibers from the vermis of the anterior as well as the posterior lobe to the vestibular nuclei. Employing the silver methods of Glees and Nauta, these authors found that lesions in lobulus II, III, IV, and V of the anterior lobe are followed by fiber degeneration in the entire dorsal halves of the lateral and inferior vestibular nuclei, but none occur in the ventral halves. There are indications of differential distribution of the fibers in a somatotopic pattern. Walberg and Jansen concluded that lobules VIII and IX of the posterior lobe also contribute to the corticovestibular projection, but apparently lobule VI does not. Whether both lobules VIII and IX or only one of them contribute was not clear. No evidence of contributions from the cortex of the cerebellar hemispheres was obtained in a limited study of these relations. The corticovestibular fibers make synaptic connections with all kinds of cells within the lateral and inferior vestibular nuclei, but Walberg and Jansen believed that the majority make contact with the giant cells. Fibers to the inferior vestibular nucleus were traced from the mandibular nerve (Torvik, 1956), the glossopharyngeal and vagus nerves (Ramon y Cajal, 1909–11), and the dorsal roots of the more anterior cervical nerves (Corbin and Hinsey, 1935; Yee and Corbin, 1939).

EFFERENT CONNECTIONS OF VESTIBULAR NUCLEI

The vestibular nuclei give rise to two systems of connections with the spinal cord, namely, a direct vestibulospinal tract and the descending medial longitudinal fascicle; connections with the midbrain are made by way of the ascending medial longitudinal fascicle; connections with the cerebellum are made through the inferior cerebellar peduncle; and connections with the reticular formation of the medulla oblongata have also been described. These have long been known from studies of preparations stained for normal fibers, by the Golgi method, and also from experimental studies employing the Marchi and Nissl methods. Much uncertainty remained, however, regarding the specific nuclei of origin as well as the distribution of many of the fibers. This has been clarified and much detail was added by application of the method for retrogressive cell changes and the techniques of Glees and Nauta for degenerating preterminal and terminal fibers by the Oslo school and by Carpenter and his co-workers in New York.

The studies of the Oslo school were presented in a series of papers and summarized by Brodal (1960) and more extensively reviewed in the monograph by Brodal, Pompeiano, and Walberg (1962). The contributions of Carpenter and his associates on the vestibular nerve and the cerebellar connections were summarized by Carpenter (1960b). Reference is made to these accounts and to the original contributions cited therein for details and for discussion of the earlier extensive but confusing literature. The principal results of the studies of the mammalian brain together with comparisons of vestibular nuclear contributions to the medial longitudinal fascicle in lower vertebrates, carried out by the Oslo school and other investigators, will be presented in the following pages.

The lateral vestibular nucleus gives origin to the direct vestibulospinal tract, as all authors agreed. A few authors also included fibers from the inferior vestibular nucleus but Brodal *et al.* (1962) regarded the tract as probably being derived exclusively from Deiters' nucleus. Carpenter, Alling, and Bard (1960) found no fibers from the inferior vestibular nucleus to the cord and they also stated that the vestibulospinal tract does not traverse this nucleus. According to Held (1892, 1893) and Ramon y Cajal (1896, 1909–11), who described the tract from Golgi preparations, and the majority of authors who employed the Marchi method, the vestibulospinal tract is ipsilateral. Russell (1897), Schimert (1938), and others followed it to the lumbar cord, while Mott (1895) and Buchanan (1937) described the vestibulospinal tract as reaching the sacral cord. According to Schimert (1938, 1941) and others the fibers end on motor cells in the medial cell groups of the ventral horn. These cell groups innervate the axial musculature.

Brodal and Pompeiano (1957), employing the modified Gudden method, sectioned the spinal cord at various levels and found that the cells originating from the vestibulospinal tract have a somatotopical arrangement in Deiters' nucleus. These cells include the giant cells of Deiters as well as medium- and small-sized elements. The tract descends in the ventrolateral funiculus of the cord. The cells whose axons end in the cervical cord are situated in the rostroventral region of the nucleus; the fibers reaching the lumbosacral cord come from cells in the dorsocaudal parts of the nucleus; and those ending in the thoracic cord are derived from cells in intermediate zones.

Fibers from cell groups *l* also descend in the ventrolateral funiculus of the cervical cord but they turn medially into the ventral funiculus of the upper thoracic cord, with many fibers continuing to the lumbosacral segments. The ventral funiculus of the cord is partly occupied by the sulcomarginal tract, which was generally regarded as the descending continuation of the medial longitudinal fascicle. The Oslo school, however, regarded the descending fibers from cell group *l* as constituents of the vestibulospinal tract that have spread into the ventral funiculus.

As already noted the interstitial nucleus of the vestibular root also sends fibers into the cord. Apparently the descending fibers from these nuclei, in part at least, occupy the ventral funiculus (Brodal and Pompeiano, 1957).

A contribution from Deiters' nucleus to the descending medial longitudinal fascicle was described by a number of authors who employed the Marchi method. P. van Gehuchten (1927) regarded this contribution as being contralateral. A. T. Rasmussen (1932) and others believed this contribution to be chiefly or exclusively ipsilateral, while Buchanan (1937) and others described it as being composed of both ipsilateral and contralateral fibers. All these authors evidently considered the interstitial nucleus of the vestibular root as part of the nucleus of Deiters defined in the broadest sense. The Oslo school considered it an aberrant part of Deiters' nucleus but described the descending fibers to which it gives rise as taking a course which differs in part from that of the tract arising from the principal part of the lateral vestibular nucleus. The descending fibers from cell group *l* described by Pompeiano and Brodal (1957a) apparently would correspond to the ipsilateral contribution of earlier authors who employed the Marchi method. The contralateral contribution possibly is represented by fibers from the interstitial nucleus of the vestibular root, although there is no certain evidence that any of these fibers cross. The effect of lesions involving the ventral funiculus on cells of group *l* and the interstitial nucleus was not regarded by Brodal and Pompeiano as evidence that the lateral vestibular nucleus contributes to the descending medial longitudinal fascicle.

Following stereotaxic lesions of the inferior as well as the lateral vestibular nuclei, Carpenter, Alling, and Bard (1960) and Carpenter (1960a) found no evidence of degenerating fibers from either nucleus to the descending medial longitudinal fascicle. These authors made no specific mention of the interstitial nucleus of the vestibular root or of cell group *l* in relation to the descending fibers, which creates uncertainty about whether or not these parts of Deiters' nucleus, broadly defined, are included in their lesions. They stated, however, that loss of large cells and dense gliosis are evident in all parts of Deiters' nucleus.

Comparison with lower vertebrates throws some light on the relations of the lateral and other vestibular nuclei to the descending as well as the ascending fasciculus longitudinalis medialis. The axons of the tangential nucleus of reptiles enter the contralateral medial longitudinal fascicle, with crossed ascending fibers probably serving ocular reflexes (Ariens Kappers, 1947); descending fibers, also crossed, probably reach the spinal cord. In birds the axons of cells of the tangential nucleus contribute to the ascending and descending medial longitudinal fascicle and form reflex pathways. The ascending fibers appear to cross and to reach the oculomotor and trochlear nuclei, according to Ariens Kappers (1947). Descending fibers, which are apparently ipsilateral, reach the abducens nucleus and spinal cord by way of the descending medial longitudinal fascicle. These were described by Wallenberg (1898) before the tangential nucleus was differentiated by Ramon y Cajal (1908). Ariens Kappers noted that it is not possible to deduce from Wallenberg's experiments whether the fibers originate in the tangential nucleus or Deiters' nucleus; however, he illustrated them as arising from the tangential nucleus. The tangential nucleus in both these groups of vertebrates gives rise to a crossed ascending fasciculus longitudinalis medialis which in birds is augmented by crossed fibers from Deiters' nucleus.

The anterodorsal part of the tangential nucleus of lizards is the terminus, by spoonlike endings, of large fibers from the posterior crista ampullaris and the papilla neglecta; similar fibers from the anterior and lateral cristae ampullares end in the ventroposterior part of the nucleus (Weston, 1936; Ariens Kappers, 1947). Ariens Kappers stated that the fibers of all three ampullary cristae and of the papilla neglecta of birds end in a large tangential nucleus by spoonlike or calyciform terminals. The part of the descending fasciculus longitudinalis medialis which originates from the tangential nucleus in lizards and birds evidently is part of the reflex pathway related to the semicircular canals and papilla neglecta.

In elasmobranchii, amphibians, and some turtles the ampullary fibers do not have spoonlike endings but terminate in a plexiform manner on polygonal cells situated laterally among fibers leading to the nucleus of Deiters (Ariens Kappers, 1947).

If the interstitial nucleus of the vestibular root of mammals gives rise to both crossed and uncrossed fibers of the sulcomarginal tract, which may be possible even though positive evidence is lacking, these fibers would correspond to the crossed and uncrossed fibers of the descending medial longitudinal fascicle of birds. The interstitial nucleus also contributes to the ascending medial longitudinal fascicle, as does the tangential nucleus of lizards and birds.

Cell group *l* of Deiters' nucleus in the cat, judging from its descending fiber connections, appears to be related to the hindlimb region of the lateral vestibular nucleus (Brodal *et al*, 1962). As already noted, cell group *l* gives rise to fibers that occupy the ventral funiculus of the cord from the upper thoracic region downward. These fibers undoubtedly were included as part of the medial longitudinal fascicle by authors who saw them in Marchi preparations and described them as being derived from Deiters' nucleus. In addition to these descending fibers cell group *l* also contributes to the ascending medial longitudinal fascicle. The descending fibers probably correspond to ipsilateral fibers from Deiters' nucleus to the descending medial longitudinal fascicle of reptiles and birds. Those from cell group *l* to the ascending medial longitudinal fascicle probably correspond to the crossed ascending fibers from Deiters' nucleus to the ascending medial longitudinal fascicle. In lizards the ascending contribution from Deiters' nucleus appears to be ipsilateral.

Cells corresponding to group *l* have not been specifically identified in lizards and birds but they probably are represented by one or another of the subdivisions of Deiters' nucleus described in birds by Ramon y Cajal (1909–11), Craigie (1928), and others. The specific peripheral connections of the relatively small number of primary vestibular fibers that end in cell group *l* of mammals are unknown. In addition to these, group *l* receives fibers from the ipsilateral vermal cortex and possibly from the fastigial nucleus (Brodal *et al.*, 1962). The significance of these connections and of the efferent fibers to the medial longitudinal fascicle is speculative.

The remainder of Deiters' nucleus, although it does not contribute fibers to the descending medial longitudinal fascicle, sends numerous fibers into the ascending fascicle, as demonstrated by Brodal and Pompeiano (1958). All types of cells in the nucleus are affected by lesions of the fascicle in the caudal part of the midbrain.

In Nauta-Gygax preparations, following stereotaxic lesions of Deiters' nucleus, Carpenter (1960a) found degenerating fibers, mostly crossed, to all three eye muscle nuclei and to the mesencephalic interstitial nucleus of Ramon y Cajal, as well as a few to the nucleus of Darkschewitsch and the nucleus of the posterior commissure. Deiters' nucleus also sends fibers bilaterally into the caudal pontine reticular formation, according to Carpenter. No fibers from this nucleus appear to project to the cerebellum.

Brodal and Pompeiano (1958) found that the medial vestibular nucleus sends fibers, chiefly crossed, into the ascending medial longitudinal fascicle. These derive from all parts of the nucleus, with a slight preponderance from the dorsomedial part. Some end in the nuclei of the trochlear and oculomotor nerves. The ventrolateral region of the caudal part of the nucleus was said to send fibers to the cerebellum. The medial nucleus gives rise to fibers that pass into the descending medial longitudinal fascicle, ipsilaterally and contralaterally, according to the experimental evidence of many authors who used the Marchi method. Brodal *et al.* (1962) regarded this nucleus as the only one for which the evidence is clear that it contributes to the descending fascicle.

To those of the Oslo school the superior vestibular nucleus appears to send all its long efferent fibers to higher levels of the brainstem, chiefly by way of the ascending medial longitudinal fascicle. Brodal *et al.* (1962) found no adequate evidence to indicate that this nucleus sends fibers to the spinal cord or to the cerebellum.

The inferior vestibular nucleus apparently does not contribute fibers to the direct vestibulospinal tract, as already noted. It probably contributes to the descending medial longitudinal fascicle, according to Pompeiano and Brodal (1957a) and Brodal *et al.* (1962), but they could not find whether the cells of origin are distributed throughout the nucleus or are localized. Carpenter, Alling, and Bard (1960) and Carpenter (1960a) found no fibers from the inferior nucleus projecting into the cord. Some degenerated fibers, according to Carpenter (1960b), extend from the inferior nucleus to the region around the solitary fascicle and its nucleus, and some continue beyond the solitary nucleus into the dorsolateral reticular formation. A few were said to distribute medially into the area between the nucleus solitarius and the dorsal motor nucleus of the vagus.

Following lesions of the ascending medial longitudinal fascicle, Brodal and Pompeiano (1957) found cell changes in all parts of the inferior nucleus except cell group *f*, where they found few cells affected. According to Carpenter (1960a) no fibers from the caudal and ventrolateral parts of the inferior nucleus appear to become part of the ascending medial longitudinal fascicle; any that do so probably originate in the rostral part only. However, fibers were said to project diffusely and bilaterally into the reticular formation of the medulla oblongata. Brodal and Torvik (1957) found retrogressed cells in the ventrolateral caudal part of the inferior nucleus following lesions of the cerebellum, which indicates that vestibulocerebellar fibers distributing medially to the nodulus, uvula, and fastigial nucleus and laterally to the flocculus arise in part from this nucleus. According to Carpenter (1960a) the cerebellar fibers from the inferior vestibular nucleus project bilaterally to the cortex of the nodulus and uvula, while a few pass into the fastigial nucleus; however, the ipsilateral fibers pass to the flocculus. After lesions of the nodulus, uvula, and fastigial nucleus, cell group *f* showed many affected cells (Brodal *et al*, 1962).

Stereotaxic unilateral lesions of the medial longitudinal fascicle near the abducens nucleus, according to Carpenter and Hanna (1962) who employed the Nauta technique, resulted in degenerated fibers to the eye muscle nuclei and midbrain and, in addition, a small number apparently projected into portions of the posteroventral nucleus of the thalamus. Such lesions of the fascicle did not permit analysis of the specific vestibular nuclear origin of fibers reaching these destinations.

Cell group *x* sends fibers into the ascending medial longitudinal fascicle (Brodal and Pompeiano, 1958) and to the cerebellum (Brodal and Torvik, 1957). According to Carpenter (1960a) predominantly ipsilateral fibers pass from group *x* to the fastigial nucleus.

Cell group *z* shows changes of uncertain character following section of the ascending medial longitudinal fascicle (Brodal *et al*, 1962) and no cell changes following destruction of the fastigial nucleus (Carpenter, 1960a). Carpenter, Alling, and Bard (1960) found that the perihypoglossal and paramedian reticular nuclei, which receive fibers from the fastigial nucleus, also send fibers to this nucleus.

Centrifugally degenerating fibers in the vestibular nerve after certain lesions of the medulla oblongata were observed by several investigators including Leidler (1913, 1914), who called them the efferent vestibular root. They apparently correspond to the crossed vestibular root fibers of Ramon y Cajal (1909–11) and of Gray (1926). P. van Gehuchten (1927) referred to them as the centrifugal vestibular nerve. Wenderowic and Klossowsky (1932) observed that descending fibers from the cerebellum also appear to enter the vestibular nerve.

G. L. Rasmussen (1946) demonstrated in the cat that fibers crossing the midline in the region of the genu of the facial nerve belong to an olivocochlear efferent bundle which passes through the vestibular ganglion and reaches the basal coil of the cochlea by way of the nerve of Oort. Subsequently G. L. Rasmussen (1953) was able to follow these fibers a short distance within the organ of Corti but not to terminations on the hair cells. An ipsilateral component which joins the crossed olivocochlear bundle before this emerges from the medulla oblongata was also found by G. L. Rasmussen (1960).

Physiological studies of anesthetized cats by Galambos (1956) led him to conclude that efferent impulses through the olivocochlear bundle may attenuate the effects on the brain of auditory stimuli. Further studies on unanesthetized animals, however, did not confirm this conception and the role of the olivocochlear bundle was said to be uncertain (Galambos, 1960).

In the vestibular labyrinth fine fibers normally present beneath the neuroepithelium disappear following section of the vestibular root (Petroff, 1955). Such degeneration also was said to follow median sagittal section between the facial colliculi of the floor of the fourth ventricle, which seems to imply that the fibers are predominantly crossed. After lesions of Deiters' nucleus or section of the vestibular root, G. L. Rasmussen and Gacek (1958) found small degenerating fibers that they traced through the vestibular ganglion, along with the olivocochlear bundle; like the fibers of this bundle, these have no connection with the cells of the ganglion. Such fibers, according to Gacek (1960), accompany the olivocochlear bundle as far as the inferior vestibular ganglion and then at that point sharply leave the efferent fascicle to the cochlea and distribute by small bundles to the ampullary cristae and the maculae of the utriculus and sacculus. Gacek was unable to follow these fibers beyond the point where they penetrate the basement membrane of the vestibular neuroepithelium.

Wersäll (1960) observed that type I hair cells of the vestibular sensory epithelium are innervated by thick myelinated fibers and the type II cells by thin fibers. All the fibers lose their myelin sheaths before or during their passage through the basement membrane of the neuroepithelium. The thick fibers divide into a small number of branches that end in calyces around the type I cells. The small fibers divide into a large number of very fine fibers that form a plexus at the base of the epithelium. Fibers from this plexus were said to end on the bases of type II cells or on the outer surface of the calyces enclosing the type I cells, with some terminating on the nerve fibers leading to these calyces (Wersäll, 1956; Engström, 1958). Some of the endings on type II cells and all on the calyces are granulated, while others on the type II cells are nongranulated. Engström (1958) regarded the granulated endings as probable efferents that represent a feedback system to the hair cells.

Dohlman, Farkashidy, and Salonna (1958) presented histochemical evidence of an efferent innervation of the vestibular receptors. An extensive distribution of dotlike granules beneath and to some extent between the hair cells of the ampullary cristae of the pigeon was demonstrated by Dohlman (1960) in silver-stained sections. These corresponded in size and distribution to the afferent and efferent terminals on hair cells described by Wersäll in the guinea pig, but Dohlman was unable to differentiate afferents from efferents. In histochemical studies Dohlman found evidence of an acetylcholinesterase activity beneath the sensory epithelial cells of the ampulla and utricle, and suggested that such activity is related to the function of the efferent fiber system.

The sources of the efferent fibers to the vestibular labyrinth have been interpreted in many ways. Carpenter, Bard, and Alling (1959), following labyrinthectomy in adult cats, described cell changes and losses in the medial, the superior, and parts of the inferior vestibular nuclei, in the interstitial nucleus of the vestibular root, and in the fastigial nucleus. Small- and medium-sized cells are involved in the medial nucleus; in the superior vestibular and fastigial nuclei both large and small cells were said to be affected, but no large cells of Deiters' nucleus showed changes. Degenerated cells were found both contralaterally and ipsilaterally. These observations seem to be indicative of efferent fibers coming from several nuclei to the vestibular labyrinth. Employing the Brodal-Gudden method on kittens (somewhat older than those found by the Oslo school to respond most favorably), Gacek (1960) obtained no conclusive results in the vestibular or related nuclei after unilateral labyrinthectomy. In fiber degeneration experiments by Gacek lesions of the superior, inferior, or medial nuclei are not followed by degenerating fibers into the vestibular nerve, but lesions of Deiters' nucleus or intramedullary lesions of the vestibular root result in degeneration of fibers that could be traced to the vestibular labyrinth. Contrary to Petroff (1955), Gacek found intact, in the chinchilla, the plexus of fine fibers beneath the neuroepithelium in protargol-stained material following intramedullary section of the vestibular root. Decalcification of the petrous bone is completed within an hour in the chinchilla — this method avoids the deleterious effects on stainability of the fibers produced by long continued action of decalcifying fluids. Using Sudan black, Marchi, and silver preparations, after midline lesions between the facial colliculi of the cat, Gacek found degeneration of the olivocochlear bundle but none in the branches of the vestibular nerve. Gacek regarded the lateral vestibular nucleus as the probable origin of the small myelinated efferent vestibular fibers, but he recognized the possibility of a system of unmyelinated fibers to the vestibular labyrinth.

The myelinated efferent fibers, as described by Gacek, appear to be entirely ipsilateral and their number approximates only about 200 in a total of 12,000 fibers in the vestibular nerve of the cat (G. L. Rasmussen and Windle, 1960). This is a small number to be divided among the five units of the vestibular labyrinth.

The conflicting observations and interpretations of various authors are difficult to reconcile but the presence of efferent fibers to the vestibular labyrinth seems certain. Their specific nucleus or nuclei of origin, as well as whether they are strictly ipsilateral or possibly both ipsi- and contra-lateral in origin, as are the efferents to the cochlea, require further investigation. The functional significance of the vestibular efferents also is in need of study by experimental methods.

Neuromuscular Spindles

Fusiform collections of small striated muscle fibers in the skeletal muscles of mammals were described by Kuhne (1863a, 1863b), who called them muscle spindles, and by other early authors in studies of mammals and the frog. Ruffini (1893, 1897–98) and Sherrington (1894) described their structure and innervation more completely in the cat. Sherrington also demonstrated experimentally that the nerve fibers then known to end in the spindles passed into the dorsal roots of the spinal nerves, which indicates the sensory nature of the organs.

The neuromuscular spindles are composed of a variable number of small striated muscle elements called intrafusal fibers, nerve fibers and their terminations on the intrafusal fibers, and a surrounding capsule of connective tissue. The intrafusal fibers are arranged in an axial bundle with a periaxial space intervening between it and the capsule. Outside the capsule a zone of perimysium separates the spindle from the neighboring ordinary skeletal muscle or extrafusal fibers, whose course is parallel with the intrafusal elements. According to Swett and Eldred (1960b) the capsule proper extends over only 30 percent to 50 percent of the length of the spindle, with each end of the capsule continuing as a sleeve around the axial bundle toward its respective pole of the spindle. The spindle length was defined by these authors as the distance from the tip of the longest intrafusal fiber at one pole to the tip of the longest fiber at the opposite pole of the spindle.

Simple and compound spindles have long been recognized. Boyd (1959) differentiated them on the basis of differences in size and innervation of the intrafusal fibers. Tandem series of two or three simple spindles were described by Cuajunco (1927), Barker (1959), Swett and Eldred (1960a), and others. Usually the spindles lie in clefts between fascicles of muscle fibers but generally not in the larger septa of connective tissue.

Swett and Eldred (1960a, 1960b) compared the distribution, numbers, and structure of the muscle spindles in the medial gastrocnemius and soleus muscles of the cat. These two muscles differ greatly in size and also in their histological, contractile, and reflex characteristics. The medial gastrocnemius of the cat was said to be 2.5 to 4 times as large in volume as the soleus. The soleus is a "red" muscle, while the gastrocnemius is a "white" muscle. Both extend the ankle, but the soleus contracts more slowly, is less subject to fatigue, and differs in other physiological respects from the gastrocnemius. According to

Swett and Eldred (1960a) large marginal strips of both muscles are devoid of spindles. Areas at either end of the gastrocnemius have no spindles and approximately 40 percent of the muscular part of this muscle lacks them. In the soleus, muscle spindles supposedly occur nearer its origin and insertion, and distribution is more widespread. Relative to the volume the soleus is more richly supplied with muscle spindles than the gastrocnemius.

The length of muscle spindles varies over a wide range. According to Tello (1906) this variation is not related to the length of the muscle since there are short spindles in long muscles, long ones in short muscles, and spindles of different length in the same muscle. Swett and Eldred (1960b) found the mean lengths of spindles of the soleus muscle in the cat to be 5.8 mm and those of the medial gastrocnemius to be 4.8 mm. The soleus spindles are only 22 percent longer, although the muscle fascicles of the soleus are approximately twice as long as those of the gastrocnemius.

The spindle length in a number of human muscles, as recorded by various authors, ranges from 0.3 mm to 13 mm. Cooper and Daniel (1956) found a range between 3 mm and 12 mm in single human spindles. In the cat and monkey Sherrington (1894) recorded lengths from 0.75 mm to 4 mm. Hagbarth and Wohlfart (1952) reported mean lengths of 2.6 mm for the soleus and 1.8 mm for the gastrocnemius of the cat. These authors evidently measured the length of the capsule part of the spindles, as Swett and Eldred (1960b) suggested. Double-linked tandem spindles have an average length of 10.2 mm in the soleus and 10 mm in the gastrocnemius, while triple-linked spindles are 15.4 mm and 14.4 mm long in the respective muscles, according to Swett and Eldred.

At the proximal pole of the spindle the intrafusal fibers are attached to the endomysium of extrafusal fibers, while individual intrafusal elements frequently are related to different extrafusal fibers. The intrafusals are gathered together in a common sheath as one organ. Distally they end on the endomysium of adjacent extrafusal fibers or become invested for a short distance by dense connective tissue, with the small tendon so formed ending in an aponeurosis; most of the small intrafusal fibers, however, end in the sleevelike distal part of the capsule (Swett and Eldred, 1960b). In tandem-linked spindles one or two intrafusal fibers, after being traced through the pole of a spindle, were found to continue into another spindle in which they develop a second zone of nuclei, while the intrafusal fiber appears to belong equally to both spindles, according to Swett and Eldred (1960a). Intrafusal fibers are also supposed to end in intermuscular septa of the tendon serving the entire muscle.

The number of intrafusal fibers in individual spindles varies. Hagbarth and Wohlfart (1952) found an average of 6 in the soleus and medial gastrocnemius muscles of the adult cat. A range of 5 to 12 intrafusal fibers in the medial gastrocnemius and 4 to 8 in the soleus of a cat weighing 1 kg was recorded by Swett and Eldred (1960b), with means of 7.4 and 6.5 for the two muscles respectively. The human hand and neck muscles have 8 to 12 intrafusal fibers in the larger spindles, but at one end of the tandem spindles small spindles with 4 or fewer intrafusal fibers often occur (Cooper and Daniel, 1956). The number of intrafusal fibers is increased in compound spindles.

Considerable variation in the size of the intrafusal fibers within individual spindles was recognized by Sherrington, Ruffini, and other early authors. Swett and Eldred (1960b) recorded diameters ranging from 7 μ to 35 μ in the soleus and medial gastrocnemius muscles of the cat.

According to Barker (1948) the intrafusal fibers have two striated polar segments, which are separated by a richly nucleated noncontractile zone called the nuclear bag. A transitional zone, the myotube of Barker, is situated between the nuclear bag and the polar segment; the myotube loses its striations as it approaches the nuclear bag. According to Boyd (1956) the large intrafusal fibers have a nuclear bag in the equatorial region of the spindle but each of the small fibers has a chain of nuclei down the middle. The large fibers reportedly extend the full length of the spindle, while the small fibers have a length equal to about one-half of the spindle. Barker (1948), Boyd (1956, 1958), Cooper and Daniel (1956), Walker (1958), and Swett and Eldred (1960b) regarded the small fibers as a second type of intrafusal fibers. Boyd noted that the intrafusal elements of simple spindles vary somewhat in size but do not fall into two distinct groups as they do in compound spindles. Barker (1959), however, on the basis of reconstruction of the spindles, concluded that the small fibers are not discrete units but join to form an open-meshed syncytium. Cilimbaris (1910) had described, in the eye muscles of sheep, anastomosis of intrafusal fibers into a pattern somewhat similar to that of the heart muscle. Cooper and Daniel (1956) stated that they never observed division of intrafusal fibers in human muscle spindles, which agrees with Boyd's (1956) observations in the cat. Swett and Eldred (1960b) described the small fibers in the spindles of the cat's soleus and medial gastrocnemius muscles as frequently appearing to fuse but whether they actually do so is uncertain.

In the soleus muscle an extrafusal fiber sometimes accompanies the axial bundle through the capsule and beyond the nuclear region and ends in the connective tissue attachment of the spindle on a large intrafusal fiber. Instances of an extrafusal fiber joining the axial bundle and terminating on the proximal end of a large intrafusal fiber also were encountered in the soleus muscle. No such connections with extrafusal fibers were seen in the spindles of the gastrocnemius. These continuations of extrafusal fibers do not have nuclear regions at the levels where such occur in intrafusal fibers. Termination of extrafusal fibers on intrafusal elements places the two in series and presumably would increase the afferent discharge from the spindle (Swett and Eldred, 1960b).

Both the sensory and the motor terminals in the spindles are of two types, Boyd (1958) noted. Annulospiral or primary endings of large sensory root fibers wind about each large and small intrafusal fiber. Secondary flower-spray endings were said to occur at variable distances toward one or both poles of the spindle and as terminals of medium-sized fibers on both large and small intrafusal fibers. In addition, diffuse endings connected by fine nerve fibers occur throughout the sensory region of the small intrafusals. These diffuse endings Boyd (1959) divided into sensory and motor groups: the sensory group disappears after section of the dorsal roots of spinal nerves leading to specific muscles, and the diffuse motor endings disappear after section of ventral roots of the nerves.

The motor fibers to the large intrafusal muscle fibers terminate as one, two, or more motor end plates in the polar halves of each muscle fiber; these end plates are similar to those of extrafusal fibers. The motor terminals on the small intrafusal muscle fibers form very small plates (often near the nuclear region), long narrow plates, or diffuse networks that extend the length of the muscle fiber (Boyd, 1959).

Leksell's (1945) important discovery that selective stimulation of the small fibers of the ventral roots of the spinal nerves does not result in contraction of muscles but instead induces firing from the muscle spindles indicated that these small root fibers are the efferents of the intrafusal muscle elements. Since these small root fibers conduct impulses at velocities of 20 meters to 44 meters per second they were called γ fibers. Electrophysiological evidence (Pascoe, 1958; Diete-Spiff and Pascoe, 1959; Boyd and Davey, 1959) indicated two types of efferent fibers to the muscle spindles, both having conduction rates in the γ fiber range. One type, called β fibers, almost certainly ends on the large intrafusal fibers of compound spindles, according to Boyd and Davey; the other type presumably ends on the small intrafusal fibers. Boyd (1959) claimed there is suggestive evidence that the large intrafusal fibers with typical motor end plates serve twitch reflexes and that small intrafusal fibers with diffuse motor endings are capable of gradual contraction. For details of structure refer to the contributions cited above and for physiological analysis of the muscle spindles refer to the monograph of Granit (1955).

According to Granit, Pompeiano, and Waltman (1959) the large ventral root or α fibers that innervate the typical extrafusal fibers also activate muscle spindles in the cat. As already noted, Swett and Eldred (1960b) sometimes found extrafusal fibers in the soleus muscle entering the axial bundle of the spindles and terminating on a large intrafusal fiber or ending in the connective tissue attachment of the spindle. Such muscle fibers presumably are innervated by branches of α fibers of the ventral roots.

Barker and Chin (1961) investigated the possibility that some fibers may branch in such a way that they innervate both intra- and extra-fusal muscle fibers, as believed by a number of authors including Denny-Brown (1932) and Häggqvist (1960). After studying numerous gold-chloride preparations of muscle spindles of the spiny anteater (*Echidna aculeata*), bat, rat, rabbit, cat, and monkey, Barker and Chin did not find any histological evidence of branching of α fibers in a way which indicated that they appeared to enter the muscle spindles. Thus, Barker and Chin concluded that in mammalian muscle the intrafusal γ efferents and extrafusal α efferents are discrete.

The occurrence and number of spindles in individual muscles or muscle groups have engaged the attention of a number of authors. Cilimbaris (1910) reported a range of 78 (inferior oblique) to 281 (external rectus) spindles in the extraocular muscles of sheep, not including the retractor bulbi and levator palpebrae superior in which there are fewer spindles. Other authors have described spindles in this muscle group in various mammals, whereas many investigators failed to find them in other species. Similar contradictions with respect to spindles in the tongue also appear in the literature. Cooper (1953) noted that spindles are present in the eye muscles of man and goat, although they are not found in the macaque and cat. This author also found spindles in the tongues of man and monkey but not in those of cats and lambs. Merrillees, Sunderland, and Hayhow (1950) described spindles as a constant feature in human extraocular muscles. The spindles vary in number from 22 to 71 in different muscles and are confined to the proximal and distal thirds of the muscles. Inoue (1960) also found spindles in human eye muscles. Wolter (1955), who employed silver techniques, described six types of sensory end organs in the striated muscles of the human eye: neuromuscular spindles; sensory endings that resemble flower buds in the interstitial connective tissue and not in contact with muscle fibers; arborial sensory endings; brushlike endings; sensory spools; and sensory end bulbs. Spindles in other muscles have been studied in many species of mammals and in man.

In a comparative study of spindles in the lumbrical muscles of the hand and foot of the opossum, dog, five species of primates, and man, Voss (1937) found interesting differences especially in the first and second lumbricals of both extremities. The number of spindles in the first lumbrical of the hand range from 3 in the opossum and dog to 9 in the lemur and mandrill, 12 in the orangutan, 46 in the chimpanzee, 51.5 (average from 4 muscles) in man. There are 6 spindles in the second lumbrical in the hand of the opossum, 5 in the dog, 10 in the lemur, 11 in the mandrill, 22 in the orangutan, 31 in the chimpanzee, and 36 in man. The range is smaller in the first and second lumbricals of the foot but the number is much larger in the chimpanzee (36 and 27) and man (36 and 23) than in the orangutan or the subanthropoids.

Comparison of the number in the first and second lumbricals of the foot of the adult orangutan (9 and 14, respectively) with the larger number in the chimpanzee and man is of interest, since the weight of the adult male orangutan and the weight of the adult male chimpanzee, which can approach 200 pounds and 150 pounds respectively, both approximate the average weight in man. The lumbricals of the foot in man were said to flex the proximal phalanx of each of the four lateral toes and probably to feebly extend the middle and distal phalanges. In man, the lumbricals of the hand together with the interossei flex the basal phalanges on the metacarpal bone and extend the terminal and middle phalanges. They also draw the fingers toward the thumb. The greater number of muscle spindles in the first lumbrical of the hand of man and the chimpanzee, as compared with the orangutan, presumably is correlated with the greater manual dexterity of man and the chimpanzee.

According to Cameron (1929) the soleus muscle of the rabbit has a greater number of spindles, relative to volume, than the gastrocnemius. In the adult cat Hagbarth and Wohlfart (1952) found 56 spindles in the soleus and 45 in the medial gastrocnemius; Swett and Eldred (1960a) found 53 spindles in the soleus and 70 in the gastrocnemius of a cat weighing 1 kg. Whether or not the differences in the results of these groups of investigators are owing to technical procedure or to other factors, the soleus muscle in the cat as in the rabbit has the larger number of spindles in proportion to its volume. The functional significance of the difference is not clear.

Freiman (1954) found the human masseter, temporal, and medial pterygoid muscles rich in spindles relative to their weight. The concentration of spindles in the medial pterygoid varies in different parts of the muscle; in the lateral pterygoid no spindles were found. After studying spindles in various mammals and man, Latyshev (1957) concluded that the finer the coordinative action of a muscle, the greater the number of spindles within it. Barker (1959) found a range of 77 to 132 spindles in the rectus femoris of the cat and 52 to 89 spindles in the tibialis anterior. The fifth interosseus of the forefoot ranges from 20 to 31 spindles. Barker concluded that the lower the spindle content of a muscle the narrower the range of variation is and that the number of spindles in a pair of identical muscles is closely equivalent, with the equivalence being closest in muscles with a low spindle count.

In terms of richness of nerve fibers and nerve endings Ruffini (1897–98) regarded the muscle spindles as second only to the eye and ear among the sensory organs. The more recent contributions have shown that the spindles are far more intricate in structure and innervation than Ruffini thought. The enumeration of spindles in various muscles of different species and their measurements are too fragmentary to estimate the total volume of the spindles in comparison with other sensory organs in any one species, but the aggregate spindle mass must be considerable.

Neurotendinous Organs

The neurotendinous organs were described by Golgi (1880) in man, dogs, cats, rabbits, and a number of submammals, and his name usually is attached to them. Rollett (1876) had previously described them less fully. Similar nerve endings in the tendons of the eye muscles were found by Marchi (1882) and the sensory nature of neurotendinous organs was demonstrated by Cattaneo (1888). Huber and De Witt (1900), Dogiel (1902, 1906), and others made important contributions regarding structural variations, distribution, and details of the terminal branching of the nerve fibers in the organs. Their embryonic development was described by Tello (1917). The earlier literature was reviewed by Elwyn (1929).

The organs of Golgi are situated, as a rule, at the junction of muscle and tendon: one end is attached to the muscle and the other is continuous with the tendon fascicles; sometimes both ends are continuous with tendons. They occur in virtually all tendons and are especially numerous in the large fasciae of the back muscles. Instead of being situated in the tendons of some muscles the organs of Golgi can occur in the septa or sheaths. Sherrington (1894) and Barker (1948) also found them at the insertions of neuromuscular spindles.

The tendon organs usually are spindle-shaped but elongated cylindrical forms are not uncommon. They range in length from 0.08 mm to 0.8 mm and in width from 0.02 mm to 0.4 mm, as reported in mammals by Golgi and other authors. In man lengths up to 3 mm and widths up to 1.5 mm have been reported (Ciaccio, 1891).

The tendon organs of mammals usually are enclosed in a lamellated capsule of varying thickness. The thickest capsules are formed of many layers of collagenous fibers separated by flattened cells. Nonencapsulated tendon organs have been described and compound organs also have been observed by a number of authors.

The nerve supply of the Golgi organs typically is by a single large myelinated fiber with unusually short internodal segments. Occasionally two or three independent fibers innervate a single organ. The fibers often divide into two or three branches which accompany nerve trunks in the intermuscular septa. The fibers always approach the Golgi organ from the muscular side and usually enter it at the center, which is sometimes at the muscular pole. The sheath of Henle becomes continuous with the capsule of the organ and the nerve fibers divide into primary, secondary, and tertiary branches which retain their myelin sheaths. The tertiary branches divide into numerous unmyelinated rami winding between and around the primary fascicles and give off side branches that also divide repeatedly, appearing as delicate ribbons with large leaflike expansions. According to Dogiel the terminal branches and plates form an enveloping network around the primary tendon bundles.

In the soleus and medial gastrocnemius muscles of the cat Swett and Eldred (1960a) found organized bundles of connective tissue extending from the aponeurotic coverings of the muscles into the muscle substance. These bundles, classified as tendon organs, differ from other more irregular projections of connective tissue by their association with nerve fibers and the presence of a thin capsule. They were found only immediately adjacent to the deep and superficial aponeuroses of the two muscles, and their areas of distribution correspond with the areas of attachment of the muscles. Fusion with or attachment to a muscle spindle was never observed.

The average length of the tendon organs is 0.81 mm in the soleus of the cat and 0.66 mm in the gastrocnemius. The organs number 45 in the soleus and 44 in the gastrocnemius, the majority in both muscles lined the aponeuroses of insertion. If one considered the tendon organs in relation to muscle volume or number of motor units they would be more numerous in the soleus, but ratios for numbers of spindles to tendon organs are 1:2 in the soleus and 1:6 in the gastrocnemius.

Ralston, Miller, and Kasahara (1960) recently described Golgi organs and other types of nerve terminations in human tendons.

Central Connections of Proprioceptors

The primary central connections of the proprioceptors, except those related to the trigeminal and eye muscle nerves, are with the spinal cord. Agduhr (1919) demonstrated that the neuromuscular spindles of some muscles of the cat may be connected by their sensory nerve fibers to two segments of the cord. Monosegmental, bisegmental, and trisegmental innervation of the spindles of the flexor digitorum sublimis and profundus muscles of the cat was found by Cuajunco (1932). In plurisegmental innervation consecutive segments of the cord are involved. The number of segments or nerves was said to have no relation to the size of the spindle or the number of intrafusal muscle fibers.

Experimental studies by Mountcastle, Covian, and Harrison (1952) and McIntyre (1953), using the method of evoked potentials, indicated that impulses carried by large fibers (13 μ to 20 μ in diameter), described as primary or nuclear bag nerve fibers, reach the cerebellum only after relay in Clarke's column of the spinal cord. McIntyre noted that impulses through fibers 6 μ to 12 μ in diameter, described as secondary or myotube fibers, project to the cerebral cortex. Responses in the cerebral cortex that are not diminished by removal of the cerebellum were obtained by Mountcastle *et al.* only when the smallest nerve fibers (1 μ to 8 μ) from the muscles had been more strongly stimulated. A possible nociceptive function for the small fibers was suggested by Mountcastle and associates. These authors stated that small fibers are only moderately represented in muscle nerves, although they are numerous in nerves going to the skin.

The neuromuscular spindles of the jaw muscles, which are terminals of fibers in the branches of the trigeminal nerve, and other proprioceptors of the teeth and gums, also served by the trigeminus, are connected with the mesencephalic trigeminal nucleus (Corbin, 1940; Corbin and Harrison, 1940).

The central connections of the muscle spindles and tendon organs of the eye muscles are in doubt. Many authors (Golgi, 1893; Clark, 1926; Weinberg, 1928; and others) believed that they are connected with the mesencephalic trigeminal nucleus. Tozer (1912), Sherrington (1918), Nicholson (1924), and others suggested that cells along the roots of the eye muscle nerves, especially the oculomotor, are related to proprioceptive fibers.

Pearson (1949a) described cells of mesencephalic V type intermingled with motor cells in the nuclei of the oculomotor and trochlear nerves of human fetuses. In the opossum, rat, and man, Pearson (1949b) found indications that the oculomotor and trochlear roots contribute fibers to the mesencephalic trigeminal root. He also described fibers from this root and processes of mesencephalic V cells that enter the base of the cerebellar vermis and hemispheres. They spread out in a thin sheet of fibers; some appear to enter the cerebellar nuclei.

The curious absence of spindles in the eye muscles of the monkey (Cooper, 1953), mentioned above, may account for certain differences in the occurrence of central cells. Whether other types of proprioceptors occur in the monkey, as in human eye muscles, appears not to have been established.

Many other histological types of receptors in muscles, joints, ligaments, and elsewhere have been described by Gardner (1944, 1956), Ralston, Miller, and Kasahara (1960), and earlier authors. These receptors probably differ functionally from the tendon organs as well as from the muscle spindles but their central connections are little understood. The muscle spindle and tendon organ impulses reach the corpus cerebelli. The increase in relative size and elaboration of structure of this division of the cerebellum appears to be closely related to the elaboration and increase of these sensory systems in the ascending vertebrate scale. In the larger mammals, as will be seen later in the book, the size of the corpus cerebelli is relatively the largest and the subfoliation of its lobules is carried furthest in species that have the best coordination of muscular activity.

SIZE AND WEIGHT OF THE MAMMALIAN CEREBELLUM

THE cerebellum of mammals varies greatly in size and weight. The breadth of the cerebellum in the masked shrew, *Sorex cinereus*, one of the smallest mammals, is approximately 5 mm whereas the breadth in the fin whale is 204 mm, according to Jansen (1953). After fixation in formalin, the weight ranges from a small fraction of a gram in the masked shrew to an average of 1230 gm in the fin whale; one cerebellum recorded by Jansen weighed 1330 gm. (The fresh cerebellum probably is somewhat heavier since Liechtenhan (1945) found the specific gravity of the human cerebellum to be 1.0452 to 1.0457 before fixation in formalin, and 1.0430 to 1.0431 after fixation.) The cerebellum of man weighs from 140 gm to 150 gm. In Ziehen's (1899) tabulation of the results from various authors the human cerebellum was recorded as having a slightly higher specific gravity than the cerebrum, but comparable determinations were not given for other species. Putnam (1928) noted that the proportion of cerebellar weight to total brain weight in different species ranges from 8 percent to 25 percent, averaging 10 percent.

The results reported by most earlier authors come within the same range. Leuret and Gratiolet (1839–57), however, gave the cerebellar weight of the rodent, *Myoxis glis*, as 32 percent of the total brain weight and that of the mouse as 50 percent of the weight of the cerebrum. Since the entire mouse brain weighs 0.37 gm or slightly more according to Ziehen's tables, the cerebellum alone would weigh about 0.12 gm. In the mole, *Talpa europea*, the cerebellum weighs 0.17 gm, representing 13 percent of the total brain weight. The cerebellum of the rabbit, *Lepus cuniculus*, weighs from 1.2 gm to 1.5 gm, or about 15 percent of the total brain weight; in the spiny anteater, *Echidna aculeata*, it weighs 1.5 gm. According to Jansen (1954) the cerebellum of the fin whale accounts for 20.2 percent, on the average, of the total brain weight. In two specimens of the dolphin, *Phocaena phocaena*, Putnam recorded weights for the cerebellum that are 15 percent and 15.75 percent of the total brain weight. She stated, however, that there is no constant relationship between body size and the ratio of cerebellar weight to total brain weight. From his observations Jansen concluded that there is no evidence that the total brain weight influences the percentage of cerebellar weight in any constant pattern.

By comparison Ziehen noted that the cerebellum of eight species of birds varies from 0.28 gm in the thrush, *Turdus merula*, to 1.05 gm in the turkey, *Meleagris gallopavo*. The range in weight of the cerebellum in relation to total brain weight is from 7.4 percent to 14.8 percent, with an average of 11.4 percent including duplicate weighings of several species by different authors. The ratio of cerebellar weight to total brain weight in birds, while not so high as in some species of mammals, remains approximately within the same limits, on the average, in these two classes of vertebrates despite the rudimentary cerebellar hemispheres of the avian brain. This must mean that a relatively more important interrelationship exists between the cerebellum and the large corpus striatum of birds than in mammals.

ALBINO RAT

DURING development, the cerebellum of the white rat (*Mus norvegicus*) passes through stages of folding of the cortex that resemble the adult pattern in small bats, shrews, and other Insectivora and the middle stages of young opossums still in the pouch. The subdivisions of the adult rat cerebellum are more readily comparable with those of birds than are those of most mammals available in sufficient numbers for adequate comparison with respect to development and adult pattern. The vermis of small adult Insectivora is much less foliated than that of birds and most mammals, and the marsupial vermis is also difficult to compare with the avian cerebellum. Since the adult rat cerebellum shows in simple form the fundamental pattern of the lobules in placental mammals and also in most marsupials, the rat cerebellum will first be described as typical of the mammalian cerebellum and its subdivisions in their various modifications.

Development

The development of the rat cerebellum was described by Aciron (1950) and myself (1952). Aciron's studies included more numerous and more closely graded early stages of cortical folding, while my studies followed later stages in greater detail. Since these accounts are important to the understanding of the adult cerebellum, they will be reviewed before the adult cerebellum is discussed.

Aciron encountered the first indication of fissure formation in the 24-mm-long embryo. At this stage a furrow has appeared in the posterior part of the cerebellum which crosses the midline; Aciron regarded this furrow as corresponding to the sulcus anonymus of Hochstetter (1929) in the human embryo. At the 36-mm and later stages of the rat Aciron recognized the continuity of the posterolateral fissure across the midline and considered the sulcus anonymus of his earlier stages as corresponding to the vermal part of this fissure. The lateral part, which evidently appears before the sulcus anonymus, was illustrated from a model of a 30-mm-long embryo as a well-defined furrow separating the flocculus from the ventrolateral part of the cerebellum. The completed posterolateral fissure was recognized by Aciron as the boundary between the flocculonodular lobe and the corpus cerebelli. I did not agree with Hochstetter's conception of the significance of his sulcus anonymus in the human embryo or with Aciron's description of the furrow he called sulcus anonymus in the rat, but Aciron's description of the formation of the posterolateral fissure is in general accord with my observations in other species.

In the 24-mm to 35-mm stages of the embryo the posterodorsal part of the cerebellum enlarges more rapidly than the rate of the anteroposterior adjustment of the cerebellar base. The border to which the choroid tela is attached becomes directed forward by the stresses of unequal growth, which results in retarded folding of the posterior part of the cortex. This in turn gives a very shallow vermal segment of the posterolateral fissure in the 35-mm-long embryo, although the fissura prima and the preculminate fissure, which have appeared in the meantime, become prominent at this stage. In subsequent development the cerebellar base elongates and the ventral part of the posterior cerebellar surface folds more deeply, which produces a more prominent posterolateral fissure.

FLOCCULONODULAR LOBE

The differentiation of the flocculonodular lobe and corpus cerebelli, as described by Aciron, is borne out by my observations in full-term fetuses and young rats. In the 21-day-old fetus and the 20-hour-old rat the posterolateral fissure extends from the lateral surface of one side of the medulla oblongata to the other as a continuous

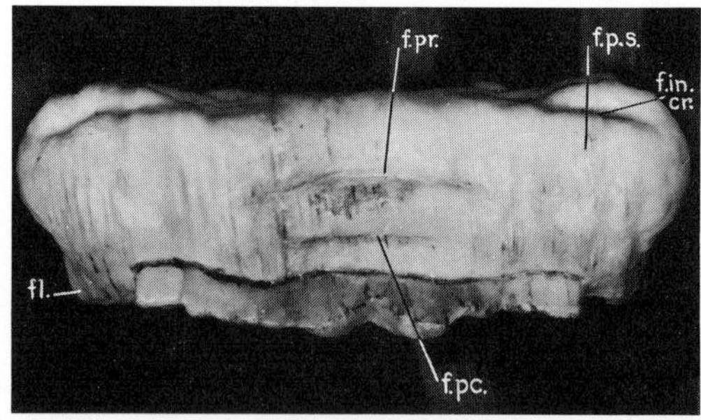

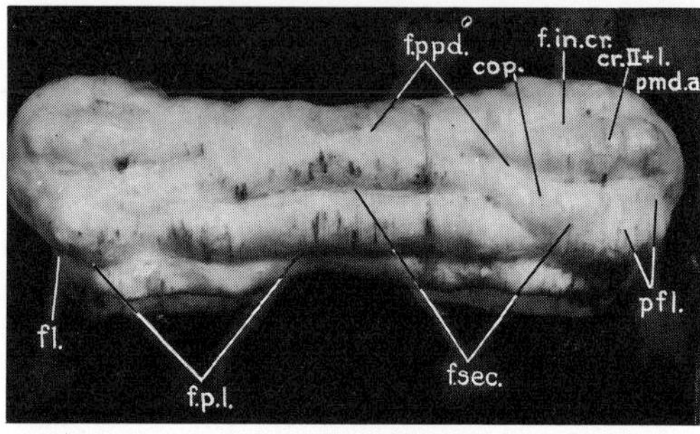

Figure 1. Model of cerebellum of rat fetus at 21 days. A. Anterior view. B. Dorsal view. (Larsell, 1952.)

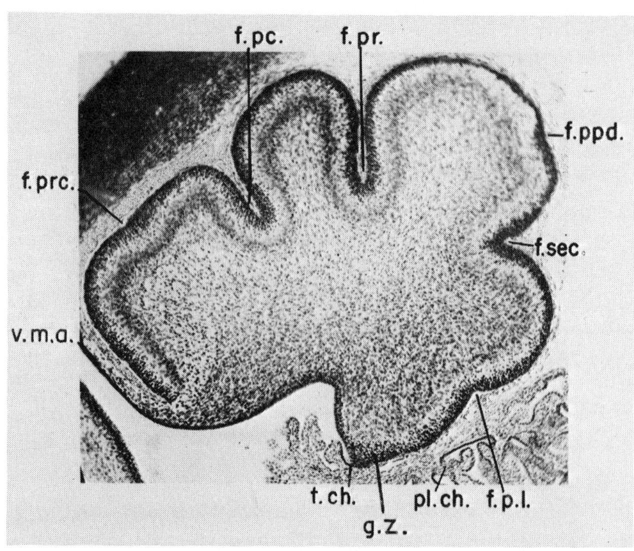

Figure 2. Midsagittal section of cerebellum of rat fetus at 21 days.

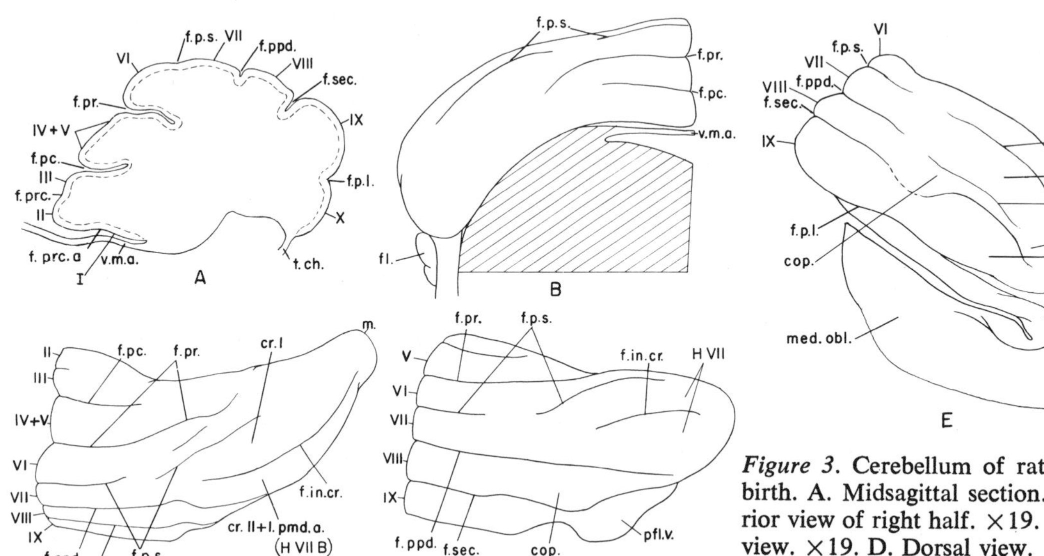

Figure 3. Cerebellum of rat 20 hours after birth. A. Midsagittal section. ×21. B. Anterior view of right half. ×19. C. Rostrodorsal view. ×19. D. Dorsal view. ×19. E. Lateral view. ×15. (Larsell, 1952.)

boundary between the two primary subdivisions of the cerebellum (figs. 1B, 3E). Medially it is shallow but on either side, between the flocculus and the corpus cerebelli, it is much deeper.

The flocculus in the full-term fetus forms a somewhat flattened swelling ventral of the posterolateral margin of the corpus cerebelli (figs. 3E, 4B). From its lower border the rhombic lip is recurved caudomedially so that a narrow cleft results between the ventricular margin of the flocculus and the rhombic lip; this cleft represents the recessus lateralis of the fourth ventricle. Rostrally, where it is continuous with the flocculus, the recurved portion of the rhombic lip is a broad triangular area, tapering caudalward, which represents the tuberculum acusticum (fig. 3E).

The nodulus, or lobule X, in the 21-day-old fetus is a prominent swelling between the posterolateral fissure and the germinal zone of the posterior cerebellar margin (fig. 2). It is connected with the flocculus on either side by a band of cortex which is separated from the corpus cerebelli by a continuation of the posterolateral fissure. The choroid tela, in the full-term fetus, extends ventrally and caudally from the ventral margin of the germinal zone. Although Aciron did not say so, it is probable that the nodulus of the rat is represented by paired rudiments at an earlier stage of development, as in man (Larsell, 1947) and in the pig (Larsell, 1954).

CORPUS CEREBELLI

Aciron found that fissuration of the corpus cerebelli begins in embryos between 28 mm and 30 mm in length by formation of transverse furrows in the medial part of the lobe. At the 30-mm stage two furrows, the fissura prima and the preculminate fissure, which are approximately equal in depth, were described and illustrated in photomicrographs of median sagittal sections of the cerebellum. The fissura prima was identified by the difference in structure of the developing cortex immediately behind

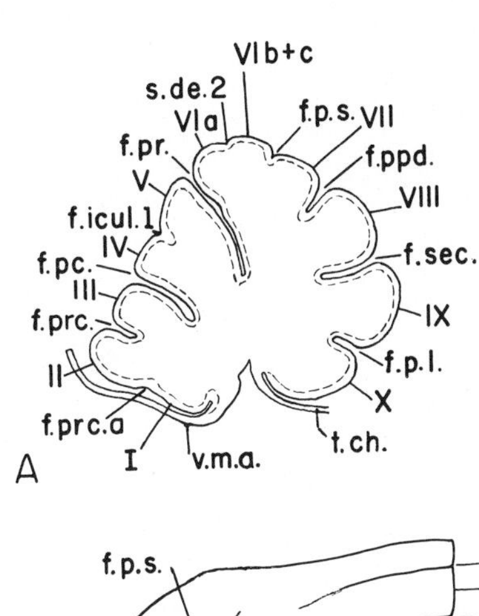

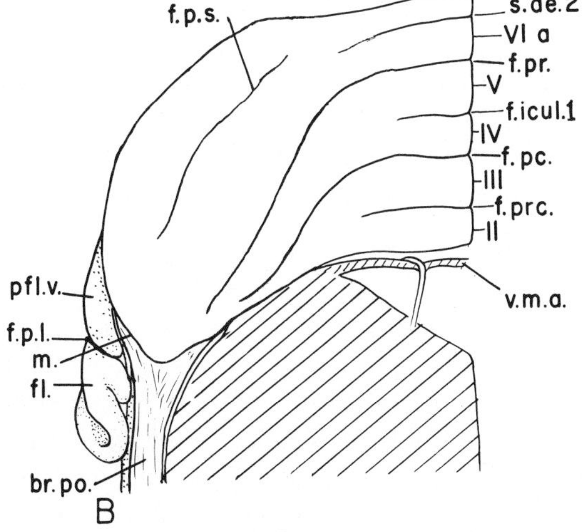

Figure 4. Cerebellum of 2-day-old rat. A. Midsagittal section. B. Anterior view of right half. ×28. (Larsell, 1952.)

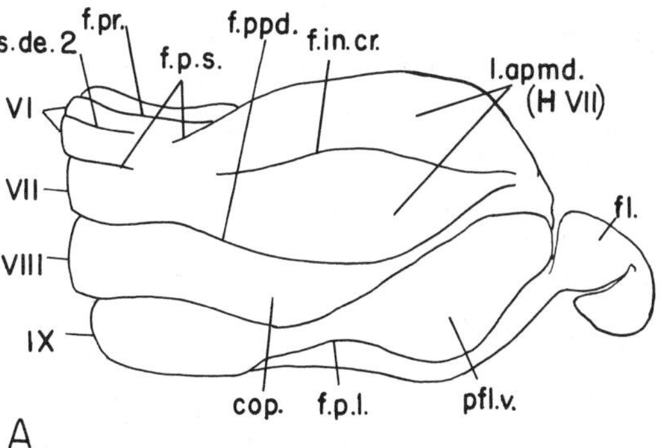

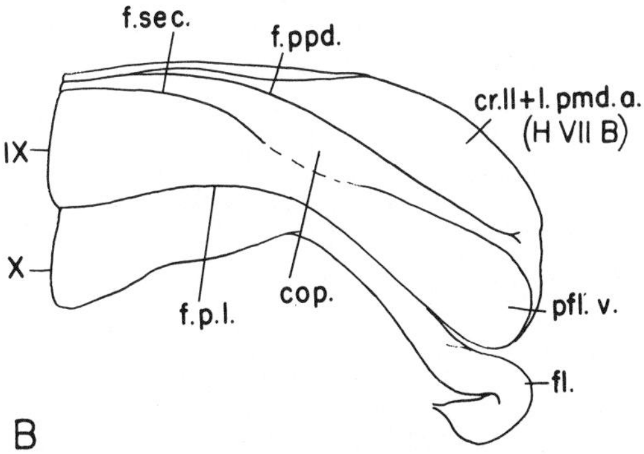

Figure 5. Cerebellum of 2-day-old rat. A. Dorsal view of right half. B. Posterior view. ×20. (Larsell, 1952.)

it. Hochstetter (1929) described similar peculiarities of the cortex situated between the fissura prima and the prepyramidal fissure in certain stages of the human embryo and named the segment involved lobus X. This should not be confused with lobule X, the nodulus.

Since the fissura prima is slightly shallower than the preculminate fissure in the earlier stages, Aciron was inclined to regard the latter as the more precocious of the two. In the full-term fetus the fissura prima is slightly deeper than the preculminate fissure, and in postpartum stages it deepens rapidly owing to accelerated expansion of the lobules that form its walls. In neonatal rats there can be no doubt that the fissura prima is the principal fissure of the corpus cerebelli and that it divides this major section of the cerebellum into anterior and posterior lobes (figs. 3A, 4A, 6A, 9A, 10A). Unlike many of the interlobular fissures, which are formed by the confluence of vermal and hemispheral furrows on either side of the vermis (figs. 5, 7, 8), the fissura prima gradually extends into the hemispheres from the vermis and is the first fissure to reach the margin of the cortex (figs. 3B, 4B, 6B, 9B, 15B). The incipient hemispheres as well as the vermis, accordingly, are included in the two primary subdivisions of the corpus cerebelli.

To determine the relative importance of other fissures

of the corpus cerebelli one must note their order of appearance, which as mentioned above varies somewhat from species to species, as does their depth in median sagittal sections, their lateral extent, and the sequence of approach of their hemispheral segments toward the margin of the cerebellar cortex. Frequently it also is necessary to follow the fissures from their position in the adult cerebellum through to that in postnatal and fetal stages. In the following description of the development of fissures and lobules in the cerebellum of the rat it should be remembered that both result from expansion of the cerebellar cortex. The lobules burgeon outward into the only available space. Their continuations with the deep part of the cerebellum become elongated and also, owing to crowding of adjacent lobules, these continuations become more or less constricted as seen in sagittal sections. The depth of the fissures increases pari passu with the outburgeoning of the lobules.

Anterior lobe. The preculminate fissure extends only a short distance from either side of the midline in the 21-day-old fetus (fig. 1A). Subsequent stages of development show that it reaches the cerebellar margin earlier

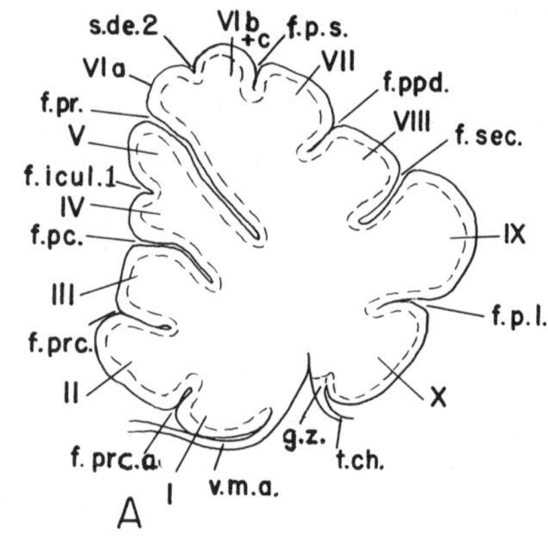

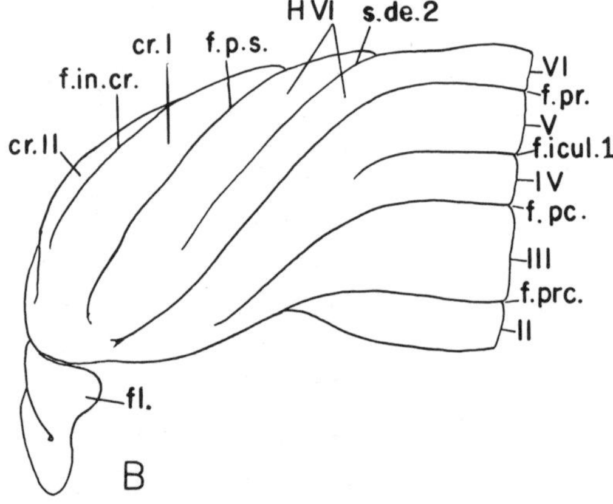

Figure 6. Cerebellum of 3-day-old rat. A. Midsagittal section. ×28. B. Anterior view of right half. ×20. (Larsell, 1952.)

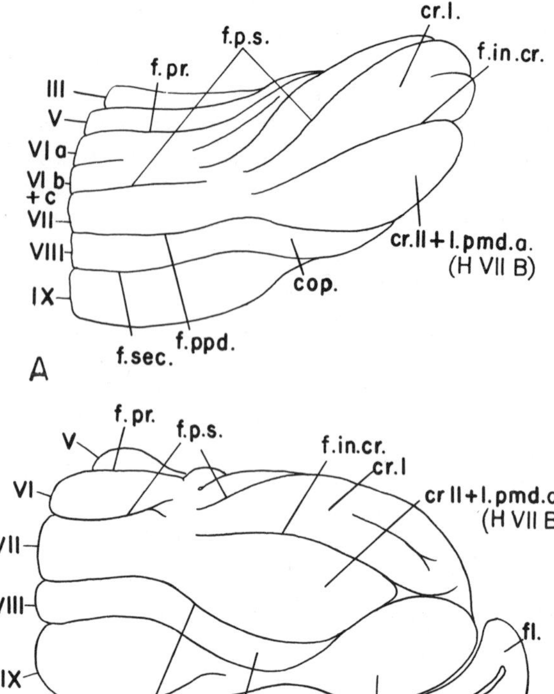

Figure 7. Cerebellum of 3-day-old rat. A. Dorsal view of right half. ×28. B. Posterior view. ×20.

than any other furrow of the anterior lobe. However, the fissura prima does appear before the preculminate fissure (figs. 9B, 10B). The preculminate fissure, accordingly, divides the lobe into dorsal and ventral segments that correspond to the only divisions represented in adult small bats and soricine shrews. The vermal parts of these segments correspond, respectively, to the culmen and the central lobule plus lingula of the human cerebellum.

The dorsal segment shows no indication of subdivision in the 21-day-old fetus but the ventral segment is divided into two parts by a shallow furrow (fig. 2). At 20 hours postpartum a second groove appears on the ventral surface of the ventral segment. The two grooves of the ventral segment were called the intracentral and the precentral fissure, respectively, in my earlier contribution on the rat (Larsell, 1952); the corresponding furrows in the cat and monkey (Larsell, 1953a) and the pig (Larsell, 1954) also were so named. Further study of these fissures and comparison with the development of the ventral part of the anterior lobe in the human embryo made it clear that the furrow in the anterior surface of the ventral segment of the rat embryo corresponds to the precentral fissure in man, while the one in the ventral surface corresponds to precentral fissure *a* (cf. figs. 3A, 4A,

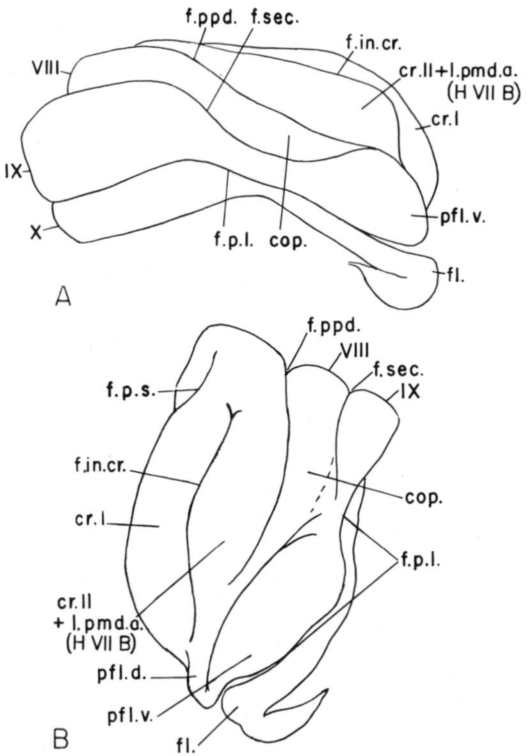

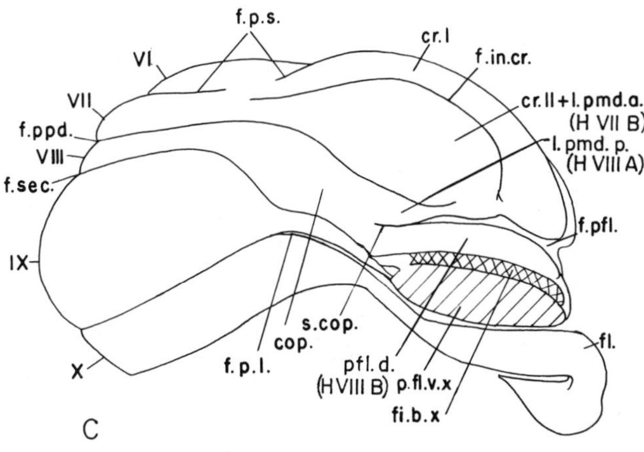

Figure 8. Cerebellum of 3-day-old rat. A. Posteroventral view of right half. ×18. B. Lateral view of left side. ×25. C. Posterolateral view of right half, after removal of ventral paraflocculus. ×22.5. (Larsell, 1952.)

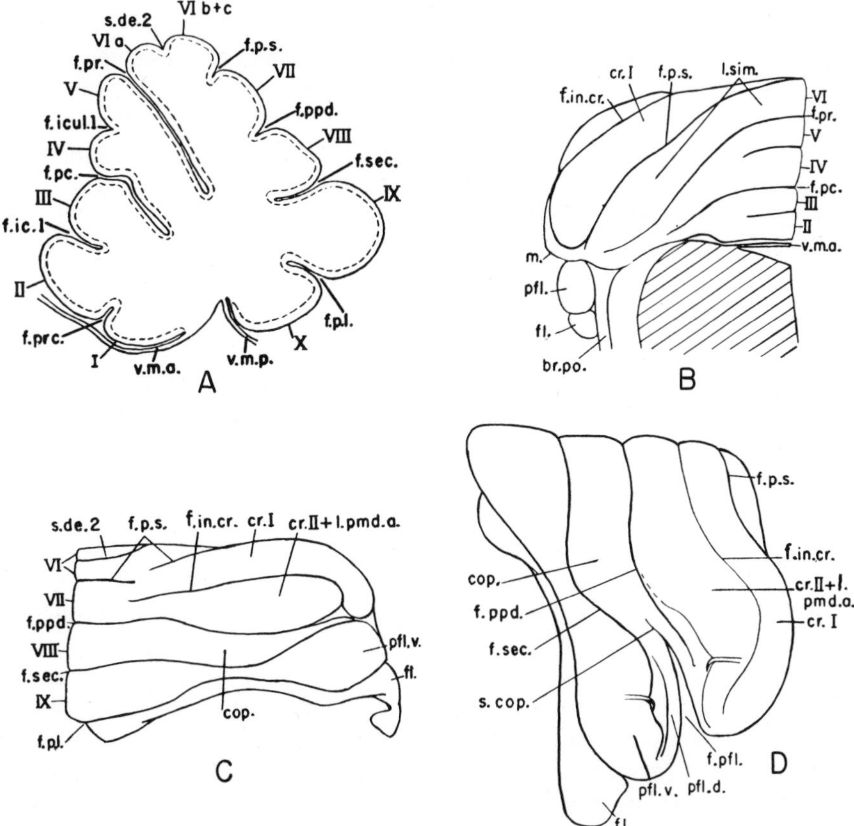

Figure 9. Cerebellum of 4-day-old rat. A. Midsagittal section. ×24. B. Anterior view of right half. ×15. C. Posterodorsal view of right half. ×15. D. Lateral view of right half. The ventral paraflocculus and crus II–paramedian lobule are shown retracted. ×22.5. (Larsell, 1952.)

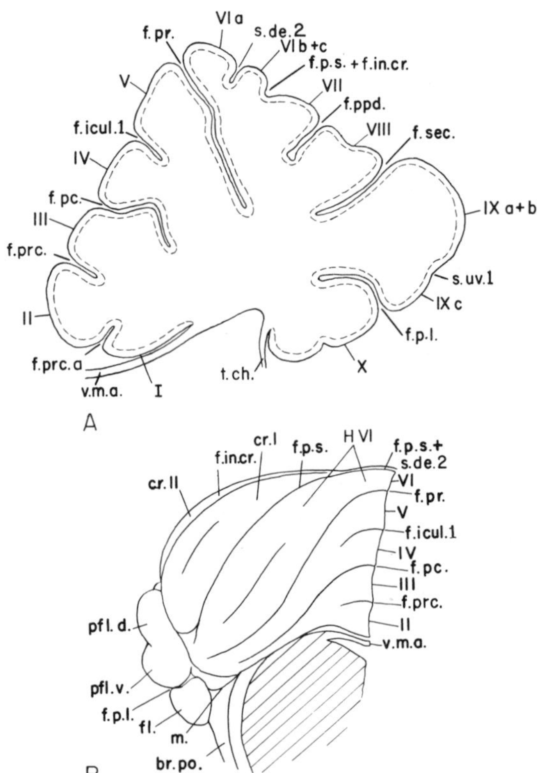

Figure 10. Cerebellum of 5-day-old rat. A. Midsagittal section. ×22.5. B. Anterior view of right half. ×15. (Larsell, 1952.)

6A). These fissures divide the anterior lobe of the rat into lobules I, II, and III, corresponding to lobuli 1, 2, and 3 of Bolk (1906) in various species. Precentral fissure *a* deepens slowly but by 3 days postpartum lobule I has enlarged sufficiently to show its characteristic form, and precentral fissure *a* is fairly deep (fig. 6A). The precentral fissure was also designated by Aciron but his figures of embryonic stages show no indication of precentral fissure *a*. In his figure of a median sagittal section of the adult cerebellum precentral fissure *a* was labeled the "fiss. praecentralis," while the deeper precentral fissure described above was not labeled. The developmental history of these fissures during the first five days postpartum in the rat clearly shows that Aciron's precentral fissure in the fetus corresponds to my precentral fissure and that his precentral fissure of the adult rat corresponds to my precentral fissure *a* of early postnatal and adult stages.

At two days postpartum the fissura prima and preculminate fissure both extend into the hemisphere, with the preculminate fissure completely dividing the anterior lobe into dorsal (or culminate) and ventral segments. The vermal part of the dorsal segment is divided by a shallow intraculminate fissure into the rudiments of lobules IV and V. The fissure extends only a short distance on either side of the midline so that the two lobules merge laterally, forming an undivided area of cortex that tapers ventrolaterally and ends between the extremities of the fissura prima and the preculminate fissure in the hemispheral part of the lobe (fig. 4B). In the ventral segment lobules II and III merge on either side at the ends of the precentral fissure. Precentral fissure *a*, not visible in the anterior view of the lobe, extends laterally as far as the lateral border of the anterior medullary velum. Lobule I lies so far behind the ventral margin of lobule II and is so small at this stage that it could be seen only by tilting the cerebellum upward in a way that exposes its ventral surface. The lobule then is visible as a rounded swelling that projects ventralward, impinging on the anterior medullary velum; it does not extend laterally into the hemisphere.

Except for differences in the depth of the fissura prima and differences in the relative size of the lobules and the form of lobule I, the anterior lobe of the 2-day-old rat corresponds to the anterior lobe and folia I–V of the 18-day-old duck embryo. Folium I of the duck embryo, however, is directly continuous rostrodorsally with the anterior medullary velum, whereas in the rat lobule I is a rounded swelling of the posterior border to which the velum is attached. Subsequent modifications of folium I in the duck, already noted, suggest the manner in which lobule I of the rat and other mammals has been transformed from a possible ancestral form resembling that of the earlier stages of the duck embryo and of most adult birds.

The hemispheres of the 2-day-old rat have enlarged considerably and the anterior surfaces are divided, by the laterally extending fissures described above, into definite hemispheral segments which I called lobules HIII and HIV + HV. Neither the fissura prima nor the preculminate fissure quite reaches the cerebellar margin. The intraculminate and precentral fissures end so far short of this margin that the hemispheral segments of lobules IV and V merge, while lobule II appears not to be represented in the hemisphere at this stage (fig. 4B). The hemisphere is larger in the 3-day-old rat but the lobules of the anterior lobe are very similar to those of the earlier stage (fig. 6).

During the fourth to tenth days postpartum the fissures continue to deepen as the lobules burgeon outward. In the 5-day-old rat the intraculminate fissure is as deep as the precentral fissure that appeared earlier (fig. 10). By 10 days postpartum lobules II, III, and V all show secondary foliation, and lobule V also has expanded dorsally and rostrally in such a manner as to dwarf lobule IV (fig. 15). At 14 days after birth the fissures have essentially the same appearance as in the adult. The lobules are fully differentiated but have not attained their ultimate growth (cf. fig. 17 with figs. 19 and 21). The common stalk (as it appears in sagittal sections) which connects lobules IV and V with the basal cerebellar mass has become elongated by the outward burgeoning of the lobules and by the increase in volume of the adjoining parts of the cerebellum. As a result the two lobules appear to be secondary divisions of a primary lobule served by one medullary ray.

Whether lobules IV and V should be regarded as secondary divisions corresponding to sublobuli 4A and 4B of Bolk (1906) and Riley (1929) or to the two divisions dorsal of the preculminate fissure in the human embryo, noted by G. E. Smith (1903c), and to lobules III and IV of Ariens Kappers, Huber, and Crosby (1936), which together were indicated as the culmen, depends on the definition of the primary lobule. If defined in terms of the primary medullary rays that branch from the deep medullary mass of the adult cerebellum, the two folds of the culmen in the rat and many other species must be considered to be secondary lobules. The appearance of the medullary rays serving these and other lobules, however, is secondary to the folding of the cortex and the formation of the fissures.

The problem of determining which fissures and lobules are primary and which are secondary is complicated by the fact that certain of the secondary ones in the adult cerebellum may appear almost simultaneously with, or just a bit later than, the primary lobules and fissures in different species. In some species a secondary fissure may appear in the vermis earlier than the primary fissure which forms one of the boundaries of the lobule subdivided in the adult, e.g., the vermal segment of the ansoparamedian fissure of the pig and other ungulates.

In the 2-day-old rat the culmen segment of the anterior lobe is divided by the intraculminate fissure, which is shallow at this stage but becomes deeper in successively later stages. The posterior superior fissure also appears as a shallow furrow in the posterior lobe and forms the posterior boundary of lobule VI (lobulus simplex of Bolk). This lobule already is subdivided by a faint furrow, which in later stages and the adult cerebellum obviously is a secondary fissure (declival sulcus 1). It is shallower than either the intraculminate or posterior superior fissures but its early appearance in lobule VI, which becomes very large in the rat, points to another difficulty in distinguishing between primary and some secondary fissures. Individual lobules develop precociously in some species and become foliated early; other lobules in the same or other species are retarded, with the primary fissures delimiting them from each of the adjacent lobules being reduced. The depth of the primary or secondary fissures and their order of appearance are related to the size ultimately attained by the subdivisions delimited by them. In the pig, lobules IV and V both are large when fully developed. The intraculminate fissure appears at about the same time in the embryo as the preculminate and precentral fissures but it becomes the deepest fissure in the anterior lobe, which causes such a deep separation between lobules IV and V that each usually has its individual medullary ray. Numerous variations in the depth of the intraculminate fissure and in the medullary rays leading to the two lobules are found in the adult cerebellum of other species.

Therefore on comparative grounds I regarded the two subdivisions of the culmen segment in the rat as lobules IV and V. Lobule IV includes the cortex from the deepest part of the preculminate fissure to the deepest part of the intraculminate fissure; lobule V includes the cortex from the depths of the latter to the deepest part of the fissura prima. So defined, both lobules have a relatively large surface.

The early division of the culmen segment of the rat into the rudiments of lobules IV and V and of the ventral segment into lobules I, II, and III is suggestive of a connection with the somatotopic relations of the dorsal and ventral parts of the culmen and of the central lobule and lingula already mentioned. It appears to represent an anticipatory differentiation of these lobules for more or less specific connections and functions.

Posterior lobe. The posterior lobe of the corpus cerebelli is more complex than the anterior lobe both in development and in adult pattern. In following the differentiation of its fissures and lobules, a natural starting point is the first of each to appear, the vermal segment of the fissura secunda and lobule IX, the uvula.

Aciron (1950) found that the fissura secunda in the 35-mm-long rat embryo is a shallow furrow in the posterior surface of the vermis. It deepens rapidly, as shown in this author's photomicrographs of later stages. In our full-term fetuses (fig. 2) the fissura secunda is nearly as deep in the median sagittal plane as the preculminate fissure but it almost disappears for a short distance on either side of the vermis. A furrow in the rudiment of the paraflocculus, corresponding to the intraparafloccular fissure of Jansen (1950) in the whale embryo, becomes confluent with the vermal furrow so that in the 3-day-old postpartum rat the definitive fissura secunda has formed (fig. 8). A similar early development of the fissura secunda from vermal and parafloccular segments also was found in embryos of the rabbit, pig, and man, as described in subsequent sections. In the course of differentiation of the rudiment of the paraflocculus into the ventral and dorsal paraflocculus the lateral segment of the fissura secunda elongates between them, ending at the lateral continuity with the other. Vermal and hemispheral segments of other fissures that were recognized in the fully differentiated cerebellum of the rat and other species also may appear in different sequence, depending on the relative development of the lobules separated by them. The fissures become confluent as cortical folding increases with further growth. As described and illustrated by Aciron, the vermal segment of the fissura secunda is the third fissure to appear in the corpus cerebelli. The lateral or parafloccular segment of the fissure, not mentioned by Aciron, is represented by a faint furrow in my full-term fetuses. In view of the subsequent confluence of these two furrows to form the definitive fissura secunda in the same manner as other fissures are formed from vermal and hemispheral segments, the two segments of the fissura secunda could be regarded as early phases of its development (figs. 3, 5, 8, 9D).

Lobule IX, the uvula, is represented in Aciron's 35-mm-long embryos by a rounded segment of cortex between the fissura secunda and the posterolateral fissure. Lobule IX expands rapidly so that in sagittal sections of the full-term fetus a caudally projecting, nearly semicircular lobule is presented (fig. 2). It tapers on either side into a narrow zone which is continuous with the incipient ventral paraflocculus (fig. 3E). In the 5-day-old rat a shallow groove, representing uvular sulcus 1, divides the lobule into folia IXa + b and IXc (fig. 12A). By 7 days postpartum this fissure has deepened greatly and uvular sulcus 2 has appeared between folia IXa and IXb. A third furrow, uvular sulcus 3, may appear by the 10-day postpartum stage differentiating folium IXd from IXc. This fissure is not always formed, however, so that lobule IX of some adult cerebella has only three subdivisions (fig. 23B).

Lobule VIII, the pyramis, is delimited from the more rostral part of the vermis by the appearance of a faint furrow representing the prepyramidal fissure in the 35-mm-long embryo of Aciron's series. The fissure deepens slowly and is still shallow in the rat 20 hours after birth (fig. 3A). A spurt of rapid growth of the cortex follows so that in the 2-day and 3-day postpartum young lobule VIII is well defined and furrows have appeared in the cortex between it and the fissura prima (figs. 5A, 7). At 3 days postpartum a furrow, the intrapyramidal fissure, appears in the posterior surface of the lobule, dividing it into two parts. The larger dorsal and anterior part reaches the external surface of the cerebellum and also faces the prepyramidal fissure. The smaller and posteroventral division forms the lower part of the anterior wall of the fissura secunda. This fissure and the two sublobules are somewhat variable in subsequent stages of development but they seem to be characteristic of the adult cerebellum. In the larger mammals, including man, lobule VIII is divided into sublobules VIIIA and VIIIB by a deep intrapyramidal fissure; sublobule VIIIB frequently is smaller than VIIIA as, for example, in man. The subdivisions in the rat seem to correspond, on a smaller scale, to those of the larger species; they may be called lamellae VIIIa and VIIIb.

The cortex situated between the prepyramidal fissure and the fissura prima (lobulus c_2 of Bolk, lobulus medius medianus of Ingvar, or lobus X of Hochstetter) is the latest part of the vermis to differentiate in the rat as in other embryos. Not only does the external granular layer appear last, but histogenetic differentiation also is retarded beneath the surface, as already noted. In the 21-day-old fetus the rostral portion of this cortex has differentiated approximately to the stage found elsewhere, but in the region immediately in front of the prepyramidal fissure the external granular layer still is thin. By 20 hours postpartum the typical pattern of the early cortex has formed here also and the cortex has begun to expand and fold. A shallow furrow has appeared about midway between the fissura prima and the prepyramidal fissure (fig. 3). Subsequent stages demonstrate that this furrow is the vermal segment of the posterior superior fissure. The two folds of cortex which this furrow separates are the rudiments

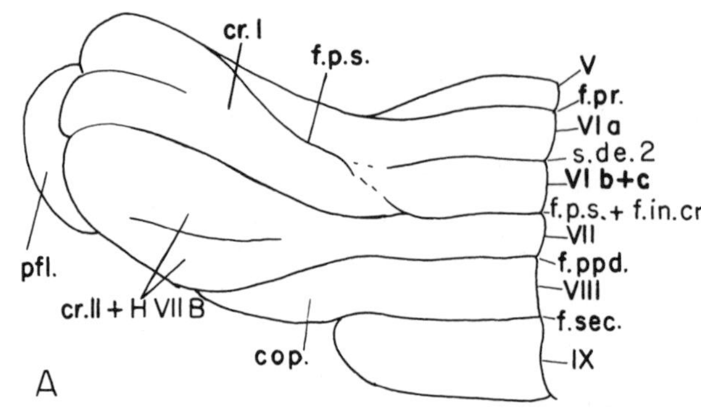

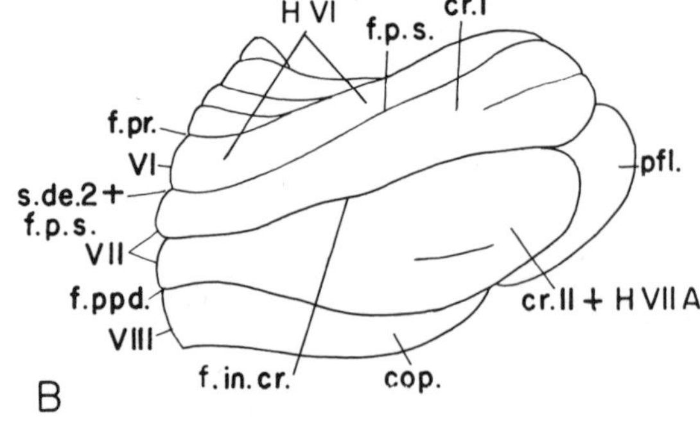

Figure 11. Cerebellum of 5-day-old rat. A. Dorsal view of left half. B. Dorsal view of right half. ×20. (Larsell, 1952.)

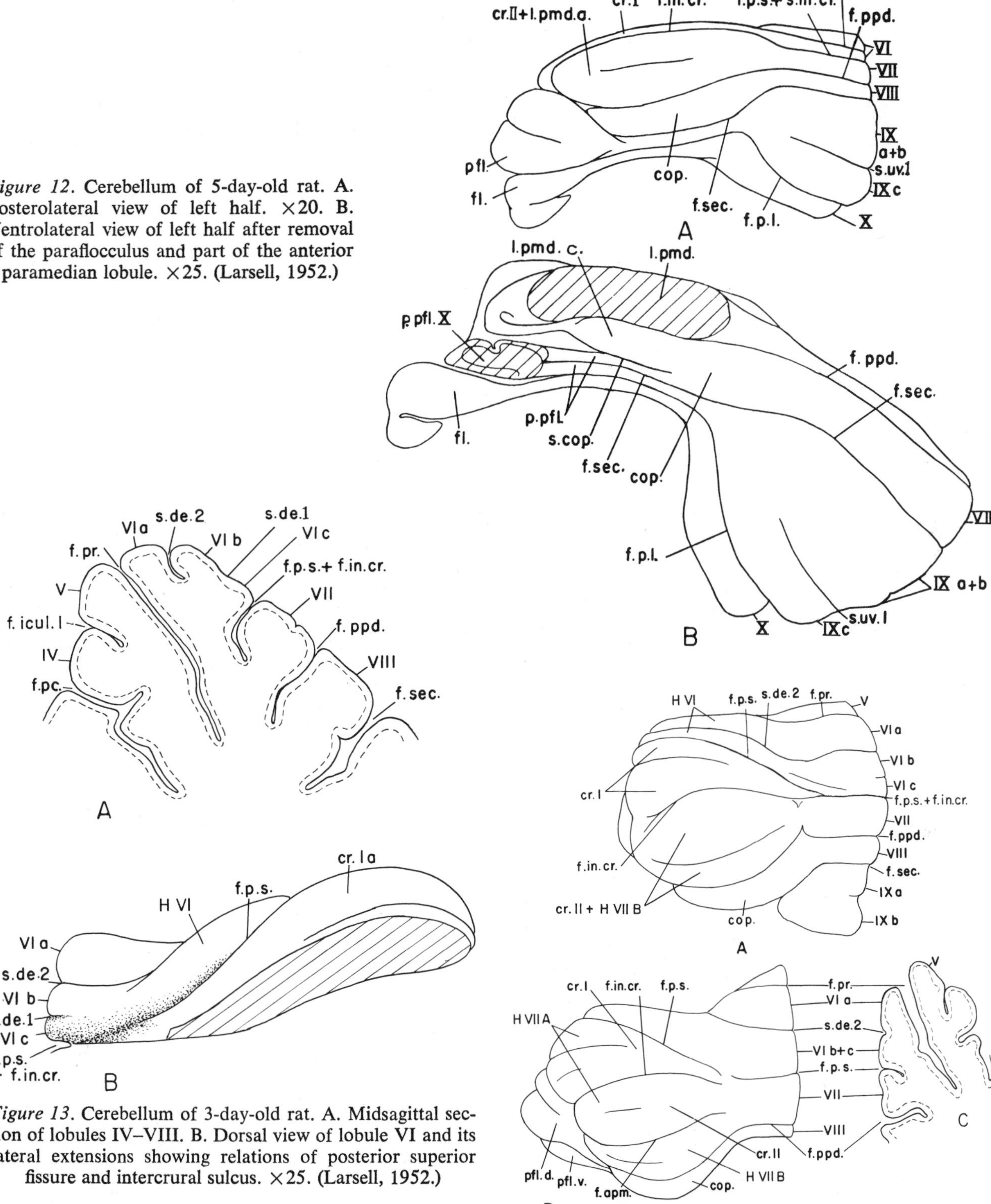

Figure 12. Cerebellum of 5-day-old rat. A. Posterolateral view of left half. ×20. B. Ventrolateral view of left half after removal of the paraflocculus and part of the anterior paramedian lobule. ×25. (Larsell, 1952.)

Figure 13. Cerebellum of 3-day-old rat. A. Midsagittal section of lobules IV–VIII. B. Dorsal view of lobule VI and its lateral extensions showing relations of posterior superior fissure and intercrural sulcus. ×25. (Larsell, 1952.)

Figure 14. Cerebellum of 7-day-old rat. A. Dorsal view of left half. ×16.5. B. Cerebellum of 8-day-old rat. Dorsal view of left half. ×16.5. C. Sagittal section of V–VII to show the features illustrated in the right-hand part of B. (Larsell, 1952.)

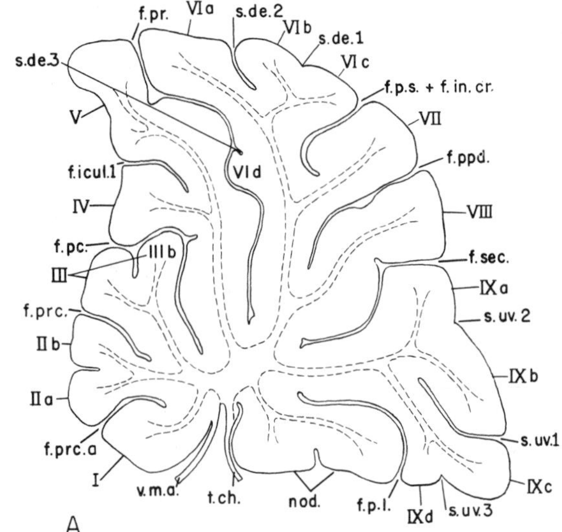

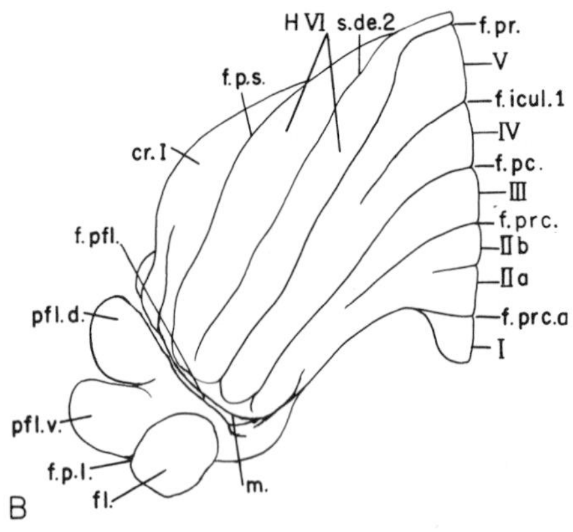

Figure 15. Cerebellum of 10-day-old rat. A. Midsagittal section. ×22.5. B. Anterior view of right half. ×15. (Larsell, 1952.)

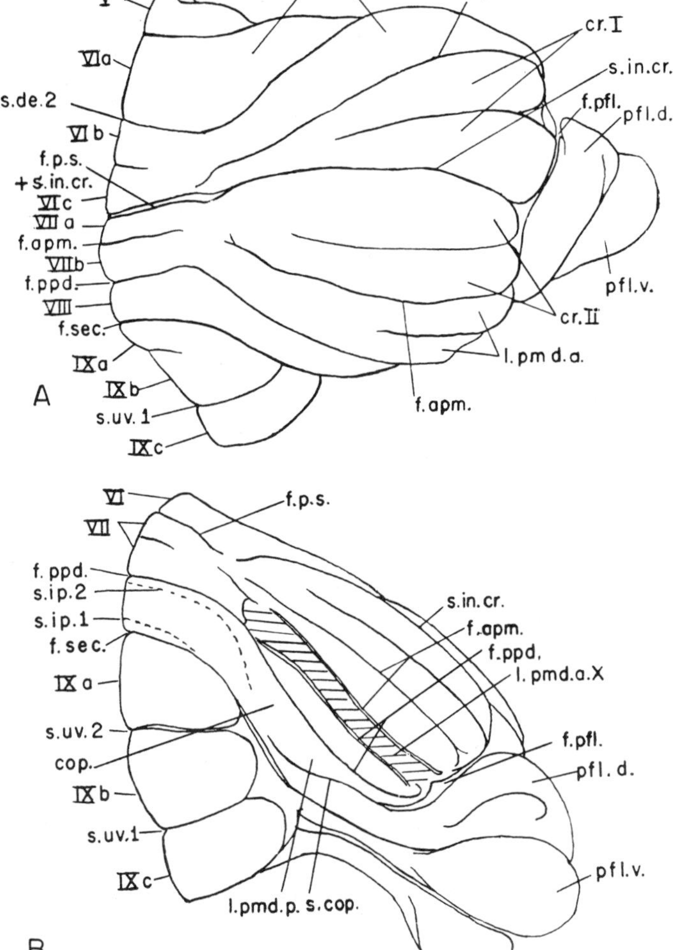

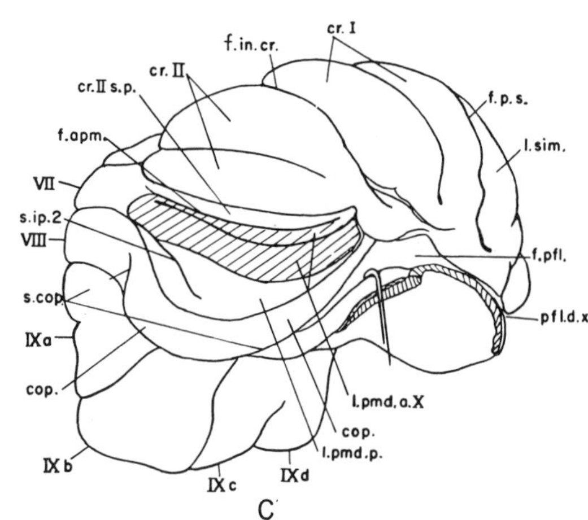

Figure 16. Cerebellum of 10-day-old rat. A. Dorsolateral view of right half. ×18. B. Posterolateral view of right half with anterior part of paramedian lobule dissected away. ×18. C. Posterolateral view of right half, tilted farther caudally than in B. The anterior part of the paramedian lobule and the dorsal paraflocculus have been largely removed and the parafloccular peduncle was retracted. ×16. (Larsell, 1952.)

of lobules VI and VII. At this stage of development the hemispheral segment of the posterior superior fissure, first noted by Aciron in the 37-mm-long embryo, is more prominent than the vermal segment. By three days after birth it has deepened still further and also lengthened so that the two segments of the fissure are almost confluent (fig. 7). As the cortex continues to expand the confluence is completed (figs. 11, 13, 14, 17).

Lobule VII, the folium-tuber vermis lobule, situated between the posterior superior and the prepyramidal fissures, shows no indication of secondary foliation until about the tenth day postpartum (figs. 15, 16). Sometimes this lobule is undivided even in the adult rat. Apparently more typical is a division of the surface into two folia by a faint furrow, which sometimes is present in the 10-day-old rat but is deeper at 14 days when present and was found in some adult cerebella but not in others. In the 14-day-old stage it has reached the lateral border of the vermis. On the basis of a detailed comparison between the developing cerebellum of the pig, rabbit, cat, and man and that of the rat, I regarded this furrow in the rat as corresponding to Bradley's sulcus *a*, and, together with its lateral continuation described below, as homologous with the ansoparamedian fissure of Jansen (1950) in the whale embryo.

The portion of lobule VII behind the vermal segment of the ansoparamedian fissure corresponds to the posterior tuber vermis (sublobule VIIB) and the anterior part corresponds to sublobule VIIA of the cat, monkey (Larsell, 1953a), and other species described below. Because of the small size and lack of subdivision of these segments in the rat I called them VIIb and VIIa, respectively. In rabbit, pig, and human embryos the posterior tuber is more distinct from the remainder of lobule VII than in the rat. In ungulates and carnivores the posterior tuber corresponds to the second segment of the tuber, as it has been called in the cat by many experimental neurologists. After the vermis assumes a sinuous form in the course of its development in the cat and pig, sublobule VIIB forms a prominent group of folia that is related laterally with the paramedian lobule of Bolk.

Lobule VI, situated between the posterior superior fissure and the fissura prima, expands more rapidly than lobule VII after the two are differentiated in the 20-hour

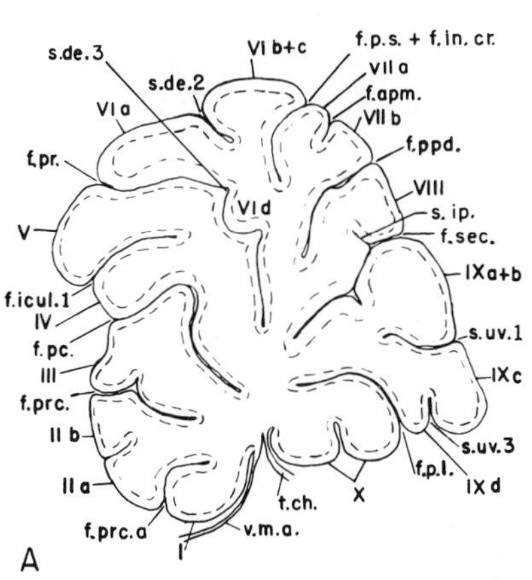

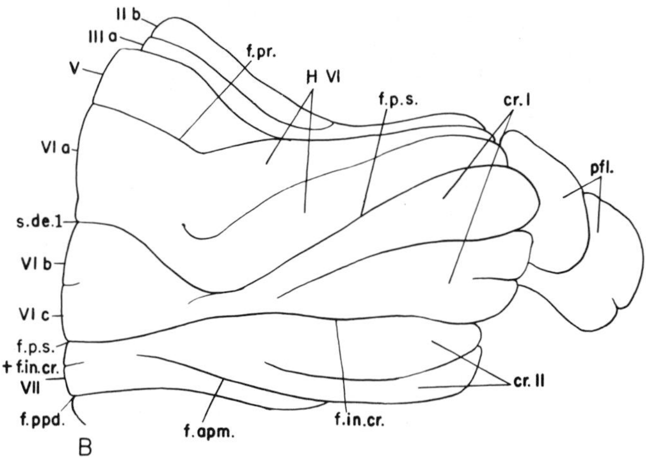

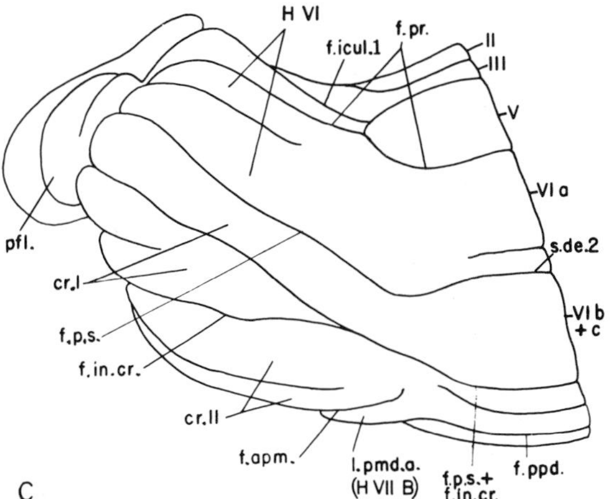

Figure 17. Cerebellum of 14-day-old rat. A. Midsagittal section. ×14. B. Rostrodorsal view of right half. ×16. C. Rostrodorsal view of left half of cerebellum of another 14-day-old rat; illustrates variation in posterior superior fissure and in lobule VI. ×16. (Larsell, 1952.)

postpartum rat. In the 2-day-old animal the lobule is subdivided by a shallow furrow into folia VIa and VIb + c (fig. 4A). In 1952, I called this furrow declival sulcus 2. It has no lateral representation until 3 days postpartum when a furrow appears in the hemispheral segment that is continuous medially with lobule VI; the furrow, however, does not become confluent with the vermal segment of declival sulcus 2 until about 5 days postpartum (fig. 11). A second vermal furrow may be encountered as early as 3 days after birth but it usually was not found until later. It may even be lacking altogether in the adult cerebellum. Frequently the posterior superior fissure and the intracrural fissure unite as they reach the vermis, forming a compound fissure between lobules VI and VII. The relations of the anterior wall of such a furrow, whether to the posterior part of the hemispheral continuation of lobule VI or to the anterior part of lobule VII, are difficult to determine in the rat.

Although declival sulcus 2 is variable in depth, thereby affecting the degree of differentiation of folia VIb and VIc from each other in embryonic stages, the three folia appear to be quite constant in the adult rat. In his illustration of a median sagittal section of the adult cerebellum of this species, Aciron interpreted as the folium and tuber vermis the folia that I designated VIb and VIc, respectively. The two segments between the folium-tuber lobule and the uvula, corresponding to my lobules VII and VIII, Aciron interpreted as belonging to the pyramis. I found no justification either in developmental stages or in the adult cerebellum for Aciron's interpretation of the pyramis as being composed of two deeply separated segments or of the two posterior folia of my lobule VI as being the folium and tuber vermis. If the declive, folium, and tuber of Aciron were regarded instead as folia VIa, VIb, and VIc, respectively, and the posteriorly adjacent subdivision of his pyramis as lobule VII, the "folium-tuber lobule," the pattern is identical with what I found in other species of mammals and also in birds. So interpreted, lobule VI of the rat is relatively large, a hypertrophy that is consonant with the importance of the trigeminus in this animal.

A furrow in the posterior wall of the fissura prima, which there is only a suggestion of in developmental stages up to 10 days postpartum, becomes well defined and constant in this growth stage and later (fig. 17). It may be called declival sulcus 3, and it delimits folium VId from the remainder of the posterior wall of the fissure. This folium is remarkably constant in the rat as is a corresponding fold of cortex in other mammals. In the larger species folium VId becomes the most prominent of several lamellae in the posterior wall of the fissura prima. In species of which appropriate embryonic stages have been available it is the first prominent fold of lobule VI to appear in this wall. Also it is identifiable in the adult cerebellum by a more or less characteristic size and form, as well as by its position in relation to other folds in the posterior wall of the fissura prima of larger mammals.

Medullary rays. In the adult cerebellum of all species, sheets of myelinated fibers radiate from the deep medullary mass, enter the individual vermal and hemispheral lobules, and ramify into their subdivisions. As seen in sagittal sections, especially of the vermis, these resemble a low tree and its branches; collectively they were known earlier as the arbor vitae, with the individual branches being called medullary rays. It is important to recognize that the rays are sections of sheets of white substance. These sheets are formed of afferent fibers from various sources that end in the cortex and of efferent fibers from the cortex that end chiefly in the deep cerebellar nuclei.

The medullary body may divide into anterior and posterior trunks of varying length, in different species; these trunks divide into medullary rays to the lobules. In other species the lobules receive direct primary branches from the medullary body; each lobule as a rule receives a principal ray which forms its core and ramifies to its subdivisions. Bolk (1906), Riley (1929), and others have defined the lobules of the adult cerebellum on the basis of the primary medullary rays.

In the developing rat cerebellum no compact medullary rays are visible in sections until the cortical folds expand superficially and the connections of these expansions with the deeper part of the cerebellum begin to become well-defined constrictions between the deep parts of the fissures. Vestibular, spinocerebellar, and olivocerebellar fibers enter the cerebellum before cortical folding begins, as also is shown in Tello's (1940) photomicrographs of the mouse cerebellum. Many of these fibers enter the early appearing commissures, but there is no indication of medullary rays until after cortical folding is well advanced. In the 19-day-old rat fetus a well-defined fascicle extends from the vestibular area of the medulla oblongata to the flocculus, with some of the fibers turning medially toward the rudiment of the nodulus. This fascicle includes vestibular root fibers and, probably, secondary fibers from the vestibular nuclei. Spinocerebellar and olivocerebellar fibers also enter the base of the cerebellum but at this stage there is no indication, in silver preparations, of medullary rays.

Newborn and early postnatal rats show rather diffuse fibers extending into the rudiments of the lobules and spreading toward the poorly defined granular layer. As the lobules expand outward and their bases become isthmuses of connection with the deeper part of the cerebellum, the fibers passing through the constricted part of each lobule become more compactly arranged; they also elongate as the lobule and its base elongate. The use of higher magnifications allows us to see growth cones at the ends of the fibers among the cells of the developing granular layer, into which the fibers fray out distally. Proximally the bands are more compact and are continuous with the deep medullary mass.

As secondary foliation of the lobules begins by a gradual localized expansion of the cortex, the fibers leading to the expanding field at first branch diffusely from the more or less compacted fibrous sheet leading to the superficial cortex. With expansion of the secondary folds their bases, in turn, become relatively constricted and elongate, and the fibers are compacted into secondary rays.

All the primary and secondary rays give off fibers along their course that pass to the unfoliated cortex lining the fissures. At the ends of the rays the fibers radiate into the rounded cortex of the lobules and their subdivisions; this radiation then becomes more apparent with the growth of lobules and the increasing numbers of fibers in the rays.

In the meantime, while afferent fibers are growing peripheralward, axons from the Purkinje cells and other large elements of the cortex, as these are differentiated, enter the incipient medullary rays and thus add to the number of fibers and lengthen the compact part of each ray. In the 10-day-old rat the medullary ray of lobule IX, the uvula, is compact almost to the tips of folia IXa, IXb, and IXc, but at the end of the compact part the fibers radiate diffusely to the expanded cortex (fig. 15A).

The same process is repeated in the formation of the medullary rays and their branches in the human cerebellum. This mode of development of the medullary rays in all mammals appears to be what one might have anticipated. It emphasizes the primary importance of cortical folding in the formation of the lobules and their subdivisions.

Hemispheral lobules. The cerebellar hemispheres are represented in the 21-day-old fetus as paired lateral expansions in which furrows already have appeared (fig. 1). The deepest of these furrows and evidently the first to be formed in the hemisphere is the parafloccular fissure, delimiting the rudiment of the paraflocculus from the remainder of the hemispheral expansion. A faint suggestion of a furrow on the anterodorsal surface, the incipient posterior superior fissure, delimits the ansoparamedian lobule of Bolk from the anterior part of the hemisphere. The ansoparamedian lobule is divided by the intercrural fissure into crus I of the ansiform lobule of Bolk and a larger posterior subdivision that represents the rudiment of crus II and the anterior part of the paramedian lobule of Bolk, both of which have not yet been differentiated from each other.

In a model of the cerebellum of the 21-day-old fetus the fissura prima does not extend into the hemisphere. Aciron's (1950) illustrations of a model of the organ in a 37-mm-long fetus show the fissures and lobules of the anterior and posterior lobes in a state almost as advanced as that in young rats 20 hours postpartum. In the latter the fissura prima extends into the hemisphere as the dorsal boundary of an incipient hemispheral representation of the culmen segment of the anterior lobe (fig. 3C, D). The preculminate fissure ends short of the hemisphere. The ventral segment of the vermal part of the anterior lobe is divided by the precentral fissure into lobules I + II and lobule III in Aciron's 37-mm-long fetus; in the 20-hour postpartum rat, as already noted, precentral fissure *a* has appeared, differentiating lobule I from lobule II. Only lobules II and III, however, continue beyond the end of the short precentral fissure and merge as undifferentiated hemispheral areas at either end of the fissure.

In the posterior lobe the hemispheral segment of the posterior superior fissure has deepened and lengthened in the 20-hour-old rat to the point where it definitely delimits an area, bounded ventromedially by the fissura prima, that corresponds to the hemispheral part of Bolk's lobulus simplex.

Aciron (1950) recognized the flocculonodular lobe and the corpus cerebelli in the rat but he employed the terminology of the human cerebellum for the vermal and hemispheral lobules, except for the paraflocculus. The hemispheral continuations of the ventral segment of the anterior lobe, including the lateral extension of lobule II, as defined above, were called the alae lobuli centralis. As will be shown later, however, the hemispheral representation of lobule II corresponds to the vinculum of the lingula in man. The area between the fissura prima and the posterior superior fissure was called the pars posterior lobuli quadrangularis, and the as yet combined crus II and paramedian lobule of Bolk, in the 37-mm-long rat fetus, was called the lobulus semilunaris inferior by Aciron. This terminology indicates the homologies of the respective lobules with the hemispheral divisions of the human cerebellum but it is unsatisfactory from the standpoint of descriptive value in the rat as well as in most other mammals below the anthropoid apes. The terminology of Bolk (1906), based primarily on the cerebellum of the primitive primate, *Lemur albifrons*, also loses its descriptive value in the rat and most other species.

It would be desirable to develop a simpler method of designating the hemispheral lobules which would indicate their individual developmental relations to specific vermal lobules, as determined by the interlobular fissures, and which also could be employed in the increasingly complex cerebellum of larger mammals, including those higher in the phylogenic scale than the rat. Such a terminology, based on the early divisions of the cortex and placing an emphasis on the interlobular fissures formed by the early cortical folds, rather than on the form of the adult lobules, is available by merely prefixing a capital H to the Roman numeral designations of the vermal lobules with which the respective hemispheral segments are continuous. The hemispheral continuation of lobule II then becomes lobule HII, that of lobule III becomes lobule HIII, and so on through the series. The flocculus will be designated by name instead of being called lobule HX since it is not a part of the hemisphere proper. For the sake of correlating this terminology with the widely used nomenclature of Bolk his terms are also frequently used.

To minimize repetition the hemispheral lobules will be described from the time they appear in the fetus to their fully differentiated form. Although the rudiments of some of the hemispheral lobules of the posterior lobe were recognizable before those of the anterior lobe, as already indicated, all will be considered in the same order as the vermal lobules.

In the 2-day-old rat the preculminate fissure extends into the hemisphere, ending near the ventral margin of the anterior lobe (fig. 4B). The hemispheral part of the lobe is divided by it into a dorsal area, continuous with vermal lobules IV and V, and a ventral area, continuous with lobules II and III. The precentral fissure deepens and gradually extends laterally and ventrally, eventually reaching the anterolateral part of the ventral cerebellar margin (fig. 6B). It divides the hemispheral part of the ventral segment of the anterior lobe into lobules HII and HIII. Lobule HII represents a hemispheral continuation only of folium IIb; folium IIa and lobule I have no hemispheral representation even in the adult cerebellum.

The intraculminate fissure also deepens and extends ventrolaterally as the cortex expands and thickens. It separates the medial part of the hemispheral portion of the culmen segment into two areas that could be regarded as the medial parts of lobules HIV and HV. The intraculminate fissure does not reach the cerebellar margin even in the adult rat; the lateral part of the culminate segment accordingly is an undivided area that represents a continuation of both lobules HIV and HV. Various stages of differentiation of the hemispheral lobules of the anterior lobe are illustrated in figures 4B, 6B, 9B, 10B, 15B.

The posterior part of the hemisphere is divided by the parafloccular fissure into the posterior division of the ansoparamedian lobule of Bolk and the rudiment of the paraflocculus, already mentioned in the 21-day-old fetus. At this stage the parafloccular fissure is relatively deep and wide laterally, but tapers medialward and ends where the swelling of the hemisphere disappears. There is no continuity with the shallow prepyramidal fissure, although in subsequent development the two appear to merge. This appearance led me (Larsell, 1952) to regard the parafloccular fissure as the lateral segment of the prepyramidal fissure. Aciron (1950) in the 37-mm-long rat fetus and G. E. Smith (1903c) in a generalized diagram of the adult mammalian cerebellum also indicated continuity between the parafloccular and prepyramidal fissures. According to Stroud (1895) regarding embryos of the cat and Bradley (1903) regarding embryos of the rabbit, sheep, and ox, the parafloccular fissure is not confluent with any vermal fissure. In most of the fetal stages of the bat, *Corynorhinus*, the parafloccular and prepyramidal fissures are not continuous; a small bridge of cortex between their ends connects a lateral extension of lobule VIII (pyramis) with the posterolateral part of the hemisphere. Late fetal and adult cerebella show an apparent confluence of the two fissures, which seems to be a result of the deepening of both by further expansion of the cortex (Larsell and Dow, 1935). The adult cerebellum of the smaller bat, *Myotis*, shows no connection between the two fissures and Scholten (1946) described them as not being continuous in adult cerebella of other mammals. In whale embryos, according to Jansen (1954), the parafloccular fissure may extend into the pyramis and divide a cortical bridge between the vermis and hemisphere into a rostral part, which connects the pyramis with the paramedian lobule, and a caudal part, which connects the pyramis with the dorsal paraflocculus. Variations in the relations of the parafloccular fissure were observed but in no instance was this fissure confluent with the prepyramidal fissure. In the newborn rat cerebellum the prepyramidal fissure ends above the parafloccular fissure and is not continuous with it (Larsell and Dow, 1935).

A restudy of the prepyramidal and parafloccular fissures and their relations in models and dissections of late fetal and neonatal rats and comparisons with models of the cerebellum of bat fetuses and with dissections of other species confirms the nonconfluence of these two fissures. Their relations could best be described in connection with the further development of the paraflocculus and the posterior divisions of the ansoparamedian lobule.

In the 21-day-old rat fetus a faint furrow in the rudiment of the paraflocculus represents the lateral segment of the fissura secunda, as already noted. This furrow divides the paraflocculus into the rudiments of the ventral and dorsal paraflocculus. The ventral paraflocculus is continuous, medially, with the rudiment of lobule IX (uvula). The dorsal paraflocculus is continuous with the ventral part of an area intervening between the medial end of the parafloccular fissure and the lateral extremity of the prepyramidal fissure, which is situated farther forward than the parafloccular fissure.

The ventral part of this area is continuous medially with lobule VIII (pyramis); the dorsal part is continuous medially with the vermal area, which subsequently becomes lobule VII, and laterally with the dorsal bank of the parafloccular fissure.

By 20 hours postpartum the cerebellar cortex has expanded sufficiently so that the vermal segment of the posterior superior fissure has appeared, delimiting lobule VII anteriorly. The vermal segment of the prepyramidal fissure has deepened and also extended lateralward toward a furrow that has appeared between the dorsal paraflocculus and the enlarging posterior division of the ansoparamedian lobule. Since this furrow becomes confluent with the vermal prepyramidal fissure by the 2-day postpartum stage, I called it the lateral or hemispheral segment of the prepyramidal fissure. This segment delimits an area, which may be called the copula pyramidis, from the part of the posterior division of the ansoparamedian lobule that later becomes the major portion of the paramedian lobule of Bolk and is continuous medially with sublobule VIIb.

The rudiment of the copula is represented in the 21-day-old fetus by the area, mentioned above, between the medial end of the parafloccular fissure and the short prepyramidal fissure (fig. 1B). In the 2-day-old rat the copula has elongated and three days after birth it shows a branch to the dorsal paraflocculus and a more dorsal one, which is continuous with the ventral lateral part of the posterior divisions of the ansoparamedian lobule, i.e., the part that becomes the paramedian lobule (fig. 8C). The medial end of the parafloccular fissure, diminishing to a thin cleft that terminates on the distal end of the copula, separates the two branches. This copular sulcus, as I named it (1952), corresponds to the shallow medial end of the parafloccular fissure in the full-term fetus. It is continuous laterally in the 3-day-old rat with a deep cleft that separates the paraflocculus from the remainder of the hemisphere and represents the parafloccular fissure, as the term usually is employed.

The lateral segment of the prepyramidal fissure ends between the dorsal branch of the copula and the posterior surface of the ansoparamedian lobule. Medially it is continuous with the vermal segment (fig. 8C).

The two branches of the copula elongate: the one to the dorsal paraflocculus becomes part of the parafloccular peduncle by the 5-day postpartum stage and the other begins to expand at this stage as the rudiment of the pars posterior or copularis of the paramedian lobule (fig. 12B). By the seventh day postpartum it has expanded to the point where it reaches the posterior inferior cerebellar surface. The pars anterior of the paramedian lobule is differentiated from crus II at this stage by the appearance of the ansoparamedian fissure. Expansion of this lobule and of the pars posterior behind it results in a deepening of the hemispheral segment of the prepyramidal fissure so that it now appears as a surface furrow which is medially continuous with the vermal segment of the prepyramidal fissure. Its relations to the parafloccular fissure are evident in a dissection of this region in the 10-day-old rat (fig. 16B, C). The prepyramidal fissure extends laterally to the posterior lateral wall of the paramedian lobule, which makes it appear to be continuous with the parafloccular fissure, but the deep part of the prepyramidal fissure ends short of the surface. The lateral part of the parafloccular fissure at this stage of growth completely separates the paraflocculus from the remainder of the hemisphere, with only the sulcus copulae remaining as a representative of its embryonic relations.

The term copula pyramidis was introduced and applied by G. E. Smith (1902, 1903a, 1903b, 1903c) to the connection between the dorsal paraflocculus and the pyramis in the adult mammalian cerebellum. Smith (1903c) stated that the term cannot be used in all mammalian cerebella. In some species the pyramis was said also to be continuous, without interruption, with the "parapyramidal area," corresponding to part of the paramedian lobule of Bolk. According to Ingvar (1918) a lamellar band passes from the pyramis to the paramedian lobule. Scholten (1946) also described such a connection. This corresponds to the cortical band, dorsal of the copular sulcus, described above in the rat. The copula of G. E. Smith appears to correspond to the branch of the elongated and somewhat widened zone immediately lateral of but continuous with lobule VIII, which passes below the copular sulcus onto the parafloccular peduncle. I have restricted the term copula to the relatively wide zone before it bifurcates into the two branches. So defined, the copula of the rat appears to correspond to the Nebenpyramiden of Henle (1871) and the wings of the pyramis of Dejerine (1901) in man, as well as to similar enlargements lateral of the pyramis in other large mammals such as the ox, horse, and camel. The anterior part of this swelling in the rat is continuous with sublobule VIIIa; the posterior part, which appears to be more specifically continuous with the dorsal paraflocculus, is continuous medially with sublobule VIIIb. In the 10-day postpartum rat the copular sulcus has extended toward the intrapyramidal fissure and the latter has lengthened lateralward; the two approach one another but do not meet (fig. 16B). Similar relations between the homologs of the two furrows are described below in larger mammals in which the two subdivisions of lobule VIII are much larger and the intrapyramidal fissure is much deeper.

A faint groove appears in the posterodorsal surface of the paraflocculus of the 21-day-old fetus. This is the lateral segment of the fissura secunda which divides the ventral from the dorsal paraflocculus. It deepens and also extends medialward as the ventral paraflocculus enlarges; by the second to third day postpartum it is confluent with the vermal segment of the fissura secunda. The dorsal and the ventral paraflocculus are continuous with each other around the lateral end of the fissure. After the ventral paraflocculus was dissected away it became evident that the two divisions of the paraflocculus are also continuous with each other beneath the fissure. In the 3-day-old rat the ventral paraflocculus is connected with vermal lobule IX by a constricted band of cortex, while the dorsal paraflocculus is continuous with the copula, which is related to lobule VIII. By the 5-day-old stage the branch of the copula leading to the dorsal paraflocculus becomes elongated and constricted; together with the closely associated and also elongated connection of the ventral paraflocculus with lobule IX, it forms the parafloccular peduncle (fig. 12B).

Although these connections with the vermal lobules have a peduncular appearance, the fissura secunda partially separates the two parts; this peduncle also is continuous, beneath the proximal part of the parafloccular fissure, with the medullary substance of the hemisphere. The peduncular connection elongates as the paraflocculus increases in size. In the 14-day-old rat the paraflocculus forms the lower lateral and anterior part of the hemisphere, with its two divisions being separated by a terminal widening of the fissura secunda (fig. 18A). As the peduncle elongates the cortex disappears except laterally and immediately adjacent to lobule IX, where it exposes a strand of fibers that is parallel with the floccular peduncle. Large folia at the distal end of the uvular part of the peduncle represent the ventral paraflocculus or lobule HIX (fig. 18B); those at the end of the parafloccular branch of the copula represent the dorsal paraflocculus or lobule HVIIIB. Probably this is related, medially, to the deep posterior part of lobule VIII which in the rat suggests sublobule VIIIb. If so the relationship would correspond to that between the dorsal paraflocculus and sublobule VIIIB in other species in which this sublobule is large. In the rat, however, it is uncertain during both growth and adult stages.

When the two folia immediately behind the ansoparamedian fissure were dissected away in the 10-day-old rat it became clear that the vermal relations of these folia are

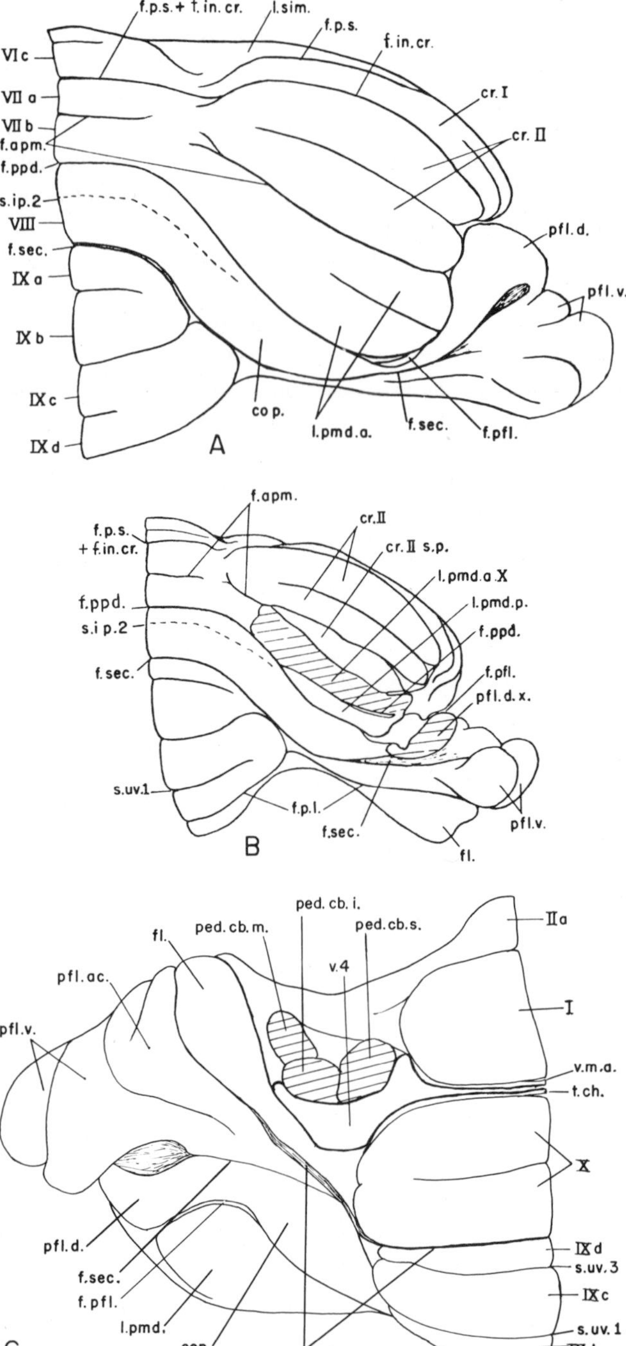

Figure 18. Cerebellum of 14-day-old rat. A. Posterodorsal view of right half. ×16. B. Posterodorsal view, with anterior part of paramedian lobule and dorsal paraflocculus removed. ×10. C. Ventral view of right half. ×16. (Larsell, 1952.)

with the posterior inferior part of lobule VII, i.e., incipient sublobule VIIb, and that crus II is continuous with VIIa. The dissection also establishes a connection, around the end of the prepyramidal fissure, with a superficially narrow but deeply extending triangular folium which is continuous with the copula pyramidis. This folium represents the expanded dorsal division of the lateral extremity of the copula mentioned above (fig. 18B). In my earlier account of the rat cerebellum (Larsell, 1952), I designated this folium as the posterior part of the paramedian lobule. Subsequent detailed comparisons with embryonic cerebella of the rabbit, pig, and cat, with the fetal and adult monkey, and with adults of other species demonstrated that this folium corresponds to the pars copularis of the paramedian lobule as defined in the monkey (Larsell, 1953a). The portion of the paramedian lobule which is continuous medially with lobule VII, as described above and which I called pars anterior in my earlier study of the rat, I labeled the pars tuberalis. The two folia into which it gradually divides probably foreshadow the pars anterior and the pars posterior of the paramedian lobule of larger species, described on subsequent pages.

Scholten (1946) stated that in the adult mammals he studied the dorsal and largest part of the paramedian lobule is joined with the caudal part of his lobulus C_1 (Bolk's lobulus c_2), but the most ventral lamellae of the lobule are continuous with the pyramis. Sholten added that in the human cerebellum the lobulus gracilis appears to be connected with the tuber, i.e., the "achterste deel" of his lobulus C_1, and with the pyramis, as is illustrated in his figures. The differences in development and lateral extent of the human lobulus gracilis and biventral lobule, as compared respectively with the pars tuberalis of the paramedian lobule and the pars copularis and dorsal paraflocculus of the rat, obscure the relations between the two lobules in man. A detailed analysis of the fetal human cerebellum at both younger and older stages than those illustrated by Scholten clearly shows that the fundamental relationships are similar in rat and man.

Crus II appears to be continuous with sublobule VIIa, as does the pars anterior of the paramedian lobule with sublobule VIIb; this indicates that the same relationships exist here as in larger mammals where the ansoparamedian fissure is distinctly continuous into the vermis. Accordingly, it seemed reasonable to call the hemispheral segment in front of the fissure crus II of lobule HVIIA and the anterior part of the paramedian lobule HVIIB.

There could be no question that the hemispheral area between the early appearing intercrural and posterior superior fissures corresponds to crus I of the ansiform lobule of Bolk. Its vermal relations are confused by the almost invariable merging of the posterior superior and intercrural fissures in the average 5-day-old rats to form a compound vermal fissure. Presumably the vermal continuation of crus I is represented in the floor and part of the anterior wall of this compound fissure. (We shall return to this point in the adult rat.) As early as the fifth day postpartum a furrow appears in the expanded lateral part of crus I that divides it into crus Ia and crus Ib.

Adult Rat

The cerebellum of the adult rat presents a relatively broad vermal region with an expanded hemisphere on either side (figs. 19, 20). The dorsal surface has, between the vermis and the swelling of the hemisphere, an anteroposteriorly directed wide and shallow depression which deepens on the posterior surface. The hemispheral and vermal lobules are continuous across the floor of the depression both on the dorsal and the posterior surfaces. The vermal and hemispheral fissures are continuous between the related vermal and hemispheral lobules of the anterior and posterior surfaces, but on the dorsal surface, as a rule, only one vermal fissure is continuous with a hemispheral fissure. When the molecular layer of the cortex is intact, the posterior superior and intercrural fissures often appear to cross the vermis together as a compound fissure. After removing the superficial part of the molecular layer and staining the surface so that the vermal and hemispheral relations of the granular layer are

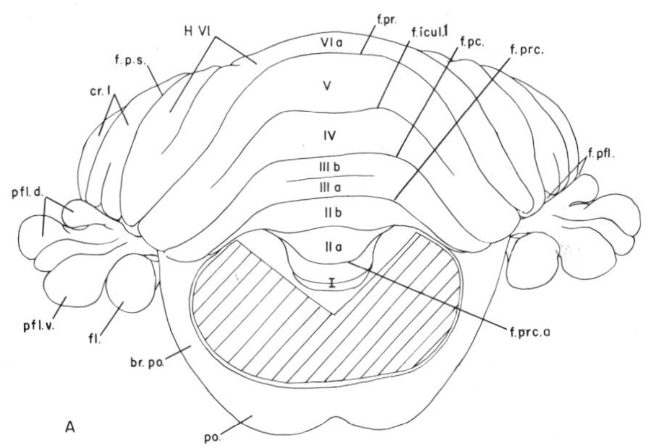

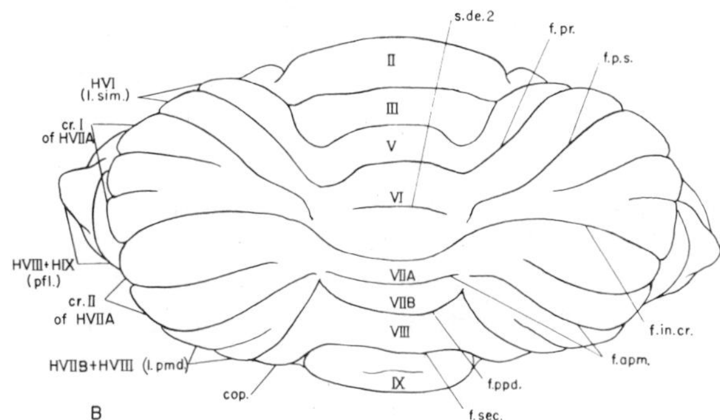

Figure 19. Cerebellum of adult rat. A. Anterior view. B. Dorsal view. ×4. (Larsell, 1952.)

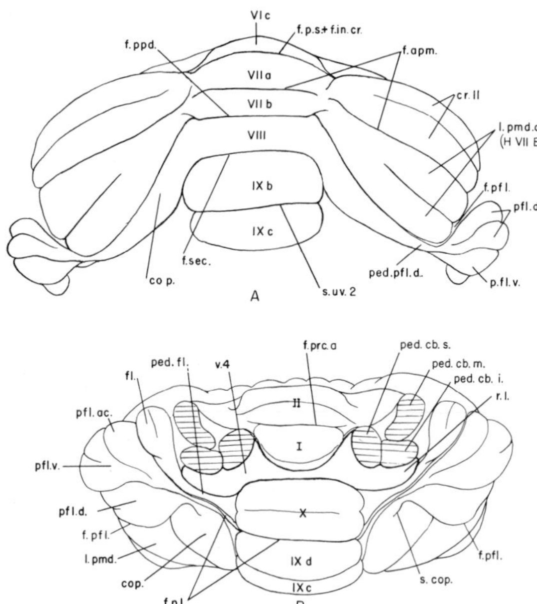

Figure 20. Cerebellum of adult rat. A. Posterior view. B. Ventral view. ×4. (Larsell, 1952.)

The cerebellum is attached to the brainstem by inferior, medial, and superior cerebellar peduncles which were also called respectively corpus restiform, brachium pontis, and brachium conjunctivum. The sectioning of

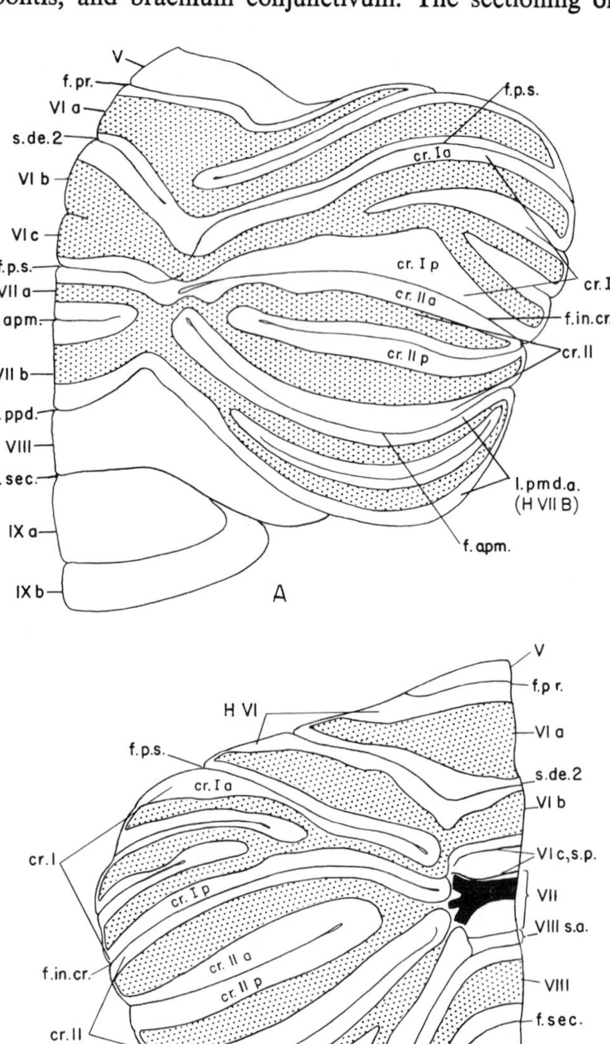

Figure 21. Cerebellum of adult rat. A. Dorsal view of right half showing one pattern of interrelations of the vermian and hemispheral lobules. The molecular layer was dissected away in a brain lightly surface-stained with borax-carmine, which exposed the granular layer shown in stipple. B. Dorsal view of left half with granular layer exposed (stippled) and lobule VII removed to the medullary base (black). The granular layer of VIb and the posterior folium of lobulus HVI is continuous with that of crus I through a gap between the lateral and medial segments of the posterior superior fissure. The medullary substance at the base of lobule VIII branches into rays to crus I, crus II, and the anterior part of the paramedian lobule. ×15. (Larsell, 1952.)

distinctly visible, one could see that the deep part of the intercrural fissure ends short of the vermal segment of the posterior superior fissure (figs. 21A, B) or is continuous across the vermis with the contralateral intercrural fissure (fig. 22B). The deep part of the posterior superior fissure may end short of the vermis or may be confluent with the vermal segment on one side and with declival fissure 2 on the other. The granular layer forms a variety of patterns across the vermis, as illustrated in figures 21A and 22B; the granular layer of crus I is sometimes continuous with that of VI alone, sometimes with VIc and VIIa, or in other instances with both.

Goodman and Simpson (1961) plotted a longitudinal paravermal zone on either side of the vermis of the rat. This zone is situated between a vermal zone, in a limited sense, and a lateral zone which is composed of the expanded part of the hemisphere. Electrical stimulation of the paravermal zone, which is about 2 mm wide, evokes a different postural pattern of limb response than what results from stimulation of the restricted vermal zone. Stimulation of the lateral zone evokes a third pattern of response. These zones appear to correspond to the cortical part of the longitudinal medial, intermediate, and lateral corticonuclear zones of Jansen and Brodal (1940, 1942) and Chambers and Sprague (1955a, 1955b). In the rat as in most other mammals, there are no externally visible boundaries between them. The vermis and hemispheres (including the paravermal zones), as topographical divisions, accordingly must serve as the basis of morphological description of the cerebellum.

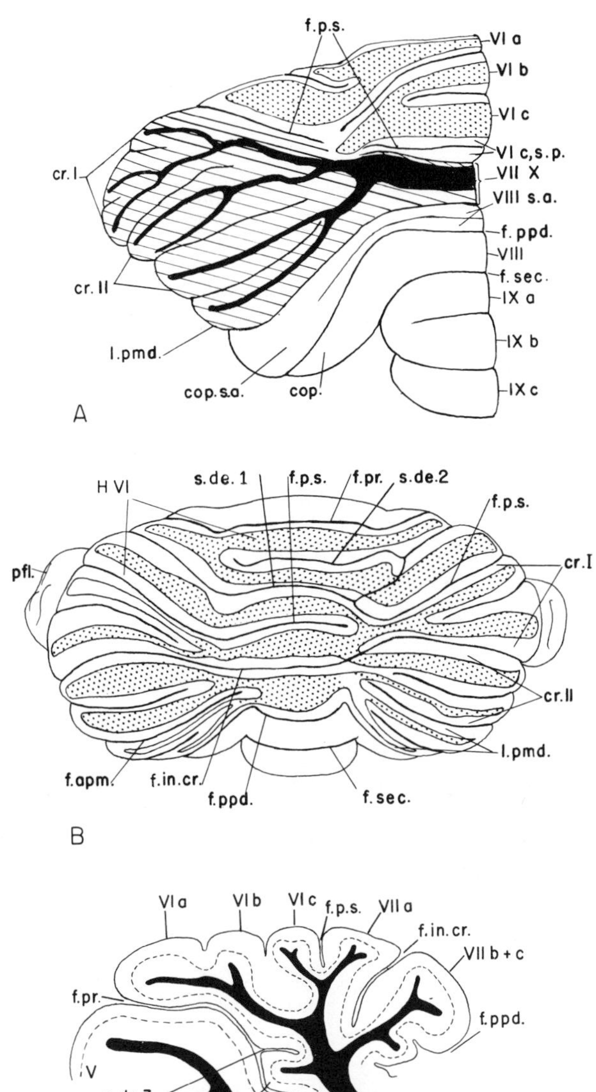

Figure 22. Cerebellum of adult rat. A. Dorsoposterior view of left half in which lobule VII, crus I, crus II, and the anterior part of the paramedian lobule were dissected down to the medullary substance (solid black). The relation of the rays from the base of lobule VII to the hemispheral lobules is illustrated. The granular layer only was exposed in lobule VI. B. Dorsal view showing atypical arrangement of the intercrural sulcus, posterior superior fissure, declival sulcus 2, and the granular layer of the intervening lobules. The molecular layer was dissected away in a borax-carmine-stained preparation. C. Midsagittal section of lobules VI and VII illustrated in B showing distinct posterior superior fissure and intercrural sulcus. ×15. (Larsell, 1952.)

these peduncles permits the exposure of the ventral aspect of the organ, as well as a better view of the flocculus and paraflocculus (fig. 20B).

The flocculus is situated ventromedial of the rostral part of the paraflocculus and is connected with the base of lobule X, the nodulus, by a band of fibers covered in part by cortex, which arches caudomedially to form a floccular peduncle. Distally the flocculus is separated from the paraflocculus by a cleft which is continuous with the posterolateral fissure. This fissure follows the lateral and laterocaudal borders of the flocculus and its peduncle to a vermal position between lobules IX and X (fig. 20B). Medially the caudomedially arching part of the flocculus and its peduncle skirts an expansion of the fourth ventricle lateral of lobules I and X, between which the ventricle forms a narrow space connecting its bilateral expansions. The choroid tela is attached to the medial and caudomedial tenial border of the peduncular part of the flocculus; this attachment then continues with the tenial margin of the nodulus.

Golgi preparations of late fetal rats show vestibular root fibers passing lateral of the restiform body to the flocculus. Other root fibers end in the vestibular nuclei while some continue through the medial part of the inferior cerebellar peduncle, i.e., through the juxtarestiform body of the adult to the fastigial nucleus. Secondary fibers from the vestibular nuclei join the root fibers in their course to the ipsilateral flocculus. Pyridine-silver preparations of the adult cerebellum show a band of primary and secondary fibers to the ipsilateral flocculus, in addition to fibers that pass medially, with some crossing the midline. The band to the flocculus is situated in the posterior and lateral part of the roof of the fourth ventricle for part of its course and then it continues forward parallel with the base of the tenia to which the choroid tela is attached. Distally this band becomes covered by the cortex of the flocculus in which the fibers terminate. The medially directed fibers form a loose fascicle at the bases of the nodulus and uvula.

In Marchi preparations of the rat and cat, after complete section of the vestibular roots or damage to these roots, Dow (1936) found degenerated root fibers to the flocculus passing lateral of the restiform body. Others pass medially between the restiform body and the spinal root of the trigeminus and terminate in the vestibular nuclei, while some continue toward the cerebellum. The latter traverse the nuclei of Deiters and Bechterew and the basal part of the fastigial nucleus and end in part in them, but some continue to the cortex of the nodulus and to the lower folia of the uvula (IXc and IXd). All root fibers terminate ipsilaterally.

Secondary vestibular fibers to the ipsilateral flocculus are divided into dorsal and ventral groups by the restiform body but these groups merge laterally and end entirely in the flocculus. Secondary vestibular fibers to the ipsilateral parts of the nodulus and uvula take the same course as the root fibers. Those to the contralateral parts of these two lobules cross the midline at their bases. Crossed fibers also continue in the base of the tenia of the fourth ventricle to the contralateral flocculus. These fibers and those of the decussation constitute a vestibular commissure which corresponds to the vestibular commissure of birds except that in embryonic stages of the avian cerebellum, at least, the commissure appears to include vestibular root fibers (Larsell, 1948; Whitlock, 1952).

Vestibular root fibers leading to the anterior lobe of the rat and cat were not found by Dow (1936) in Marchi preparations, although Ingvar (1918) had described such fibers to the lingula of the cat. Dow (1939) observed that single-shock electrical stimulation of the acoustic nerve of the cat evokes action potentials in the lingula as well as in both flocculi and in the nodulus, uvula, and fastigial nuclei, but not elsewhere. The observations of Ingvar with respect to vestibular root fibers to the lingula were thus confirmed. After a lesion of the juxtarestiform body of the rat, Dow (1936) found degenerated secondary vestibular fibers to the lingula as well as to the other lobules reached by primary fibers. Since vestibular fibers reach the lingula, a part of the corpus cerebelli, as well as the flocculonodular lobe, the question of differentiation of the two primary divisions of the cerebellum may be raised.

Considering all the vestibulocerebellar fibers, Dow (1936) estimated that the ipsilateral secondary fibers are about three times as numerous as the primary fibers. When the contralateral secondary fibers were included, all the secondary fibers amounted to five times the number of root fibers.

The distribution of the spinocerebellar tracts of the rat was studied by Anderson (1943) in Marchi preparations, following lesions of the spinal cord. Anderson noted that both ventral and dorsal tracts distribute to the culmen (lobules IV and V), central lobule (III), and lingula of the anterior lobe. As labeled, the lingula corresponds to lobule I, but it is not clear whether lobule II is included in Anderson's lingula or in the central lobule; apparently he regarded it as part of the latter. A few ventral tract fibers were found in the medial part of the lobulus simplex (lobule VI), but no degenerated fibers of this tract were seen in any other parts of the vermis, flocculus, paraflocculus, or hemispheres. Dorsal tract fibers were present in lobules VI and VIII as well as in the anterior lobe; in addition a few were found in the medial parts of the uvula (lobule IX) and the paramedian lobule (HVIIIA?). None were seen in any other part of the vermis, flocculus, paraflocculus, or cerebellar hemispheres. In the vermis they are distributed ipsilaterally and contralaterally in a ratio of about three to one. The ventral tract fibers are reportedly distributed in a narrow band near the midline of the vermis, while the majority of dorsal tract fibers are distributed in the lateral parts of the vermis.

Cerebellar afferent fibers from the external cuneate nucleus do not appear to have been described in the rat. In the rabbit and cat Brodal (1941) found that the external cuneate nucleus sends fibers chiefly to the anterior lobe and, in smaller numbers, to lobules VIII and IX; lobules VI and VII (the declive and tuber vermis) receive a very small number of fibers. Although the external cuneate nucleus receives fibers from the upper thoracic and cervical segments of the cord that ascend in the cuneate fascicle, Brodal inferred that lobuli 1 and 2 of Bolk (corresponding to lobules I and II) also receive cuneocerebellar fibers. Whether or not the nodulus receives such fibers could not be decided.

Dow (1939) demonstrated that all parts of the cerebellar cortex of the rat, including the flocculus, are activated by electrical stimulation of the inferior olive. In young cats and rabbits Brodal (1940a) showed by the Brodal-Gudden method that all parts of the cortex receive fibers from the inferior olive, but that localization from the various subdivisions of the olive to subdivisions of the cortex is remarkably sharp.

Assuming that the lingula of the rat receives vestibular fibers, as in the cat, in addition to olivary and spinal fibers, it differs from the nodulus and flocculus as a result of its spinal afferents. Whether the subdivision (IXc + d) of the uvula, which receives vestibular afferents, also shares other afferents to lobule IX is not specifically known, but Dow (1942b) indicated that there is overlapping of spinocerebellar fibers in the zone, adjacent to the posterolateral fissure, in which the vestibular fibers terminate. Undoubtedly olivocerebellar fibers also reach the inferior part of lobule IX. In larger mammals folia IXc and IXd are continuous laterally with the accessory paraflocculus; a similar relationship probably is present in the rat but it is more difficult to demonstrate.

The afferent connections of the flocculonodular lobe apparently include only vestibulo- and olivo-cerebellar fibers, whereas all other cerebellar lobules that receive vestibular afferents have spinal and other fibers in addition. Other subdivisions of the corpus cerebelli receive afferents from proprioceptive and exteroceptive systems, in addition to olivocerebellar fibers.

The flocculonodular lobe of the rat and other species represents the primary and major concentration of vestibulocerebellar fibers; these fibers are the first to reach the cerebellum, as Tello (1940) has also shown in the mouse embryo. Furthermore, the fibers from the inferior olive to the flocculonodular lobe originate in the rostral part of the medial accessory olive (Brodal, 1940a), which Kooy (1917) noted is phylogenically the oldest part of the olivary complex.

The vermis of the anterior lobe, including lobules I and II (lingula) of the cat and rabbit, receives fibers from the lateroventral parts of the dorsal and medial accessory olives; lobule IX (uvula) receives fibers from the dorsomedial cell column and from nucleus β of the olivary complex (Brodal, 1940). Presumably the distribution is similar in the rat. In addition, the anterior lobe of the rat, including lobule I, receives numerous spinocerebellar fibers; lobule IX (uvula), in addition to olivocerebellar and vestibular fibers, also receives spinocerebellar fibers (Anderson, 1943). No spinocerebellar fibers, however, end in the flocculonodular lobe.

Because the afferent connections of the flocculonodular lobe are restricted to the vestibular system and the most primitive part of the olivary system, in contrast with the corpus cerebelli and its subdivisions, there is justification for regarding it as a functionally distinctive division of the cerebellum. This conception is supported by the experimental studies of Dow (1936, 1938) on the rat, cat, and monkey and by those of authors cited in subsequent sections. This theory is also in accord with the early differentiation of the flocculonodular lobe in the ontogenetic development of the rat.

Cerebellar afferents from the reticular nuclei and other sources were demonstrated experimentally by Brodal and his co-workers in the cat. Although these afferents have been less completely studied in the rat, they undoubtedly exist. Electrophysiological studies by Dow and Anderson (1942) demonstrated activation of the cerebellum of the rat as a result of stimulating exteroceptors, proprioceptors, inferior olive and pons, as well as of the acoustic nerve.

The morphological features of the cerebellum of the rat are fully differentiated by 14 days after birth; with further development the lobules enlarge and the fissures deepen. Additional description of the rat cerebellum, as needed, will be combined with a comparison of the cerebellum of birds, which will be limited to the vermal lobules of the rat and the folia of the median part of the avian cerebellum. The small cerebellar hemispheres of birds do not have subdivisions that can be compared with the hemispheral lobules of the rat. Both the vermis and the hemisphere of the rat, excluding the paraflocculus, present in simple form the same pattern of lobules found in most other mammals. The comparison of the vermal lobules with the folia of birds therefore is applicable to mammals in general. Monotremes have peculiarities in their vermal pattern that do not readily fit into that of marsupials and placental mammals but comparison with the bird cerebellum, on the one hand, and with the rat cerebellum, on the other hand, also clarifies the pattern in monotremes.

In addition to their morphological features the somatotopic pattern of the folia of birds, as demonstrated by Whitlock (1952), provides another valuable criterion for determining homologies in comparison with mammals. The fiber tract connections of some of the vermal lobules have been described in the rat but the cerebellum of this animal is less favorable for precise localization of areas activated by exteroceptive and proprioceptive impulses than is that of larger species. The results of Snider and Stowell (1942, 1944), Stowell and Snider (1942a, 1942b), Adrian (1943), Hampson, Harrison, and Woolsey (1952), and others on cats and monkeys apparently could be transferred to the rat, since the distribution of afferents in the cortex is possibly more diffuse in this species. Assuming that the areas activated by exteroceptive and proprioceptive impulses correspond to those of the cat and monkey, one could then make direct comparisons with the areas found by Whitlock in birds.

Before comparing the folia of birds with the vermal lobules of the rat one should review the principal factors that affect foliation of the cerebellar cortex: i.e., relative body size; specialization, atrophy, or hypertrophy of parts of the body or of the extremities; methods of progression; and the relative importance of sensory organs and their cerebellar connections.

A general survey of the physical characteristics of the various species of birds, the cerebellum of which has been described in volume I (1967), indicates that the pigeon is the most suitable bird for comparison with the rat. Young adult pigeons weigh approximately 200 gm to 225 gm, while 117- to 365-day-old male albino rats weigh 223 gm to 320 gm, according to Donaldson (1915). Since the pigeon is an excellent flier and also walks well, it is less specialized with respect to methods of progression than most birds. The extremities of the rat are unspecialized and locomotion could be regarded as typically mammalian. The bodies of the pigeon and the rat have no special features, in contrast with many other species of their respective classes. The eyes, however, are relatively much larger in the pigeon and visual acuity undoubtedly is much greater than in the rat. Availability of sufficient material for adequate comparison also is important. While comparison of the avian cerebellum with that of the rat will be based chiefly on the pigeon some features of the cerebellum of other species also will be considered.

Median sagittal sections of the cerebellum of the pi-

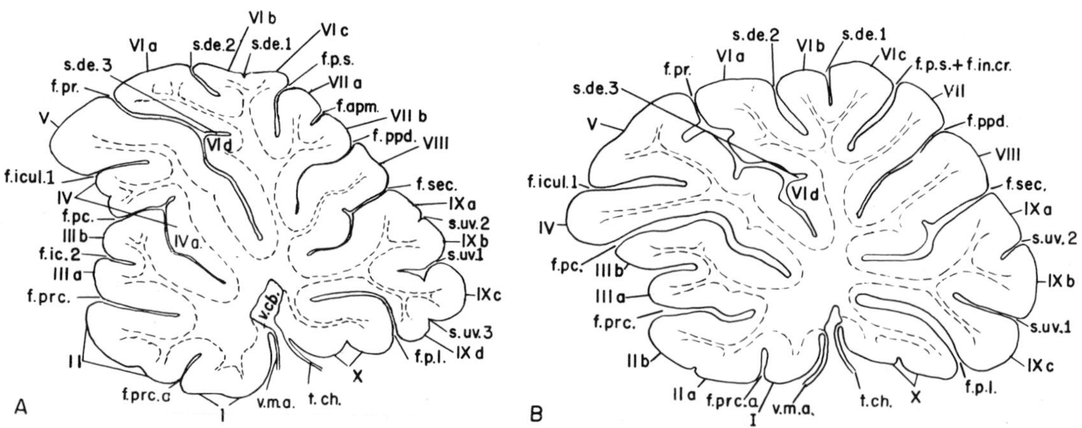

Figure 23. Cerebellum of adult rat. Midsagittal sections illustrating variations of the folial pattern, especially of lobules VI and IX. A. Dissection. ×7.5. B. Weigert-stained section. ×10. (Larsell, 1952.)

geon (fig. 26A) and the adult rat (fig. 23) show a striking similarity in the pattern of some, but not all, of the individual fissures; the vermal lobules of the rat when compared with the fissures and folia of the pigeon also show a distinct likeness to each other. In other birds resemblances are even more striking in some respects but certain other features are more or less modified by special patterns that probably are related to body size or to differences in sensory or motor equipment.

Lobule I of the rat differs greatly in appearance from folium I of the pigeon and most other birds. In the adult rat the entire rounded surface of lobule I is formed by the molecular layer of the cortex; the anterior medullary velum is attached above the posterior border of the cortex immediately rostroventral of the fastigium (fig. 23). In the pigeon and most other birds, by contrast, only the dorsal surface of folium I is cortical. The ventral surface, facing the ventricle, is formed by a thin medullary layer that gradually disappears rostralward. The anterior medullary velum, as already noted, is attached to the tapering tip of the folium and continues as a thin membrane to the midbrain. These morphological relations differ so greatly from those of lobule I of the rat that at first glance there appears to be little basis for homologizing folium I of birds with lobule I of the rat.

The development of folium I of the duck appears to present a transition form between the more typical avian folium I and lobule I of the smaller mammals. In the duck embryo until about 18 days of incubation the development of folium I is similar to that of the chick embryo (Larsell, 1948) and other species described by Saetersdal (1956). The duck embryo at 18 days incubation, however, presents a rostral enlargement of folium I and a ventral displacement of the attachment of the anterior medullary velum. By the adult stage (fig. 26B) the granular and molecular layers have turned ventralward and caudally in such a way that the anterior surface and the forward part of the ventral surface are formed by the molecular layer and the anterior medullary velum is attached to the now caudally directed tip of the recurved part of the folium. Continuation of such a process of caudal folding of the originally rostral part of the folium accompanied by increase of medullary substance and condensation into a central core would result in a structure similar to lobule I of the rat and many other mammals. Folium I in the turkey, *Meleagris gallopavo*, has the same form as in the adult duck. In the lingula of the adult human cerebellum the cortical layer faces dorsally, like that of folium I of most birds, and the anterior medullary velum is continuous beneath the tip of the cortex with the medullary layer of the lingula.

Lobule II is relatively large in the rat and is subdivided into IIa and IIb by a shallow furrow (fig. 23B). Folium II of the pigeon is undivided but in the eagle, horned owl, and some other species of birds it is more deeply divided than lobule II of the rat. In the adult human cerebellum a small lobule, called the sublobulus centralis anterior by Ziehen (1903), sometimes is interposed between the lobulus centralis (lobule III) and the lingula of Ziehen and other authors. The development of the ventral part of the anterior lobe in the human fetus makes it evident that Ziehen's sublobulus centralis anterior represents one of the numerous variations in the pattern of the human lingula and corresponds to lobule II of subhuman mammals. The relatively large and well-differentiated lobules I and II of most mammals and the corresponding folia of birds together represent the two atrophic lobules called the lingula in man. The term as used in the human cerebellum includes two atrophic lobules which correspond to lobules I and II of the rat and other mammals and to folia I and II of birds. They also correspond to lobuli 1 and 2 of Bolk (1906) in mammals.

Experimental evidence of functional representation of the tail in the "lingula" of the spider monkey (Chang and Ruch, 1949) and the cat (Hampson, Harrison, and Woolsey, 1952) has already been mentioned. In *Ateles*, where the long tail is of great importance in the animal's activities, the tail muscles were divided by Chang and Ruch into two groups, the intrinsic muscles and the basal tail muscles. The latter include muscles that have their origin from the pelvis and produce lateral and ventral movements of the tail. The muscles of the dorsal basal part of the tail represent the caudal continuation of the multifidus spines and the longissimus dorsi muscles. The intrinsic muscles are confined to the tail both in origin and insertion.

In his experiments on the spider monkey, Marchi found that degenerated fibers of the ventral spinocerebellar tract after section of the cord at the second caudal segment, as illustrated in Chang and Ruch's figures, are more numerous in the ventral segment (lobule I) but are also present in lobule II. Lobule I is unusually large in *Ateles* (Larsell, 1953a) and has a hemispheral extension. As described below, lobule I is relatively large in other species that have long and functionally important tails. In the pig, as an example of a species with a small tail, lobule I is very small. Experimental evidence is lacking but there are indications that lobule I may be functionally related to the intrinsic tail muscles and perhaps may also receive exteroceptive impulses from the tail. On this basis the large size and hemispheral representation of the lobule in *Ateles* can be correlated with the remarkably prehensile tail. The manifold functions of this organ must involve the intrinsic muscles as well as the exteroceptors, especially those on the underside of the tip of the tail in this species.

In the rat, according to Greene (1935), the caudal muscles have their origin in part from the pelvic bones and in part from the sacral and caudal vertebrae. The internal abductor of the tail originates from the lower half of the medial surface and ventral border of the ileum and inserts by tendons along the ventral surface of the tail. The external abductor originates from the medial surface of the ascending ramus of the pubic symphysis and inserts along the lateral surface of the base of the tail. The remaining muscles take origin from the vertebrae – the flexor caudae longus includes slips from as high as lumbar 5 – and insert by tendons on more caudally situated vertebrae. As in *Ateles* the tail muscles of the rat could be divided into basal and intervertebral groups. Both groups also correspond in principle to the more strongly developed tail musculature of birds, already described.

Lobules I and II are large in the spider monkey (Larsell, 1953a) and both are relatively large in the rat and other mammals that have well-developed tails. In the pig, on the other hand, lobule I is very small. Experimental evidence of functional representation of the tail in the lingula has already been cited; both lobules apparently are included in the lingula by Hampson, Harrison, and Woolsey (1952) and also by Chang and Ruch (1949). The more abundant degeneration of fibers in lobule I in the experiment of Chang and Ruch, in which the spinocerebellar tract was sectioned at the second caudal level, seems to suggest that the afferent fibers from intrinsic tail muscles and from exteroceptors of the tail reach the large lobule I predominantly. The small tail of the pig if correlated with the small lobule I lends support to this conception. In the rat, electrophysiological evidence of the presence of neuromuscular spindles in the intrinsic tail muscles recently has been presented by Steg (1962). The hairless tail of this species probably also serves exteroceptive functions. Anderson (1943) found ventral spinocerebellar fibers to lobule I in Marchi preparations of the rat, although the lesions of the cord are so far forward that the fibers do not necessarily derive from the tail segments of the cord. On the basis of evidence, lobule I seems to be functionally related to the muscles and skin of the greater part of the tail, rather than to the muscles and skin of its base.

With reference to the basal tail muscles of the rat, i.e., those having their origin on the bones of the pelvis, there is no experimental evidence relating to specific representation in the lingula. According to Paramore (1910), the caudopelvic muscles of pronograde mammals form an integral part of the mechanism regulating the internal pressure of the body. This author compared the pelvic muscles in several species of mammals. In the rabbit and hare the pubococcygeus is but feebly developed or is absent; in the guinea pig it is present only as a thin muscular sheet. Yet in the squirrel both pubococcygeus and iliococcygeus are almost as well developed, relative to species size, as in carnivores. The author ascribed this fact to the climbing habit of the squirrel, which requires support from below for maintenance of internal pressure. The squirrel also has a relatively large tail, and sagittal sections of the cerebellum show relatively large lobules I and II.

Elftman's (1932) analysis of the caudopelvic muscles in the great apes and man and their participation in forming the pelvic floor is suggestive of their interrelationship when correlated with the comparative anatomy of lobules I and II. This author described the chief muscles that strengthen the floor of the pelvis as falling into three groups: the first group includes the pubocaudalis (pubococcygeus), the iliocaudalis (iliococcygeus), and the coccygeus. These muscles originate from the pubis, ilium, and ischium, and insert chiefly into the tail in species possessing this appendage. The pubococcygeus and iliococcygeus constitute the major part of the levator ani in man but retain an insertion into the tip and sides of the coccyx, in addition to insertions into the coccygeal raphe and the aponeurosis of the sacrococcygeal ligament. The coccygeus retains the insertion into the coccyx and the fourth and fifth sacral vertebrae. Elftman found that in man variability is one of the principal characteristics of the pelvic musculature.

The muscle group in most mammals, in addition to forming an integral part of the pelvic wall, is of great importance in flexing and abducting the tail. In the great apes lacking a tail and in man in whom the tail is reduced to a coccyx, the tail-moving function of the three muscles is lost and the muscles are atrophied; the pubococcygeus (which supports the pelvic viscera) is the only one that remains consistently strong, although not as muscular as in the tailed monkeys. The reduction in size and the more tendinous structure of the iliococcygeus and coccygeus in apes and man appear to be correlated with the disappearance of the tail.

The important basal tail muscles of the spider monkey are represented in the great apes and man by the shortened and transformed muscles of the pelvic diaphragm. The large caudopelvic muscles of birds, which are especially well developed in the peacock and turkey (Porta, 1908), could be correlated with the large folium II of birds. Folium I probably is functionally related to the interspinales muscles between the successive free caudal vertebrae and between the last of these and the pygostyle. Activation from stimulation of the tail feathers was recorded chiefly from folia III and IV, possibly because of the difficulty of exploring folia I and II due to their position. These comparisons appear to justify the conclusion that folia I and II of birds and lobules I and II of mammals are functionally related, respectively, to the two groups of tail muscles and the integument innervated from the same spinal segments. The loss of the tail and the modifications of the basal muscles in the higher primates appear to be correlated with atrophy of the lingula, which in the human embryo and in the adult is represented by rudiments of lobules I and II.

Since the hindlimb is related somatotopically to lobules III and HIII in the cat and monkey and, presumably, in the rat, the spinocerebellar fibers to these lobules probably originate in the lumbar and upper sacral segments of the cord ($L_2 - S_3$ in man). The muscles of the pelvic diaphragm receive their nerve supply from S_3, S_4, and S_5 in man, and cutaneous fibers from these segments reach the perianal region (Keegan and Garrett, 1948). If one assumed a similar but relatively greater and modified innervation of corresponding structures in the rat and other tailed mammals, it would not seem unreasonable to postulate the existence of spinocerebellar fibers from these segments of the cord to lobule II. Some fibers from more caudal segments also may be included, as in *Ateles.*

Lobule III of the rat, corresponding to lobulus 3 of Bolk, bears a stronger resemblance to folium III of the eagle, horned owl, and cormorant than to that of smaller birds. It is separated from lobule II by a deep furrow, the precentral fissure, and is divided into folia IIIa and IIIb by a shallower furrow. Folium III of the pigeon cerebellum sometimes shows secondary foliation; in the chicken, grouse, and duck foliation is less evident (fig. 26).

The furrow above lobule III of the rat clearly is the preculminate fissure as is shown by its development and its resemblance to this fissure in other mammals. The division dorsal to it was labeled lobulus 4 by Bolk, who subdivided it in many mammalian species into sublobuli 4A and 4B in recognition of the deep fissure that divides the cortex into two groups of lamellae. In many mammals this fissure penetrates as deeply as a number of the other principal vermal clefts, as is also shown in a number of Bolk's figures.

G. E. Smith (1903c), although describing only four lobules in the human anterior lobe, recognized two lobules above the preculminate fissure; his "third" and "fourth" lobules corresponded to Bolk's sublobuli 4A and 4B. The development of this part of the anterior lobe in the rat and other mammals and the similarity of it to the corresponding region of the avian cerebellum led me to designate as lobule IV the subdivision immediately above the preculminate fissure and as lobule V the more extensive subdivision whose dorsoposterior surface faces the fissura prima. The two are separated by a furrow, intraculminate fissure 1, which remains relatively shallow in the adult rat as compared with the fissura prima and the preculminate fissure; it is nearly as deep, however, as the precentral fissure. If the dorsal wall of the preculminate fissure is included as part of lobule IV, this lobule has a considerable expanse of cortex (fig. 23).

There are rather striking similarities between lobules IV and V of the rat and the similarly named folia in the pigeon. In both species lobule IV projects well beyond the general anterior surface of the cerebellum, and its exposed surface is considerably expanded. Folium V is subfoliated into Va and Vb in the pigeon and all other birds described except for the hummingbird. In the rat cerebellum illustrated in figure 23A the corresponding lobule is expanded distally but is not subfoliated. In the specimen represented in figure 23B, a slight subfoliation is evident.

Folia IV and V of the pigeon are relatively much larger than lobules IV and V of the rat, which is no doubt correlated to the large wing area and wing muscles of the pigeon as compared with the skin and muscles of the forelimb of the rat. In addition to activating folia IV and V by stimulation of tactile receptors in the wing or of the wing nerves, Whitlock (1952) plotted more limited loci of activation, in both folia, which had been induced by stimulation of the leg. Folia III and IV also were activated by stimulation of the tail, and folium V was involved to a slight degree. Evidently the distribution of fibers carrying impulses from the leg and the tail is more diffuse in the anterior lobe of the pigeon than in experimental mammals, as represented by the cat and monkey. The electrophysiological studies of Snider and Stowell (1942, 1944), Dow and Anderson (1942), Adrian (1943), and Snider (1943) on exteroceptive and proprioceptive distribution to the anterior lobe of mammals were summarized by Dow and Moruzzi (1958).

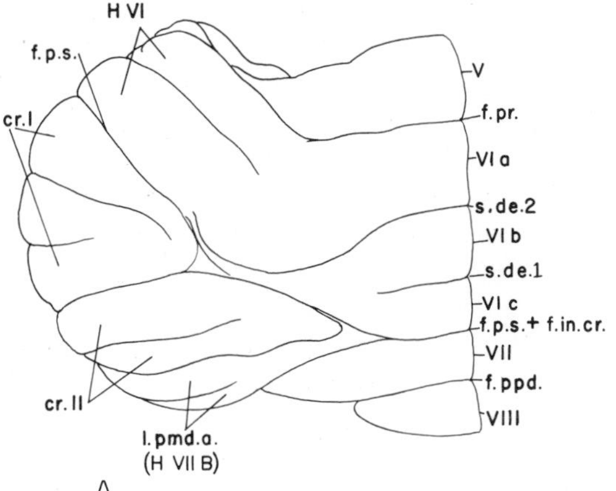

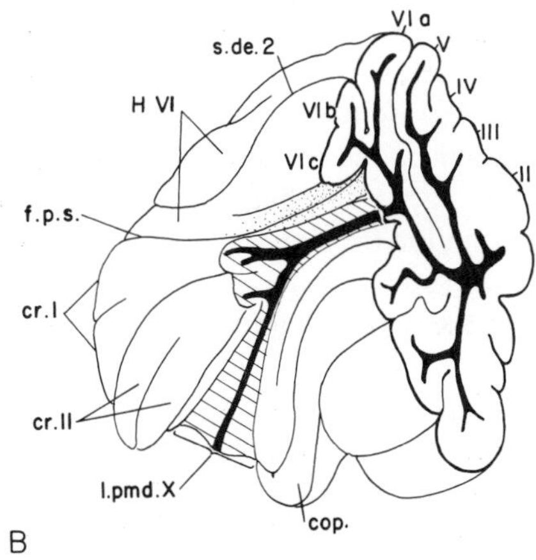

Figure 24. Cerebellum of adult rat. A. Dorsal view of left half. B. Posteromedial view of same specimen with lobule VII, medial portions of crus I and crus II and anterior part of the paramedian lobule dissected down to medullary substance. The relations of the medullary substance of the lobules named to the medullary rays, as shown in midsagittal sections, are illustrated. ×12. (Larsell, 1952.)

Posterior lobe. Vermal lobules VI, VII, VIII, and IX of the adult rat are remarkably similar to folia VI–IX of the pigeon, with respect both to form and subfoliation and to activation by exteroceptive stimulation from corresponding parts of the body and to stimulation of nerves to these parts.

Lobule VI is a well-defined segment delimited caudally by the posterior superior fissure (fig. 23). Usually in the rat a hemispheral furrow, the intercrural fissure, is confluent with the vermal segment of the posterior superior fissure (fig. 24) and forms a compound fissure that already has been described in developmental stages of the cerebellum. The external surface of the lobule is divided by two furrows, declival sulci 1 and 2, into three folia indicated as VIa, VIb, and VIc (fig. 24B). Folium VI of the pigeon and some other birds presents three similar subdivisions (fig. 26). The posterior wall of the fissura prima of the rat presents a characteristic folium, designated VId, which was found as a similar fold, or as a lamella in the larger species, in all except the smallest mammals. There are uncertain suggestions of a similar fold in some pigeon cerebella but in general it does not form a distinct cortical fold in birds.

The electrophysiological experiments on birds (Whitlock, 1952) and mammals (Snider and Stowell, 1944) demonstrate that the anterior part of folium VI and lobule VI, in the respective groups of animals, is activated by stimuli mediated by the trigeminal nerve. The morphological correspondence of the two subdivisions, coupled with experimental results, can leave no doubt about their homology. The relatively large size of the lobule in the rat undoubtedly is correlated with the importance of the trigeminal nerve in this animal.

Lobule VII of the rat, which lies immediately behind lobule VI, is bounded posteriorly by a deep furrow that clearly represents the prepyramidal fissure on the basis of both development and comparative anatomy. In young and adult stages of some specimens the lobule shows no evidence of subfoliation. In others, a shallow furrow extends slightly beyond the midline on either side and divides its surface into two approximately equal areas. This furrow, as more fully described in connection with the paramedian lobule, appears to be the vermian representation of the ansoparamedian fissure and to correspond to sulcus *a* of Bradley (1903). In the rat, lobule VII when unfoliated shows an apparent similarity to folium VII of the horned owl, bantam chicken, hummingbird, and some pigeon cerebella. When secondary folia are present in the rat lobule VII resembles folium VII of the grouse, barn owl, and cormorant. This similarity of lobule VII of the rat to folium VII of birds, in addition to the evidence that these segments of birds and mammals are activated by visual and auditory stimuli (Whitlock, 1952; Snider and Stowell, 1944), leaves no doubt that the two primary divisions are homologous.

Lobule VIII, the segment behind the prepyramidal fissure in the rat (fig. 25), obviously corresponds to folium VIII of birds by reason of both its position between the readily recognizable prepyramidal and secunda fissures and its similarity in form. In the domestic fowl, the grouse, duck, cormorant, horned owl, and eagle, the surface of lobule VIII is subfoliated, a feature which is only suggested in some of the rat brains; in the anterior wall of the fissura secunda of the rat, however, a constant sulcus is present (fig. 23). In the pigeon such a sulcus is

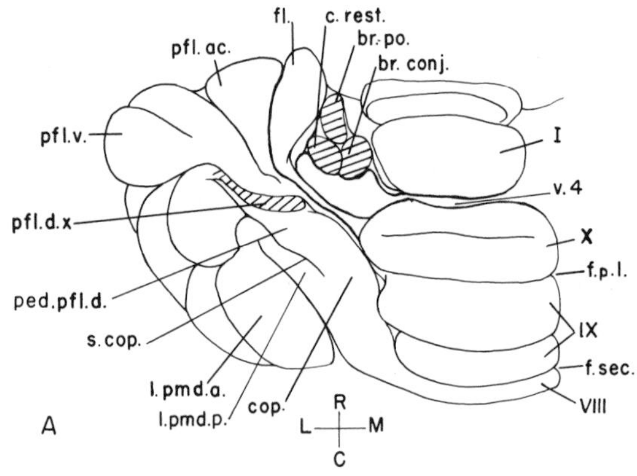

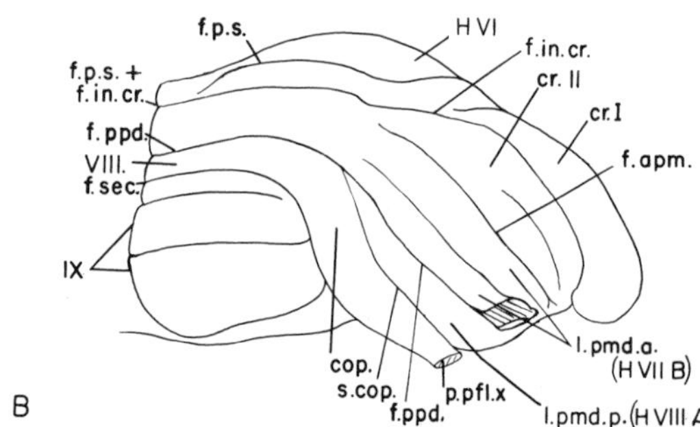

Figure 25. Cerebellum of adult rat. A. Ventral view of vermis and right hemisphere with part of dorsal paraflocculus removed. B. Posterolateral view of atypical cerebellum of adult rat in which the posterior part of paramedian lobule is exposed on the cerebellar surface. The distal folium of the anterior paramedian lobule has been dissected away, showing the connection by a narrow band of marginal cortex between the posterior and anterior parts of the paramedian lobule. ×7. (Larsell, 1952.)

only suggested by a rostral arching of the anterior wall of the fissura secunda. It is apparent in the developing duck and chick, while in most adult birds it seems to be represented by the deeper one of several shallow sulci that are present in the bantam chicken, grouse, duck, and eagle. Lobule VIII of the cat and monkey, like folium VIII of birds, is activated by auditory and visual stimuli.

Lobule IX, the uvula, of the rat obviously corresponds to folium IX of birds. As shown in figures 18A and 23A it consists of four folia that reach the surface. These clearly correspond to subfolia IXa, IXb, IXc, and IXd of the adult pigeon (fig. 26A). In many avian species folium IXc is not divided so that only three subfolia were found as is sometimes true in the rat (fig. 23B). Furthermore, the uvular furrow pattern of the rat is almost identical with that of birds. Folium IXb is delimited from folium IXc by the deep uvular sulcus 1; folium IXa is separated from folium IXb by the shallower uvular sulcus 2; and folium IXc is sometimes divided in the rat, as well as in some species of birds, by the still shallower uvular sulcus 3. In some species of birds even the secondary furrows from the deep portions of the principal fissures are very similar to those in the rat, as may be seen by comparing uvular sulcus 1 of the grouse with the corresponding furrow in the rat.

Folium X, the nodulus, of birds shows various degrees of folding on itself in different avian species (fig. 26). In the embryonic chick and duck cerebellum and in the adult stage of some birds, it is a thickened plate, one side of which is covered by cortex while the other side is ventricular. In other species, e.g., the grouse, the adult stage is represented by a completely formed folium entirely covered by cortex except at its ventricular base, where the choroid tela is attached to its posterior border. In the adult rat lobule X resembles folium X of the grouse more than that of other birds, but in its development the stages of transformation from an unfolded condition are shown. A shallow groove on the ventral surface divides the nodulus of the adult rat into two folia, as already noted (fig. 23).

In birds the folia, except X and the posterior portion of IX, and the furrows as far caudally as uvular sulcus 1, continue on the lateral surface of the cerebellum toward the rudimentary cerebellar hemisphere. The fissures reach various levels of the incipient hemisphere in different species of birds and extend well ventralward in some of the larger species so that the rudimentary hemisphere is foliated. Only the posterior portions of the uvula and the nodulus, however, are represented by lateral extensions, the "avian paraflocculus" and the flocculus, respectively.

The surface features of the vermal portion of the avian

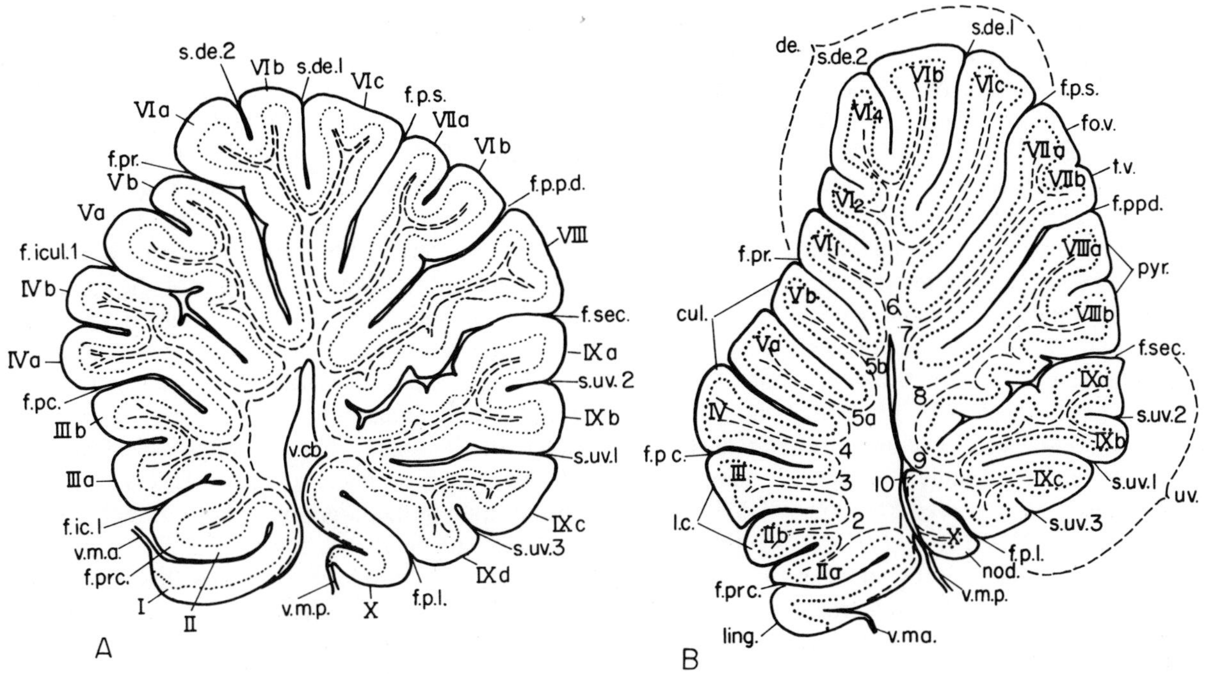

Figure 26. A. Midsagittal section of cerebellum of pigeon. Weigert series. ×7. (Larsell and Whitlock, 1952.) B. Midsagittal section of cerebellum of wild mallard duck (*Anas platyrhynchus*). ×7. (Larsell, 1948.)

cerebellum are more difficult to identify with corresponding ones in the rat than is true of the fissures and folia as seen in sagittal section. This is owing to the domelike form of the organ in birds and the rapid lateroventral slope of the folia toward the cerebellar base on each side, in contrast with the lateral extension of the vermal lobules of the rat into the expanded hemispheres. After comparing vermal portions of figures 26A, B with figures 19 and 20 one found many points of similarity.

The homologies between the individual folia of birds and vermal lobules of the rat, based on morphological evidence, are substantiated by fiber tract connections. In the Marchi experiments on the pigeon, Whitlock (1952) followed spinocerebellar fibers to folia II–VIb, VIII, and IX, with some possibly passing to folium I. Anderson (1943) previously had obtained virtually identical results in the rat, although they were reported in terms of lingula, central lobule, culmen, declive, pyramis, and uvula. Using the Marchi method, Whitlock found trigeminocerebellar fibers in birds distributed to folia V and VI and tectocerebellar fibers distributed to folia VI, VII, and VIII. In the experiments with the aid of the oscillograph, the areas of activation by stimuli from different parts of the body were virtually identical in birds and mammals with respect to the vermal segments involved when compared with the results of Snider and Stowell (1942, 1944) and Adrian (1943) on the cat, monkey, and other mammals.

Using electrophysiological methods, Adrian (1943) demonstrated an ipsilateral somatotopic distribution of tactile and proprioceptive impulses to the anterior lobe and part of the declive or lobulus simplex of the posterior lobe of the cat, monkey, and other mammals. Snider and Stowell (1942, 1944) similarly demonstrated the distribution of tactile impulses and found activated areas not only in the anterior lobe and the lobulus simplex but also in the paramedian lobule (HVIIB + HVIIIA) for the forefoot and hindfoot. These authors, in addition, discovered that visual and auditory impulses also evoke action potentials in the cerebellar cortex (Snider and Stowell, 1942, 1944; Stowell and Snider, 1942a, 1942b). There were responses to clicks in the posterior part of lobule VI and HVI and in lobules VII and VIII. Responses to photic stimuli of one eye were maximal in three areas including, respectively, lobule VI, the anterior part of lobule VII, the posterior part of lobule VII, and part of lobule VIII. Photic responses were modified by certain drugs but Pupilli and Berger (1956) observed activation of lobules VI and VII in the unanesthetized cat. After injection of chloralose, photic responses could be recorded from part of lobule HVIIA.

A similar somatotopic pattern was demonstrated by

Hampson, Harrison, and Woolsey (1952) by stimulation of the cortex of the vermal lobules; these authors included the lingula as being functionally related to the tail. Developmental and other considerations already noted appear to justify dividing the lingula into lobules I and II.

The electrophysiological evidence, reviewed in extenso by Dow and Moruzzi (1958), leaves little room for doubt that with respect to both afferent and motor functions lobule III is related to the hindlimb and its subdivisions, lobule IV to the shoulder and elbow, and lobule V to the forelimb and paw or hand. Lobules VI and HVI are related to the neck and head; lobules VII and VIII to vision and hearing; the area activated by photic impulses probably occupies lobule VII, primarily, while that for auditory impulses probably occupies the pyramis (lobule VIII). Visual and occasionally other somatic afferent impulses have also been recorded from lobule HVIIA. The paramedian lobule (HVIIB + HVIIIA) is activated somatotopically and bilaterally by impulses from the face, forelimb, and hindlimb, with considerable overlapping of the areas. It also represents motor cortex, similarly arranged.

According to Brodal (1954), the pyramis and uvula (lobules VIII and IX) receive dorsal spinocerebellar and external cuneate nucleus fibers, as well as fibers from the pons. Brodal regarded the spinal cord and the cerebral cortex as the chief systems acting on these lobules. The ventral part of the uvula (IXc and d) receives some primary and secondary vestibular fibers, as demonstrated by Dow (1936). Stimulation of lobules VIII, IX, and HVIIB–HVIII was said to produce responses similar to those obtained from the anterior lobe.

These patterns of sensorimotor cortex undoubtedly are transferable to the cerebellum of the rat and other mammals, both small and large, which are described here. The relative differentiation and size of individual lobules varies with the relative importance of the sensory systems and, apparently, with the mass and functional differentiation of the muscle groups served by each lobule. The number of cortical folds is less in the smaller species than in the larger ones, both in marsupial and in placental mammals. As individual lobules differentiate, however, they do so in correlation with the functional importance in each species of the sensory and motor organs to which they are related. They may appear in varying sequences in different species, according to the degree of development of motor and sensory organs that have cerebellar connections.

MONOTREMATA

THE cerebellum of the platypus, *Ornithorhynchus anatinus*, was briefly described and illustrated by G. E. Smith (1899). Ziehen (1897) described the organ in *Echidna* and, less fully, in *Ornithorhynchus*. His interpretations of fissures and lobules differed so widely from those of G. E. Smith that two fundamentally different patterns of division of the organ resulted. A wax model reconstruction of the anteater cerebellum was described and illustrated by de Lange (1918), and Hines (1929) described the cerebellum of the platypus, comparing it with the organ in the anteater, pigeon, and opossum. The brainstem and cerebellum of *Echidna* were described by Abbie (1934) and, more recently, Dillon (1962) briefly compared the cerebellum of the platypus and anteater with the organ in the bandicoot and rat, with special reference to the principal fissures and lobules.

G. E. Smith labeled the deepest fissure of the cerebellum the fissura prima. In monotremes it is situated in the posterior part of the organ and, according to Smith, divides the cerebellum into a very large anterior lobe and much smaller medial and posterior lobes, which are located behind the fissura prima.

The fissura prima of G. E. Smith was called the fissura horizontalis magna by Ziehen (1897) in *Echidna* and the deepest sulcus by Hines (1929). In *Ornithorhynchus*, however, the corresponding deep fissure was called the fissura secunda by Hines. She interpreted the fissura prima in both the platypus and the anteater as being a shallower fissure in the anterior part of the organ. In *Echidna*, a furrow situated posteroventrally and much shallower than her fissura secunda of *Ornithorhynchus* was called the fissura secunda or *z* of Ingvar. The fissura prima of Hines in the platypus appears to correspond to Ziehen's sulcus cerebellaris anterior superior in *Echidna*. A doubtfully corresponding fissure, in the anteater, which will be discussed later, was interpreted as the fissura prima by Hines. Abbie (1934) and Dillon (1962) defined the fissura prima as had G. E. Smith, but their interpretations of the region behind this fissure differ from G. E. Smith's as well as from each other's.

As subdivided by G. E. Smith, Abbie, and Dillon the monotreme cerebellum differs so greatly from that of marsupials and placental mammals that there is little resemblance in the relative size of the primary lobes and their subdivisions. On the basis of Hines' interpretation of the fissura prima, the anterior lobe corresponds more closely in relative size to that of other mammals, and the subdivisions behind the fissure would compare with the lobules of other authors, which had been interpreted differently on the basis of the significance attached to the individual fissures of this part of the cerebellum.

The state of confusion which still prevails regarding the monotreme cerebellum probably could be clarified if adequate embryonic material were available. Lacking this, we need to make do with a close comparison between the cerebellum of birds and the cerebellum of the rat, as representatives of a relatively simple placental type. The development of the cerebellar subdivisions and fissures has already been described in birds (Larsell, 1967) and the rat, and the subdivisions have been homologized. A supplement to the morphological comparisons is the somatotopic localization in individual folia or corresponding lobules that was demonstrated experimentally in birds by Whitlock (1952) and in mammals by Snider and Stowell (1942, 1944), Stowell and Snider (1942a, 1942), Adrian (1943), Hampson, Harrison, and Woolsey (1952), and others. It seemed reasonable to assume that the experimental results obtained in birds and placental mammals are applicable to monotremes, so far as morphological homologies of the cerebellar subdivisions can be reasonably well established. A brief summary of the phylogenic relationships of monotremes and of the features of body form and motor and sensory equipment will afford some insight with respect to the probable correlations involved in the presumptive somatotopic pattern.

The monotremes or Prototheria, according to Romer (1955), are an offshoot of advanced mammal-like reptiles, the Therapsida. Another branch of the therapsids divided into the Metatheria (marsupials) and the Eutheria (placental mammals). The monotremes, although definitely mammalian, lay shelled eggs as do reptiles. The shoulder girdle is reptilian in that it retains the interclavicle and paired clavicles. In marsupials and placental mammals the interclavicle disappears but among the more generalized species the clavicle remains, articulating with the sternum. In birds the clavicles and interclavicles are fused, forming the furcula or wishbone (Romer). Complex modifications of the forelimb muscles are associated with these skeletal changes.

Romer noted that the pelvic girdle of mammals and ancestral mammal-like reptiles is modified from the reptilian type in association with the different limb posture and changed musculature. A pair of marsupial bones also extends forward and supports the body wall in monotremes and marsupials. The pelvic girdle of Archosauria and their avian descendants is modified from the reptilian type in adaptation to the bipedal habit of these groups.

These anatomical features of the shoulder and pelvic girdles of monotremes and the comparisons with higher mammals and birds are mentioned because they have a bearing on the interpretation of the anterior lobe of the monotreme cerebellum. The anterior lobe of present-day reptiles, such as the Crocodilia, is relatively small, while in birds and the rat (representing placental mammals) it forms a large but not predominant division of the cerebellum. The amazingly large anterior lobe of monotremes, as interpreted by G. E. Smith (1899), Abbie (1934), and Dillon (1962), and the small size of the more posterior lobules, with their various names, require examination in the light of body structure and sensory equipment of monotremes, in comparison with experimental mammals such as the cat. Also the results of electrophysiological studies that demonstrate somatotopic localization of activation in specific lobules of mammals and corresponding folia of birds must be taken into consideration in interpreting the lobules of the anterior lobe as well as those in the remainder of the cerebellum.

Externally the body of monotremes does not differ greatly from that of unspecialized placental mammals such as the rat. The tail of *Ornithorhynchus* is elongated (having 20–21 caudal vertebrae) and beaverlike; it is covered with fur, as is the rest of the body. The dorsal part of the body of *Echidna* is covered with strong, pointed spines between which are coarse hairs. The tail of the anteater is short and the caudal vertebrae are reportedly represented by flattened nodules. The legs of the platypus are short, the feet have five clawed digits that are also webbed, and the limbs are equally adapted for burrowing and swimming. The limbs of the anteater are short and powerful. Five toes on each foot end in very strong claws, enabling the animal, which is entirely terrestrial, to burrow rapidly into the ground or dig into the termite or ant hills that supply its food.

Both species were said to be chiefly nocturnal. They have small eyes and lack the auditory pinna. According to Abbie (1934) vision is poor in *Echidna* and the auditory division of the acoustic nerve represents about one-third of the volume of the combined bundles.

Abbie found that the trigeminal nerve is large in both species, with many trigeminal fibers passing directly to the cerebellum in *Echidna*; however, the trigeminal system is larger in the platypus than in the anteater. The chief sensory trigeminal nucleus is reportedly very large and is divided incompletely into medial and lateral parts, which send fibers to the cerebellum and the pons. Hines (1929) described fibers from the dorsolateral part of this nucleus in *Ornithorhynchus* as forming a considerable fascicle in the inferior cerebellar peduncle.

Instead of vibrissae, which are lacking in monotremes, the snout and beak of the platypus were said to have numerous specialized receptors of the tactile type, which are supplied by the trigeminal nerve. According to Abbie, the snout of *Echidna* is smooth but hard and apparently has no specialized receptors, but the trigeminal nerve is hypertrophied, although less so than in *Ornithorhynchus*, and the snout probably is extremely sensitive. Since the long tongue of this species is used in gathering food, this organ is probably richly supplied with receptors of the exteroceptive type, in its mucosa, which are related to the trigeminus. G. E. Smith (1899) regarded the broad expanse of skin covering the ducklike beak of the platypus as the principal organ of touch in this species.

Although activation of the cerebellum by stimulation of cutaneous receptors had not yet been demonstrated experimentally, Abbie (1934) postulated a physiological extension of the surface area of the body of *Echidna* which he believed to be associated with the spines. He assumed that tactile sensibility is of great importance in both species of monotremes.

Cerebellum

The cerebellum of *Ornithorhynchus* and also of *Echidna* has morphological features that resemble the organ of birds and mammals more than that of any

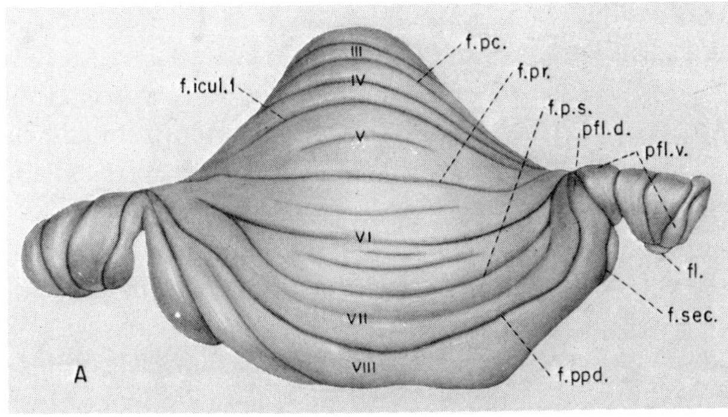

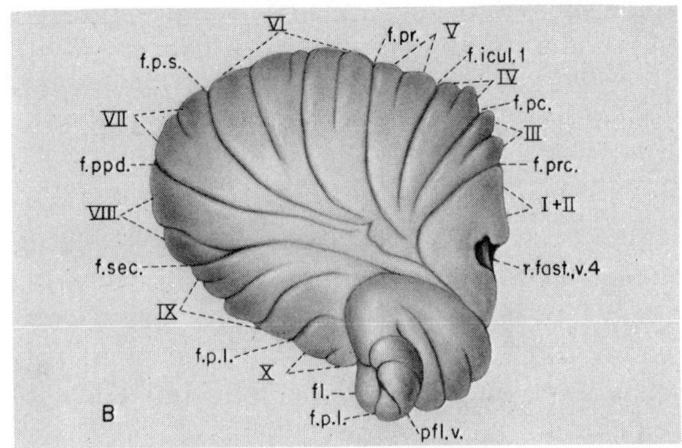

Figure 27. Cerebellum of *Ornithorhynchus anatinus.* A. Dorsal view. B. Lateral view. (Redrawn and modified from Hines, 1929.)

present-day reptile. The cerebellar hemispheres of *Ornithorhynchus* and *Echidna* seem greatly reduced when compared with small marsupials and placentals. This feature and the superficial pattern of fissures and lobules, especially in the platypus, give the cerebellum a more avian than mammalian aspect (fig. 27).

I did not have material for a personal study of the cerebellum of *Ornithorhynchus* but I closely examined an *Echidna* cerebellum (fig. 28) both grossly and microscopically. Some features of this specimen differ from the descriptions of Abbie (1934) and Dillon (1962); other features that were not mentioned or obscured in the descriptions of other authors clarify the morphology of the organ in the anteater. Therefore my observations on the *Echidna* cerebellum are presented in comparison with those of other authors who had more abundant material.

Since a comparison with the cerebellum of *Ornithorhynchus* is of great importance I reinterpreted the descriptions of this species by Hines (1929) and her comparisons of it with *Echidna.* Many changes in the conception of cerebellar morphology have occurred during the more than three decades since the appearance of the monograph by Hines on the platypus brain. The numerous photomicrographs and drawings of sagittal sections of the brain and cerebellum, supplemented by many figures of surface features of the cerebellum, make possible a reinterpretation when these figures are compared with this organ in *Echidna,* birds, the rat, and other mammals.

The posteroventral part of the *Echidna* cerebellum constitutes a flocculonodular lobe, not unlike that of placental mammals. The corresponding part of the cerebellum of *Ornithorhynchus* also is the flocculonodular lobe but in some respects it resembles this lobe in birds more than in mammals. The remainder of the cerebellum of both species corresponds to the corpus cerebelli.

FLOCCULONODULAR LOBE

Beginning with the posterior ventral part of the *Echidna* cerebellum, three folds of cortex are situated behind a small cerebellar ventricle and the fastigial recess (figs. 29, 30). The most caudal of the three is separated from the remainder of the posterior part of the organ by a relatively deep fissure which corresponds to the posterolateral fissure of birds and other mammals (fig. 30). The three folia together correspond to folium X of birds and to lobule X of mammals. For the sake of conformity with the terminology of the vermal segments of mammals, I called this and other divisions of the vermal part of the

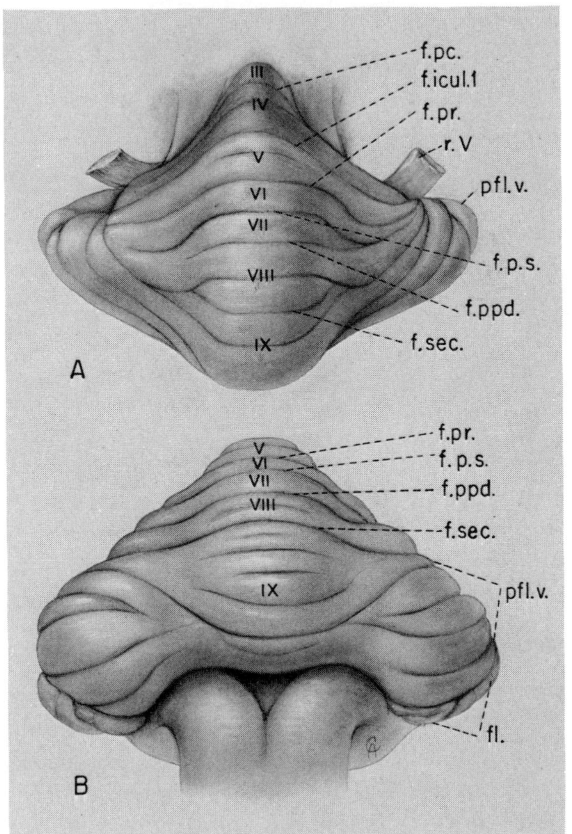

Figure 28. Cerebellum of *Echidna aculeata.* A. Dorsal view. B. Posterior view.

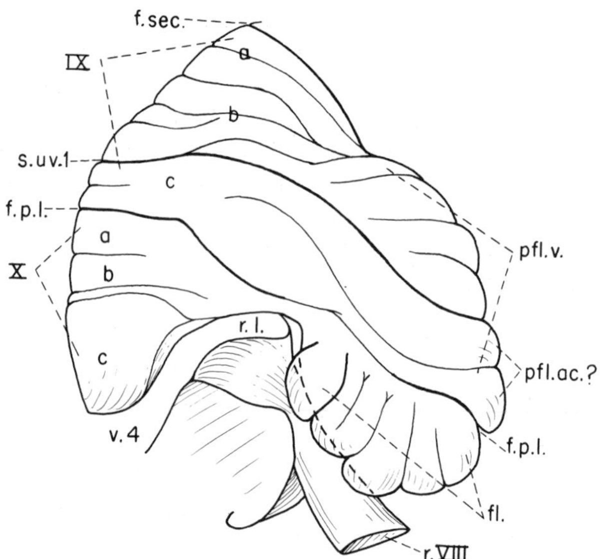

Figure 29. Cerebellum of *Echidna aculeata.* Dorsolateral and posterior view of right half.

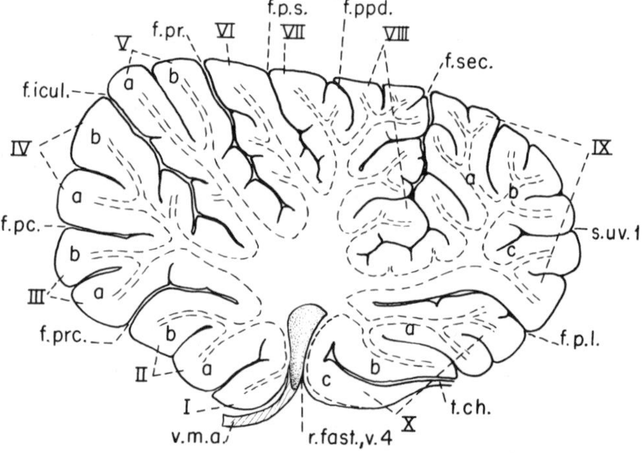

Figure 30. Cerebellum of *Echidna aculeata.* Midsagittal section.

monotreme cerebellum lobules rather than folia, although many of them have a greater resemblance to avian folia than to mammalian lobules.

The three subdivisions in *Echidna* may be called folia Xa, Xb, and Xc. They are relatively larger and more deeply separated than the folia of the nodulus of birds and mammals and do not altogether correspond to these folia. In her figure of a nearly median sagittal section of the cerebellum of *Echidna* Hines (1929) included three folds in the nodulus. Abbie (1934) illustrated three similar folds but regarded only the one immediately behind the fastigial recess as the nodulus – the other two he erroneously called the uvula.

Ziehen (1897) illustrated three similar folds in *Echidna*; the one corresponding to Xc is directed ventrocaudally but ends bluntly behind the fastigial recess. Dillon (1962) labeled as the nodulus two folds that appear to correspond to Xa and Xb; the more anterior fold and a smaller one which he illustrated in front of it were called, respectively, the lobulus ventralis and lobulus carnalis.

Folium Xc, illustrated in figures 29 and 30, tapers caudalward beneath Xb and is continuous with the choroid tela. No attachment of the choroid tela to any part of the ventral surface of the cerebellum was mentioned or illustrated by any of the authors cited above – indeed the choroid tela was entirely ignored. The fastigial recess shows up in the figures of Ziehen and Abbie and indistinctly in Hines' figure. Because of their importance as morphological landmarks, the fastigial recess and the attachment of the choroid tela merit special attention.

In *Ornithorhynchus* G. E. Smith's (1899) figure shows three cortical folds between a well-defined fastigial recess and a furrow that corresponds to the posterolateral fissure of *Echidna* (fig. 31A). The ventral part of the anterior fold, labeled nodulus, has an anteriorly tapering process, but whether or not the choroid tela is attached to it is not clear. Hines' photomicrographs showing sagittal sections of the cerebellum of a less mature platypus cerebellum show folium Xc descending nearly vertically behind the fastigial recess, except for a slight turn forward and a blunt end (fig. 31B). The granular layer of the folium faces the recess which, in this cerebellum, continues dorsocaudally as a narrow rudimentary cerebellar ventricle. A thin superficial layer, which appears to be fibrous, continues beneath the cerebellar ventricle from the medullary ray leading to folia Xa and Xb and seems to fray out in the medullary layer of Xc. The choroid tela of the fourth ventricle extends forward as far as the rostroventral surface of folium Xc in some of the sections but one could not be certain with the low magnification of these photomicrographs about the attachment of the tela.

There seems to be no question that folia Xa, Xb, and Xc are related and that together they constitute one lobule. Only the posterior folium, apparently corresponding to Xc, was included by Dillon (1962) in the nodulus. The two folds that apparently correspond to Xb and Xc were designated lobule 7; Dillon's nodulus was called lobule 6. I found no justification in the descriptions or figures of other authors for dividing the region between the fastigial recess and the posterolateral fissure of the platypus into the two lobules and their subdivisions of Dillon. After examining the *Echidna* cerebellum illustrated in figures 28, 29, and 30, and the figures of other authors I found that I disagreed with Dillon's interpretation of the corresponding region of the anteater.

Apparently there is considerable variation in this region of the monotreme cerebellum, but this also is true of other mammals, including man. Unless close attention is directed to the fastigial recess and to the true posteroventral cerebellar margin, as determined by the attachment of the choroid tela, interpretations frequently are difficult. According to my interpretations, the nodulus is larger and has more prominent folds in monotremes than in birds; it does not differ enough from small marsupials and placental mammals to justify further subdivision, except in the relative depth of the furrows between the folia and in the forward position of folium Xc.

The three folia of lobule X are continuous by a short peduncle with the flocculus, as illustrated in figure 29. Since the noduli of Abbie and Dillon, taken together, correspond to this lobule as I defined it, my observations correspond to the combined interpretations of both these authors.

The posterolateral fissure is deep in the vermal part of the *Echidna* cerebellum and becomes shallower between the peduncle and the accessory paraflocculus, which will be discussed again later. It forms a deep cleft between the distal part of the flocculus and the accessory paraflocculus described below (fig. 29).

By comparing the three subdivisions of lobule X in monotremes with folium X of birds, we can learn something about the manner of their development and their relationships. Folium Xc of *Echidna* and *Ornithorhynchus* is similar in many respects to the nearly vertically elongated (as seen in median sagittal sections) nodulus of the eagle, horned owl, and some other species (fig. 26). The distal part of the nodulus expands caudalward and, in some species, doubles forward on itself, forming a ventral fold (Larsell, 1948; figs. 10, 11, 13, 15). In the grouse the dorsal and ventral folds fuse into one compact lobule, to the anterior ventral part of which the choroid tela is attached. The comparison must not be pressed too closely but folia Xa and Xb of the monotreme cerebellum could be regarded as corresponding on an enlarged scale, involving secondary foliation, to the posteriorly directed part of the nodulus of many birds.

In the *Echidna* cerebellum illustrated in figure 29, folium Xc turns caudalward, as already noted, instead of forward as does the part giving attachment to the tela in birds. If one considered folium Xc, however, on an enlarged scale, as corresponding to the vertical part of the avian nodulus, then the general pattern of lobule X is similar to that of folium X of birds. Variations in the form, foliation, and point of attachment of the tela are so numerous in the mammalian and human adult cerebellum that the comparisons made above did not seem too farfetched.

The flocculus of *Echidna* is so situated beneath the posterolateral margin of the hemisphere that it forms a relatively large lobule comprising five or six folia (fig. 29). It was similarly illustrated in the anteater by Hines and Abbie. In *Ornithorhynchus* the flocculus of Hines is a small lobule situated behind the laterally projecting paraflocculus of this species (fig. 27), which resembles the relations of the flocculus and the avian paraflocculus in birds. Hines described direct vestibular fibers to the cerebellum of the platypus as ending in the cortex of the nodulus, uvula, and flocculus and in the lingula of the anterior lobe. This distribution corresponds to that in the flocculonodular lobe and the lingula of experimental mammals.

The flocculus, nodulus, and connecting peduncle of *Echidna* together correspond to the flocculonodular lobe of the rat. In *Ornithorhynchus* the nodulus is more directly continuous with the flocculus, with little or no constriction occurring between them, as in the flocculonodular lobe of birds.

CORPUS CEREBELLI

Identification of the subdivisions of the corpus cerebelli is so dependent on the correct interpretation of the fissura prima and fissura secunda that these fissures must be examined first. In *Echidna* Hines (1929) described and labeled the most prominent and deepest fissure of the cerebellum, which opens onto the posterodorsal surface, as the "deepest sulcus." A shallower fissure, opening onto the anterior dorsal cerebellar surface and corresponding to Ingvar's sulcus *x* of birds, was regarded as the fissura prima by Hines. A shallow furrow in the posterior part of the organ was labeled fissura secunda or sulcus *z* of Ingvar. In *Ornithorhynchus*, however, the fissure corresponding to the deepest sulcus of *Echidna* was called the fissura secunda and a shallower but nevertheless quite deep furrow opening onto the dorsal surface was interpreted by Hines as the fissura prima. On the ground that the fissura prima always is the deepest fissure in the cerebellum, Abbie (1934) contended that the posterior deep fissure of *Echidna* is the fissura prima. Dillon (1962) also named it the fissura prima in the platypus as well as in the anteater. Abbie designated as the fissura secunda the furrow identified above as the posterolateral fissure; Dillon, in both species, so named a furrow that corresponds to Ingvar's sulcus *z*. As already noted in birds and the rat, sulcus *z* of Ingvar is uvular sulcus 1.

The interpretations of the fissura prima advanced by G. E. Smith, Abbie, and Dillon in monotremes divide the cerebellum into anterior and posterior divisions so unequal in size, even if the flocculonodular lobe is included in the posterior division, that the pattern of the organ would be entirely different from that of birds and mammals. These authors emphasized this difference in comparison with other mammals. However, there are no differences in body form or in sensory or motor equipment of monotremes, as compared with other mammals or with birds, that can be correlated with such disparities in the primary lobes of the corpus cerebelli, if you consider these lobes and their subdivisions from the functional point of view. Abbie (1934) emphasized the importance of the trigeminal nerve in relation to the cerebellum of *Echidna* and noted that ventral spinocerebellar fibers also enter the organ anteriorly. He also mentioned tectocerebellar fibers from the superior and inferior colliculi entering the organ by way of the anterior medullary velum. Hines (1929) had also emphasized the trigeminal contribution in the platypus and described the tectocerebellar tract, apparently for the first time (1925) in any mammal. Pathways for exteroceptive impulses to the cerebellum thus were established in monotremes many years before cerebellar responses to such impulses were demonstrated experimentally in laboratory mammals. The distribution of these fibers within the cerebellum, however, remained unknown.

Dillon (1962), in his analysis of the lobules of monotremes, apparently ignored the subsequently accumulated electrophysiological evidence, both in birds and mammals, of somatotopic activation in specific segments of the cerebellar cortex by exteroceptive and proprioceptive impulses. Although similar experimental evidence of somatotopic localization has not been presented with respect to monotremes, the results with birds and mammals are so strikingly similar in cerebellar subdivisions homologized by morphological methods that in all probability they can be transferred to the subdivisions of the monotreme cerebellum, if these can be shown to correspond to the folia of birds or the lobules of experimental mammals.

Comparing the morphological features of the monotreme cerebellum (figs. 27, 31) with those of birds and of the rat (representing placental mammals), we found that the deep anterior fissure that opens onto the dorsal surface in *Ornithorhynchus* corresponds to the fissura prima of birds, marsupials, and placental mammals. Hines (1929) also regarded this furrow as the fissura prima in the platypus, but the anterior furrow so designated by her in *Echidna* probably is the intraculminate fissure, as will be pointed out later. In *Ornithorhynchus* the fissura prima is the deepest cerebellar fissure, except for the fissura secunda. In most higher mammals it is the deepest fissure of the organ but there are exceptions, which will be discussed later. The depth of this or any other fissure is not a sufficient criterion for identification.

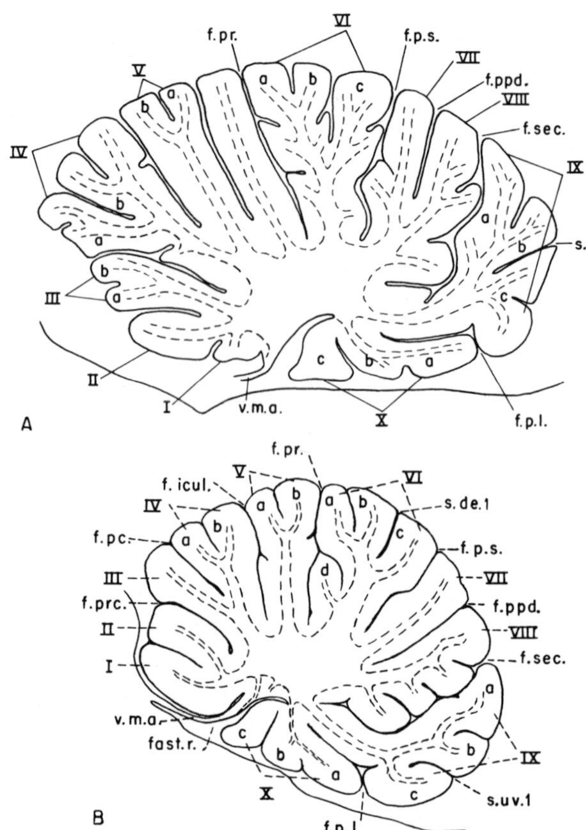

Figure 31. Midsagittal sections of cerebellum of *Ornithorhyncus*. A. (G. E. Smith, 1899.) B. (Hines, 1929.)

In birds the fissura prima is relatively shallow but extends widely on the lateral surface of the corpus cerebelli. The corresponding fissure in the platypus and anteater is much deeper than that in birds but it has similar morphological relations and extends into the lateral part of the corpus cerebelli in a similar position (figs. 27, 28A).

On comparing the various fissures that authors labeled as prima and secunda in monotremes with my own observations in *Echidna*, birds, and other mammals, I decided that the anterior deep fissure so labeled in figure 31 must be regarded as the fissura prima. It corresponds to Ziehen's anterior superior sulcus in this species and to Hines' fissura prima in *Ornithorhynchus*. The developmental history of the furrow similarly situated in birds, opossum, and placental mammals shows that in most species it is the first to appear in the corpus cerebelli. As already noted the relative depth of fissures in the rat is determined by the ultimate size of the lobules between which they are situated. In the adjustments during growth that result in the adult position and expansion of some of the lobules, their connections with the deep part of the cerebellum are elongated and the delimiting fissures are deepened accordingly.

When comparing the fissura secunda of birds and the rat with the furrows in the posterior part of the monotreme cerebellum I found that the one called fissura secunda in *Ornithorhynchus* (fig. 31) and deepest sulcus in *Echidna*, by Hines, appears to be homologous with the avian and mammalian fissura secunda. Its walls in monotremes are more foliated than those of other fissures, as is true of the fissura secunda of the larger birds, especially, and its lateral continuation forms the anterodorsal boundary of the ventral paraflocculus, as in birds. In the platypus it separates the ventral paraflocculus from a lateral continuation of lobule VIII which appears to represent an incipient dorsal paraflocculus. Whether this folium is continuous around the end of the fissure with the ventral paraflocculus, as in placental mammals, is not clear in *Echidna* or from Hines' figures of *Ornithorhynchus*.

The fissura secunda of *Echidna*, as labeled in figure 30, corresponds to the deepest sulcus of Hines in this species and to this author's fissura secunda of *Ornithorhynchus*. The depth of the fissure was attributed to the large size attained by lobule IX, the uvula, in both species. Comparing the fissura secunda of *Echidna* with that of birds one found the foliation of the walls of the fissure to be more prominent both in birds and monotremes than is true of other fissures. When lobule IX was compared with folium IX of birds and with IX of the rat, the subdivisions into IXa, IXb, and IXc were found to correspond. These divisions are relatively larger in *Echidna* and involve tertiary foliation. We shall return to lobule IX, but note that the embryonic development of this region in birds, opossum, rat, and other placental mammals supports the interpretations set forth. Lacking embryonic material from monotremes, we could not regard the apparent X homologies as established for these two species, but they appear to be the most probable explanation of the morphological features described.

If one regards the posterior deep fissure as the fissura secunda, lobule IX (the uvula) together with lobule X (the nodulus) corresponds to G. E. Smith's posterior lobe of the cerebellum in other mammals. The segments between the fissura secunda and fissura prima, as defined above, would correspond to G. E. Smith's lobus medius. The differing medial and posterior lobes of Ingvar were based on this author's misinterpretation of folium IXa as the pyramis. Aside from the depth of the fissura secunda in monotremes there is no more reason for dividing the cerebellum behind the fissura prima of these species into two lobes than there would be in birds and other mammals. Therefore I divided the corpus cerebelli into anterior and posterior lobes, corresponding to those of birds and the rat.

Anterior lobe. From the few available descriptions and illustrations of the monotreme cerebellum the anterior lobe, as defined above, seems to vary considerably in the relative size and configuration of its lobules and in the depth of the intervening fissures. The numerous variations that also occur in other mammals, as will be shown later, are a subject of comment by several authors. Each species has a more or less distinctive general pattern of lobules and fissures but variations that apparently occur in the early folding of the embryonic cortex result in differences in the size of the lobules and the depth of fissures in the anterior lobe of the individual cerebellum.

The description of the anterior lobe in *Echidna* was restricted to my own observations in this species, but comparisons were made with the accounts of other authors. The anterior lobe of *Ornithorhynchus* was described as reinterpreted from the description, photomicrographs, and other illustrations of Hines (1929) and from the figures of G. E. Smith (1899). Interpretations in both species were based on the comparison with the anterior lobe of birds, rats, and other mammals and with the descriptions and illustrations of the monotreme cerebellum published by other authors. Although the reinterpretations must be considered to be more or less subjective, an attempt was made to give due weight to the various factors that affect the development of the anterior lobe of birds, rats, and other mammals.

If the subdivisions labeled III and IV in figure 30 were regarded as individual lobules the anterior lobe of *Echidna* is divisible into five lobules. The preculminate fissure between lobules III and IV is relatively shallow as is the corresponding fissure in many birds. Folia III and IV of birds, however, have individual medullary rays. After comparing a large series of mammals with a considerable number of birds along with the available illustrations of the monotreme cerebellum, I found it justifiable to regard the two divisions as corresponding to folia III and IV of birds and to lobules III and IV of mammals in general.

Lobules I and II of *Echidna* resemble these lobules in the rat (fig. 23) except that lobule I is less completely transformed from the pattern of folium I of the duck (fig. 26B). Lobule I expands around a medullary ray which is a continuation of the medullary layer forming the anterior wall of the cerebellar ventricle and the fastigial recess. This layer is similar to that which continues into folium I of birds. In *Echidna* the folding of the cortex of the lobule is complete, in contrast with the partially folded folium I of the duck, and the medullary ray has become the core of the lobule. Lobule II is subdivided into folia IIa and IIb by a deeper furrow than that in the corresponding lobule of the rat or in folium II of most birds.

In Ziehen's (1897) figure of a median sagittal section of the cerebellum of *Echidna* (hystrix?) two much larger subdivisions, each having a distinct medullary ray, occupy a corresponding position; a smaller fold of cortex, lacking a ray, lies immediately in front of the fastigial recess. Whether the more dorsal of the larger folds should be regarded as lobule III or as an enlarged folium IIb, compensating for a relatively small lobule III, cannot be determined from this figure alone. Such variations occur in other mammals. The small fold in front of the fastigial recess I regarded as a reduced lobule I. Hines' (1929) figure of *Echidna aculeata* is similar, in general, with respect to the corresponding region, which she called the lingula. Abbie's illustration of a median section through the cerebellum shows a somewhat similar pattern but a layer of cortex appears to be situated between the fastigial recess and the medullary ray leading to folium IIa (called the lingula by Abbie) and continuing with the anterior medullary velum. In his corresponding figure of *Echidna* Dillon (1962) subdivided into three parts the region immediately rostral of a narrow zone which appears to be a medullary band continuous with the anterior medullary velum. These divisions appear to correspond, respectively, to lobule I and folia IIa and IIb of figure 30.

After studying this region in *Ornithorhynchus*, as illustrated in Hines' photomicrographs, one can see a small fold of cortex, immediately rostral of the fastigial recess, that tapers toward the anterior medullary velum. It covers a thin medullary layer which is continuous with the velum. Two larger folds are situated dorsorostrally. Identification of these three cortical segments cannot be made with any assurance but they appear to correspond to lobules I and the two divisions of lobule II of *Echidna*. Whether the more ventral of the two larger folds should be regarded as lobule I or as folium IIa is uncertain. In many placental mammals the anterior medullary velum is continuous with a fold of variable size behind the principal part of lobule I but it is so closely related that I regarded it as folium Ia. The interpretations suggested above are entirely hypothetical but, as interpreted, the lobules fall into the pattern characteristic of birds, rats, and other mammals.

Lobule III is separated from lobule II by a deep precentral fissure in *Echidna* (fig. 30). A shallower furrow divides the lobule into folia IIIa and IIIb, as in rats and larger birds. The precentral fissure is relatively deep also in *Ornithorhynchus* but lobule III is not divided in the small cerebellum (fig. 31B). The preculminate fissure, separating lobules III and IV, has already been mentioned in both species. In Hines' figures of sagittal sections of a platypus cerebellum, apparently more advanced in development than that illustrated in figure 31B, the preculminate fissure is deep and the medullary rays of the two lobules are separated almost to the medullary body. In these figures lobule III is not subdivided but lobule IV is relatively larger.

Lobule IV is separated from lobule V by a deep intraculminate fissure in *Echidna*. This furrow appears to correspond to the one that Hines called the fissura prima in the anteater. As illustrated in this author's figure and also that of Abbie, it is shallower than the fissure which I regarded as the fissura prima, but in figure 30 it is slightly deeper.

Saetersdal (1956) pointed out that in chicken, pheasant, and pigeon embryos the intraculminate fissure appears earlier and becomes deeper than the preculminate fissure. My own observations in later embryos of several species of birds and in adult birds indicated that the intraculminate fissure always is the deeper of the two, as it is in the monotreme cerebella illustrated in figures 30 and 31. Some of the illustrations of Hines, both of *Echidna* and *Ornithorhynchus*, show a deeper fissure in the position corresponding to the preculminate fissure. Whether this divides the anterior lobe of the embryo into dorsal, or culminate and ventral segments, as in the rat and other mammals, is a question which cannot presently be answered. A similarly early division does not appear in the developing bird cerebellum.

Lobule IV in the *Echidna* and *Ornithorhynchus* cerebella illustrated in figures 27 and 28A is divided superficially into folia IVa and IVb. It is more closely related to lobule III than to lobule V (fig. 30), whereas in marsupials and most placental mammals the reverse is true. In some species lobule IV is distinctly separated from both III and V.

Lobule III of experimental mammals is the principal hindlimb area of the anterior lobe. Lobule IV together with lobule V constitutes the forelimb area – both III and IV + V are subdivided somatotopically with reference to the segments of each limb. In birds the wing, leg, and to a lesser extent the tail are represented in folium IV but only the leg and tail are represented in folium III. Except that lobules III and IV of monotremes share a primary medullary ray, they are more similar to folia III and IV of birds than to lobules III and IV of mammals, in which lobule IV is more closely related to lobule V in most species.

Lobule V is so well defined, both on the external cerebellar surface and in sagittal sections, that there is no mistaking it as a distinct segment either in *Echidna* or *Ornithorhynchus*. A furrow of variable depth divides it into two superficial folia in both species (figs. 30, 31). Posteriorly the lobe is delimited by the fissura prima. It closely resembles folium V of the pigeon and many other birds but it is less deeply divided than is this folium in the eagle, duck, and horned owl. The principal somatotopic relations of folium V are to the wings; in experimental mammals lobule V is related to the upper extremity, as already noted. Since lobule V of monotremes corresponds morphologically to the dorsal part of the culmen of birds and other mammals, presumably it also corresponds functionally.

Dillon (1962) included the three divisions that I called lobules III, IV, and V in *Echidna* and *Ornithorhynchus* in his central lobule. The subdivisions situated between the fissura prima, as I defined it, and the fissura secunda (Dillon's fissura prima) collectively were called the culmen by Dillon. Neither fissures or medullary rays, which were both well illustrated in Dillon's figures, nor presumptive somatotopic correlations provide any basis for the disparity between the size of the central lobule and culmen, as interpreted in monotremes by Dillon, and these divisions in the marsupial or rat cerebellum. The relative size of the central lobule and culmen, as interpreted in monotremes, is so much greater than in either birds or other mammals that there appears to be no possible correlation between these lobules and any corresponding differences in the body form, appendages, or sensory equipment of the platypus and anteater, as compared with experimental animals.

Posterior lobe. Both similarities and differences could be noted after comparing the subdivisions of the cortex between the fissura prima and the posterolateral fissure in *Echidna* with the corresponding region in the rat and bird. The subdivision immediately behind the fissura prima resembles folium VI in the four-day-old chick and also in the young adult bantam fowl, except that in the latter it is expanded distally. In the grouse the distal expansion is divided into two subfolia by a shallow furrow. The anterior subfolium of a similar division in the pigeon, duck, eagle, and other species is subdivided so that three superficial subfolia of folium VI are presented (fig. 26). These appear to correspond to folia VIa, VIb, and VIc of the rat, with which they have already been compared (Larsell, 1967). In the small platypus cerebellum illustrated by Hines (fig. 31B) the cortical segment immediately behind the fissura prima is larger than in the anteater and is divided into three superficial folia as in the rat and some of the birds mentioned above. It also shows a fold in the posterior wall of the fissura prima which corresponds to folium VId of the rat. In Hines' figures of the larger platypus cerebellum a large segment in a corresponding position has subdivisions that can be similarly interpreted. G. E. Smith's figure of the platypus cerebellum shows a large subdivision similar in most respects to what I called lobule VI in the small cerebellum of Hines. An elongated segment, similar to lobule VI of *Echidna*, however, is interposed between it and lobule V as labeled (fig. 31A). To determine whether this should be considered as an enlarged and anomalous folium VId, or as a subdivision of lobule V, one would need to compare it with many platypus cerebella. The furrow between this segment and lobule V, as labeled, is shallower than that behind the segment, but the segment has an independent medullary ray. In placental mammals folium VId is quite constant, as a rule, but I found variations ranging from the typical form that only faces the fissura prima to enlarged sublobules that branch from lobule VI at the position of VId and extend to the external cerebellar surface (fig. 192). Bolk's (1906) and Riley's (1929) figures show similar variations in some species of the corresponding fold of the posterior wall of the fissura prima. A large sublobule which could be similarly interpreted is shown in some of Jansen's (1950, 1954) figures of the finwhale cerebellum and in my observations in the porpoise.

Irrespective of the relations of the interposed segment in some specimens of platypus, the large lobule VI of this species as compared with *Echidna* probably is correlated with the rich sensory innervation of the ducklike beak and, perhaps, the larger head of *Ornithorhynchus.* If the body of *Echidna* has the special cutaneous innervation postulated by Abbie (1934) the fibers from the cutaneous endings that reach the cerebellum would be distributed in the anterior lobe, if the pattern in birds and experimental mammals also prevails in monotremes.

Lobule VI, as defined in *Echidna*, is delimited caudally by a fairly deep fissure from a group of folia whose identities are puzzling. In both the small and the large cerebellum of *Ornithorhynchus* a corresponding furrow, which appears to represent the posterior superior fissure, separates lobule VI from an elongated segment which is similar to folium VII in the pigeon and some other birds and to lobule VII of the rat. In many birds folium VII is divided to various extents; in the eagle two completely separated subfolia VIIa and VIIb exist. A shallow groove partially divides lobule VII in some rats. If the segment so labeled in figures 27 and 31 of *Ornithorhynchus* was considered as lobule VII, the fissure which delimits it from lobule VIII (the next segment in the series) corresponds to the prepyramidal fissure. In *Echidna* this furrow is relatively shallow and lobule VII is small.

Lobule VIII of both *Echidna* and *Ornithorhynchus* is more foliated than in birds and the rat and it is relatively larger than in most birds. A lateral continuation of the superficial folium of *Ornithorhynchus* tapers to the narrow connection of the paraflocculus with the principal mass of the cerebellum (fig. 27). In *Echidna* a lateral continuation of lobule VIII reaches a corresponding position but in this species there is no constriction between the principal cerebellar mass and the paraflocculus (fig. 28). The lateral continuation of lobule VIII in both species could be regarded as a rudimentary dorsal paraflocculus.

Since folia VII and VIII of birds and lobules VII and VIII of experimental mammals are both activated by visual as well as auditory impulses, the two lobules in monotremes presumably also are functionally related to the organs of vision and hearing.

Lobule IX, the uvula, is the largest subdivision of the cerebellum in *Echidna*. It is situated between the posterolateral fissure and the fissura secunda. The similarly situated subdivision in Ziehen's figure of *Echidna* also is the largest and is subdivided as in figure 30. In Hines' figure of a sagittal section of *Echidna* a similar large division is delimited by the uvulonodular sulcus and the deepest sulcus. As already noted these correspond, respectively, to the vermal part of the posterolateral fissure and the fissura secunda. The expanded part of the lobule is divided into folia IXa, IXb, and IXc, each being further subdivided, so that the term lamellae would be appropriate in *Echidna*. An elongated pedunclelike connection, as seen in sagittal section, joins the expanded part of the lobule with the deep part of the cerebellum.

Lobule IX of *Ornithorhynchus* is relatively smaller than in *Echidna* but it is similarly subdivided into folia IXa, IXb, and IXc; only IXc, however, is subdivided in the figure of G. E. Smith of the large cerebellum (fig. 31A). An elongated connection with the deep part of the cerebellum, like the similar but relatively shorter connection in the rat, apparently has resulted from adjustments for space.

The subdivisions of the lobule in both species correspond to folia IXa, IXb, and IXc of birds, and to IXa, IXb, and IXc of the rat. Uvular sulcus 1, separating IXb and IXc in both species, was called the fissura secunda or fissure *z* by Hines in *Echidna*, following Ingvar's (1918) terminology in birds and other mammals. Comparison with lobule IX of the platypus makes it evident that the uvula of these authors corresponds to folium IXc.

A posterolateral view of the *Echidna* cerebellum (fig. 29) shows folium IXc continuing laterally with an elongated lobule, faintly subdivided into two folia, which is delimited from the remainder of the paraflocculus by a lateral continuation of uvular sulcus 1. This lobule appears to represent an enlarged version of the avian paraflocculus. I favored the position of regarding it as also corresponding to the accessory paraflocculus of placental mammals.

Cerebellar hemisphere. The lateral continuations of lobules IV–IX of *Echidna* extend ventrolaterally, while those situated posteriorly also turn forward (fig. 28). Together they form a small lateral hemisphere of which, in accord with Abbie, the paraflocculus constitutes the largest part. A band of fibers, the brachium pontis, extends dorsally and posteriorly from the pons, distributing to the underside of the hemisphere. The pons, as described by Abbie, consists of a large nuclear mass covered by a thin capsule of fibers. The pontine decussation occurs in the anterior part of the pons but is inconspicuous. Comparing the lateral hemisphere of the anteater with that of the chicken, as defined by Brodal, Kristiansen, and Jansen (1950), one found that the *Echidna* hemisphere is much larger owing to the much greater volume of the ventral paraflocculus. The principal distribution of pontine fibers in the chicken is to folia VI, VII, and VIII, with the unfoliated cortex probably being included. The paraflocculus receives a large number of fibers, chiefly from the ipsilateral lateral pontine nucleus. Pontine fibers also reach the anterior lobe and the medial parts of the folia of the posterior lobe. It was thought that the lateral extremities of subfolia Va and Vb are probably richer in pontine fibers than the medial parts. Some fibers also appear to reach the lateral part of folium IV, as indicated in a diagram. According to Whitlock (1952) destruction of the cortex of the rostral folia of the posterior lobe in the pigeon was followed by chromatolysis of cells in the pontine nuclei, ipsilaterally and contralaterally.

Assuming that the pontine fiber distribution is similar in *Echidna*, but more abundant as indicated by the larger pons and brachium pontis, one could make some interesting comparisons. The accessory paraflocculus, mentioned above, which is probably homologous with the avian paraflocculus, would have pontine connections. The large size of the ventral paraflocculus of *Echidna* (fig. 28), representing the lateral continuation of lamellae IXa and IXb in expanded form, also suggests a greatly increased number of fibers from the pons. Since lobule IX and its lateral continuations are situated behind the fissura secunda, as defined above, pontine fibers probably reach the equivalent part of the posterior lobe of G. E. Smith in marsupials and placental mammals. Presumably they reach the lateral parts of lobules VIII, VII, and VI, corresponding to G. E. Smith's medial lobe of these mammalian groups. They probably also reach the lateral parts of lobules V and IV belonging to the anterior lobe. The lateral extension of lobules IV and V into the hemisphere is suggestive of the hemispheral parts of these lobules in the rat, but in *Echidna* the intraculminate fissure extends to the cerebellar margin (fig. 28A).

Without experimental studies in *Echidna* this suggested distribution of pontine fibers is hypothetical. It is based, however, on the experimental studies of birds by Brodal, Kristiansen, and Jansen (1950) and Whitlock (1952), and in part on my own observations in normal cell and fiber preparations of penguins, in which the brachium pontis is relatively large.

In *Ornithorhynchus*, according to Hines (1929), the cerebellar folia continue lateralward until they merge into a small band which this author called the pons, but which undoubtedly is the brachium pontis. G. E. Smith's (1899) figure of a ventral view of the platypus brain shows a similar band from the cerebellum, which expands ventromedially into a pons. According to Hines there is no lateral hemisphere in the platypus; the lateral parts of the folia, however, probably correspond to the small hemisphere of birds. A lateral projection, continuous with folia behind the fissura secunda, was called the paraflocculus by Hines. It is similar in some respects to the avian paraflocculus, but whether it includes a homolog of the accessory paraflocculus of *Echidna* and also folia that correspond, in part, to the ventral paraflocculus of the anteater could not be determined from available descriptions or illustrations.

CEREBELLAR NUCLEI

Echidna aculeata has two cerebellar nuclei, a medial and a lateral one, on either side of the midline. The medial nucleus, according to Abbie (1934) is by far the smaller of the two. In Hines' (1929) description of the medial and and lateral cerebellar nuclei in *Ornithorhynchus*, she stated that the lateral nucleus is divided by a notch into the anterior and posterior parts. The medial nucleus was described as a solid ellipsoid which extends farther caudalward than the lateral nucleus. Abbie did not mention the division of the lateral nucleus in *Echidna*, and I failed to note any. The bilateral medial nuclei of the platypus, according to Hines, are interconnected by a commissure.

The medial nucleus of both species appears to correspond to the medial nucleus of reptiles and to the fastigial nucleus of higher mammals. The lateral nucleus corresponds to the nucleus lateralis of reptiles plus a rudiment of the nucleus lateralis (dentatus) of higher mammals. The notch mentioned by Hines probably indicates the zone of transition from the homolog of the reptilian nucleus lateralis to the portion that corresponds to the mammalian nucleus lateralis (dentatus). The latter, in higher primates, becomes the dentate nucleus. The homolog of the reptilian nucleus lateralis probably corresponds to the nucleus interpositus of placental mammals.

According to both Hines and Abbie, the lateral nucleus gives origin to an efferent system of fibers, the brachium conjunctivum, which Hines followed to the midbrain and its tegmentum and to the thalamus in *Ornithorhynchus*. My observations in *Echidna* indicated that brachium conjunctivum fibers originate from all parts of the nucleus. Fibers from the medial nucleus appear to radiate ventroanteriorly and ventroposteriorly.

Cells of various sizes were recognizable in both the medial and lateral nuclei of *Echidna*, but with intergradations and little evidence of grouping. Hines was unable to differentiate a large-celled and a small-celled division of the medial nucleus in *Ornithorhynchus*.

FIBER TRACTS

Primary vestibular fibers in *Ornithorhynchus*, according to Hines (1929), pass to the nodulus, uvula, flocculus, and lingula, with some also reaching the medial nucleus. Secondary fibers from the vestibular nuclei also reach the cerebellum and its medial nucleus. Hines regarded these as arising from the nucleus of Bechterew and the nucleus of Deiters. In view of the origin of such fibers in the medial and inferior vestibular nuclei of the opossum (Voris and Hoerr, 1932) and the cat (Brodal and Torvik, 1957), it is probable that in monotremes the secondary fibers have a similar source and only traverse the lateral and superior vestibular nuclei.

The trigeminal nerve is greatly hypertrophied in monotremes, and even more so in *Ornithorhynchus* than in *Echidna*, according to Abbie. The root fibers form descending and ascending tracts in the medulla oblongata. The ascending tract terminates chiefly in the sensory nucleus of the trigeminus, but a large number of fibers, as seen in protargol series of *Echidna*, continue into the cerebellum, with some accompanying the ventral spinocerebellar tract through the anterior medullary velum. Abbie described the trigeminal nerve as sending fibers to the cerebellum "by every conceivable pathway," including the anterior medullary velum. As seen in protargol preparations many of the fibers entering anteriorly pass into a commissural mass in the anterior ventral part of the cerebellum. Others continue farther dorsalward but are lost in the confusion of fibers. The sensory trigeminal nucleus gives rise to secondary fibers, many of which also take a dorsal course but then disappear. The chief sensory trigeminal nucleus is divided into lateral and medial parts in the platypus (Hines) and *Echidna* (Abbie). According to Hines the connections of the lateral division with the cerebellum are very greatly developed.

Experimental methods were not used to examine the distribution of trigeminocerebellar fibers in either species, but on the basis of somatotopic distribution of trigeminal fibers in birds and placental mammals distribution would be to lobule VI. The relatively large size of this lobule in the platypus thus appears to be correlated with the unusually abundant exteroceptive innervation of the beak.

Spinocerebellar connections are but sketchily mentioned in monotremes and I can add little. Hines spoke of spinocerebellar fibers in the lateral funiculus of the cord in the platypus but added that the localization of entrance of the "ventro-spino-cerebellar systems" was not ascertained. In *Echidna* a fascicle that appears to correspond to the anterior part of the ventral spinocerebellar tract of crocodilians enters the cerebellum through the anterior medullary velum. The fibers could be followed only a short distance within the cerebellum; some of them appear to enter the anterior ventral commissural mass. Hines included fibers from the lateral funiculus of the cord in the restiform body. These possibly represent a dorsal spinocerebellar tract or they may be part of the ventral tract, as in crocodilians.

Olivocerebellar fibers are included in the restiform body by both Hines and Abbie, as are fibers from the gracile and cuneate nuclei; Abbie added others, including probable fibers from the lateral reticular nucleus. Since cerebellar fibers from the region of the dorsal nuclei in experimental mammals have been shown by experimental methods to have originated in the external cuneate nucleus, it would not be surprising if some similar differentiation, probably incipient, of the nuclear origin of such fibers exists in monotremes. The gracile and cuneate nuclei of experimental mammals give rise to the medial lemniscus, without any fibers passing to the cerebellum.

A tectocerebellar system was described by Hines, in the platypus, as comprising rostral and caudal divisions from the superior colliculus and a ventral division from the region of the mesencephalic trigeminal nucleus. Abbie described the tectocerebellar tract in *Echidna* as originating from both the superior and the inferior colliculi. The ventral division of Hines probably corresponds to mesencephalic trigeminal fibers that enter the cerebellum through the anterior medullary velum in other species, including man (Pearson, 1949b).

HISTOLOGY

Histologically the cerebellar cortex of monotremes appears to be typically mammalian. The molecular and granular layers are separated by Purkinje cells arranged as a single layer. Our protargol preparations of *Echidna* were unsatisfactory for details of finer structure but Hines, in *Ornithorhynchus*, described climbing fibers on the Purkinje cells and axons of basket cells around the cell bodies. Many fibers seem to end about the "ghosts" of cells in the granular layer. With our technique no collaterals of Purkinje cell axons were observed, but others found some in submammals.

MARSUPIALIA

The marsupial cerebellum has been described in various species by a number of authors using a variety of terminologies. Ziehen (1897) used descriptive terms. In the same way that G. E. Smith divided the cerebellum of other mammals, he (1903a, 1903b) divided the marsupial cerebellum into lobus anticus, lobus medius, lobus posticus, and lobus flocculi. Bradley (1904) divided the cerebellum of *Didelphis azarae* into five transverse lobules that correspond to his divisions in other mammals. Ingvar (1918) divided the cerebellum of the kangaroo into anterior, medial, and posterior lobes, but his dorsal boundary of the posterior lobe differs from the fissura secunda of G. E. Smith, with the posterior and medial lobes of the two authors differing accordingly. Ingvar recognized that the flocculus is continuous with the nodulus and regarded the paraflocculus as a lateral projection of the uvula. The subdivisions of the principal lobules were named according to the terminology of Bolk (1906), with modifications in some instances. Obenchain (1925) employed the terminology of G. E. Smith in describing the cerebellum of the marsupial shrew, *Caenolestes obscurus*, as did Voris and Hoerr (1932), for the most part, in the opossum, *Didelphis virginiana*. A slightly modified version of the nomenclature of Bolk was applied by Riley (1929) to the cerebellum of the kangaroo, *Macropus*, and the Tasmanian wolf, *Thylacinus*. The cerebellum is divided into anterior and posterior lobes by the fissura prima and the lobules of the vermis are based on the primary medullary rays. My own studies on the developing and adult cerebellum of the opossum led to the division of the organ into the flocculonodular lobe and the corpus cerebelli. The latter is divided into anterior and posterior lobes, corresponding to those of Riley except that the posterior lobe excluded the nodulus, which is part of the flocculonodular lobe.

In marsupials, as in other mammals, the cerebellum varies in complexity with the body size of the species. The cerebellum is large and shows considerable foliation in the larger species of the kangaroos; it is less complex in the opossum and in the smaller marsupials only three to five fissures and their intervening cortical folds were found. The simplest cerebellum of any adult mammal, according to G. E. Smith (1903b), is that of the marsupial mole, *Notoryctes typhlops.* Although this species is larger in body size than the soricine shrews and other small Insectivora and small Chiroptera, it has a cerebellum which is less folded than that of the smallest shrews and bats. Phylogenic factors probably are involved but the adaptations of *Notoryctes* for its special mode of life also must be taken into consideration. We shall return to the marsupial mole after describing the cerebellum in less specialized marsupials.

The cerebellum of the opossum has been described most fully, with respect to both development and adult structure. Also its fiber tract connections are best known of the marsupials. Therefore my earlier observations on development will be reviewed first, and then supplemented by a study of additional pouch-stage young opossums. Following this, the adult cerebellum will be more completely described. The cerebellum of some other species, both smaller and larger than *D. virginiana*, will then be described from the literature and from my own observations of the organ in the kangaroo.

OPOSSUM

Development

Late in the tenth day of intrauterine development of the opossum (*Didelphis virginiana*) embryo (stage 29 of McCrady, 1935), the roof of the rostral part of the rhombencephalon is thin and shows no indication of the metencephalon. Ascending fibers of the trigeminal root, however, extend toward the future cerebellar region, as

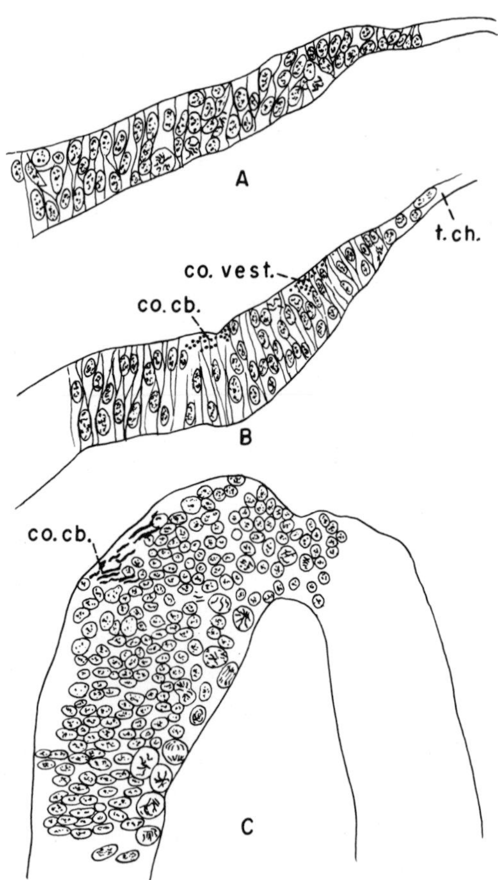

Figure 32. A. Midsagittal section through the cerebellar region of the neural tube in opossum embryo of McCrady's stage 30, early eleventh day. B. Midsagittal section of cerebellar anlage in a more developed opossum embryo of McCrady's stage 30. C. Transverse section of cerebellar anlage in opossum embryo of McCrady's stage 30. ×144. (Larsell, 1935.)

do similar fibers of the acoustic nerve root. These ascending fibers are visible beneath the external limiting membrane of the rostral part of the rhombencephalon, but none reach its roof at this stage. The number of mitotic figures in the future cerebellar region is about the same as in neighboring parts of the neural tube.

At McCrady's stage 30 (early eleventh day) sagittal sections show only a plate, in the cerebellar region, which is continuous with the midbrain rostrally and with the choroid tela of the rhomboidal fossa caudally (fig. 32). Numerous mitotic figures indicate rapid proliferation of cells. In a more advanced embryo, also assigned to stage 30, the plate has thickened into the rudiment of the metencephalon and a slight dip rostrally indicates the inception of the constriction between this and the midbrain. A small fascicle of trigeminal root fibers and one of vestibular root fibers now cross the midline, the former at the anterior border of the metencephalic plate and the latter farther posteriorly (fig. 32B). These represent the commissura cerebelli and the commissura vestibularis respectively, with the commissura cerebelli later becoming augmented by spinocerebellar fibers. A transverse series of a stage 30 embryo shows thickening of the dorsal part of the lateral wall of the neural tube in the metencephalic region, with numerous mitotic figures in the neuroepithelial layer and immediately above it (fig. 32C). The proliferated cells migrate into the mantle layer of His or the migration layer of Bergqvist and Källén (1953). Thus a paired rudiment of the cerebellum is formed. The cerebellar rudiment represents the rostralmost part of the columna dorsalis of these authors, which is situated within the dorsal part of the first rhombomere (Bergqvist and Källén, 1954). The posterior margin of the cerebellum of the opossum, as it becomes cellular, evidently is formed by expansion of the columna dorsalis. This margin is continuous ventrolaterally with the margin of the rhombic lip. The vestibular commissure takes its course parallel with the cerebellar margin and the later development and fiber connections of the marginal zone indicate vestibular relationships. Vraa-Jensen (1956) regarded the vestibular nuclei, except for Deiters' nucleus, as being derived from the columna dorsalis in the chick. Hugosson (1957), however, considered the vestibular nuclei of the mouse, chick, and other embryos that he studied as being derived from the dorsolateral column. According to Hugosson this column is formed by division of the earlier intermediate column into ventrolateral and dorsolateral columns. The margin of the rhombic lip, with which the posterior margin of the cerebellum is continuous, is included in the columna dorsalis.

At stage 30 of the opossum embryo, cell proliferation in the roof of the metencephalon has resulted in thickening of this region anteriorly (fig. 32C), and in the initiation of fusion of the bilateral rudiments of the cerebellum across the midline. The fusion continues and soon the cerebellum becomes a massive arch above the fourth ventricle. In embryonic and early pouch stages of young opossum the thicker bilateral halves of the organ are partly separated by a median sagittal ventricular groove corresponding to that in the frog.

At stage 31 (late eleventh day) the lower lateral wall of the zone of continuity of the upward arching cerebellum with the medulla oblongata has begun to bulge outward and a lateral pocket of the ventricle represents the incipient recessus lateralis (fig. 33). The fascicles of trigeminal and vestibular fibers that decussate in the roof of the cerebellum can be followed in successive sections to the respective commissures. At stage 33 (late twelfth day) the ventricular surface of the cerebellar region shows the recessus lateralis in a position lateral to the level where the cerebellum begins to arch dorsalward and medially from the alar lamina of the floor of the ventricle (fig. 34). The anterior and dorsal walls of the recess thicken but the lateral wall becomes reduced to a membrane which is continuous with the choroid tela of the fourth ventricle.

A slight groove has appeared on the anterolateral cerebellar surface at stage 32 (early twelfth day). It extends from beneath the lateral bulge of the lower cerebellar wall upward and medially, parallel with the cerebellar margin and the vestibular fascicle, but disappears dorsomedially. This groove is the incipient lateral segment of the posterolateral fissure. It marks the beginning of differentiation of the cerebellum into the corpus cerebelli and the flocculonodular lobe but only the margin which becomes the flocculus and its peduncles represents this lobe – the nodulus differentiates later. The thickened bilateral cell masses, already described, become the corpus cerebelli; the flocculus and remainder of the flocculonodular lobe are formed from cells that proliferate in the marginal zone.

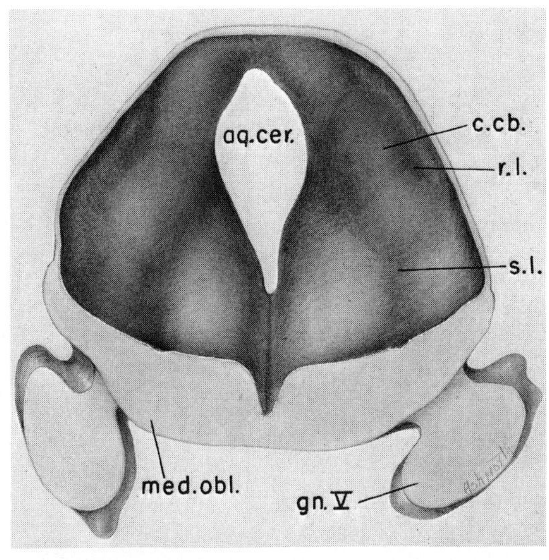

Figure 34. Drawing made from a graphic reconstruction of the cerebellar region of opossum embryo of McCrady's stage 33, late twelfth day, as seen from caudal aspect. ×40. (Larsell, 1935.)

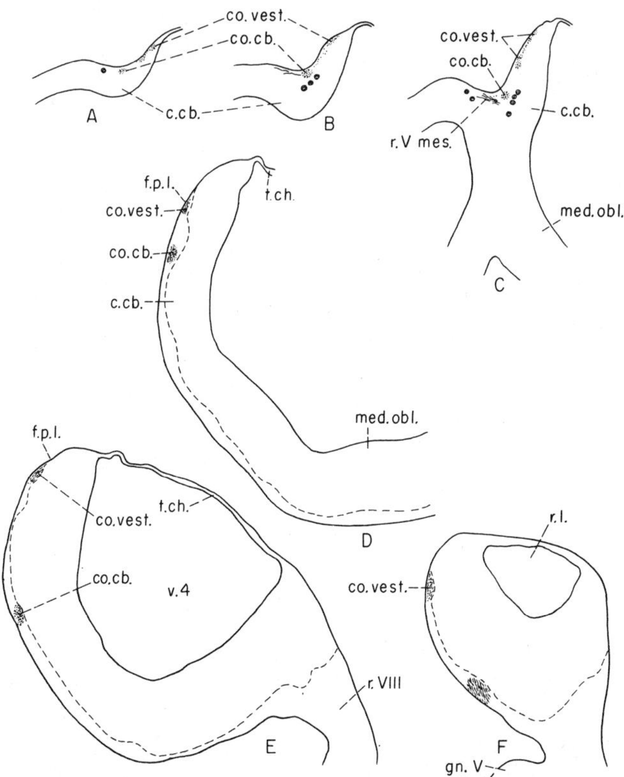

Figure 33. Outlines of sagittal sections through cerebellar region of opossum embryo of McCrady's stage 31, late eleventh day. A. Midsagittal section. B–E. Sections at successively more lateral levels of corpus cerebelli. F. Section through part of the flocculonodular lobe. ×65. (Larsell, 1935.)

At stage 31 (early eleventh day) a few large cells have appeared in the anterior part of the cerebellar base and in the adjacent part of the midbrain. At stage 34 (early thirteenth day) such cells are quite numerous; they are rounded or pear-shaped and have a large, vesicular nucleus. In the midbrain these cells evidently represent the mesencephalic V nucleus, among which fibers of the mesencephalic V root occur. Those in the cerebellum I regarded (Larsell, 1935) as a stage in the differentiation of Purkinje cells. The subsequent studies of Tello (1940) in the mouse embryo and of Baffoni (1954) in the cat embryo have shown that Purkinje cells have a very different origin. The large cells found in the cerebellum of the opossum embryos, of pouch-stage opossum, and of adult opossum, along the mesencephalic V root to its emergence from the medulla oblongata, must be considered mesencephalic V cells such as those found by Pearson (1949a, 1949b) in human and other mammalian embryos.

In stage 33 a fascicle of spinocerebellar fibers reaches the cerebellum (fig. 35) but does not appear to cross the midline. At stage 34 (early thirteenth day) spinocerebellar fibers decussate, augmenting the trigeminal fascicle of the commissura cerebelli (figs. 36, 37). Pyridine-silver series of the pouch stage of young opossums show secondary trigeminal fibers, arising from cells dorsomedial of the principal part of the chief sensory V nucleus, that also pass to the cerebellar commissure. The trigeminal root fibers of embryonic stages presumably remain but cannot be differentiated from other intermingled fibers. Presumably both trigeminal and spinal fibers

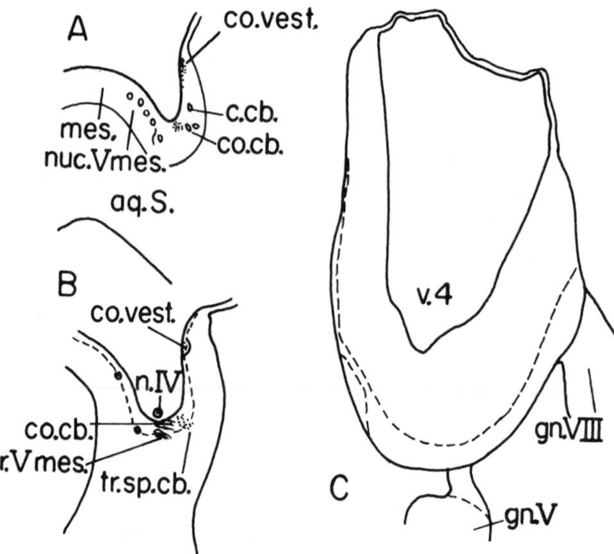

Figure 35. Outlines of sagittal sections through the cerebellar region of opossum embryo of McCrady's stage 33, late twelfth day. A. Midsagittal section. B–C. Sections through corpus cerebelli. ×65. (Larsell, 1935.)

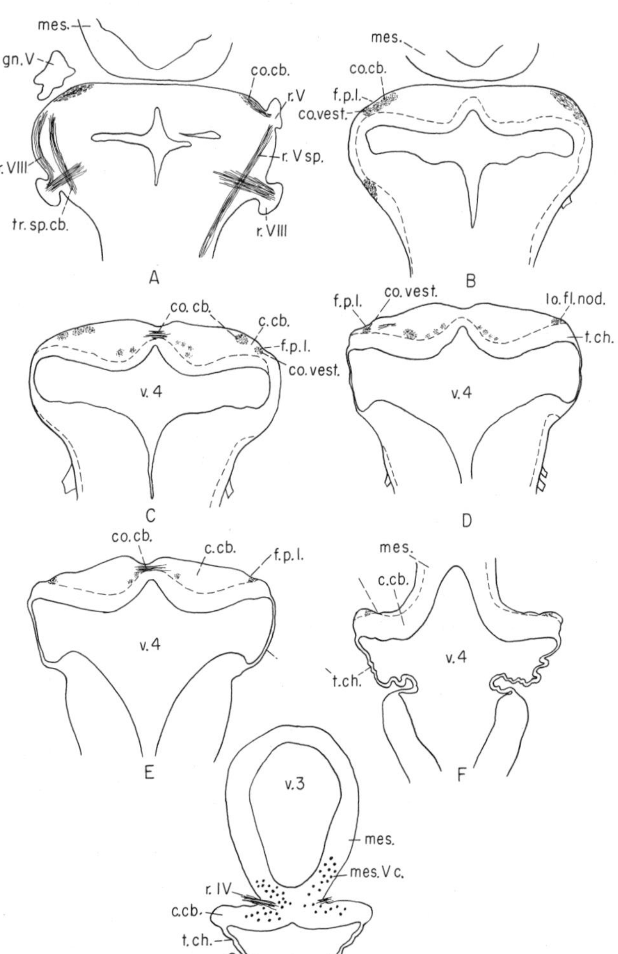

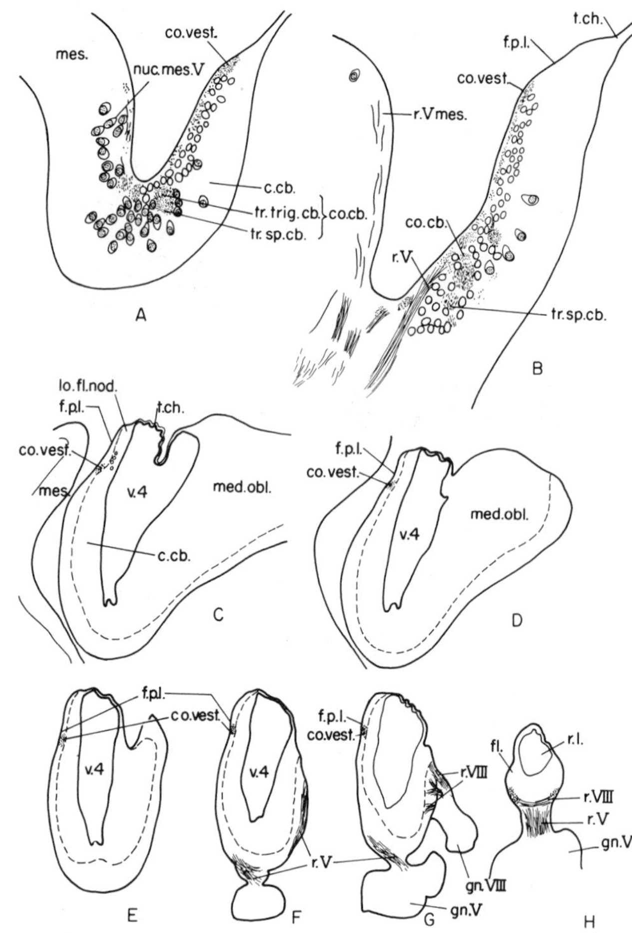

Figure 36. Outlines of sagittal sections through cerebellar region of opossum embryo of McCrady's stage 34, early thirteenth day. A. Paramedian section. B–E. Sections at successively more lateral levels of corpus cerebelli. F–H. Sections through floccular region. A, B ×86. C–H ×24. (Larsell, 1935.)

terminate ipsilaterally as well as contralaterally in the corpus cerebelli.

With continued growth of the cerebellum the recessus lateralis becomes more prominent and its dorsal wall thickens as the rudiment of the flocculus (figs. 38, 39). This is continuous ventroposteriorly beneath the lateral recess with a caudally tapering part of the rhombic lip, whose ventral border flares out slightly, and with the roots of the VIII nerve entering the medulla oblongata immediately beneath this border in early pouch stages of opossum. It is difficult to relate this feature of the devel-

Figure 37. Outlines of horizontal sections through cerebellar region of opossum embryo of McCrady's stage 34, early thirteenth day. A. Sections through level of V and VIII roots. B–F. Sections at successively more dorsal levels. G. Section through level of IV root. ×24. (Larsell, 1935.)

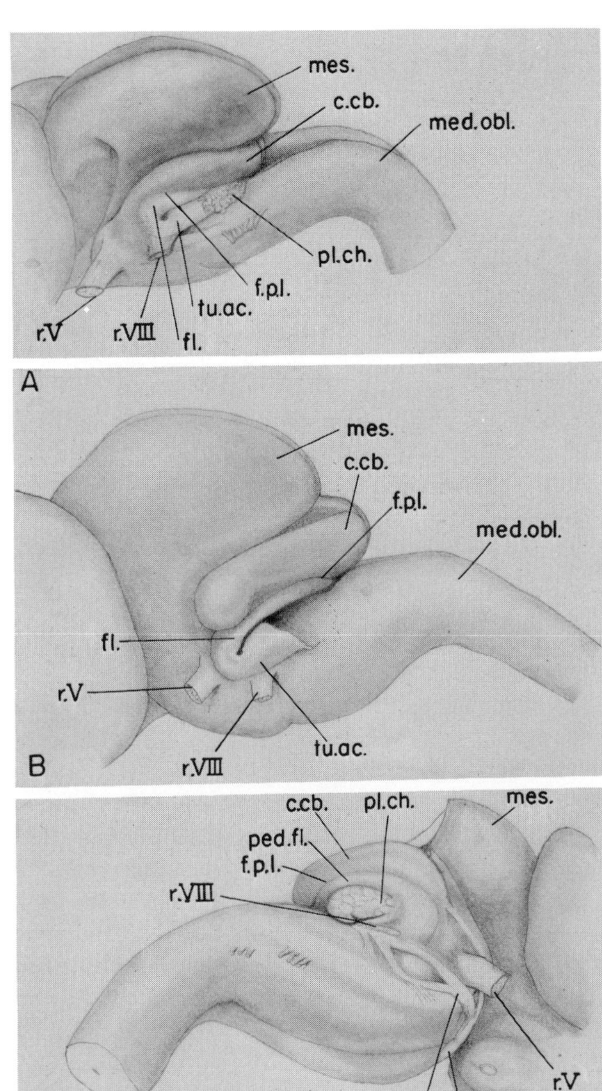

Figure 38. Cerebellum and adjacent parts of pouch-stage opossum. A. Lateral view of 18-mm C.R. length, 8 days after birth. B. Lateral view of 27.75-mm C.R. length, 18 days after birth. C. Ventrolateral view of 22-mm C.R. length, 13 days after birth. ca. ×13. (Larsell, 1935.)

oping rhombic lip to structures of this region in the adult opossum. In part, at least, it appears to correspond to the corpus pontobulbare of Voris and Hoerr (1932).

The rudiment of the flocculus increases in size and the posterolateral margin of the cerebellum, which is continuous with it, also thickens. The lateral segment of the posterolateral fissure deepens but has not reached the midline in day 8 of the pouch-stage opossum (fig. 40). In day 19 of the pouch-stage opossum, the fissure crosses the midline and is continuous from one side of the cerebellum to the other (fig. 41). The medial segment of the fissure appears with the differentiation and growth of the nodulus. G. E. Smith (1903c) illustrated the confluence of the "postnodular and floccular fissures" in a pouch-stage specimen of *Dasyurus,* which forms a continuous fissure corresponding to the posterolateral of the terminology here employed. G. E. Smith recognized that the

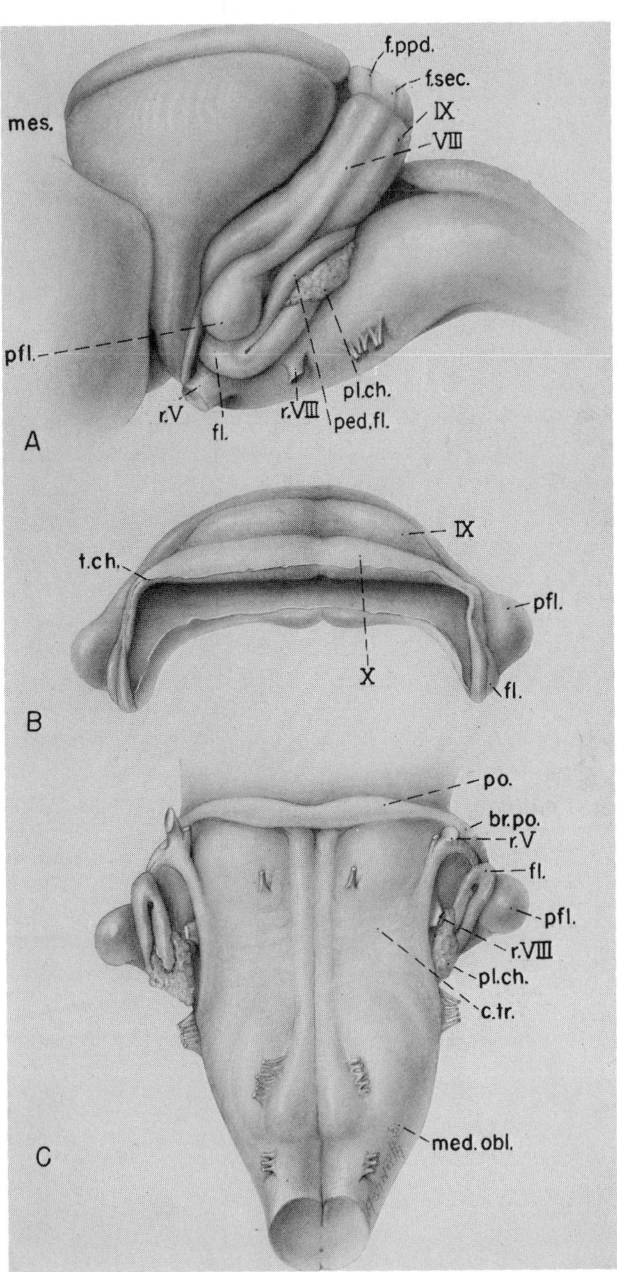

Figure 39. Cerebellum and adjacent parts of pouch-stage opossum of 36-mm C.R. length, 26 days after birth. A. Dorsolateral view. ca. ×13. B. Ventral view of cerebellum. ca. ×9.5. C. Ventral view of medulla oblongata, pons, flocculus, and paraflocculus. ca. ×9.5. (Larsell, 1935.)

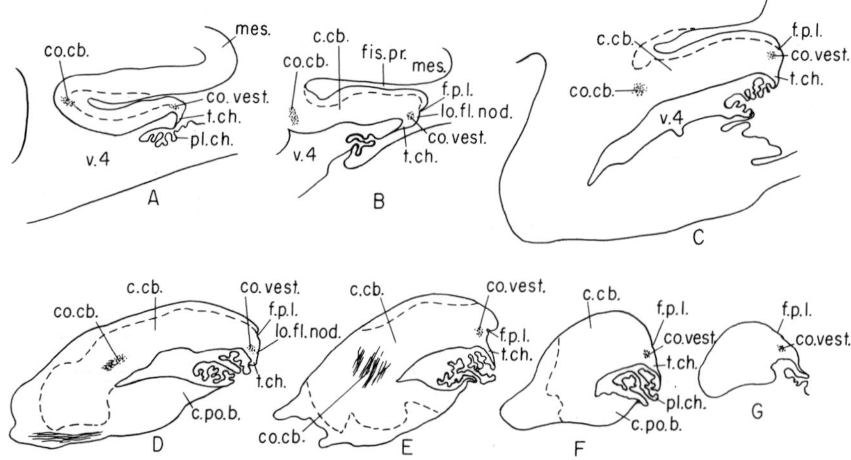

Figure 40. Outlines of sagittal sections through cerebellum of pouch-stage opossum of 18-mm C.R. length, 8 days after birth. A. Midsagittal section. B–G. Successively more lateral sections. ×24. (Larsell, 1935.)

postnodularis is the most precocious, although the shallowest, of the three early vermal fissures and that it divides the region behind the fissura secunda into uvula and nodulus. He grouped the two lobules together as his lobulus posticus. The nodulus develops as a thickening of the rhombic lip on either side of the midline (fig. 39B); the bilateral rudiments presently fuse and eventually expand, forming an unpaired vermal lobule. On day 26 of pouch-stage opossums a slight constriction still remains in the median sagittal plane, which still indicates incomplete fusion. The two flocculi, the thickened margin of the cerebellum between them, and the nodulus constitute the fully differentiated flocculonodular lobe (fig. 39B). The choroid tela is attached to the ventral borders of these units as, at earlier developmental stages, it was attached to the posterior and posterolateral margins of the cerebellum.

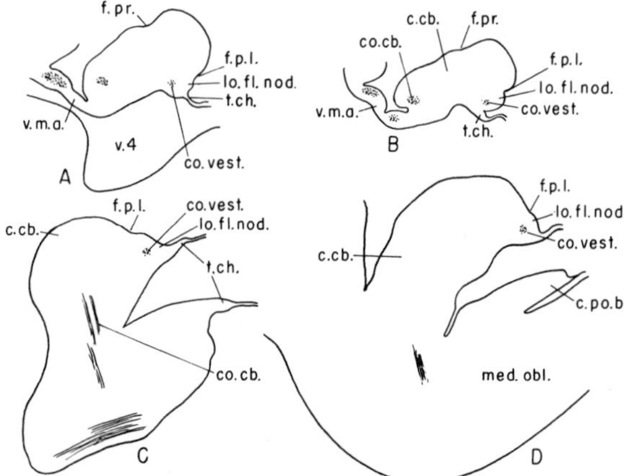

Figure 41. Outlines of sagittal sections through cerebellum of a pouch-stage opossum of 28.5-mm C.R. length, 19 days after birth. A–D ×24. (Larsell, 1935.)

The corpus cerebelli, in the meantime, has increased in volume. By day 8 of the pouch stage, it has elongated anteroposteriorly and by day 19 it has thickened and begun to fold (figs. 40, 41). A transverse furrow, the fissura prima, divides the median (vermal) part into anterior and posterior lobes, but it does not yet extend to the lateral part of the corpus cerebelli. A slight notch in the dorsal surface of the cerebellum in day 8 of the pouch stage may represent an earlier appearance of this fissure, but this is uncertain. Rapid growth of the anterior and posterior lobes deepens the fissura prima and the two lobes differentiate into subdivisions delimited by shallower fissures.

The anterior lobe divides into dorsal, or culminate and ventral segments separated by the preculminate fissure. This stage of differentiation is described in a pouch stage of *Dasyurus viverrinus* by G. E. Smith (1903c), but the opossum material available to me did not include this particular phase of cerebellar development. The dorsal or culminate segment elongates but does not foliate until a considerably later stage. The ventral segment has two divisions in day 27 of the pouch stage. The more dorsal of these, immediately beneath the preculminate fissure, becomes lobule III, the central lobule. The larger ventral division, delimited from lobule III by the precentral fissure in the marsupial pouch stage, was called the lingula by G. E. Smith, while no mention of subdivision was made. In day 42 of the pouch stage of opossum this division is differentiated into lobules I and II and separated by a well-defined precentral fissure *a*. Lobules II and III both are subfoliated and the culminate segment shows early folia that in the adult can be assigned to lobules IV and V (fig. 42).

The culminate segment in day 42 of the pouch stage of opossum shows a large anterior ventral fold, facing the preculminate fissure, and three smaller folds, one facing anteriorly on the cerebellar surface with the other two facing the fissura prima. The large anterior ventral fold subfoliates in subsequent growth and becomes lobule IV; the remainder of the culminate segment undergoes further folding and constitutes lobule V, as more clearly shown in the adult cerebellum.

Differentiation of the posterior lobe begins with lobule IX, the uvula, and progresses dorsalward and anteriorly (fig. 42). Sagittal sections of the cerebellum from day 27 and day 31 of pouch stages show lobule IX delimited dorsally by the fissura secunda, while a shallower furrow delimits a low lobule VIII, the pyramis. The fissura secunda appears earlier than the prepyramidalis, but stages

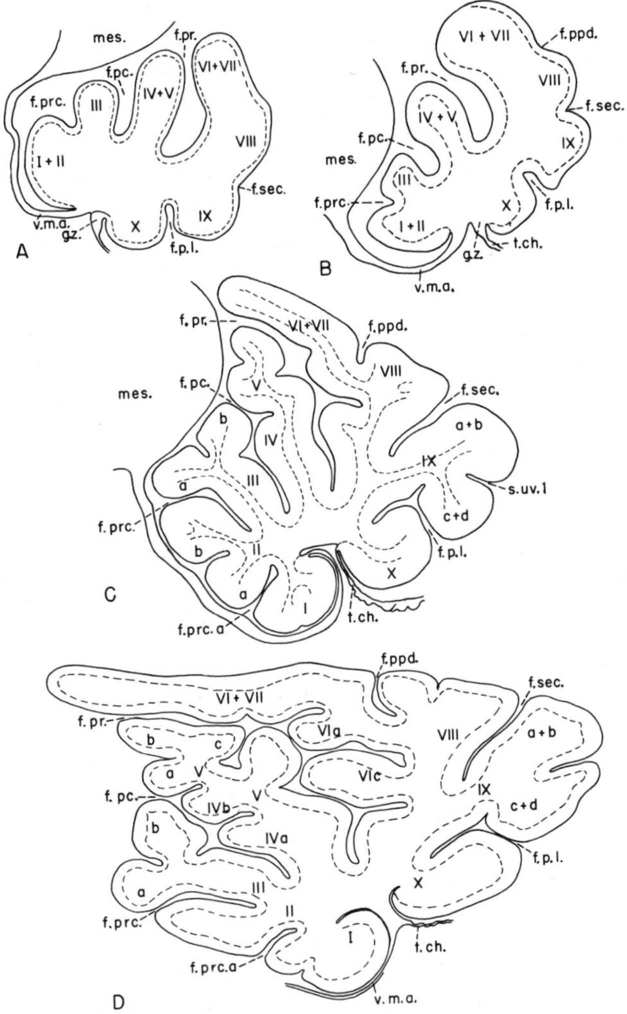

Figure 42. Midsagittal sections through cerebellum of pouch-stage opossum. A. 27 days after birth. B. 31 days after birth. C. 42 days after birth. D. 48 days after birth.

that would determine its sequence with reference to the preculminate fissure are lacking; there are indications that the eventually deep preculminate fissure is the earlier of the two, as G. E. Smith found in *Dasyurus* and some other marsupials in the pouch stage. The anteriorly elongated part of the posterior lobe (lobulus impendens of Ziehen) remains unfoliated as late as day 48 of the pouch stage. We shall return to this part of the corpus cerebelli in the adult cerebellum, in which it is relatively still more elongated and also shows four or five shallow furrows.

The corpus cerebelli extends lateralward on either side, forming rudimentary cerebellar hemispheres. In day 8 of the pouch stage these lie beneath the caudally projecting posterior part of the midbrain (fig. 38A). They have expanded considerably by day 13 of the pouch stage and the posterolateral surface of each shows a shallow furrow, the incipient parafloccular fissure. This fissure is prominent in day 26 of the pouch stage and delimits a rounded paraflocculus from the more medial part of the hemisphere. At this stage it appears to be directly continuous with the prepyramidal fissure (fig. 39A).

Adult Cerebellum

The flocculonodular lobe of the adult opossum is well defined and the posterolateral fissure is prominent although shallower than many of the fissures in the corpus cerebelli (figs. 43, 44, 45). The continuation of the fissure on either side of the nodulus, where it divides the pedunclelike connections of the nodulus with the flocculi, is the shallowest part; between the flocculus and the corpus cerebelli the fissure deepens, completely separating the greater part of the floccular expansion from the corpus cerebelli. The fissura prima in the opossum is unusually deep in comparison with that in most other mammals; this is a result of the forward elongation of the posterior lobe as the lobulus impendens of Ziehen.

The ventral and dorsal segments of the anterior lobe were recognizable in more expanded form rather than during the pouch stage. Lobule I, in the ventral segment, is relatively large and is divided from lobule II by a relatively deep precentral fissure *a* (figs. 44, 45). Lobule II is divided into two folia, IIa and IIb. The two lobules correspond to the lingula of Voris and Hoerr (1932). Presumably they are functionally related to the tail, with the prominence of lobule I probably being correlated with the prehensile capacity of this organ in the opossum, which also appears to be true in the spider monkey, *Ateles*. Lobule III of the opossum is large and subdivided. The culminate segment is greatly expanded, compared with the late pouch stages, and has five folia and the beginning of a sixth. The furrow labeled intraculmi-

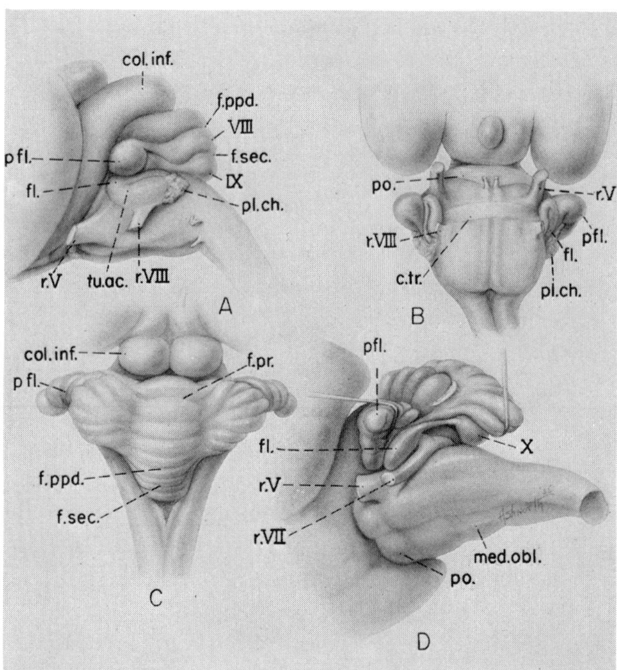

Figure 43. A. Lateral view of cerebellum and adjacent parts of pouch-stage opossum of 42-mm C.R. length, 30 days after birth. ×5. B. Ventral view of medulla oblongata, pons, flocculus, and paraflocculus of the same specimen as A. C. Dorsal view of cerebellum and adjacent parts of adult opossum. ×2. D. Ventrolateral view of cerebellum and adjacent parts of adult opossum. The caudal folia of the left cerebellar hemisphere have been dissected away to expose the parafloccular peduncle to the pyramis and the uvula, and the paraflocculus has been pulled forward to expose the flocculus and its connection with the nodulus. The nodulus has been exposed by separating the cerebellum and the bulb. ×2. (Larsell, 1936a.)

nate fissure 1 in figure 45 is more prominent in some other specimens. It appears to correspond to the fissure so named in the rat and other species, and is interpreted as dividing the culminate segment into lobules IV and V. Folium Ve corresponds in relative position and size to the folium so named in other species. Comparing the anterior lobe of the large specimen of *Didelphis virginiana* with that of *Didelphis azarae* (fig. 45B) as described and illustrated by Bradley (1904), one notes that Bradley's lobule A_1, which corresponds to lobule I, is relatively larger and more elongated rostralward, with a consequent deepening of the precentral fissure *a* (Bradley's fissure *c*). His lobule A_2, corresponding to lobules II and III, evidently is based on the elongated medullary ray, which divides at some distance from the larger mass of the medullary body. Apparently this is owing to the rostrally more elongated ventral part of the anterior lobe in Bradley's specimen, as compared with *virginiana*. The culminate segment (lobule B of Bradley) has two large subdivisions that correspond to lobules IV and V, but are separated by a more prominent and relatively deeper furrow which corresponds to intraculminate fissure 1. A large folium, facing the fissura prima, in *D. azarae*, apparently corresponds to folium Ve of my specimens. Fissure I of Bradley corresponds to the preculminate fissure.

The rostral surface of the anterior lobe of *D. virginiana* (fig. 44) shows lobule I projecting into the fourth ventricle, but it is limited to the median part of the cerebellum. Lobule II tapers lateralward on either side of the midline to a narrow strip of cortex into which lobule III also tapers. Lobules IV and V turn ventrolaterally but merge at the ends of the intraculminate fissure, forming a ventral continuation which can be assigned to the cerebellar hemisphere as lobule HIV + V. In Bradley's figure of the anterior surface of the cerebellum of *D. azarae* only lobules III, IV, and V are visible. The intraculminate fissure extends to the preculminate fissure and completely separates lobules IV and V, each of which is partly subdivided by a shallow furrow. This cerebellum evidently was more massive than that of *D. virginiana*.

As in their developmental stages the lobules of the posterior lobe will be described by beginning with lobule IX. In adult *D. virginiana* this lobule was divided into two folds by a relatively deep uvular sulcus 1. Both folds have shallow furrows indicating the beginning of subfoliation into IXa and IXb and IXc and IXd, respectively (fig. 45). In comparison with many other species the lobule is relatively small, but the fissura secunda is unmistakable when followed through the pouch stages of opossum to the adult. As illustrated by Voris and Hoerr the uvula has three subdivisions while in Bradley's figure of *D. azarae* only two are shown in the lobule ventral of his fissure *d*, which corresponds to the fissura secunda in other species. The lobule between the fissura secunda and Bradley's fissure III which, in most species described by this author corresponds to the prepyramidal fissure, is a caudally elongated but dorsoventrally narrow fold having little resemblance to lobule VIII, the pyramis, of my specimens or to this lobule as illustrated by Voris and Hoerr.

Lobule VIII, the pyramis, of *D. virginiana* (figs. 44B, C, 45A) comprises two folds of cortex separated by a relatively deep furrow, and is present by day 42 of the pouch stage as a shallow groove. The prepyramidal fissure of this pouch stage is represented in the adult by a wide but shallower furrow which corresponds to the suprapyramidal fissure of Voris and Hoerr. The pyramis of the opossum accordingly is composed of two cortical folds, with the furrow between them representing the intrapyramidal fissure. In *D. azarae*, fissure *a* of Bradley in the median sagittal section appears to correspond to the

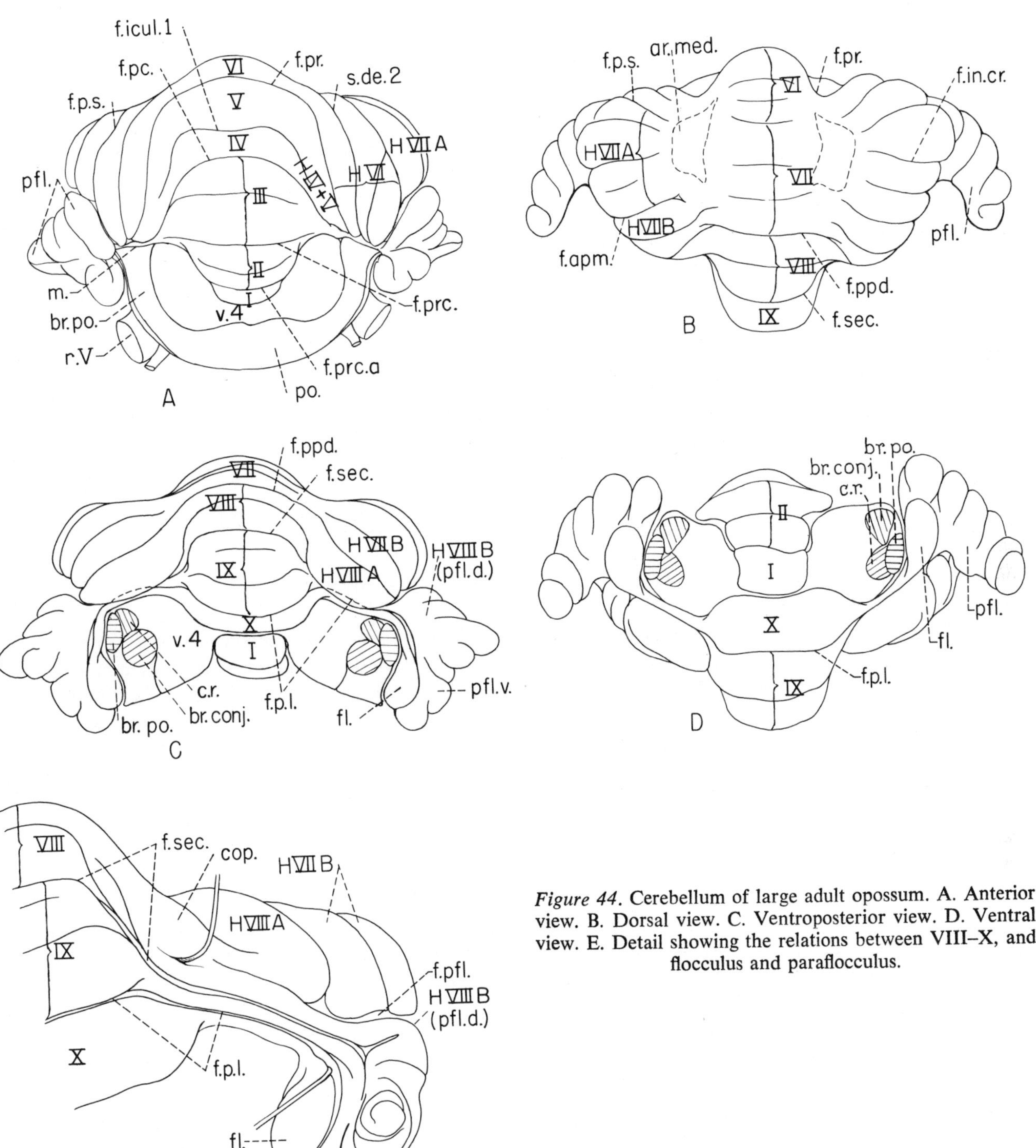

Figure 44. Cerebellum of large adult opossum. A. Anterior view. B. Dorsal view. C. Ventroposterior view. D. Ventral view. E. Detail showing the relations between VIII–X, and flocculus and paraflocculus.

prepyramidal fissure as described above. Bradley's fissure *a* in other species corresponds to the ansoparamedian fissure, which also appears to be true in this author's figure of the dorsal surface of the cerebellum of *D. azarae*. Possibly fissure *a* of the median sagittal section represents a compound furrow including the prepyramidalis, with the dorsally directed deep branch of the cleft representing the vermal part of the ansoparamedian fissure in the anterodorsal wall of the prepyramidal fissure, as in many species of placental mammals described in

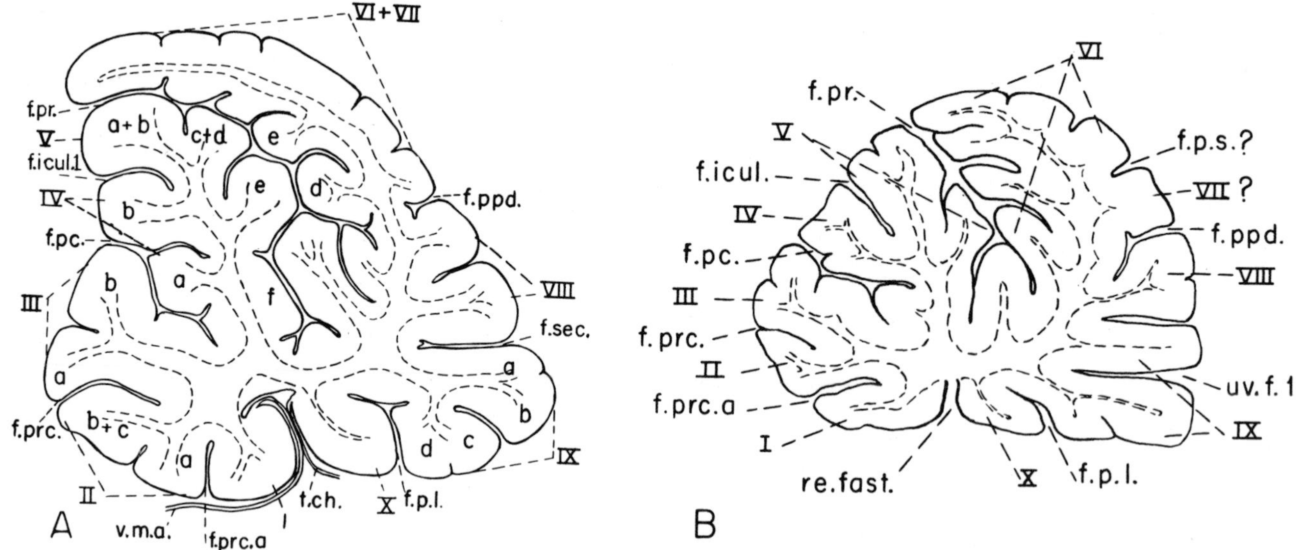

Figure 45. A. Midsagittal section of cerebellum of large adult opossum. ×6. B. Midsagittal section of cerebellum of *Didelphis azarae.*

subsequent sections. If so, lobule VIII of *D. azarae* would include two subdivisions, as in *D. virginiana.*

The rostrally projecting part of the posterior lobe (lobulus impendens of Ziehen) has six low cortical folds, separated by five shallow furrows, in the large cerebellum illustrated in figures 44 and 45A. Other specimens show only five folds, which are usually more prominent, and four deeper furrows. Since the vermal furrows end short of the medullary areas between vermis and hemispheres they cannot be related, individually, to individual hemispheral fissures with any certainty. If the three anterior folds of cortex were regarded as corresponding to the superficial folia of lobule VI, then the remainder of the dorsal surface, as far posteriorly as the prepyramidal fissure, would represent lobule VII. The ventral surface of the lobulus impendens, facing the fissura prima, is more deeply folded. As in other species it was regarded as part of lobule VI, while folia VId and VIe were individually identifiable; the large folium in the lower posterior wall of the fissura prima probably corresponds to VIf of other species but is relatively much larger (fig. 45A). The rostrally projecting part of the posterior lobe (lobule C of Bradley) is less elongated and more massive in *D. azarae*, as illustrated by Bradley. If lobule VII was regarded as being crowded caudalward so that VIIB is pushed into the anterodorsal wall of the compound fissure which Bradley's fissure *a* appears to represent, then the pattern of lobules VI and VII would be essentially the same as in *D. virginiana.*

The cerebellar hemisphere of the opossum is divided into simple lobules that correspond rather closely to the hemispheral lobules of the rat. However, a medullary area devoid of cortex intervenes between the medial parts of most of these lobules and the vermal lobules. The extent of the medullary area varies in individual cerebella; in the large specimen illustrated in figure 44B it is more extensive than in others.

Lateral of the fissura prima on the anterior surface of the cerebellum two fusiform folds, the more medial of which is continuous dorsomedially with the anterior fold of lobule VI, represent lobule HVI, the hemispheral part of Bolk's lobulus simplex (fig. 44A). The furrow delimiting the more lateral fold from the remainder of the hemisphere corresponds to the posterior superior fissure of the rat but is not continuous with a vermal furrow. The three or four folds behind this fissure correspond to lobule HVIIA. They differ somewhat in the two hemispheres, but the intercrural fissure, as labeled on the right side of figure 44, subdivides the lobule into parts that correspond to crus I and crus II of Bolk. The posterior part of the hemisphere is separated from lobule HVIIA by the ansoparamedian fissure and forms lobule HVIIB, corresponding to the anterior part of the paramedian lobule of Bolk. The dorsal subdivision of lobule VIII (sublobule VIIIA) is continuous ventrolaterally with an expanded hemispheral segment which is concealed beneath lobule HVIIB but represents lobule HVIIIA, the posterior part of the paramedian lobule. In posteroventral view the lateral continuation of sublobule VIIIA is seen to expand as the copula, from which a branch continues to the ventral surface of HVIIIA (fig. 44E). Another afferent branch of the copula, which is a continuation from sublobule VIIIB and upon which the copula is superposed, extends to the dorsal paraflocculus or lobule HVIIIB. The ventral paraflocculus which is connected with lobule IX by the ventral part of the parafloccular peduncle may be regarded as lobule HIX. An accessory paraflocculus could not be certainly identified in the opossum.

HEMISPHERAL LOBULES

The margin of a thin zone of unfoliated cortex could be seen in rostral view of the adult cerebellum in the opossum (fig. 44A). It covers the brachium pontis as this peduncle enters the cerebellum, and is continuous medially with lobules II and III of the vermis, forming a small triangular area which may be regarded as an incipient lobule HII + HIII. Lobules IV and V merge laterally, forming a small hemispheral culminate lobule or lobule HIV + HV. The hemispheral fissures and lobules of the posterior lobe are difficult to identify in the formalin-hardened cerebellum, but when further hardened in alcohol, the shrinkage produced intensifies the fissures and differentiates the principal ones from the secondary ones. The posterior superior fissure forms the caudal boundary of a group of two elongated folia that sometimes expand to three as they approach the anterior cerebellar margin. This group represents lobule HVI (fig. 44A). The two principal folia are separated by a furrow which has the same relations as declival sulcus 1 of the rat except that it lacks continuity with a vermal segment. Such continuity also is lacking with respect to the posterior superior fissure (fig. 44B).

Although sublobules VIIA and VIIB were not identifiable in the vermis, as is also true of lobule VI, the pattern of the hemisphere behind the posterior superior fissure is so similar, in alcohol-treated cerebella, to that of the rat and other small species that division into lobules HVIIA and HVIIB, the ansiform and paramedial lobules of Bolk respectively, appears to be justified. Compared with the cat – an animal approximately the same size as or somewhat smaller than the opossum – these lobules have few subdivisions just as is the case with all others in the opossum. Lobule HVIIA comprises three to four large folia that are divided into two groups by a deeper and more prominent furrow than the others behind the posterior superior fissure. This furrow was interpreted as the intercrural fissure (fig. 44B) and the two groups of folia were regarded as corresponding to crus I and crus II. The ansoparamedian fissure, as labeled in figure 44B, is deeper and more prominent than those immediately adjacent to it and delimits two folia that correspond to the paramedian lobule of the rat and some other species in position and lateral elongation. The pars copularis of the paramedian lobule has already been mentioned in connection with lobule VIII.

CEREBELLAR NUCLEI

According to Voris and Hoerr (1932), the opossum has three cerebellar nuclei: the nucleus fastigii, the nucleus interpositus, and the nucleus dentatus. In the later pouch stages of opossums (figs. 46, 47) I found three corresponding masses (Larsell, 1936a). Foltz and Matzke (1960) described the nuclei in the adult opossum as comprising a well-defined medially situated nucleus fastigii and a lateral mass which is incompletely subdivided into nucleus interpositus and nucleus lateralis (dentatus).

In *Ornithorhynchus*, as already noted, Hines (1929)

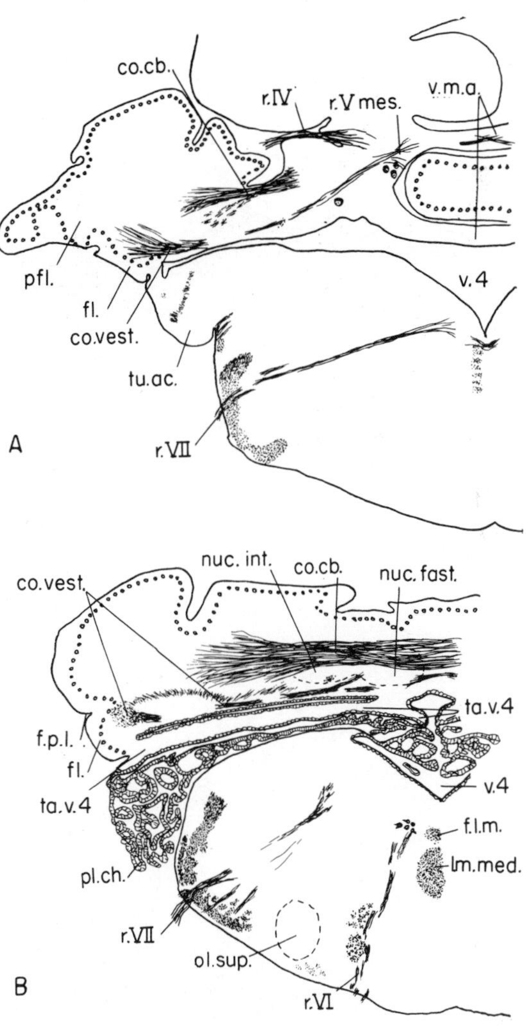

Figure 46. Transverse sections through cerebellum of pouch-stage opossum of 40-mm C.R. length, ca. 29 days after birth. A. Section through rostral part of cerebellum. B. Section just caudal of fastigium. Pyridine-silver method. ×30. (Larsell, 1935.)

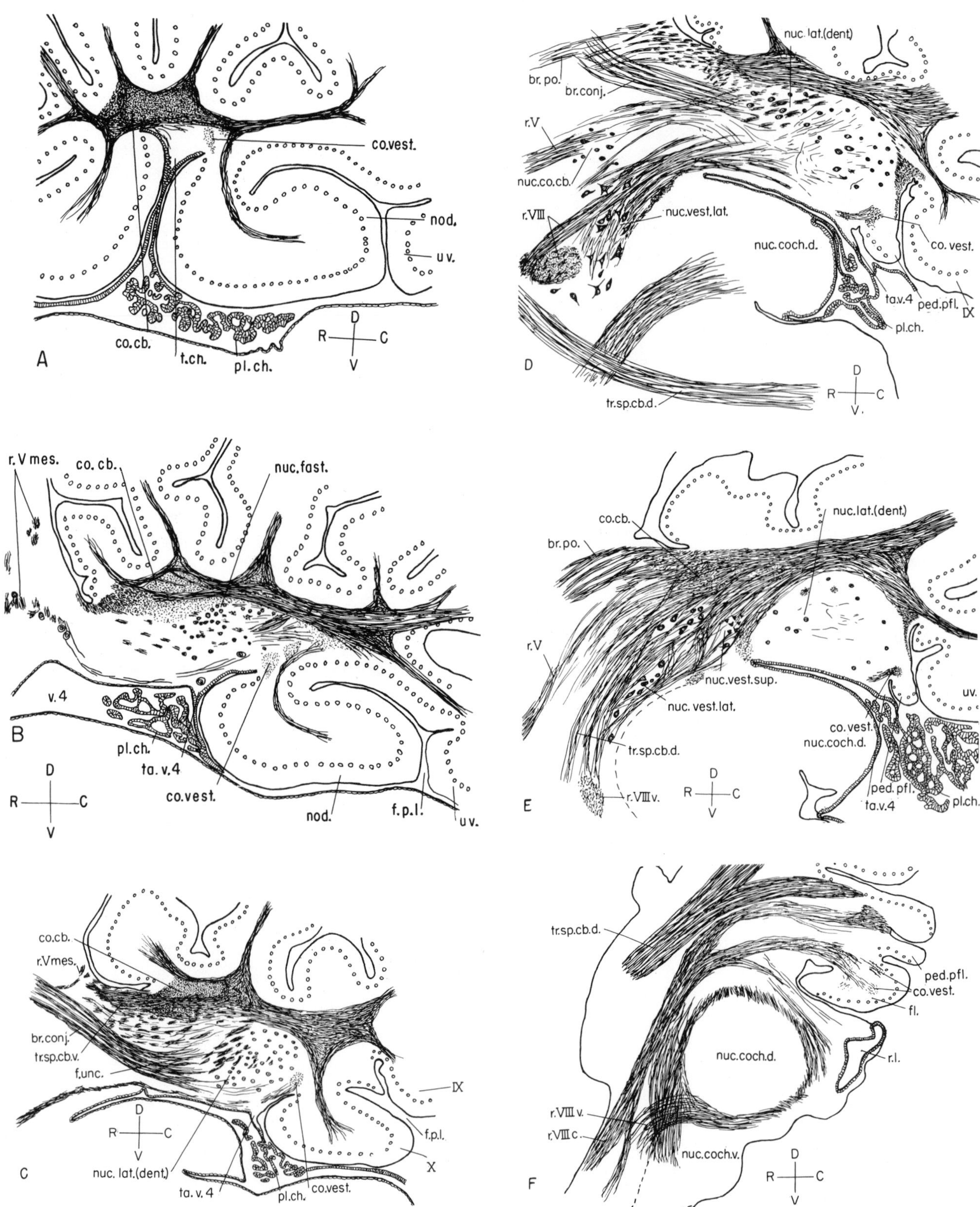

Figure 47. Sagittal sections through basis cerebelli of pouch-stage opossum of 56-mm C.R. length, 40 days after birth. A. Midsagittal section. B. Section lateral to A. C. Section through lateral part of nodulus. D. Section through nodular peduncle. E. Section through floccular peduncle. F. Section through flocculus. (Larsell, 1936a.)

found only two nuclei, a medial and a lateral one; also only two occur in the spiny anteater (Abbie, 1934). These evidently correspond to the nucleus medius and nucleus lateralis of reptiles, although the lateral nucleus in monotremes may include a part related to the small cerebellar hemisphere. Brunner's (1919) designation of the most lateral of the three nuclei in subanthropoids as the nucleus lateralis is more appropriate than the nucleus dentatus because of differences in form and because the nucleus dentatus proper of anthropoids includes a large cell mass which is poorly or not at all represented in the cerebellum of lower Eutheria. The nucleus lateralis of reptiles and the greater part of the similarly named nucleus of monotremes probably correspond more closely to Brunner's nucleus interpositus than to his nucleus lateralis. For the sake of specificity and to avoid confusion between the nucleus lateralis of reptiles and the nucleus lateralis of mammals, as widely used, I designated the latter the nucleus lateralis (dentatus).

The fastigial nucleus is elongated anteroposteriorly and is relatively narrow. Medium-sized to fairly large cells are numerous in the middle and posterior parts of the nucleus; small cells are scattered throughout. Fibers from the vestibular tract pass into it and the bilateral nuclei are interconnected by a commissure. The nucleus interpositus is separated from the fastigial nucleus by bundles of fibers but it is closely related to the nucleus lateralis (dentatus). In the zone of junction of the two, numerous medium-sized cells occur. A mass of fibers partly separates them. The nucleus lateralis (dentatus) forms a rounded mass of cells in the opossum from which a ventrolateral projection extends toward the paraflocculus. The central part of the nucleus includes numerous large, pale-staining cells.

CEREBELLAR CONNECTIONS

Afferent fibers. The trigeminal root fibers that form the beginning of the commissura cerebelli of the embryo are supplemented by more numerous fibers from the dorsomedial region of the superior sensory trigeminal nucleus. Presumably this part of the nucleus corresponds to the one in the platypus that Hines (1929) described as dorsolateral; a large number of fibers come from this part of the nucleus and pass into the cerebellum. Stokes (1909) recognized that in the adult opossum the intertrigeminal component of the cerebellar commissure forms a prominent part of the cerebellum. Within the cerebellum the trigeminal fibers soon are lost in the silver and Weigert series; presumably they reach the cortex of the posterodorsal wall of the fissura prima, while some probably are distributed in the anteroventral wall.

Two spinocerebellar tracts were evident. The ventral tract, which appears early in the embryo, was recognizable as a distinct bundle of the commissure in early stages (fig. 35), but as the number of fibers increases it merges with the trigeminal fascicle (fig. 36A). The spinocerebellar tract distributes principally to the anterior lobe. As illustrated by Voris and Hoerr (1932) in transverse sections, part of the ventral tract appears to enter the cerebellum by way of the restiform body. The dorsal spinocerebellar tract enters the cerebellum through the restiform body. In the sagittal pyridine-silver series of pouch-stage opossum it was followed to the anterior lobe, the uvula, and the pyramis (fig. 47).

Olivocerebellar fibers leave the medial side of the inferior olivary complex and cross the raphe of the medulla oblongata to enter the cerebellum through the restiform body. A smaller number of fibers pass dorsalward and appear to enter the cerebellum ipsilaterally, as described by Voris and Hoerr (1932). Dorsal and medial accessory olives and a lateral mass corresponding to the chief olivary nucleus of higher mammals were described by Kooy (1917) in the opossum. Presumably these distribute to the cerebellum in the same way as those found in higher mammals by Brodal (1940a).

The tectocerebellar tract was observed in the opossum by Tsai (1925) and by Voris and Hoerr (1932). Subsequently I described it (Larsell, 1936a) as originating at various levels of the optic tectum and entering the cerebellum as a compact fascicle which is soon lost among the fiber masses of the corpus cerebelli. I was unable to differentiate the several divisions of the tectocerebellar system described by Hines (1929) in *Ornithorhynchus*, and the distribution of the fibers in the cerebellum could not be followed.

The mesencephalic root of the trigeminus, as it passes into the midbrain, gives off fibers that enter the base of the cerebellum. A few large cells of the mesencephalic trigeminal type are scattered among the fibers in the cerebellar base and similar cells accompany the mesencephalic trigeminal root as far as its emergence from the medulla oblongata. Pearson (1949b) found even more numerous mesencephalic trigeminal cells and fibers in the base of the cerebellum of the human fetus.

Pontocerebellar fibers, constituting the brachium pontis, form a considerable mass in the opossum although the pons is relatively small and entirely pretrigeminal (fig. 39C). Most of the pontine fibers pass into the principal mass of the hemisphere but some turn lateralward and enter the paraflocculus.

Vestibular root fibers cross the median sagittal plane of the cerebellar plate in the 11-day-old opossum embryos so that they form a vestibular commissural fascicle (fig. 32B). As the cerebellum grows and its subdivisions become differentiated, the vestibular root fibers are distributed to the flocculus, nodulus, and the portion of the uvula adjacent to it, as well as to the fastigial nucleus. Vestibular root fibers appear to reach the lingula in company with spinocerebellar fibers. Those that appear to be of vestibular origin are smaller in size and stain differently in pyridine-silver preparations than those of spinal origin. Ingvar (1918) had described, from Marchi preparations, direct vestibular fibers to the lingula of the cat. Subsequently Dow (1939) obtained action potentials in the lingula of the cat by stimulation of the vestibular nerve. The vestibulocerebellar or secondary vestibular tract of the opossum originates, according to Voris and Hoerr (1932), only from the medial and inferior vestibular nuclei – the superior vestibular nucleus does not contribute fibers, as I (Larsell, 1936a) thought was true in the pouch stage. Brodal and Torvik (1957) found cellular degeneration only in the medial and inferior nuclei of cats, never in the superior or lateral vestibular nuclei, which confirms the observations of Voris and Hoerr in the opossum with respect to the origin of the secondary vestibular tract.

Other cerebellipetal fibers, such as those found by experimental-anatomical methods, especially in the cat by Brodal and his co-workers, undoubtedly are present in the opossum. However, in preparations stained for normal fibers these tracts could not be identified.

Efferent paths. The brachium conjunctivum and a fastigiobulbar tract, or uncinate fascicle of Russell, were described from Weigert and reduced silver preparations by Voris and Hoerr (1932) and myself (1936a). Recently Foltz and Matzke (1960) described the efferent paths from Marchi preparations. According to these authors the cerebellifugal fibers that constitute the brachium conjunctivum arise chiefly if not entirely from cells of the ipsilateral nucleus interpositus and nucleus lateralis (dentatus). The brachium is typically mammalian, decussating in the midbrain and dividing into a crossed ascending and a crossed descending limb. Just prior to decussation the brachium gives off a small number of fibers to the ipsilateral mesencephalic tegmental nuclei. Most of the fibers in the tract arise from the lateral (dentate) nucleus; these fibers continue forward in the ventral half of the fascicle and cross in the ventral part of the decussation. They were said to terminate chiefly in the contralateral nucleus ruber and the nucleus ventralis, the pars principalis of the thalamus. Fibers from the nucleus interpositus occupy the dorsal half of the brachium conjunctivum and cross in the intermediate part of the decussation. These fibers were said to end in the contralateral red nucleus for the most part, while some ascend in the field of Forel and the zona incerta.

The fastigial nucleus gives rise to three fascicles: a crossed ascending limb of the uncinate fascicle and a crossed and uncrossed descending limb of this fascicle. The ascending limb crosses within the cerebellum and ascends dorsomedial of the brachium conjunctivum, as the latter leaves the cerebellum. In front of the decussation of the trochlear nerve it intermingles with the dorsomedial margin of the brachium conjunctivum and continues as a well-defined fascicle at the lateral border of the periaqueductal gray substance. The crossed descending component of the uncinate fascicle was said to take origin principally from the fastigial nucleus but also, to a lesser extent, from the nucleus interpositus. It decussates within the cerebellum and terminates in the vestibular nuclei and upper cervical cord. The uncrossed descending component, or direct fastigiobulbar tract, ends ipsilaterally in the same general areas as the crossed component.

MARSUPIAL MOLE

The cerebellum of the marsupial mole (*Notoryctes typhlops*) was described by G. E. Smith (1903b), who believed it represented the simplest form of the organ in mammals. According to him, the cerebellum is divided into four folds of unequal size by three principal furrows: the fissura prima, the fissura secunda, and the fissura postnodularis. The fissura prima separates the anterior lobe from Smith's medial lobe and the fissura secunda delimits the latter from his posterior lobe, which comprises the uvula and nodulus. The two segments of the posterior lobe, so defined, are separated by the postnodular fissure. The flocculus and paraflocculus are grouped together as the floccular lobe, which was described as a small irregular appendage having a shallow furrow between the two component parts. The parafloccular fissure separates the floccular lobe (as defined by Smith) from the principal mass of the cerebellum. The following description is my interpretation of G. E. Smith's text and illustrations in terms of the concepts of cerebellar morphology set forth in this volume. My conclusions (fig. 48) are based on a close comparison of G. E. Smith's description with my own observations on the adult cerebellum of other small mammals, especially the Insectivora and Chiroptera, and on developmental stages of the opossum, bat, and rat, as described in other sections. It should be emphasized that the basic pattern of the marsupial cerebellum is identical with that of Eutheria and its complexity is correlated in both animal groups with body size and relative functional importance of the various organs having cerebellar connections. No specific primitive feature not shared to a greater or less degree by the lower orders of placental mammals could be singled out in marsupials.

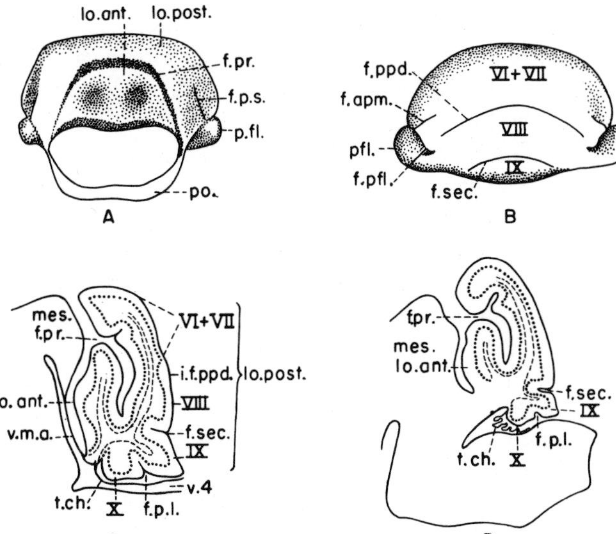

Figure 48. Cerebellum of marsupial mole (*Notoryctes*). A. Anterior view. B. Posterior view. C. Midsagittal section. D. Lateral sagittal section. (G. E. Smith, 1903b.)

The marsupial mole approximates 150 mm in length (Regan, 1937). It burrows about three inches beneath the surface but does not leave a permanent tunnel. According to Troughton (1947) the limbs are short and stout and the hands and feet have five digits adapted for digging. The nails of the third and fourth fingers are greatly enlarged and, reportedly, function as a combined pick and shovel in "dredging" a way through sand which is thrown up behind by the flattened nails of the feet. The animal emerges to breathe more freely at intervals of a few feet to many yards. The mole's progression on the surface was described as a shuffling with a peculiar sinuous action that leaves a triple track made by the body and the paired limbs; the latter evidently do not elevate the body from the ground. The snout is protected by a horny shield; there is no external ear, only a small opening beneath the fur leading to the auditory mechanism; the eyes have degenerated and disappeared. The tail is rudimentary and is covered by leathery skin. The animal is so specialized that its relationships to other families of marsupials was doubted but certain features of foot structure and of dentition point to a common early origin with the Paramelidae (Troughton).

The postnodular fissure of G. E. Smith in *Notoryctes* obviously corresponds to the vermal segment of the posterolateral fissure of the opossum and other mammals. In the pouch and adult stages of opossums continuity of the posterolateral fissure from one side to the other of the cerebellum is very evident, as already noted, and it also is shown in G. E. Smith's figures of pouch specimens of *Dasyurus* and *Trichosurus* and of adult *viverrinus*. The bat fetus has a continuous posterolateral fissure (Larsell and Dow, 1935) but in adult *Myotis* the furrow almost disappears along the parafloccular peduncle and reappears between the small flocculus and the paraflocculus (Larsell, 1936b). In the soricine shrews, which have a very small flocculus closely apposed to the parafloccular peduncle, the continuity of the posterolateral fissure is not in doubt (fig. 57). The flocculonodular lobe is distinctly delimited from the corpus cerebelli in all these species as well as in all other mammals including the monotremes.

G. E. Smith designates as "ala noduli" lateral extensions of the nodulus, one on either side, which are continuous with the flocculus of *Notoryctes*. The paraflocculus was described as being continuous with his lobus medius by means of a narrow zone between the parafloccular fissure and a shallow groove which appears to correspond to the lateral part of the posterolateral fissure of shrews and bats. Possibly the groove is represented by the furrow labeled fissura secunda in G. E. Smith's figures 7 and 15, in which it was said to delimit the nodulus from his lobus medius, a relationship which I have not found in other mammals. He designated the narrow zone of cortex the copula pyramidis.

The lobus flocculi of G. E. Smith reportedly forms a curved band of gray substance which bends forward around the middle cerebellar peduncle. The shallow groove on its surface, already mentioned, divides it into a smaller ventral part or flocculus that is continuous medially with the ala noduli; and a dorsal part, the paraflocculus, that is continuous by means of the copula pyramidis with the lobus medius. The shallow groove of G. E. Smith evidently corresponds to the lateral segment of the posterolateral fissure. The floccular lobe, as described by him in higher mammals, is not a morphological unit since the flocculus clearly is part of the flocculonodular lobe and the paraflocculus is differentiated from the posterolateral part of the corpus cerebelli. There can be little doubt that the cerebellum of *Notoryctes* also is divided into a flocculonodular lobe and corpus cerebelli in the same manner as in birds and other mammals.

The corpus cerebelli of *Notoryctes* is divided into anterior and posterior lobes by a deep and prominent fissura prima (fig. 48C). The anterior lobe forms a dorsorostrally directed, nearly semicircular fold which is covered dorsally and caudally by the posterior lobe (fig. 48A, C). On its anterior surface a suggestion of a transverse furrow, beneath which the molecular layer is thickened, probably represents the preculminate fissure in rudimentary form. The lobe, however, is undivided and, while it is much more deeply separated from the posterior lobe by the fissura prima, it corresponds to the stage of differentiation represented in the pouch stage of *Didelphis* and *Dasyurus* and in the bat and mole fetuses prior to, or at the earliest stages of, formation of the preculminate fissure.

The posterior lobe of the corpus cerebelli comprises all of the cerebellum between the posterolateral fissure and the fissura prima. It is subdivided by the fissura secunda, the prepyramidal fissure (suprapyramidal of G. E. Smith), and a furrow in the posterodorsal wall of the fissura prima illustrated but not mentioned by G. E. Smith. The fissura secunda is prominent in the median region but disappears laterally (fig. 48). It forms the dorsal boundary of the uvula, which corresponds to lobule IX of the opossum, Insectivora, Chiroptera, rat, and other species. The prepyramidal fissure, the occurrence of which marks an advance in differentiation of the posterior lobe, compared with the soricine shrews, is shallow, as in the 18-mm C. R. length *Corynorhinus* embryo among the bats and in the 21-day-old rat fetus. It is variable, however, in *Notoryctes*; sometimes, as in the specimen illustrated in figure 48, it was said to be indicated only by a notch in the granular layer. Ventral of this notch the molecular layer is thickened as is this layer of young alligators where fissures eventually appear. The cortical segment between the fissura secunda and the incipient prepyramidal fissure is very similar to the corresponding segment in the 27-day-old opossum in the pouch, the 21-day-old rat fetus, and the 18-mm C.R. length bat fetus. This part of the lobe in *Notoryctes* is the pyramis or lobule VIII. It is continuous with the triangular area, between the parafloccular fissure and the lateral part of the fissura secunda, which G. E. Smith called the copula pyramidis.

Since folium VIII of birds and lobule VIII of experimental mammals are activated by auditory impulses, the rudimentary corresponding lobe of *Notoryctes* probably receives similar fibers but in smaller numbers. Absence of the external ear points to a reduction of the auditory sense in this species.

The remainder of the posterior lobe, rostral of the more or less rudimentary prepyramidal fissure, is elongated and arched forward but its dorsal surface has no indication of foliation. The rostral region is expanded and arches forward and ventrally in a flangelike manner, which results in a considerable area of cortex (fig. 48B, C). A similar elongation and a rostral enlargement were found in the soricine shrews but a furrow corresponding to the vermal segment of the posterior superior fissure also was recognizable. No suggestion of this fissure appears in G. E. Smith's figures of the *Notoryctes* cerebellum but the ventral surface of the dorsorostral elongation is notched by a furrow, already mentioned, which probably corresponds to declival sulcus 3 of the rat and other species. If one regards the enlarged anterior part of the posterior lobe, including the cortex of the dorsoposterior wall of the fissura prima as far as the bottom of this fissure, as corresponding to lobule VI of the opossum, rat, and other species, but without a definite boundary on the dorsal surface, then this part of the cerebellum could be correlated with the sensory importance of the snout of *Notoryctes*, which probably is the principal exteroceptive organ. It appears justifiable to assume that the expansion and relatively advanced differentiation of lobule VI, except for the absence of demarcation on the dorsal cerebellar surface, are related to termination in this lobule of large numbers of afferent trigeminal fibers.

The elongated but thin stretch of cortex between the indeterminate posterior boundary of lobule VI and the prepyramidal fissure must be regarded as the undifferentiated homolog of lobule VII. Presumably the reduction of this part of the cerebellar cortex should be correlated with the lack of vision in the marsupial mole.

A short furrow on the lateral anterior surface of the hemisphere (fig. 48A), which is designated fissura postlunata by G. E. Smith, corresponds in position to the hemispheral segment of the posterior superior fissure of adult shrews and young rats. It partially delimits an area of cortex which corresponds to lobule HVI of the rat, opossum, and other mammals. A short furrow on the posterolateral hemispheral surface of *Notoryctes* appears to be homologous with the ansoparamedian fissure of the young rat and adult shrews. There is no indication of further subdivision of the hemisphere (fig. 48B).

G. E. Smith compared the cerebellum of *Notoryctes* with that of *Perameles* on the premise that this bandicoot is one of the most generalized mammals known. It has a slender body and a long, tapering, prehensile tail, which is used for gripping branches when climbing. *Perameles* is larger than the marsupial mole. Its total length including the tail approximates 500 mm, but this mole is smaller and less sturdily built than *Didelphis virginiana*. The kangaroolike hindlimbs are longer than the forelimbs and are adapted for digging, scratching, and leaping. The forelimbs and hands are used in climbing and other activities.

The cerebellum of *Perameles* (fig. 49) as illustrated in the median sagittal section by G. E. Smith (1903a) is a diagrammatic version of the organ in the adult opossum, except for the relative proportions of some of the subdivisions. The anterior lobe is subdivided by two deep fissures and often also by two or three shallow furrows. The prepyramidal fissure in *Perameles* may be lacking in the posterior lobe but it is reportedly more constant than in *Notoryctes* and to become confluent with the paraflocu-

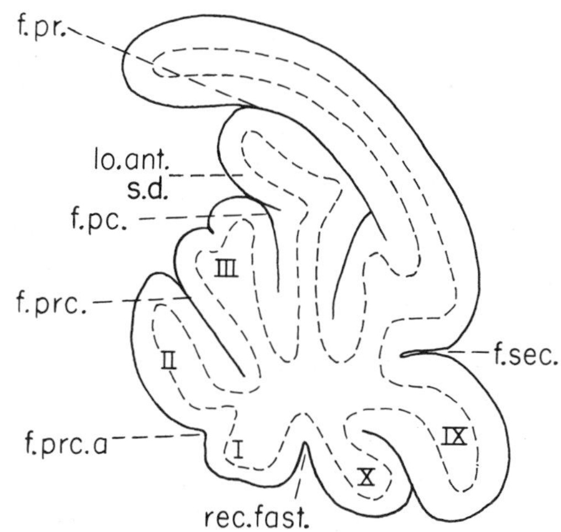

Figure 49. Cerebellum of *Perameles.* Midsagittal section. (Redrawn and modified from G. E. Smith, 1903b.)

lar fissure (G. E. Smith, 1903b). Constant parapyramidal fissures also were said to occur and a furrow corresponding to the ansoparamedian fissure, as labeled in figure 48B, sometimes is present. The paraflocculus is separated from the flocculus by a definite "fissura floccularis" (lateral segment of the posterolateral fissure), and the uvula (lobule IX) is relatively larger and is divided from the nodulus by the "postnodular fissure."

This description applies equally well to the cerebellum of the opossum except that the lobules are more subfoliated in the adult *Didelphis.* The two deep furrows of the anterior lobe of *Perameles* represent the preculminate and precentral fissures. The subdivision between them corresponds to lobule III, but is relatively larger in *Perameles,* probably in correlation with the elongated, kangaroolike legs of the bandicoot. Lobules I and II, as labeled in figure 49, correspond closely to these lobules of the opossum except that lobule II is undivided. Lobule I in the bandicot is relatively well differentiated, as in the opossum, and probably is functionally related to presumably well-developed intrinsic muscles of the prehensile tail. Presumably lobule II is related to the basal tail muscles and perhaps to those of the marsupium.

The culminate segment is expanded distally in *Perameles,* with a shallow furrow between the anteroventral part of the expansion and the posterior wall of the preculminate fissure apparently representing the intraculminate fissure. Division of the culminate segment into lobules IV and V is thus foreshadowed. Since the lobules of the anterior lobe correspond morphologically to those of the opossum and the rat, as well as to those of larger marsupial and placental mammals, they probably also correspond in fiber connections and functional significance.

The part of the posterior lobe extending dorsally and rostrally above the fissura secunda is relatively more elongated than in the opossum but, except for the presence of a shallow prepyramidal fissure in some specimens, as described by G. E. Smith, it is unfoliated. This may mean that the entire lobulus *c* of Bolk is a generalized area serving touch, vision, and hearing, with the initial specialization of the posterior part as the rudiment of lobule VIII serving auditory impulses. In the larger cerebellum of the opossum, as already noted, lobule VIII is well differentiated and the anterior part of lobulus *c* is foliated into rudimentary lobules VII and VI. The anterior part of lobule VI is activated by trigeminal impulses, lobule VII by optic impulses, and lobule VIII by auditory impulses, but there is overlapping, especially at the borders of each lobule.

In reviewing and evaluating G. E. Smith's comparison of the cerebellum of *Notoryctes* with that of *Perameles,* one must consider the functional factors that had been experimentally demonstrated in placental mammals but were unknown six decades ago. This author believed that the cerebellum of the marsupial mole represents a morphological stage through which the developing organ of other mammals passes before becoming further differentiated and subdivided. Because it remains small and relatively simple in adult *Notoryctes* the cerebellum of this species was regarded as the most primitive among the mammals, rather than as a regressive type.

The anterior lobe of the *Notoryctes* cerebellum is the most atypical division, as compared with other Marsupials and placental mammals. In *Orolestes* and *Caenolestes,* described below, this lobe is divided into dorsal and ventral segments, as it is in the much smaller soricine shrews which include the smallest species of mammals. The anterior lobe of the small bats, with their special modifications of forelimbs and hindlimbs, is similarly divided. It would be of interest to know if the corresponding part of the cerebellum of small marsupial mice, such as *Planigale subtilissima* (with a head-body length of 45 mm and a tail length of 50 mm) or *Planigale ingrami* (with a head-body length of 63 mm and a tail length of 54mm), is also subdivided. One might well expect to find the most generalized type of cerebellum in this group of Marsupialia.

The anterior lobe of *Notoryctes* does not differentiate beyond that represented in the 19-day-old pouch stage of opossum, the 15-mm C.R. length bat embryo, and the 22-mm-long fetus of the placental mole, *Scapanus.* Since the anterior lobe is functionally related to the extremities, as shown in experimental placental mammals, the arrest of development in the marsupial mole presumably is related to some modification of the functional capacities of the appendages. The three tracks made in progression on the surface of the ground and the peculiar motion, mentioned above, suggest that the legs are unable to raise the weight of the body. By contrast the placental moles not only dig extensive permanent tunnels at an amazingly rapid speed, but also are rather clumsily supported by their legs in running above ground. In these moles the anterior lobe is divided into culminate and ventral segments, and the latter is subdivided into lobules I, II, and III. Aside from the increased foliation of the cerebellum characteristic of placental mammals, the great differences between the anterior lobe of *Notoryctes* and the Talpidae strongly point to a relationship with the functional capacity of the extremities.

The posterior lobe of *Notoryctes* also seems to be arrested in development, but at a later stage than the anterior lobe and unequally with respect to the individual rudimentary lobules. As already noted, these attain a degree of differentiation which can be correlated with the relative importance of the sensory systems related to each.

Although the development of the cerebellum of *Notoryctes* is the simplest in mammals with respect to its subdivisions in general, it is probably not the most primitive but rather is modified in accordance with the needs of a marsupial adapted to a very specialized mode of life. The differentiation of the posterior lobe is as advanced as in *Perameles*, and apparently more so with respect to its anterodorsal tip. Whether the relative reduction and lack of subdivision of the anterior lobe should be considered regressive is dependent on the character of this lobe in smaller marsupials and in the possibly common ancestor of *Notoryctes* and the Paramelidae.

MARSUPIAL SHREWS

These South American marsupials (*Caenolestes obscurus* and *Orolestes inca*) have a head-body length of 113 mm to 135 mm with a long and slender tail. Osgood (1925) described *Caenolestes* as having long hindlegs and as probably being active and roving. This animal is terrestrial in habit, feeding on insects. Vision appears to be limited but the olfactory and cochlear centers of the brain are large, according to Obenchain (1925), as are the trigeminal roots. The brain, including the cerebellum, of these two species was described by Obenchain (1925); her use of descriptive terms for the cerebellum followed the nomenclature of G. E. Smith.*

The cerebellum of the two species (figs. 50, 51) is virtually identical in general structure and except for a definite preculminate fissure, which is lacking in the marsupial mole, is intermediate in pattern between the cerebellum of *Notoryctes* and that of *Perameles*. It has a rounded external surface, with the dorsal part overhanging the optic tectum in a hoodlike manner. The ventral part of the organ extends caudalward above the greater part of the fourth ventricle. Small lateral lobes, delimited from the median or ventral part of the organ by faint depressions in the general surface, were believed to represent the cerebellar hemisphere. In *Caenolestes* a large mushroom-shaped pedunculated mass projects from beneath the lateral lobes and beyond them, on either side, as the paraflocculi (fig. 50A). These were regarded by Obenchain as the dorsal components of the floccular lobes of G. E. Smith. The ventral components are formed by small flocculi; they are hidden from view except for their anterior tips and each is separated from the paraflocculus by the floccular fissure. The parafloccular fissure separates the paraflocculus from the medial part of the cerebellum, cutting down to the floccular peduncle. The paraflocculus and parafloccular fissure of *Orolestes* were not specifically described. The lateral view of this cere-

*The opportunity to review the sectional brains of *Caenolestes* and *Orolestes* was kindly afforded me by Dr. Obenchain.

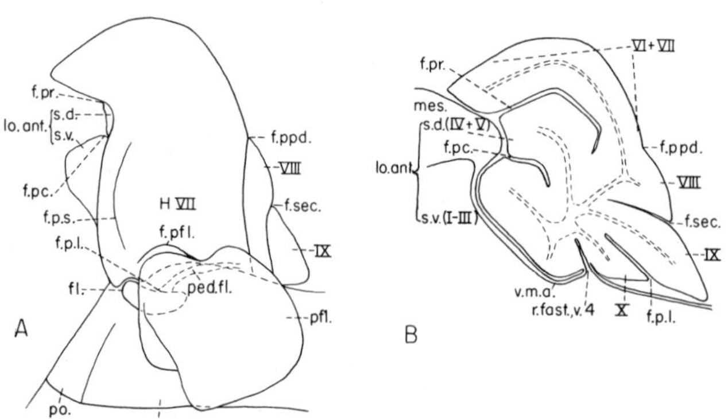

Figure 50. Cerebellum of *Caenolestes obscurus*. A. Lateral view. B. Midsagittal section. (Redrawn and modified from Obenchain, 1925.)

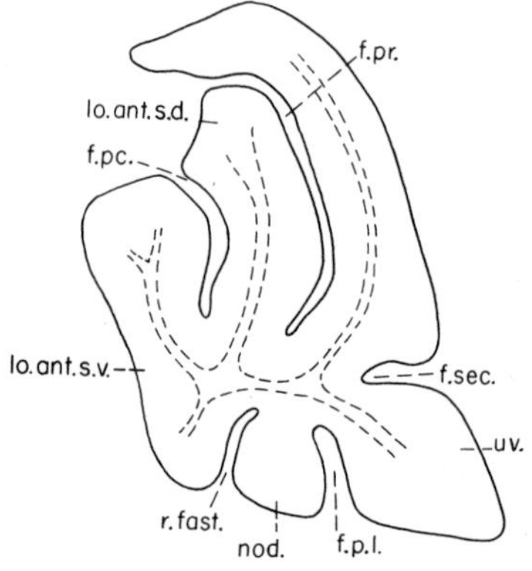

Figure 51. Cerebellum of *Orolestes inca*. Midsagittal section (Redrawn and modified from Obenchain, 1925.)

bellum, illustrated in figure 50A, however, shows a dorsocaudally tapering furrow in the ventral posterior part of the principal cerebellar mass. This is similar to the incipient parafloccular fissure of the late rat fetus. The small posteroventral area which it delimits anteriorly is suggestive of the parafloccular rudiment of the rat fetus. If this is the paraflocculus in *Orolestes* there is great disparity in development of this lobule in the two marsupial shrews.

In the median sagittal section the fissura prima is shown as a deep, arched cleft beneath the dorsal hood (figs. 50B, 51). The rostral part of the cerebellum beneath and in front of this fissure is the anterior lobe of the corpus cerebelli. In both species it is divided into dorsal and ventral segments by a relatively deep preculminate fissure. The dorsal or culminate segment is more elongated in *Orolestes* than in *Caenolestes* but in neither species is it subfoliated. The ventral segment has a wide, shallow depression on its anterior surface, which seems to be the incipient precentral fissure. Obenchain divided the ventral segment into the pars preculminata and the lingula, with each having a distinct medullary ray. Interpreted according to the terminology of this volume the lingula corresponds to lobules I and II, the pars praeculminata to lobule III, and the culmen to lobules IV and V. Lobules I and II and IV and V, respectively, are not differentiated from one another as they are in the rat and in larger species of marsupials.

The posterior lobe of the corpus cerebelli has a well-defined fissura secunda which delimits the uvula (lobule IX) from the upward and forward arching part of the vermis. In *Caenolestes* a shallow prepyramidal fissure divides this part of the vermis into lobule VIII (the pyramis) and the forward arching portion which corresponds to lobules VII and VI, but there is no indication of differentiation of these from each other. *Orolestes* has no prepyramidal fissure and the entire surface between the fissura secunda and fissura prima lacks any sign of foliation (fig. 51).

Continuity between the large paraflocculus of *Caenolestes* and the pyramis or the uvula remain obscure, as do the relations of the parafloccular fissure to the prepyramidal fissure. If the above suggested interpretation of the parafloccular fissure in *Orolestes* is valid, the rudimentary paraflocculus which it delimits is continuous medially with the zone that is differentiated into the pyramis of *Caenolestes*.

The nodulus (lobule X) is delimited from the uvula by a relatively deep "postnodular fissure" which corresponds to the vermal segment of the posterolateral fissure of other species. The small, concealed flocculus appears to have a peduncle but its relations with respect to the nodulus are not indicated. Obenchain combined the flocculus and paraflocculus as the floccular lobe of G. E. Smith, but probably a distinct flocculonodular lobe exists as in other marsupials.

The only indication of a hemispheral fissure was found on the rostrolateral surface and it appears to represent the hemispheral segment of the posterior superior fissure (fig. 50A). This delimits an anterior area, which could be regarded as a rudimentary lobule HVI, from a broader lateral zone in which no furrows are present. This zone apparently corresponds to lobule HVII before it is subdivided even to the extent found in the smallest soricine shrews (fig. 50A).

According to Obenchain the deep cerebellar nuclei are represented by a pair of large oval cell masses that almost meet at the midline. Indications of separation into medial or fastigial and lateral or interpositus + lateral (dentate) masses were said to be slight.

KANGAROOS

The kangaroo family, or Macropodidae, comprises the rat-kangaroos, wallabies, walleroos or rock-kangaroos, and the kangaroos proper, which are the largest of the group. These marsupials are herbivores, while the large wallabies and kangaroos are grazers. The hindlimbs are much longer and larger than the forelimbs and are adapted for hopping. The tail is long in most species and muscular; in the rat-kangaroos it is prehensile. The smallest and most primitive species is the musky rat-kangaroo, *Hypsiprymnodon moschatus*, which has a head-body length of 30 cm and a tail length of 15 cm. The largest is *Megaleia rufa*, which attains a head-body length of 1.6 meters. Old males of some of the large kangaroos were said to attain a standing height of nearly two meters.

Macropus has a relatively small head and short neck, but the body is large and heavy, with the abdominal part being more massive than the thoracic region. The powerful hindlimbs have greatly elongated feet. The forelimbs are disproportionately small and short but the paws are well developed and can be pronated and supinated to a considerable degree; this enables them to function almost as hands and actually have some measure of unilateral independence (Riley, 1929). The long tapering tail has a heavy and muscular root. When the animal is sitting or standing the tail along with the hindlimbs supports the body. In fighting, the forepaws were said to scratch at the opponent's head while the hindlimbs were used to kick. The body is supported by one leg and the tail or, when both legs are used, by the tail alone. The ears are long; the eyes, situated well forward, have overlapping fields of vision and limited but conjugate movements (Riley,

1929). The diurnal kangaroos undoubtedly have better vision than the nocturnal opossums and rat-kangaroos.

Progression is by a series of leaps by action of the powerful hindlimbs; the elongated feet were said to serve as springs. In rapid movement the tail is used as a balancer and rudder; some authors believed that it also takes part in the initial thrust when leaping. The forelimbs are not used in jumping, not even when landing. However, while grazing they are used to support the upper part of the body and the tail is then used to push the body forward (Troughton, 1947). Ordinary jumps may be from less than two meters to more than three meters in length, but leaps as high as three meters with lengths of eight to twelve meters have reportedly been made by individuals of the larger species.

Cerebellum

The cerebellum of the kangaroos (figs. 52–55) is much larger and its fissures and subdivisions are more prominent than in the opossums. The vermis and hemispheres are separated anteriorly and posteriorly, by a distinct paravermian sulcus which is a result of the rostral and caudal expansion of the hemispheres. On the dorsal surface a broad, depressed medullary area intervenes between the cortex of much of the vermis and that of many of the hemispheral lobules. Lateral of each hemisphere, and separated from it by a prominent paraflocculular fissure, a large group of folia forms the paraflocculus (fig. 53).

The anterior lobe of the corpus cerebelli is relatively larger than in the opossum and the posterior lobe is more massive and does not extend so far forward. The fissura prima, as a result, opens onto the anterior part of the dorsal surface (fig. 52). The posterolateral fissure is relatively deep and the flocculonodular lobe is well defined (fig. 54).

CORPUS CEREBELLI

Anterior lobe. The vermal lobules of the anterior lobe are prominent (fig. 52). Lobule I is large in sagittal section but narrow from side to side, and it projects ventralward into the fourth ventricle. No portion of it has a ventricular surface owing to the interposition of the anterior medullary velum, which is attached in front of the fastigium (fig. 55). Precentral fissure *a*, which delimits lobule I from lobule II, is deep. In the median sagittal section lobule I shows four principal folia that merge on the lateral surface into a medullary band which merges with a similar band leading to lobule II. As seen in sagittal section (fig. 55) the medullary ray of lobule I has a separate origin from the ventral part of the central medullary body. The cortical fold nearest the fastigium, labeled Ia,

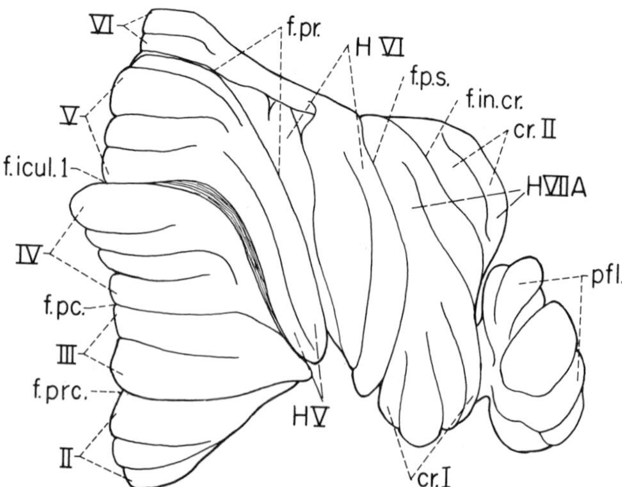

Figure 52. Cerebellum of large kangaroo (*Macropus*). Anterior view. Most of lobule II and all of lobule I hidden from view.

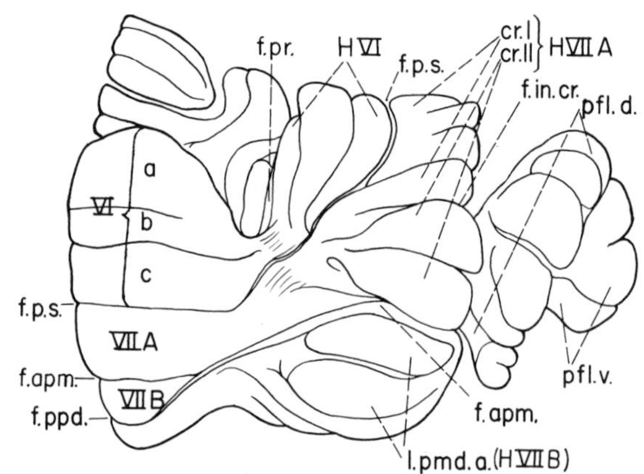

Figure 53. Cerebellum of kangaroo. Same specimen as in figure 52. Dorsal view.

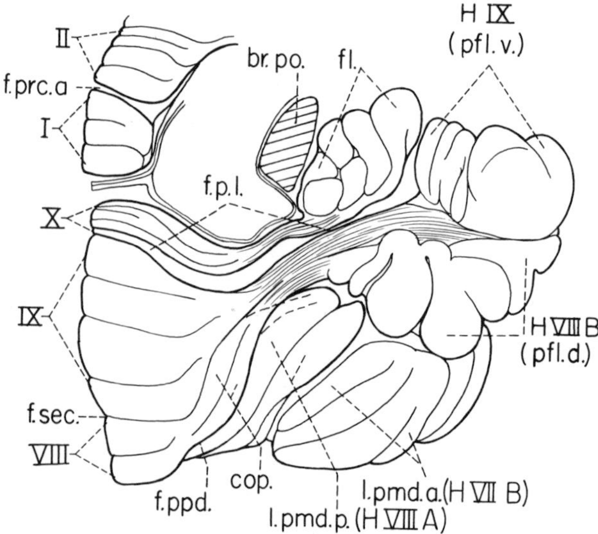

Figure 54. Cerebellum of kangaroo. Same specimen as in figure 52. Ventral view.

may receive a small separate ray, or its ray may branch from the principal ray of the lobule.

Lobule II is divided into lamellae IIa and IIb, which are separated by a shallow furrow that does not reach the lateral cerebellar margin. Lamella IIb is much wider horizontally than lamella IIa. The precentral fissure, between lobules II and III, is prominent and extends to the cerebellar margin of either side (fig. 52).

Lobule III comprises two lamellae, IIIa and IIIb, which are separated by a relatively deep fissure and are both subfoliated. The lobule extends so far laterally on both sides that it seems to have a small hemispheral representation. Together with lobules I and II it forms approximately fifty percent of the area of the anterior lobe as seen in median sagittal section (fig. 55). Ingvar's (1918) photograph of such a section of the cerebellum of *M. robustus*, a smaller but more heavily built species, shows that a relatively smaller proportion of the anterior lobe is formed by the corresponding lobules. Lobule III is smaller but lobule IV of the culmen is relatively larger than in other species of large kangaroos, which are similarly illustrated.

The culminate segment of *Macropus* and most other Macropodidae is divided into lobules IV and V by intraculminate fissure 1 (figs. 52, 55). This fissure is variable in depth; the two lobules, accordingly, are deeply separated in some cerebella and less deeply in others. They share a large primary medullary ray of variable length which divides into two longer branches, one for each lobule. Riley (1929) divided the culmen, his lobulus 4, into sublobuli 4A and 4B in *Macropus*; in the Tasmanian wolf he illustrated a similar division of the segment but he did not label the subdivisions. The figures of Dillon (1963), who called the culmen lobe 4, show the two divisions in *Wallabia elegans*, *Megaleia rufa*, and *M. major*, but in *Setonix brachyurus* and *W. rufogrisea* the culmen is not subdivided except into superficial folia. In *Potorus tridactyla* the culmen resembles that of the opossums, especially *Didelphis azarae* in which rudimentary lobules IV and V were recognizable. Whether the undivided culmen in *Setonix* and *W. rufogrisea* represents the usual pattern in these species, or is a variation of it, could not be determined from a single cerebellum of each. In Ingvar's illustration of *M. robustus*, lobules IV and V as defined here are large and deeply separated. In the larger placental mammals lobule IV presents many variations, but was recognizable in all, as it was in most marsupials and small placentals.

In the *Macropus* cerebellum as seen on the anterolateral surface, intraculminate fissure 1 turns ventrolaterally between the ventrolateral continuation of lobule V and a similar continuation of lobule IV. The latter forms a small lobule HIV, most of which is hidden from view by the larger lobule HV as represented in figure 52. In median sagittal section lobule IV is elongated and divides into two terminal sublamellae, with its fissural surfaces also being foliated. Lobule V is considerably larger and more foliated (fig. 55).

The fissura prima, separating the anterior and posterior lobes, is less deep, relatively, than in the opossum, due to the more vertical position of the dorsal part of the posterior lobe. Both its anterior and posterior walls have large folia and sublamellae (fig. 55).

Posterior lobe. The fissura secunda is the most prominent landmark of the posterior lobe and is its deepest fissure (fig. 55). It corresponds to the fissura secunda of the opossum, other marsupials, and placental mammals in its morphological relations. There can be no question that the segment that it delimits dorsally is the uvula, corresponding to lobule IX of other species (fig. 54). This lobule in the kangaroo has the characteristic pattern found in birds and other mammals. In sagittal section uvular sulci 1, 2, and 3 divide it into four surface folia (fig. 55) that correspond to the much smaller folia IXa, IXb, IXc, and IXd of the opossum and to the lamellae similarly designated in large placental mammals. Additional folia on the fissural surfaces give the lobule a large size as compared with the opossum. Dorsal of the fissura secunda a shallower furrow delimits a smaller lobule. The furrow is the prepyramidal fissure and the segment which it delimits dorsally is lobule VIII, the pyramis. In Riley's (1929) figure of a median sagittal section of the kangaroo cerebellum the corresponding fissure is deeper and the lobule, designated c_1, is larger. Ingvar's (1918) photographs of the cerebellum of *robustus* show that the pyramis includes two fairly large subdivisions having a common medullary ray. Laterally lobule VIII is continuous with the paraflocculus, with a slight fusiform swelling of the lateral folia that lead to the paraflocculus representing the copula pyramidis (fig. 54).

The area of cortex between the prepyramidal fissure and the fissura prima, corresponding to Bolk's lobulus c_2, is divided by four well-defined furrows and some shallower ones into a series of segments whose interpretation presents difficulties because of the general similarity between the furrows and the cortical folds, respectively. If the next furrow above the prepyramidal fissure was regarded as the ansoparamedian fissure and the more prominent one beyond it was interpreted as the posterior superior fissure, then the entire segment of cortex would fall into the general pattern of other larger mammals, but with relatively shallower fissures. In figure 53 the lobules and fissures were labeled according to this interpretation of the two fissures. The segment between the prepyrami-

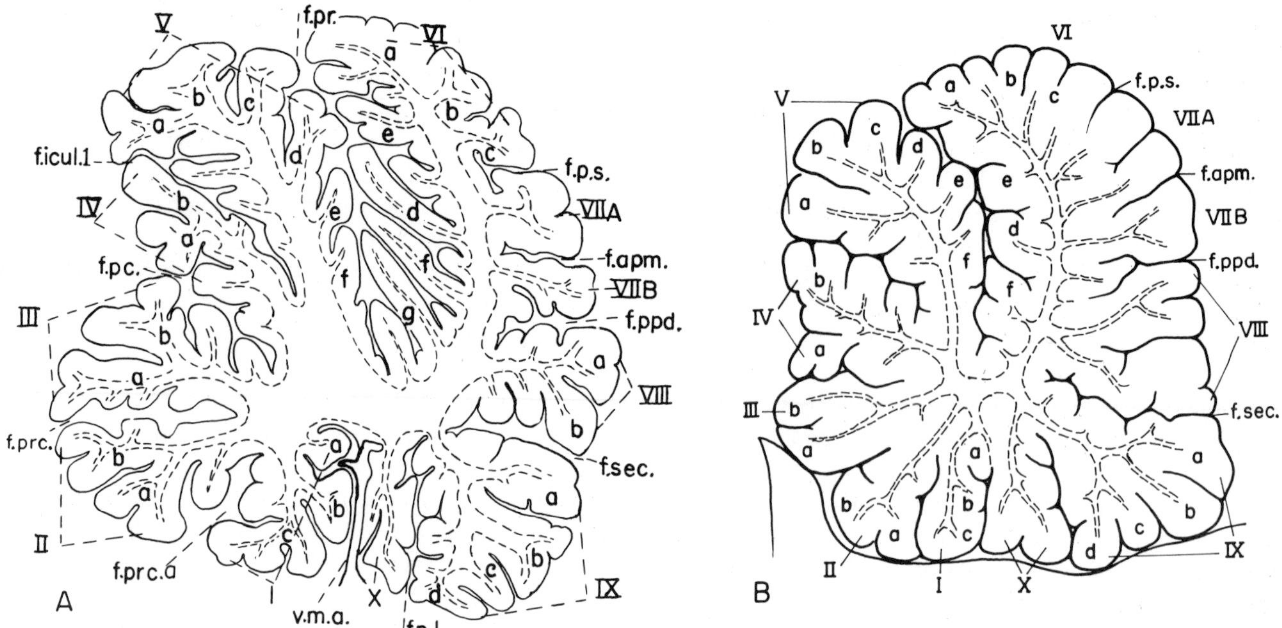

Figure 55. Cerebellum of *Macropus robustus.* A. Large specimen; sagittal section at one side of the midline. B. Midsagittal section of another specimen.

dal and the posterior superior fissures appears to correspond to lobule VII and is subdivided into lamellae VIIa and VIIb. The segment between the posterior superior fissure and the fissura prima then becomes lobule VI, the declive. The latter has three principal superficial folds that apparently correspond to folia or lamellae VIa, VIb, and VIc of the rat and larger placental mammals. These lamellae, together with those in the posterior wall of the fissura prima, several of which are much more elongated in the large species of *Macropus* than in *M. robustus*, give lobule VI an extensive cortical surface (fig. 55).

HEMISPHERAL LOBULES

The hemispheral representation of the individual lobules of the vermal part of the posterior lobe is more apparent in the kangaroo than in the opossum, although the large medullary area of the dorsal surface separates the lobe into discontinuous vermal and hemispheral parts, so far as the cortex and fissures are concerned. The connections of the subdivisions of the medullary substance were revealed by dissection. Folia VIa, VIb, and VIc, however, converge laterally into a narrow unfoliated band which takes a lateralorostral direction and expands on the rostral surface of the hemisphere into three broad folia (fig. 53). These constitute lobule HVI, the hemispheral continuation of the declival lobule, which corresponds to the hemispheral portion of Bolk's lobulus simplex. A large folium in the posterior wall of the fissura prima, which is continuous with folium VIe of the sagittal sections, extends lateralward as a fissural fold of lobule HVI. Folia VId, VIf, and VIg end laterally in the depths of the fissure.

The hemispheral lamellae and fissures apparently related to lobule VII disappear at the medial margin of the medullary area so that they cannot be followed in direct continuity. Lateral of the medullary area, however, distinct segments that appear to correspond to crus I and crus II constitute lobule HVIIA (fig. 53). Crus I includes two elongated folia that expand and subfoliate on the lateral cerebellar surface. An elongated folium which may correspond to crus Ia of other mammals, described below, is exposed when the posterior superior fissure is spread open, with the folium forming the outer portion of the caudal wall of the fissure. The intercrural fissure is deep but ends short of the medullary area. Crus II is subdivided by a deep fissure into two parts.

The paramedian lobule (HVIIB + HVIIIA) of the kangaroo is large and distinct (fig. 54). It comprises six or seven folia that may be divided into two groups, an anterior one of four or five cortical folds and a posterior one of two folds. Their vermal relations are obscure because the intervening fissures do not cross the paravermian sulcus. A deep ansoparamedian fissure separates lobule HVIIB from lobule HVIIA, the ansiform lobule (fig. 53). The caudal folium of the posterior group is connected with the copula pyramidis by a bridge of cortex that is exposed by dissection. This folium apparently corresponds to the pars copularis of the paramedian lobule of the rat and other species.

The paraflocculus is represented by a series of rounded folia that are connected with the pyramis and the uvula by a short medullary peduncle (fig. 54). The dorsal paraflocculus (HVIIIB) comprises a group of large folia on the dorsal division of the parafloccular stalk and a distal group which extends forward to the rostral surface of the cerebellum (fig. 54). Lateral of crus I the dorsal paraflocculus arches ventralward and is continuous with the ventral paraflocculus. The latter turns posteromedially as a series of large folia on the lateral portion of the ventral division of the parafloccular peduncle. The fissura secunda, prominent in the vermis, disappears for a short distance on the posterior surface of the peduncle but reappears as a prominent cleft between the dorsal and the ventral paraflocculus.

FLOCCULONODULAR LOBE

The flocculonodular lobe was described last in the kangaroo because of its relatively small size. Lobule X, the nodulus, is delimited from lobule IX by a rather deep vermal segment of the posterolateral fissure. A fibrous floccular peduncle extends from either side of the nodulus to the flocculus, which is relatively large and foliated (fig. 54). The flocculus is separated from the paraflocculus, in typical fashion, by a deep lateral segment of the posterolateral fissure. Rostrally the flocculus lies lateral of the middle cerebellar peduncle and projects forward from beneath the paraflocculus so that it is visible in an anterior view of the cerebellum.

CEREBELLAR NUCLEI AND FIBER TRACTS

The cerebellar nuclei of the kangaroos are on a larger scale than those of the opossum to which they probably correspond. The fiber tracts presumably also are similar to those of the opossum and placental mammals. The brachium pontis is much more prominent in the kangaroo than in the opossum and a branch entering the paraflocculus is visible after dissection. The superior and inferior cerebellar peduncles are well defined.

Somatotopic Relations

Experimental studies with reference to somatotopic relations of the cerebellar lobules have not been reported in marsupials. The afferent and efferent somatotopic patterns, established by electrophysiological methods in the cat, monkey, and other placental mammals by Snider and Stowell (1942, 1944), Stowell and Snider (1942a,b), Adrian (1943), Hampson, Harrison, and Woolsey (1952), and others, whose contributions have been reviewed in extenso by Dow and Moruzzi (1958), probably also prevail in marsupials.

The large lobules I and II of most marsupials can then be correlated with the large tail, whose distal part is prehensile in many species and whose basal part is heavily muscled. Lobule III of species that employ only the large hindlimbs, aided by the tail, in progression appears small in proportion to the appendages. Stimulation of lobules VIII (the pyramis), IX (the uvula), and the posterior part (lobule HVIIIA) of the paramedian lobule of Bolk also produces motor effects in experimental placental mammals. In addition to spinocerebellar fibers to all the lobules of the anterior lobe, the vestibular fibers to the lingula, probably lobule II chiefly, must be important in the kangaroos. In addition to spinocerebellar fibers to lobules VIII and IX, as in the opossum, the kangaroos probably have auditory and visual connections with lobule VIII, as demonstrated in placental mammals by electrophysiological methods (Snider and Stowell, 1944). Pontine connections with all parts of the vermis of the cat, except the nodulus, have been demonstrated by Brodal and Jansen (1946) with experimental-anatomical methods. Vestibular fibers to the base of lobule IX were found in the opossum (Larsell, 1936a) and to the part of this lobule adjacent to lobule X, the nodulus, in the cat and rat (Dow, 1936). Lobule IX is very large in sagittal section in the Macropodidae; this is especially so for lamellae IXc and IXd.

If one compared the modes of progression and the relative size and functional significance of the limbs, tail, and other organs that are known to have cerebellar connections in placental mammals and correlates these features, as described by Regan (1937), Troughton (1947), and others with the vermal subdivisions of the different species, a somatotopic relationship similar to that in placental mammals clearly emerges. In Macropodidae the relative size of the vermal lobules and the number of secondary folia of each vary not only with the size of the species but also with the relative size and functional importance of the organs, which are somatotopically related to each. A species-related functional factor, accordingly, is added to the factor of size.

INSECTIVORA

THE cerebellum of the hedgehog, *Erinaceus europaeus*, and that of the mole, *Talpa europaea*, were illustrated and briefly described, with reference to its lobules, by Bolk (1906). *Talpa* was included in Ingvar's (1918) analysis of lobules and W. E. L. Clark (1928, 1932) described the organ in Macroscelidae, *Blarina brevicauda*, and other shrews. According to Clark the cerebellum of *Blarina* is the simplest in the insectivores that he investigated. Many features of the organ are very similar in the various families of Insectivora but others differ sufficiently to warrant a description of the cerebellum of representatives of the principal families. Some of the smaller shrew-mice of the genus *Sorex* that are related to *Blarina* have an even simpler cerebellum than does the latter species. For comparative purposes, therefore, I shall begin with my own observations on several species of Soricidae.

SORICIDAE

The shrew-mice (*Sorex cinereus, Sores pacificus, Blarina brevicauda*) are small animals with slender bodies, very small limbs, an elongated pointed snout, much reduced eyes, and small external ears usually concealed by fur. *S. cinereus*, the masked shrew, is one of the tiniest of mammals, having a body weight of 3.5 gm to 5.5 gm (Burt and Grossenheider, 1952). *S. pacificus* and *B. brevicauda* are larger, with the latter species weighing 12 gm to 23 gm. The tail is long in the masked shrew but short in *Blarina*. The eyes appear to serve merely as light-sensitive organs, at least in *Blarina* (Palmer, 1954). The vision of *S. cinereus* may be better since this species has 900 small nerve fibers in the optic nerve, compared with less than 450 in the same nerve of *Blarina*, as counted by Hyde (1957). Hearing, touch, and smell were said to be well developed. The long flexible snout, which is innervated by an enormous trigeminal nerve, appears to serve as the principal sensory organ. *S. cinereus*, according to Palmer, depends more on touch than on smell in finding food. With respect to hearing, Nelson observed that *Blarina* is extremely sensitive to sudden sounds.

Cerebellum

The cerebellum of the Soricidae presents a rounded nearly smooth surface posterodorsally (figs. 56B, 57B, 58B). The vermis is broad and is flanked on either side by a small hemisphere. An irregular rostrocaudally elongated medullary area is surrounded by a narrow zone in which the granular layer is superficial and extends caudolaterally from the tapering posterior end of the medullary area. This strip and the medullary area together separate the molecular layer of the vermis from that of the hemisphere on either side. A small triangular medullary area also is situated on either side of the uvular portion of the vermis in *S. cinereus*. The rostral part of the vermis, as seen from above, tapers anteriorly and turns ventralward forming a hooked projection which ends above the midbrain. The anterior surface of the vermis beneath this hook constitutes the posterior wall of a recess which is enclosed on either side by the rostral part of the hemisphere. The cerebellum is divided into flocculonodular lobe and corpus cerebelli; the latter is subdivided into anterior and posterior lobes.

Anterior lobe. The cerebellum of *S. cinereus* is the simplest, from the viewpoint of form and fissuration, of any mammal except that the anterior lobe of the corpus cerebelli has a deep fissure not present in the marsupial mole. This fissure divides the lobe into nearly equal dorsal and ventral segments (fig. 56A) that correspond to the dorsal and ventral divisions of the lobe in the 21-day-old rat fetus. The dorsal segment is larger than the ventral one in *Blarina* (fig. 58E) and it extends into the hemisphere in all these species. The lateral tip of the ven-

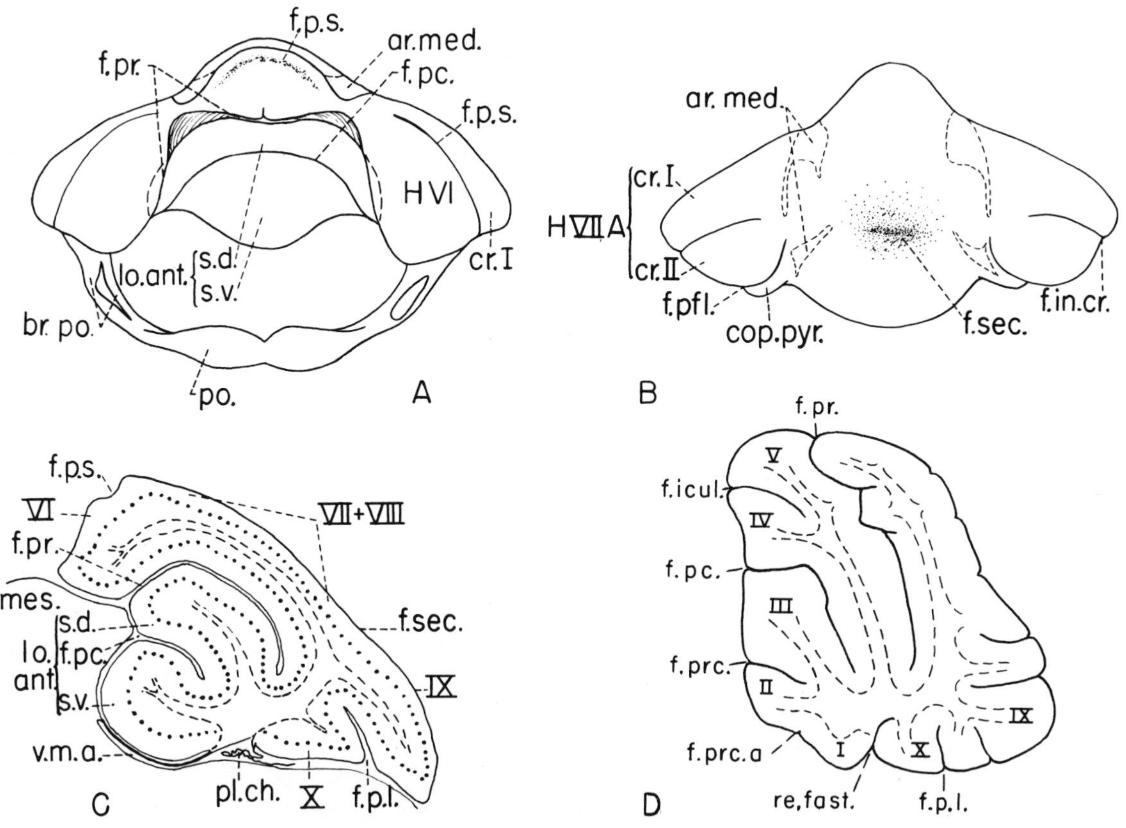

Figure 56. Cerebellum of masked shrew (*Sorex cinereus*). A. Rostral view. B. Dorsal view. ×9. C. Midsagittal section. Bodian method. ×16. D. Cerebellum of *Erinaceus*, midsagittal section. (W. E. L. Clark, 1932.)

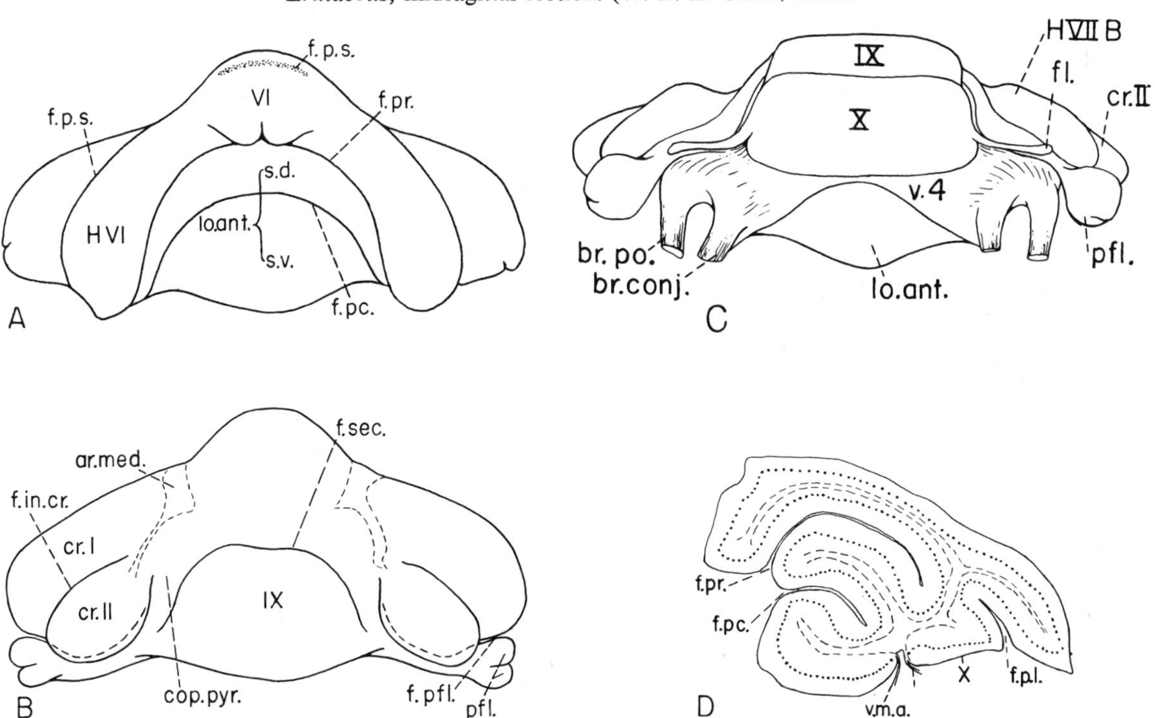

Figure 57. Cerebellum of masked shrew (*Sorex pacificus*). A. Anterior view. B. Dorsal view. C. Ventral view. D. Midsagittal section.

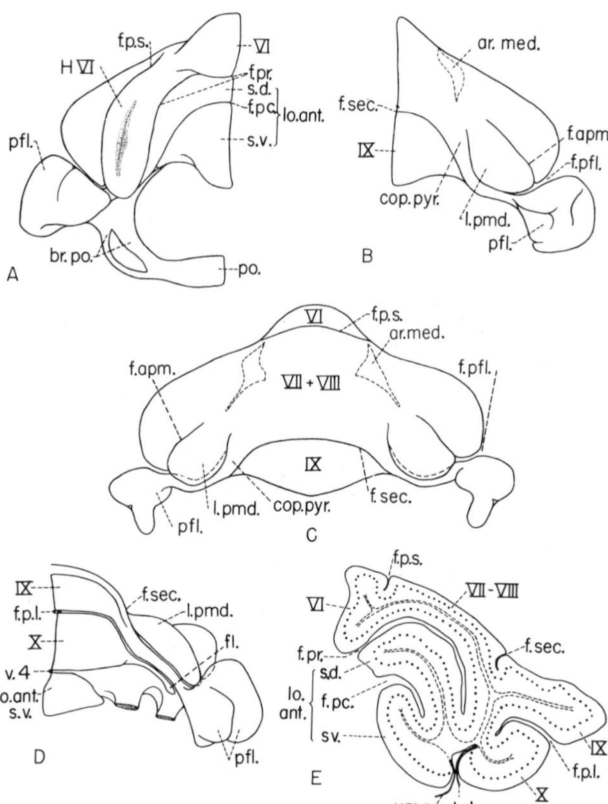

Figure 58. Cerebellum of masked shrew (*Blarina brevicauda*). A. Anterior view. B. Posterior view. C. Dorsoposterior view. D. Ventral view. E. Midsagittal section.

tral segment may also be regarded as hemispheral but there is no real boundary between vermis and hemisphere. The ventral segment corresponds to the subdivision in the 21-day-old rat fetus and in certain stages of the fetal placental mole, rabbit, pig, and human cerebellum, described in later sections, from which lobules I, II, and III are differentiated. The dorsal segment corresponds to that in other fetuses which differentiates into lobules IV and V.

Posterior lobe. The vermal part of the posterior lobe forms an anteroposteriorly elongated arched plate (figs. 56C, 57D). In the masked shrew the only indication of the fissura secunda is a wide shallow depression in the posterior part of the dorsal surface and a slight thickening of the underlying cortex (fig. 56B, C). These features and the branching of the medullary layer beneath the thickened cortex differentiate a caudally projecting subdivision of the vermis which is delimited ventrally by the posterolateral fissure (fig. 56C). Comparison with the Pacific shrew and *Blarina* indicates that this subdivision of the vermis is the uvula or lobule IX. In these two species the fissura secunda forms a definite and typical fold in the cortex and also arches posterolaterally, on either side, toward the caudal margin of the corpus cerebelli (figs. 57B, 58B, C).

Rostral of the incipient fissura secunda of *S. cinereus* the vermis forms a curved plate above the arched fissura prima, the anterior part of which is thickened; it dips in front of the dorsal segment of the anterior lobe and extends farther rostrally above the midbrain than in the other two species (fig. 56C). A broad shallow furrow delimits the rostral and more expanded portion of this plate from the remainder. The cortex beneath this furrow is so slightly thickened in the cerebellum illustrated in figure 56 that it is doubtful if it is an incipient fissure. In other specimens, however, the underlying cortex is more typical of fissure formation. The fissure may be dorsally instead of rostrally situated, according to the degree of curvature of the rostral part of the vermis. The position of this furrow and its apparent relations to the posterior superior fissure of the hemisphere, described below, seem to justify the interpretation that it is the vermal segment of the posterior superior fissure. The corresponding furrow of the Pacific shrew and of *Blarina* is a typical shallow fissure (figs. 57A, 58B). It extends farther laterally, and in *Blarina* a broad shallow groove connects this fissure with the hemispheral segment of the posterior superior fissure. The segment of vermis between this fissure and the fissura prima, including the dorsoposterior wall of the fissura prima, corresponds to lobule VI of other species. Its differentiation in *S. cinereus*, in which other vermal lobules are so poorly represented, and its more pronounced representation in the Pacific shrew and *Blarina* are without question correlated with the large trigeminal nerve of the shrews. A secondary trigeminocerebellar tract from the principal sensory nucleus of the trigeminus has been demonstrated in the masked shrew and *Blarina* (Hyde, 1957). Neurophysiological evidence, already cited, has shown that the corresponding part of the vermis of birds and other mammals is activated by stimulation of the trigeminus. Therefore, it should not be a matter of surprise that the preponderantly trigeminal portion of the vermis of the shrews is differentiated prior to many of the other lobules, since the trigeminus is the principal sensory nerve which has cerebellar connections in these animals.

The elongated area of cortex between the posterior superior fissure and the fissura secunda of *S. pacificus* and *B. brevicauda* must be regarded as including lobules VII and VIII, which are undifferentiated from each other in these species (figs. 57B, 58C). In the masked shrew the corresponding area ends caudally at the incipient fissura secunda. This expanse of cortex, which is considerable, presumably is the principal visual and auditory area of the shrews. Its failure to increase by folding and fissure formation probably is related to the rudimentary vision of the shrews and, compared with the small bats, with the much less acute auditory sense.

HEMISPHERAL FISSURES AND LOBULES

A narrow furrow on the anterior surface of the hemisphere of the masked shrew extends from the cerebellar margin toward the vermis. It is flanked on either side by an inward folding of the molecular layer which penetrates deeply enough to produce a zone much more lightly stained than the adjacent unfolded cortex, in which the deeply staining granular layer lies nearer the surface. There appears to be little question that this furrow is the hemispheral segment of the posterior superior fissure. It delimits a broad area which represents lobule HVI and is bounded medially by the fissura prima (fig. 56A). Lobule HVI tapers toward the vermis and is continuous with lobule VI by a narrow nexus. A wide gap intervenes between the vermal and hemispheral segments of the posterior superior fissure. In *S. pacificus* and *Blarina* the hemispheral part of the posterior superior fissure reaches farther medially (figs. 57A, 58A). Lobule HVI is more elongated and relatively narrower than in the masked shrew; however, in *Blarina* a wide but shallow depression suggests that its anterior surface is folded (fig. 58A).

The remainder of the hemisphere, except for the paraflocculus, corresponds to the ansoparamedian lobule of Bolk. It is delimited from the vermis anteriorly by a broad medullary area and posteriorly by a narrow zone in which the granular layer emerges to the surface. In *S. cinereus*, the ansoparamedian lobule is divided into anterior and posterior parts by a furrow similar to the posterior superior fissure, as described above. The anterior subdivision, which represents crus I, continues onto the anterior cerebellar surface (fig. 56A). In microscopic sections the posterior division is more extensive than the dorsal superficial appearance indicates because much of its surface faces ventrally. The posterior division includes crus II and the paramedian lobule (fig. 56B); the first suggestion of a furrow between the two is represented by a thickening of the cortex of the ventral surface in *S. cinereus* whereas a distinct ansoparamedian fissure is developed in *Blarina* (fig. 58B, C). Crus I is relatively larger in *S. pacificus* and *Blarina* (figs. 57A, 58A). The cortex of the combined crus II and the paramedian lobule is continuous with that of crus I lateral of the superficial granular area and with the vermal cortex of lobule VII + VIII medial of this area, as is also less strikingly apparent in the masked shrew. Whether or not this fact has any significance is conjectural. The separation of the vermal and hemispheral parts of the cortex, however, suggests that they may represent areas having distinct connections without overlap.

The paraflocculus is connected by an elongated slender peduncle with a tapering area which lies medial of the parafloccular fissure in all three species and between this fissure and the fissura secunda in *S. pacificus* and *Blarina*. This area is continuous medially with the posterior part of lobule VII + VIII (figs. 57B, 58C). The significance of the small medullary and granular area at the base of the parafloccular fissure of *S. cinereus* is obscure.

FLOCCULONODULAR LOBE

The flocculonodular lobe comprises a large nodulus and a rudimentary flocculus. Bradley (1903) and Bolk (1906) were doubtful of the presence of a flocculus in the European shrew, *S. vulgaris*. In the three species I have studied the flocculus has a triangular attachment to the posterior lower border of the nodulus and extends lateralward behind the parafloccular peduncle as a small elongated mass of granules accompanied by a slender fibrous peduncle (figs. 57C, 58D).

CEREBELLAR NUCLEI AND FIBER TRACTS

The cerebellar nuclei of *S. cinereus* are represented (1) by a mass of cells on either side of the midline which is the nucleus fastigii; (2) by a prominent mass in the medullary substance of the ventromedial part of the hemisphere, which is the nucleus lateralis (dentatus); and (3) by more scattered cells between the lateral and medial cell groups, which must be regarded as the nucleus interpositus. A ventral zone of cells connects the three nuclei.

Hyde (1957) found a very large trigeminocerebellar tract in *Blarina* and *Sorex*, which have a relatively large trigeminal nerve and tract. The snout of these species undoubtedly represents the principal sensory organ.

TALPIDAE

The moles (*Scapanus townsendii*, *Scalopus aquaticus*) have a cylindrical body on which the forelimbs are placed so far forward that the head appears to rest on the shoulders. The snout is long and naked, apparently constituting the principal sensory organ of these species. The eyes are minute and almost hidden by the fur, which presumably greatly reduces vision. The ears open at the level of the skin and have no conches. The forelimbs are muscular and terminate in broad, shovel-shaped feet with the palms directed outward. The scapula is as long as the humerus and radius together which adapts the forelimbs for digging. Moles were said to swim through the soil, excavating their tunnels with astonishing speed. The feet are long and narrow and the relatively small hindlimbs are

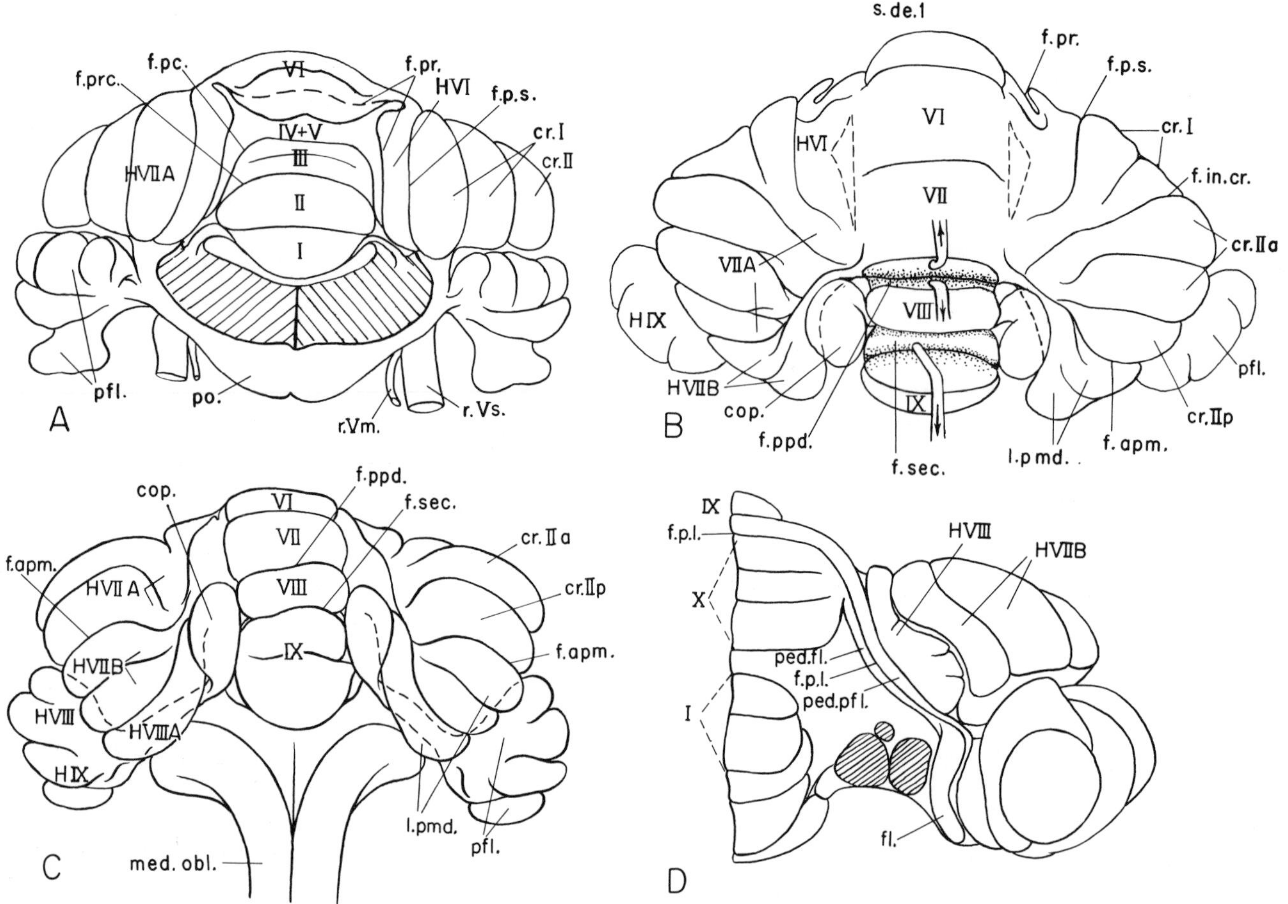

Figure 59. Cerebellum of mole (*Scapanus*). A. Anterior view. B. Dorsal view. C. Dorso-posterior view. D. Ventral view, showing the floccular and parafloccular peduncles connecting lobules X and IX with the flocculus and paraflocculus, respectively.

used to push the excavated soil behind the body. Moles sometimes come to the surface and run with a clumsy gait. The toes of *Scalopus* are webbed.

Scapanus townsendii, the largest of the moles, attains a length of 200 mm to 225 mm, including the tail which is 50 mm long or more (Palmer, 1954). The weight of this species ranges from about 173 gm to 170 gm. *Scalopus aquaticus* attains a length of 145 mm to 203 mm including to 20-mm- to 35-mm tail. This species weighs 42.5 gm to 57 gm.

Cerebellum

The cerebellum of the mole has a similar general pattern to that of the elephant shrews but it is larger and more foliated than that in *Elephantulus*. The hemispheres, especially, are not only larger but also present all the principal lobules that are typical of higher mammals (fig. 59). These lobules are separated by rather deep fissures and are subfoliated. An elongated medullary area on either side of the dorsal part of the vermis partly separates the hemispheral from the vermal cortex (fig. 59B). The dorsally visible part of the vermis is elongated rostrally and caudally, while the anterior end overhangs the posterior part of the midbrain; the caudal part of the vermis covers the fourth ventricle. Nearly all the fissures of the dorsal part of the vermis are shallow, in contrast with the deeply penetrating fissures of the ventral part. A typical posterolateral fissure divides the cerebellum into the corpus cerebelli and the flocculonodular lobe (fig. 59D). The entire organ is more elongated anteroposteriorly and somewhat flattened dorsoventrally, in comparison with other species.

CORPUS CEREBELLI

In a 22-mm C.R. length fetus of *Scapanus townsendii* the posterolateral fissure has appeared at the midline, delimiting a small nodulus from the corpus cerebelli (fig. 60). The latter is divided into anterior and posterior lobes by a shallow fissura prima. The anterior lobe is undivided but the posterior lobe has a caudal projection,

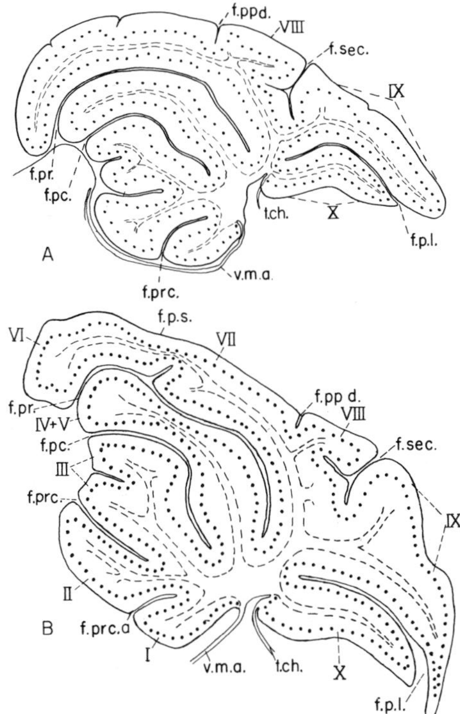

Figure 60. A. Midsagittal section of cerebellum of young adult mole (*Scapanus*). B. Midsagittal section of cerebellum of adult mole (*Scalops aquaticus machronoides*). Weigert stain.

dorsal of the posterolateral fissure, and a forward projection dorsal of the fissura prima. A larger fetus, apparently near term, shows a deep fissura prima and much larger rostral and caudal projections of the posterior lobe; the anterior lobe is divided into dorsal and ventral segments, as in adult soricine shrews, by the preculminate fissure (fig. 61).

Anterior lobe. The ventral segment of young and adult *Scapanus* has three subdivisions that correspond to lobules I, II, and III of the rat and other small mammals (figs. 59A, 62A). Lobules I and II are relatively large in comparison with the corresponding lobules of *Elephantulus* (fig. 63), especially when the comparative length of the tails of the two species is taken into consideration. The naked tail of *Scapanus* possibly is relatively more important as a tactile organ, and the basal muscles may be modified somehow to serve the backward push of the hindlimbs. These suggestions, however, are speculative and lack any basis of anatomical observation. Lobule III is divided by a furrow of variable depth which ends short of the lateral margins. A similar but deeper division of the preculminis of W. E. L. Clark (1932), corresponding to lobule III, is illustrated by him in *Rhynchocyon.* The ventral segment of the anterior lobe in *Scalopus aquaticus* is divided into three lobules similar to those of *Scapa-*

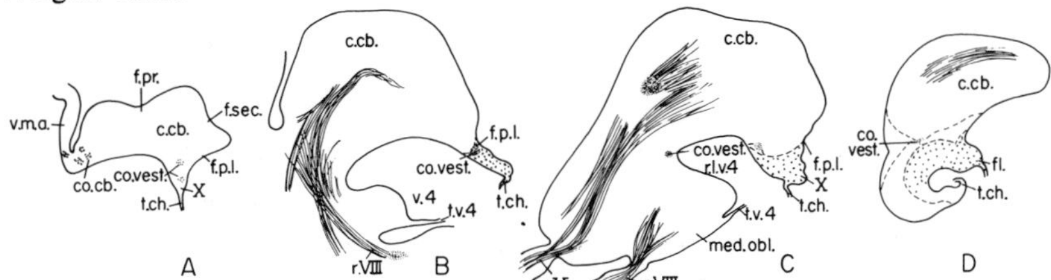

Figure 61. Sagittal sections through cerebellum of 22-mm-long fetal mole (*Scapanus townsendii*). A. Midsagittal section. B–D. Sections successively farther laterally. ca. ×17. (Larsell, 1934.)

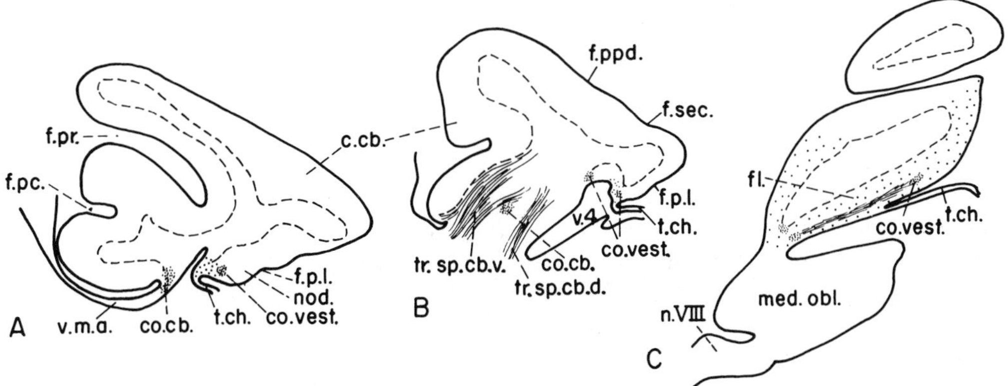

Figure 62. Sagittal sections through cerebellum of a newborn mole (*Scapanus townsendii*). A. Midsagittal section. B, C. Sections farther laterally. (Larsell, 1934.)

nus but lobule I is smaller, possibly in correlation with the shorter tail of this species (fig. 62B).

The culminate segment of *Scapanus* is greatly elongated rostralward, beneath the overhanging dorsorostral part of the posterior lobe (fig. 62A). It is undivided but measurements of the outline of its surface, in median sagittal section, from the deepest part of the preculminate fissure to the deepest part of the fissura prima, in comparison with similar measurements of lobule III, the central lobule, demonstrate that the culmen has a much larger area of cortex; this is further increased by the greater width of the culminate segment. The functional requirements of the powerful shoulder and the modified forelimb of the mole thus appear to be met without folding of the somatotopically related culminate segment. In *Scalopus* this segment is similar but its ventral part is more expanded than in *Scapanus* (fig. 62B). Bolk's (1906) figure of the cerebellum of the European mole, *Talpa europaea*, in sagittal section, shows four divisions, designated lobuli 1, 2, 3, and 4, that correspond, relatively, to lobules I–III and the culminate segment, as described above in the American moles. The culminate segment of all, although undivided, corresponds to lobules IV and V of the rat and other species in which an intraculminate fissure has appeared. As already noted, W. E. L. Clark's (1932) figure of the large macroscelid shrew, *Rhynchocyon*, shows subdivision of the terminal part of the culmen (fig. 64).

Posterior lobe. The lobules of the vermal part of the posterior lobe, except lobule IX, the uvula, are poorly defined in the moles (fig. 60). The caudal projection of the posterior lobe in the late fetus, mentioned above, becomes the uvula. The rostral projection expands forward, above and beyond the anterior lobe, from which it is separated by the deep fissura prima (fig. 61). Lobule IX, the uvula, is separated in the adult from the rostrally projecting part of the lobe by a relatively deep fissura secunda (fig. 60). The lobule is divided by a transverse furrow into two folds with the ventral one being subdivided in the larger specimens of *Scapanus*. The furrow between the two principal folds appears to correspond to uvular sulcus 1 of the rat. In *Scalopus* and the smaller specimens of *Scapanus* this fissure is shallower and the posterior division of the lobule is elongated, tapering to a thin edge in *Scalopus* (fig. 62B).

Rostral of the fissura secunda a second furrow represents the prepyramidal fissure. This is deeper in *Scapanus* than in *Scalopus* (fig. 62). It separates lobule VIII, the pyramis, from the anterior part of the posterior lobe. In both species a fold in the lower part of the anterior wall of the fissura secunda appears to represent a part of the pyramis which probably corresponds to the posterior subdivision of this lobule in the opossum and to a similar deep fold in the rat. The furrow dividing it from the dorsal part of the lobule corresponds to the intrapyramidal fissure of the rat.

The rostrally elongated portion of the posterior lobe in front of the prepyramidal fissure corresponds to Bolk's lobules c_2 and to Clark's pars suprapyramidalis. It presents little indication of foliation in either species. Some specimens of *Scapanus*, however, have a shallow furrow, beneath which the cortex is thickened, probably representing an incipient vermal segment of the posterior superior fissure. In *Scalopus* the rostral end of Bolk's lobulus c_2 is thickened and slightly hooked, as in soricine shrews; a shallow depression on the dorsal surface, beneath which the cortex is slightly thickened, suggests the posterior superior fissure (fig. 62B). If this shallow furrow in the two species be regarded as the posterior superior fissure, in incipient form, the anterior part of Bolk's lobulus c_2 and the posterior surface of the fissura prima together correspond to lobule VI of the rat and other species. The fissural surface is more folded in *Scapanus* but in both species a folium, more prominent in *Scapanus*, corresponds in relative position and even in form to folium VId of the rat and other mammals. The elongation of the anterior end of lobule VI in *Scapanus* and the elongation and enlargement of lobule VI in *Scalopus* probably are correlated with the importance of the snout in these species.

The posterior part of Bolk's lobulus c_2 corresponds to lobule VII of the rat. Its poor differentiation from lobule VI in the moles and the absence of a folded lobule formation can be correlated with the imperfect vision of these animals.

HEMISPHERAL LOBULES

Many of the hemispheral lobules of the mole are difficult to relate to those of the vermis, especially in brains preserved in formalin and dissected in water. In these, some of the hemispheral fissures become very faint as they approach the lateral border of the vermis. In alcohol-hardened brains, however, the fissures could be followed farther medialward. Lateral of the fissura prima a broad folium on each side represents the hemispheral declival lobule or lobule HVI (fig. 59A). The posterior superior fissure is deep on the rostral cerebellar surface but becomes shallow on the dorsal surface and disappears as a definite furrow lateral of the vermis.

The ansoparamedian lobule of Bolk in *Scapanus* is definitely divided into ansiform and paramedian lobules (fig. 59B, C, D). The ansiform lobule, or lobule HVIIA, includes five folia that are divided into an anterior group of two and a posterior group of three by a deep furrow representing the intercrural fissure. The anterior two folia constitute crus I and the posterior group crus II. The two crura converge medially toward lobule VII but are separated from it by the medullary area (fig. 59B).

A group of three folia situated caudal of and, in part, beneath crus II is delimited from the ansiform lobule by a deep furrow corresponding to the hemispheral segment of the ansoparamedian fissure of other species. The two anterior folia of this group are directed medially toward the posterior part of lobule VII (fig. 59C). In their relations they correspond to the pars anterior plus pars posterior of the paramedian lobule of the rat and other species. The posterior folium is continuous medially with the copula pyramidis which, in the mole, forms a pear-shaped elevation immediately lateral of lobules VIII and IX. The copula, which is labeled as the paramedian lobule in Bolk's and Ingvar's figures of the cerebellum of *Talpa europea*, is continuous medially with the anterior part of lobule VIII (fig. 59C). In some specimens only a shallow groove occupied by a blood vessel intervenes between the superficial surfaces of lobule VIII and the copula; in others a deeper furrow separates them. The copula becomes constricted between the lateral surface of lobule IX and the paramedian lobule and divides into lateral and medial parts. A broad folium is attached to the lateral division and passes beneath the posterior part of the superficially visible paramedian lobule. This folium has every indication of corresponding to the pars copularis of the paramedian lobule of the rat and other species. The medial division of the copula is continuous with the parafloccular peduncle which also has a medial connection with the submerged fold of lobule VIII.

The paraflocculus is connected with lobule IX as well as with lobule VIII. No continuation of the fissura secunda along the parafloccular peduncle has been identified, however, and a satisfactory differentiation of a dorsal and a ventral paraflocculus could not be made. A distinct division of the brachium pontis passes into the paraflocculus.

FLOCCULONODULAR LOBE

Lobule X, the nodulus, is a flattened plate which extends caudalward, completely hidden by the uvula. A slender fibrous peduncle connects it with the flocculus which is a flattened and elongated lobule situated between the brachium pontis and the paraflocculus (fig. 59D). The posterolateral fissure is prominent between the nodulus and the uvula and also laterally between the flocculus and the paraflocculus. A less conspicuous groove marks its position between the floccular and the parafloccular peduncle. The flocculonodular lobe is well defined and the flocculus is relatively a great deal larger than in the shrews.

MACROSCELIDIDAE

The cerebellum of the elephant or jumping shrews was described by W. E. L. Clark (1928, 1932), primarily with G. E. Smith's terms but also with some of the terms of Bolk (1906) and Ingvar (1918). Comparison with the vermal lobules, especially of soricine shrews and of moles, and comparison of the extremities and other organs to which these lobules are functionally related, respectively, made it possible to interpret the macroscelid cerebellum in terms of the nomenclature of this volume.

The Macroscelididae are adapted for swift movement over rocky or open ground. The hindlimbs are elongated for hopping, and rapid progression is accomplished by a series of jumps. In walking the forelimbs also may be used. These animals were said to be able to disappear quickly in soft soil or sand by digging. The body is chubby and the head has an elongated flexible and sensitive snout. Most species are 100 mm to 125 mm in head-body length and like other hopping animals have long tails. They are diurnal insectivores, with large eyes and external ears. The long-nosed elephant shrew, *Rhynchocyon*, is much bigger and has relatively larger forelimbs.

The cerebellum of *Elephantulus myurus*, described by W. E. L. Clark, is similar in most respects to that of soricine shrews. The anterior lobe, however, is relatively larger and the ventral segment is divided into three folds (fig. 63) that correspond to lobules I, II, and III of the moles. The culminate segment is undivided and is separated from the ventral segment by a deep preculminate fissure as in soricine shrews and moles. The furrow that W. E. L. Clark seemed to have inadvertently labeled the culminate segment in his figure showing the cerebellum in sagittal section does not agree with the description that says it forms the anterior boundary of the culminate segment. The apparently mislabeled fissure corresponds to the precentral fissure of the rat, mole, and other small mammals; the subdivision between it and the preculminate fissure represents lobule III, the central lobule. The two folds, separated by a shallow furrow, that lie anterior of the central lobule correspond to lobules I and II of the mole, rat, and other small species.

In the larger elephant shrew, *Rhynchocyon*, the anterior lobe is relatively massive and bulges forward beneath the posterior part of the midbrain (Clark, 1933). It has four principal lobules, as in *Elephantulus*, but lobule II is subdivided by a shallow furrow; lobule III is subdivided by a deeper one, and the culmen is also divided into terminal folds (fig. 64). These folds are no larger than the subdivisions of lobule III, as illustrated by Clark, but

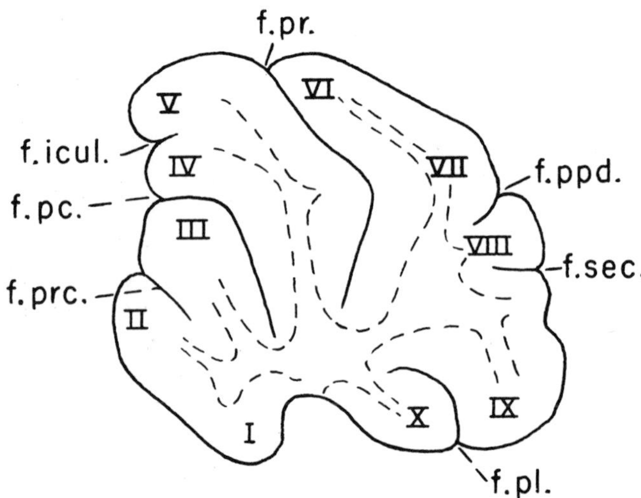

Figure 63. Cerebellum of *Centetes ecaudatus.* Midsagittal section. ×12. (Redrawn from W. E. L. Clark, 1932.)

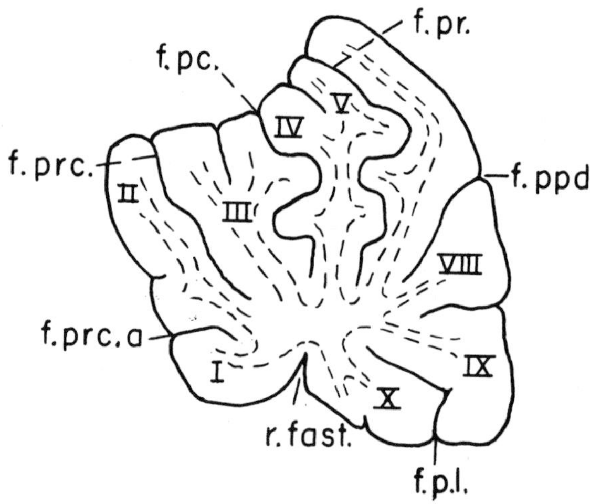

Figure 64. Cerebellum of *Rhynchocyon.* Midsagittal section. (Redrawn from W. E. L. Clark, 1932.)

they may be interpreted as the rudiments of lobules IV and V which, in the rat and other species, are relatively larger and are separated by a deeper intraculminate fissure. The greater relative size of the anterior lobe and its subdivisions in *Rhynchocyon* and the greater folding of the lobules, as compared with *Elephantulus*, appear to be correlated with the more powerful, larger limbs and tail required by the heavier body.

The posterior and inferior parts of the cerebellum of Macroscelididae apparently could be divided into the posterior lobe of the corpus cerebelli and the flocculonodular lobe as in other mammals, but W. E. L. Clark included the uvula and nodulus in the posterior lobe as defined by G. E. Smith. Reviewing the posterior part of the cerebellum of *Elephantulus* from the standpoint of the divisions in soricine shrews and moles, I noticed that the vermal part of the posterior lobe of the corpus cerebelli includes the uvula, pyramis, and declive of W. E. L. Clark. The declive and pyramid were said to be separated by a faint furrow called the fissura suprapyramidalis, with the pyramid forming a poorly defined fold below this fissure. It is not clear whether this fold, alone or including the dorsal segment of W. E. L. Clark's uvula, corresponds to the pyramis of the mole and other species. In the opossum the pyramis comprises two cortical folds and in the mole a submerged fold in the floor of the fissura secunda has lateral continuations to the paraflocculus. Whether this submerged fold is related to the pyramis or to the uvula could not be determined in adult cerebella of the mole.

The declive of W. E. L. Clark is elongated and unfoliated in *Elephantulus* but its anterior part, as illustrated, is expanded somewhat as in soricine shrews. It seemed permissible to identify this expanded part and the posterodorsal wall of the fissura prima as lobule VI. The remainder of the dorsal surface of W. E. L. Clark's declive then would correspond to lobule VII. In the same way, the pyramis represents lobule VIII and the uvula, lobule IX (fig. 63).

In *Rhynchocyon*, as illustrated, the corresponding part of the cerebellum is more deeply folded (fig. 64). Lobule VI, as interpreted in *Elephantulus*, has a prominent fold in the posterior wall of the fissura prima which appears to correspond to folium VId of the rat, mole, and other species. According to W. E. L. Clark the suprapyramidal (prepyramidal) fissure is absent but the uvula has two large subdivisions. In view of these statements the inferior part of the posterior lobe of the corpus cerebelli was difficult to interpret in terms of the nomenclature of this volume.

The flocculus and the nodulus are present in both *Elephantulus* and *Rhynchocyon*, apparently in typical relations, but whether they form a typical flocculonodular lobe is not clear.

According to W. E. L. Clark, the lateral lobules of the cerebellum of *Elephantulus* are divided into three folds, approximately equal in size, by well-defined but incomplete fissures. The pyramis was said to be connected by a simple copula pyramidis to the paraflocculus which is divided by a horizontal fissure into two folia, with the dorsal one being somewhat the larger. In *Rhynchocyon* the lateral lobe reportedly is divided into five folia on its exposed surface, and the pyramis is connected by a broad copula pyramidis with the paraflocculus. Apparently the lateral lobe and its subdivisions of *Elephantulus* correspond fairly closely to these divisions in *Blarina*, as does the paraflocculus; in *Rhynchocyon* the lateral lobe corresponds more closely to that of the moles, while the paraflocculus apparently is smaller than in moles. The descriptions are too brief, however, to justify closer comparison of the lobules.

W. E. L. Clark (1932) briefly described the cerebellum of a number of other Insectivora. In all, the general pattern seen in Macroscelididae is represented but with variations in individual families and species. The larger the species the more prominent are the subdivisions that correspond to those of Macroscelididae.

CHIROPTERA

THE small bats (*Myotis californicus caurinus, Corynorhinus rafinesquii townsendii, Tadarida cynocephala*) belonging to the Microchiroptera fall within the general range of size and weight of the soricine shrews. The various species of the little brown bat, *Myotis*, weigh from 4 gm to 9.5 gm; the big-eared bats of the genus *Corynorhinus* vary from 9 gm to 14.5 gm (Palmer, 1954). *Tadarida* has a flattened head and body whose combined length (87.5 mm to 100 mm) is about the same as that of *Corynorhinus*; in addition it has a free tail 29 mm to 63 mm in length. *Myotis californicus caurinus* and *Corynorhinus rafinesquii townsendii* are among the smallest representatives of their respective genera. The forelimbs are greatly modified and lengthened in the bats and the fingers are elongated and joined together by a membrane. The hindlimbs are small.

The Microchiroptera are nocturnal insectivores that find their prey and avoid objects by an ultrasonic auditory system which includes receptors in flaps of naked skin on the snout of some species or in the skin of the external ears and membranous wings of others. Progression is chiefly by flight but bats can climb on rough surfaces and can shuffle along the ground by their hooklike thumbs and straddled legs (Regan, 1937). The ears of *Corynorhinus* are much larger than those of *Myotis*, the snout is broader and its skin is more folded. *Tadarida* occupies an intermediate position with respect to these features.

Cerebellum

The cerebellum of Microchiroptera is small and has a simple pattern of lobules and fissures. This pattern could be described most simply by following the development of the lobules in *Corynorhinus* and comparing the adult cerebellum of this species with the cerebellum of *Myotis* and *Tadarida*. Division of the cerebellum of the small bats into the flocculonodular lobe and corpus cerebelli was described by Larsell and Dow (1935) and Larsell (1936b). The cerebellar arch is massive across the midline by the 12-mm C.R. length stage of the *Corynorhinus* embryo (fig. 65A). The posterolateral fissure dividing the cerebellum into the flocculonodular lobe and the corpus cerebelli is prominent but no other fissures have appeared at this time.

CORPUS CEREBELLI

A fetus of 13-mm C.R. length shows a slight indentation on the rostral surface of the corpus cerebelli (fig. 68A). This is the first indication of the fissura prima. A similar slight groove on the posterior surface represents the fissura secunda (figs. 66, 67), which at the 15-mm stage of the fetus is as deep as the fissura prima (fig. 68B). The latter divides the corpus cerebelli into anterior and posterior lobes, while the fissura secunda differentiates the posterior lobe into lobule IX, the uvula (lobulus *b* of Bolk), and a rostral segment, which Bolk (1906) called lobulus *c* in bats as well as in adult mammals in general. The early differentiation of the uvula probably is related to the flying habit of the bats since in birds the corresponding segment also is delimited very early in cerebellar development and becomes very large.

Anterior lobe. By the 16-mm fetal stage of the embryo (fig. 69) both the anterior lobe and lobulus *c* of Bolk have expanded to such an extent that the fissura prima is the deepest furrow of the cerebellum (fig. 68C). At this stage the preculminate fissure has appeared, dividing the anterior lobe into two segments that correspond to those of the 30-mm-long rat fetus described by Aciron (1950) and to the culminate and ventral segments of soricine shrews. In subsequent stages of the bat the preculminate fissure deepens and the two segments of the anterior lobe grow in volume but do not subdivide (fig.

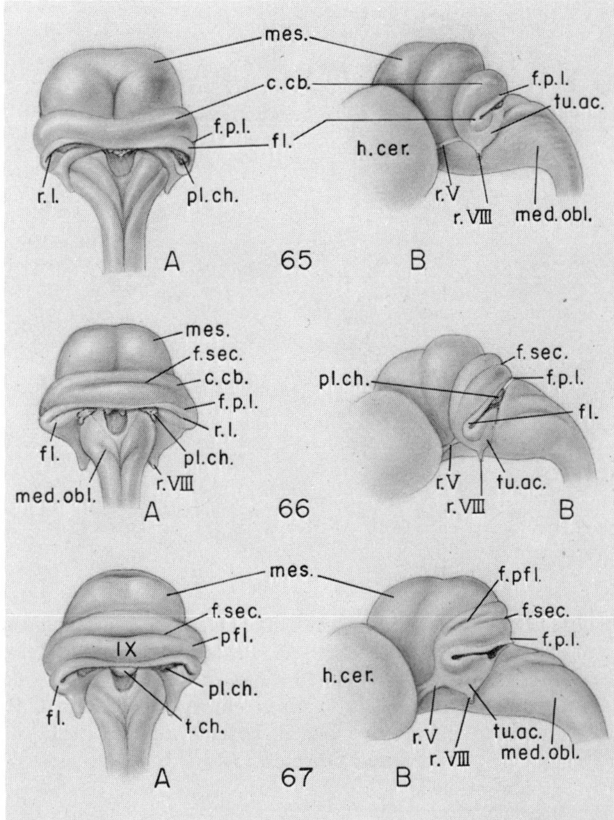

Figure 65. Brainstem and cerebellar anlage of *Corynorhinus* embryo of 12-mm C.R. length. A. Posterior view. B. Lateral view. (Larsell and Dow, 1935.) *Figure 66.* Brainstem and cerebellar anlage of *Corynorhinus* embryo of 13-mm C.R. length. A. Posterior view. B. Lateral view. (Larsell and Dow, 1935.) *Figure 67.* Brainstem and cerebellar anlage of *Corynorhinus* embryo of 14-mm C.R. length. A. Posterior view. B. Lateral view. (Larsell and Dow, 1935.)

68D, E). The preculminate fissure of adult *Corynorhinus*, as of *Myotis* and *Tadarida* (fig. 76A), extends ventrolaterally on either side to a depression between the anterior lobe and the hemisphere, and then joins the fissura prima there. As seen in median sagittal sections of fetal and adult cerebella the two segments of the anterior lobe project rostrally as elongated folds of cortex similar to those of the soricine shrews but they are relatively longer in the adult bats (figs. 77, 79). The ventral segment, as in the shrews, corresponds to the part of the anterior lobe that differentiates into lobules I, II, and III in the moles and rat and in embryos of other mammals described later on. The ventrocaudal part of the ventral segment of the free-tailed *Tadarida* has a small swelling which appears to correspond to folium I, or possibly folia I and II combined, of the hummingbird, although the remainder of the ventral segment is lacking in this bird. The dorsal segment in the bats corresponds to that of the rat and other fetuses in which it differentiates into lobules IV and V.

The anterior lobe of *Vespertilio murinus*, as illustrated by Bolk, also has only two segments, both of which are more massive than those in the three species described here. Furthermore, the dorsal segment is larger than the ventral one. In the large fruit bats of the genus *Pteropus*, illustrated by Bolk (1906) and by Riley (1929), the anterior lobe has a very different aspect and the two principal subdivisions have a great deal of foliation.

Posterior lobe. The posterior lobe enlarges more rapidly than the anterior lobe (figs. 67–75). The portion of the vermis between the fissura prima and fissura secunda, corresponding to lobules VI–VIII (Bolk's lobulus *c*), has begun to expand dorsorostrally prior to the 16-mm stage of the fetus. In the 18-mm-long fetus it forms an elongated lobule, on the posterodorsal surface of which the prepyramidal fissure was recognizable (fig. 70). At this stage the fissure terminates medially and rostrally of the end of the parafloccular fissure. At the 19-mm and later stages of the fetus and in adult *Corynorhinus* the prepyramidal and parafloccular fissures are superficially confluent (fig. 71). The prepyramidal fissure of *Myotis* ends beneath the posterior lateral part of the hemisphere and a shallow depression continues from it to the parafloccular fissure. In *Tadarida*, which has a more flattened cerebellum the prepyramidal fissure ends slightly medially and rostrally of the parafloccular fissure (fig. 76B), as in the 18-mm-long fetus of *Corynorhinus* (fig. 70).

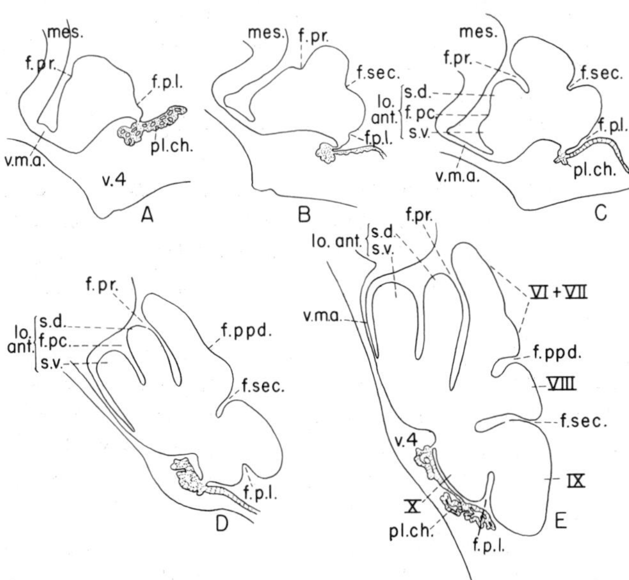

Figure 68. Midsagittal sections of cerebellum of *Corynorhinus.* A. Embryo of 13-mm C.R. length. B. Embryo of 15-mm C.R. length. C. Embryo of 16-mm C.R. length. D. Embryo of 18-mm C.R. length. E. Embryo of 22-mm C.R. length. ×25. (Larsell and Dow, 1935.)

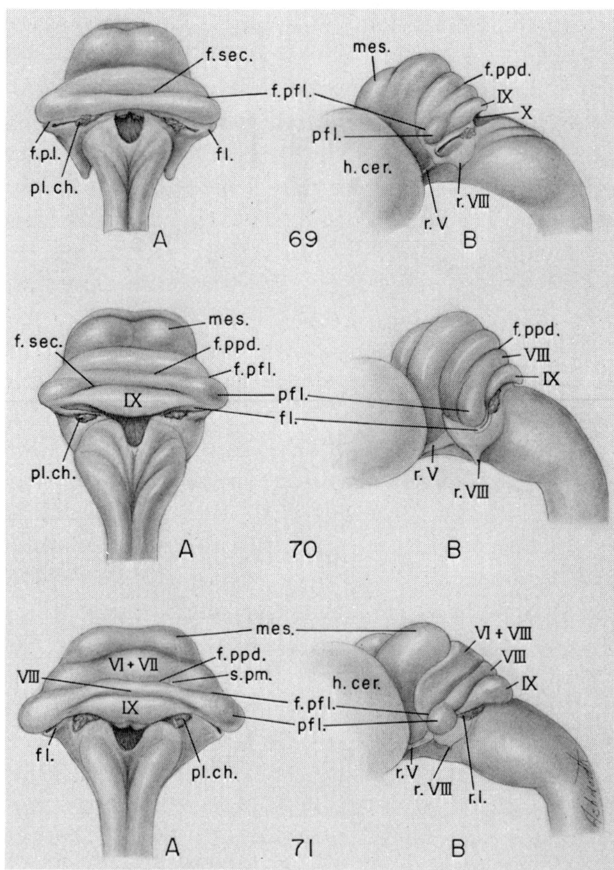

Figure 69. Brainstem and cerebellar anlage of *Corynorhinus* embryo of 16-mm C.R. length. A. Posterior view. B. Lateral view. (Larsell and Dow, 1935.) *Figure 70.* Brainstem and cerebellar anlage of *Corynorhinus* embryo of 18-mm C.R. length. A. Posterior view. B. Lateral view. (Larsell and Dow, 1935.) *Figure 71.* Brainstem and cerebellar anlage of *Corynorhinus* embryo of 19-mm C.R. length. A. Posterior view. B. Lateral view. (Larsell and Dow, 1935.)

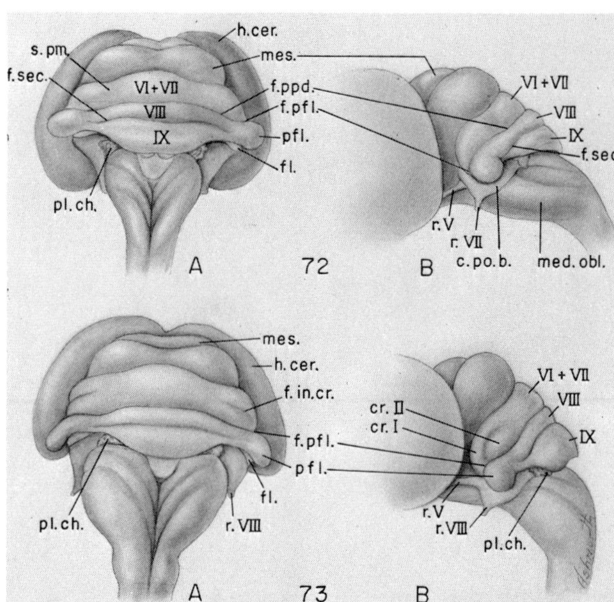

Figure 72. Brainstem and cerebellar anlage of *Corynorhinus* embryo of 21-mm C.R. length. A. Posterior view. B. Lateral view. (Larsell and Dow, 1935.) *Figure 73.* Brainstem and cerebellar anlage of *Corynorhinus* embryo of 22-mm C.R. length. A. Posterior view. B. Lateral view. (Larsell and Dow, 1935.)

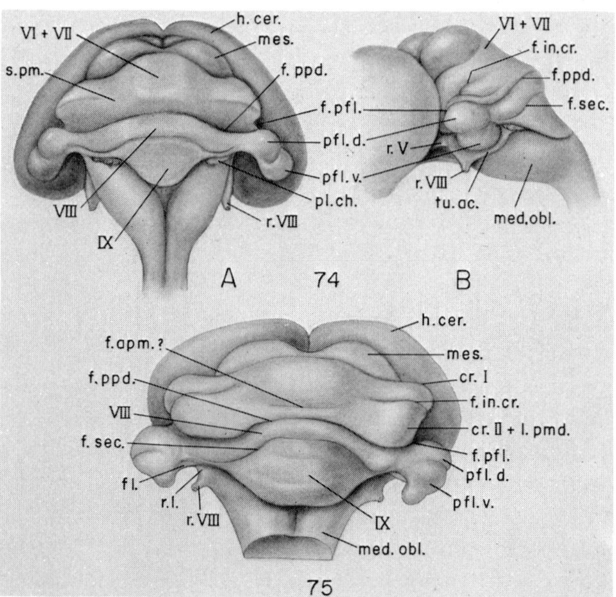

Figure 74. Cerebellum of young *Corynorhinus*. A. Posterior aspect. B. Lateral aspect. ca. ×5. (Larsell and Dow, 1935.) *Figure 75.* Cerebellum of adult *Corynorhinus*. Posterior aspect. ca. ×5. (Larsell and Dow, 1935.)

The variations appear to be due to differences in form and size of the cerebellum of the three species. The prepyramidal fissure differentiates lobule VIII (lobulus c_1 of Bolk) from the more rostral part of the vermis, Bolk's lobulus c_2.

Rostral of the prepyramidal fissure in the 21-mm and 22-mm fetuses, a shallow furrow has appeared which was designated sulcus *a* in our earlier description of the development of the bat cerebellum (Larsell and Dow, 1935). It was tentatively interpreted as corresponding to the posterior superior fissure. In adult *Corynorhinus* a short furrow, which was also designated *a* in our earlier contribution, is separated from the prepyramidal fissure by a narrow zone of cortex. A faint furrow occupies a similar position in the young of this species. Further consideration makes it evident that this furrow is situated too far caudally to represent the posterior superior fissure. More probably it is the incipient vermal segment of the ansoparamedian fissure (fig. 75). A similar furrow is lacking in the *Tadarida* cerebella available but in *Myotis* a thickening of the cortex is evident in the corresponding

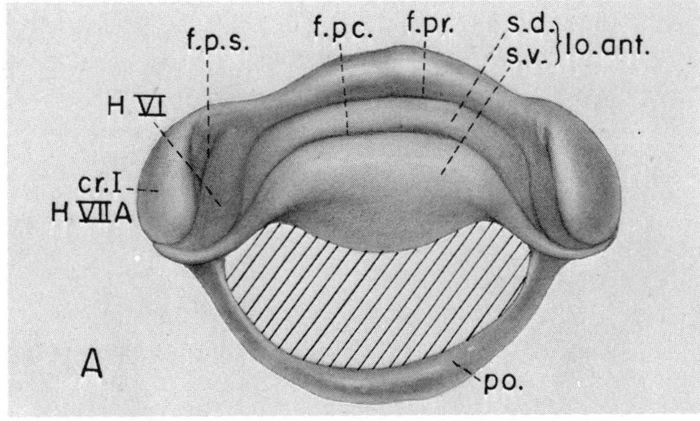

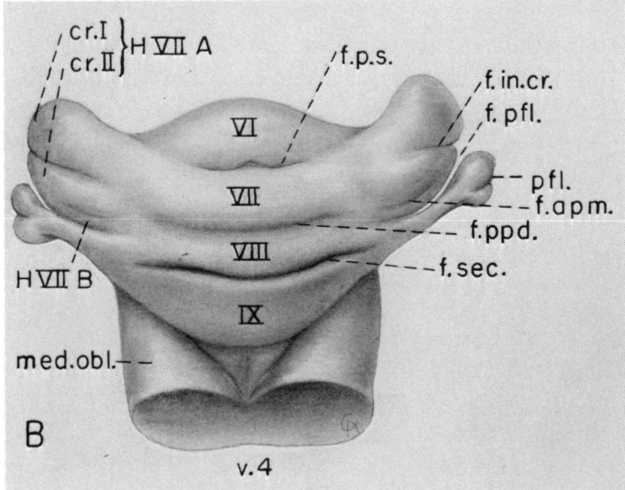

Figure 76. Cerebellum of *Tadarida* sp. A. Anterior view. B. Dorsoposterior view.

position. A 21-mm-long *Corynorhinus* fetus, the cerebellum of which was more advanced than that of the 22-mm-long specimen, presents a slight furrow, farther dorsorostrally, which corresponds in position more nearly to the posterior superior fissure of *Tadarida* and also to a second thickening of the cortex in *Myotis*. Sulcus *a* of the 22-mm-long fetus evidently has been carried dorsorostrally by elongation of lobulus c_2 of Bolk. In *Tadarida*, which has less arching of the dorsal cerebellar surface than does *Corynorhinus*, the vermal segment of the posterior superior fissure extends laterally and rostrally; it is continuous with the deep hemispheral segment of the fissure, described below, by a shallow groove passing between the vermis and the hemisphere (fig. 76B).

Bolk's figure of *Vespertilio murinus* shows two fissures and three segments, none of which were named, in lobulus *c*. The posterior furrow of this figure, however, appears to correspond to the prepyramidal fissure of *Corynorhinus* and *Tadarida*, while the anterior one appears to correspond to the posterior superior fissure (fig. 77). If these interpretations are correct lobulus *c* of Bolk may be subdivided into lobules VI, VII, and VIII in the bats as in most other mammals, except that in *Myotis* lobules VI and VII corresponding to lobulus c_2 present only the earliest phase of differentiation, namely, a thickening of the cortex along the line of the delimiting fissure of the larger species. Sections of *Myotis* cerebella, stained by methods revealing fibers, show a branch of the medullary sheet of lobulus *c* to the region of cortex situated between the prepyramidal fissure and the more posterior of the two zones of thickened cortex mentioned above. Lobule VIII (lobulus c_1 of Bolk) is well defined in all three species (figs. 75, 76B, 79). The rudimentary lobule VI of *Corynorhinus* and *Tadarida* is elongated rostralward but is not enlarged by dorsoventral expansion as in the shrews. The greater prominence of this lobule in the shrews probably is related to the comparatively greater importance of the trigeminocerebellar connections.

In these three species of bats lobule VIII is differentiated and in two of them there is a suggestion of lobule VII. By contrast in the soricine shrews these lobules are absent. This is very interesting in terms of functional relationships being a factor correlated with hypertrophy or atrophy of individual lobules of the cerebellum. Since the smaller shrews compare rather closely in size and weight with the small bats, while *Blarina brevicauda* outweighs all three species of bats, the factor of body size can be eliminated in comparing foliation. How much significance should be attached to the relative phylogenic position of the two groups is problematical. Vision is greatly reduced in both groups. The auditory sense and its centers are extraordinarily important in the nocturnal bats, who prey on insects in flight, and who depend on ultrasonic echoes to avoid obstacles. Thus the outstanding difference between the bats and shrews is with respect to sensory equipment which is connected with the region of the cerebellum under consideration. The corresponding region of birds (folia VII and VIII) and other mammals (lobules VII and VIII) has been demonstrated by elec-

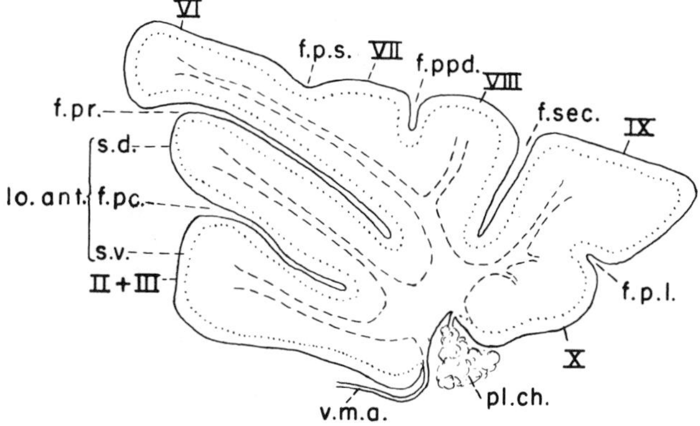

Figure 77. Cerebellum of *Tadarida* sp. Midsagittal section.

trophysiological methods, as already mentioned, to respond to visual and auditory stimuli. It seems reasonable to regard the differentiation of lobule VIII in the small bats as related to the great development of the auditory function.

The uvular segment, lobule IX, of the posterior lobe, which is situated between the posterolateral fissure and the fissura secunda, is relatively large in the bat fetus from the time when the fissura secunda was first recognizable (figs. 66–73). It increases rapidly in volume and projects caudalward, crowding the nodulus into the fourth ventricle. When the nodulus begins to expand, at about the 18-mm stage of the fetus, the uvula overlaps it posteriorly and greatly deepens the medial segment of the posterolateral fissure. Continued caudal growth of the uvula carries the nodulus with it, which in late fetal and adult stages gives the appearance that uvula and nodulus are subdivisions of a larger lobule. The developmental stages of *Corynorhinus* and the analysis of fiber tract connections in adult *Myotis*, however, clearly show the relations of uvula and nodulus to the corpus cerebelli and flocculonodular lobe, respectively. The uvula of the bat corresponds in all respects to lobule IX of the rat, and the nodulus corresponds similarly to lobule X.

HEMISPHERAL LOBULES

The rudiment of the hemisphere shows no indication of subdivision until the 14-mm C.R. length stage of the embryo. At approximately this stage the parafloccular fissure appears on the lateral surface and extends medially to a point rostral of the lateral extremity of the fissura secunda (fig. 67B). The paraflocculus, so delimited from the rest of the hemisphere, remains connected with the portion of the vermis immediately above the fissura secunda by a narrow strip of cortex between the two fissures; it also is continuous, ventral of the end of the fissura secunda, with lobule IX. In the 16-mm-long fetus the paraflocculur fissure is deeper and extends ventrally on the rostrolateral surface of the hemisphere, and the paraflocculus now projects slightly beyond the general lateral surface (fig. 69). With continued growth the paraflocculus is increasingly separated, as an expanded projection, from the remainder of the hemisphere while its connection with the vermis gradually becomes an elongated peduncle (figs. 72–75). The fissura secunda meanwhile extends lateralward into the proximal part of the paraflocculus but in such a manner that the connection between the uvula and the paraflocculus is gradually attenuated into a narrow peduncular band, while the connection between the paraflocculus and the pyramis remains relatively broad. In the 21-mm-long fetus and in young and adult *Corynorhinus* the paraflocculus is divided into pars dorsalis and pars ventralis by a furrow which had been previously called the lateral sulcus of the paraflocculus. The two divisions probably represent the dorsal and the ventral paraflocculus, respectively, but no continuity between the fissura secunda and the lateral sulcus of the paraflocculus is in evidence (figs. 72–75).

In addition to its connection with the paraflocculus, the pyramis of the 16-mm-long and later embryos is connected with the hemisphere immediately rostral of the paraflocular fissure (figs. 69, 70B). This connection has disappeared superficially in the 19-mm-long and larger fetuses as well as in the adult, owing to the confluence of the prepyramidal and parafloccular fissures, but a shallow portion of the now continuous fissure represents the same continuity in the adult cerebellum of *Corynorhinus*. In the more flattened cerebellum of *Tadarida* the prepyramidal and parafloccular fissures do not join and a band of cortex connecting pyramis and hemisphere in front of the parafloccular fissure is evident (fig. 76B). *Tadarida* also shows that the hemispheral portion so connected is the rudimentary lobule HVIIB or anterior paramedian lobule, described below. The relations of the lateral part of the pyramis to the paraflocculus, behind the parafloccular fissure and the incipient paramedian lobule, are similar to those of the copula pyramidis of the rat and mole, already described, as well as to those of the rabbit and human fetuses described below. A slight enlargement comparable to the copula is apparent.

After differentiation of the paraflocculus the hemisphere enlarges rapidly. By the 21-mm stage of the fetus the portion rostral of the parafloccular fissure has grown into a rounded ansoparamedian lobule of Bolk (fig. 72A). In the 22-mm-long fetus the intercrural sulcus subdivides this lobule into crus I and a caudal mass which represents crus II and the paramedian lobule of Bolk (fig. 73A). The intercrural sulcus is prominent in adult *Corynorhinus* but is less so in *Tadarida* (figs. 75, 76). In *Myotis* there is no superficial furrow (fig. 78),

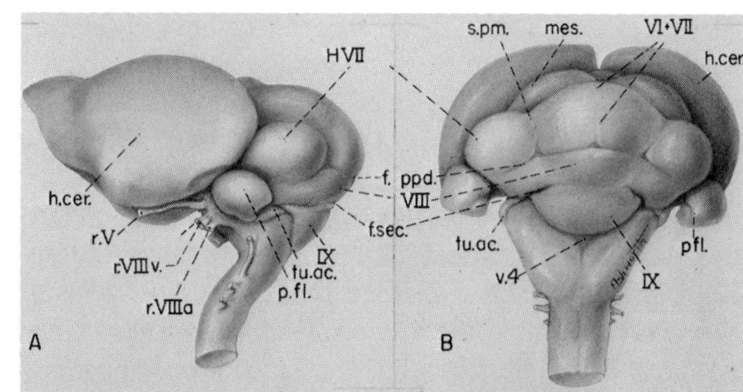

Figure 78. Brain of *Myotis*. A. Lateral view. B. Posterior view. ca. ×5. (Larsell, 1936b.)

but its position is indicated in sections by a thickening of the cortex. Crus I extends laterally beyond crus II and also forms the lateral portion of the anterior surface of the hemisphere. In adult bats a prominent furrow, the hemispheral segment of the posterior superior fissure, delimits this rostral portion of crus I from a narrower area of cortex that is bounded medially by the fissura prima: this represents lobule HVI. The boundary between crus II and the paramedian lobule is not visible superficially in *Myotis* and *Corynorhinus* but is shown in sections of both species by a thickening of the cortex that is less pronounced in the smaller bat. In *Tadarida* a faint furrow in the corresponding position represents the hemispheral segment of the ansoparamedian fissure although no indication of the vermal segment was found in this species (fig. 76B). Crus I, crus II, and the incipient paramedian lobule of the small bats constitute lobule HVII.

A shallow paravermian sulcus appears in late fetal stages of *Corynorhinus* and is also present in the adult stage of all three species (figs. 72, 74, 78). It results from a gradual spreading apart and enlargement of the hemisphere and of lobules VI and VII, without corresponding growth of the intervening cortex. In adult *Myotis* a cortical layer is entirely lacking in the deepest part of the sulcus and the medullary layer appears at the surface. On either side of the deepest portion of the sulcus the granular layer appears at the surface; farther laterally as well as medially the molecular layer also appears. This gap in the cortex on each side of the vermis presumably indicated a boundary of areas receiving certain groups of afferent fibers and perhaps also of areas giving rise to certain efferent groups. Similar areas between vermis and hemisphere that are devoid of cortex already have been mentioned in the opossum and shrews. They also occur in the rabbit and other species.

FLOCCULONODULAR LOBE

At the 12-mm stage of the *Corynorhinus* fetus the rudiment of the flocculus is already formed by the rhombic lip folding around the lateral recess of the fourth ventricle (fig. 65). As the rhombic lip turns upward and caudally it also projects laterally. The rostral portion of the lateral projection, situated in front of and above the lateral recess of the fourth ventricle, represents the flocculus; the ventrocaudal continuation beneath the tip of the lateral recess becomes the tuberculum acusticum and probably part of the pontobulbar body. The vermal region behind and below the posterolateral fissure begins to swell at about the 16-mm fetal stage, forming the rudiment of the nodulus (fig. 69). In the 18-mm-long fetus this rudiment is large in the median plane but becomes hidden from the surface view by the great expansion of the uvula. The flocculus, which is relatively large in the earlier fetal stages, is gradually covered by growth of the paraflocculus. In late fetal stages of *Corynorhinus* and in the adult cerebellum of all three species the flocculonodular lobe is entirely hidden from view. A model of part of the cerebellum of adult *Myotis* shows a small flocculus beneath the paraflocculus. It is connected with the nodulus by a slender stalk consisting entirely of fibers, as shown in pyridine-silver series. The posterolateral fissure is recognizable medially and laterally but in late fetal stages of *Corynorhinus*, as in adult *Myotis*, it is shallow almost to the point where it seems to disappear beneath the lateral part of the corpus cerebelli. The flocculus is distinct although closely related to the uvula (79A).

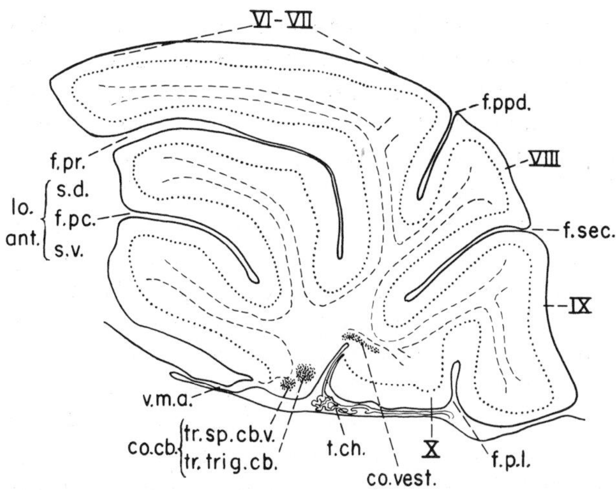

Figure 79. Cerebellum of *Myotis.* Midsagittal section. Pyridine-silver stain. ×30. (Larsell, 1936b.)

CEREBELLAR NUCLEI

The deep nuclei and fiber tracts of the cerebellum of mammals in general are discussed later in this volume. Because of their small size, their primitive position in the mammalian series, and other peculiarities, a brief description of these features of the bats is presented according to the findings in the silver and iron-hematoxylin series of *Myotis.*

The cerebellar nuclei are three in number, including a nucleus medius or fastigii, nucleus interpositus, and nucleus lateralis (dentatus) (figs. 80–82). The nucleus fastigii is an ovoid mass of large cells among which smaller cells are intermingled. It receives numerous vestibular fibers as well as fibers from the vermal cortex. Probably the medial and inferior vestibular nuclei only are involved, since Voris and Hoerr (1932) found in the opossum vestibulocerebellar fibers arising exclusively from these nuclei, and Brodal and Torvik (1957) demonstrated by experimental methods in the cat that vestibular fibers to the flocculus and nodulus are limited in origin to these nuclei. The nucleus interpositus comprises a mass of cells which is penetrated by numerous fiber bundles, some of which partly divide it into two cell groups. Small cells are scattered among large ones throughout the nucleus. The nucleus lateralis (dentatus) comprises a rounded mass of large and small cells that extends laterally and arches downward with the ventral curvature of the corpus cerebelli around the dorsal part of the medulla oblongata. A ventrolateral projection from the main mass of the nucleus continues into the proximal part of the connection between the paraflocculus and the remainder of the corpus cerebelli. This projection could be called the pars parafloccularis of the nucleus lateralis (dentatus). It forms the lateral roof of the rhomboidal fossa and is separated from the ependyma only by a few myelinated fibers (Larsell, 1936b).

FIBER TRACTS

The bat has a relatively small ventral spinocerebellar tract (figs. 80, 81), which reaches the trigeminal roots and arches upward to enter the cerebellar base by way of the lateral portion of the anterior medullary velum. This part of the velar region is not distended by numerous fibers as in higher mammals and scarcely deserves the term superior cerebellar peduncle. There is a gradual transition from the thin medial part of the velum to the massive dorsolateral wall of the rostral part of the rhomboidal fossa. Many of the ventral spinocerebellar fibers enter the commissura cerebelli but their distribution to the subdivisions of the cerebellum could not be ascertained in pyridine-silver preparations.

The dorsal spinocerebellar tract lies near the dorsolateral surface of the medulla oblongata and reaches the

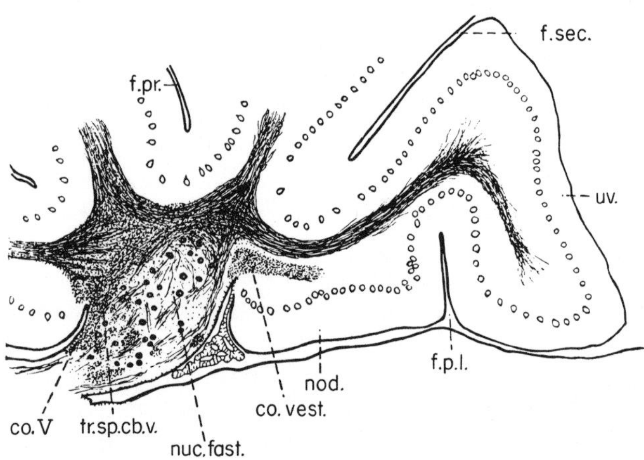

Figure 80. Cerebellum of *Myotis.* Sagittal section through the fastigial nucleus, showing the relations of the cerebellar commissures. Pyridine-silver stain. ×57. (Larsell, 1936b.)

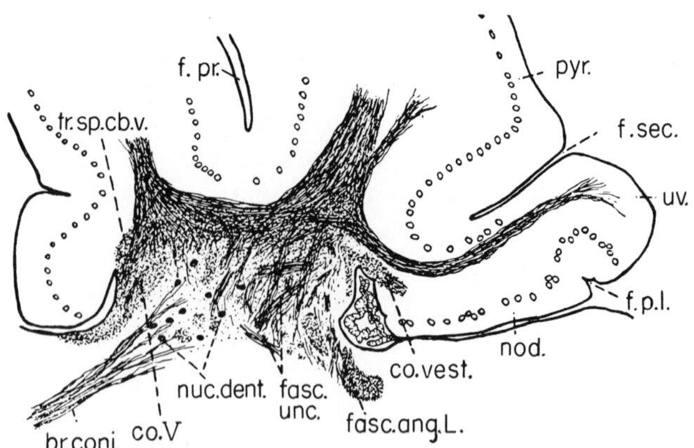

Figure 81. Cerebellum of *Myotis* through the nucleus lateralis (dentatus). Pyridine-silver stain. ×57. (Larsell, 1936b.)

cerebellum through the caudal part of the cerebellar base. This part of the cerebellar base, in *Myotis*, is more sharply demarcated from surrounding structures than any other and may appropriately be designated the inferior cerebellar peduncle. The dorsal tract arches upward in front of the fastigial nucleus, its fibers then being lost among the others of the medullary substance (fig. 82).

Trigeminocerebellar fibers arise chiefly from the dorsomedial part of the superior sensory nucleus of the trigeminus and enter the cerebellar commissure (Larsell, 1936b). Similar fibers arise from other parts of the superior nucleus also. Many of the secondary trigeminal fibers are distributed ipsilaterally in the corpus cerebelli but a considerable number decussate in the cerebellar commissure (fig. 83). So far as they could be differentiated from other fibers in the medullary layer they appear to pass to the rostral apical region of the corpus cerebelli. In transverse pyridine-silver series trigeminal fibers appear to pass also to the posterior part of the corpus cerebelli. The oscillographic evidence of tactile representation of the face in the upper part of the paramedian lobule of the monkey (Snider, 1943) points to trigeminal connections with this lobule which in *Myotis* shows the first indication of differentiation from the remainder of the hemisphere. The relatively small medullary rays of *Myotis* are more favorable than those of larger mammals for following the course of individual fiber systems, but I was unable to trace trigeminal fibers beyond the principal ray which distributes to the subdivisions of the posterior lobe.

A tectocerebellar tract emerges from the ventrocaudal border of the tectum (fig. 84) and passes beneath the principal part of the cerebellar commissure. Some of the fibers appear to cross with the commissure while others appear to be distributed to the ipsilateral vermal cortex of the posterior lobe of the corpus cerebelli – un-

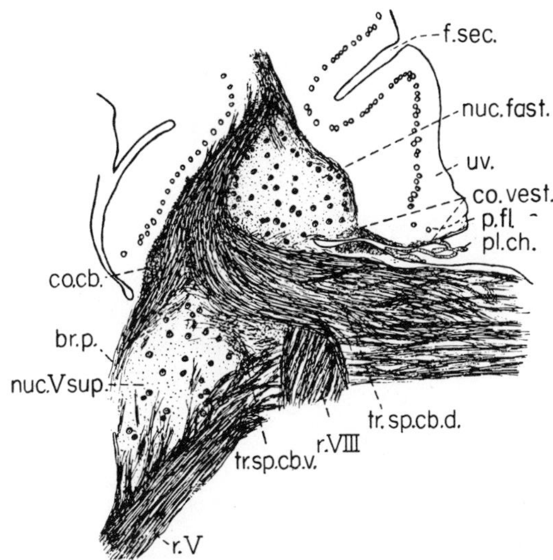

Figure 82. Cerebellum of *Myotis.* Sagittal section through superior fifth nucleus and lateral part of the fastigial nucleus. Pyridine-silver stain. ×42.5. (Larsell, 1936b.)

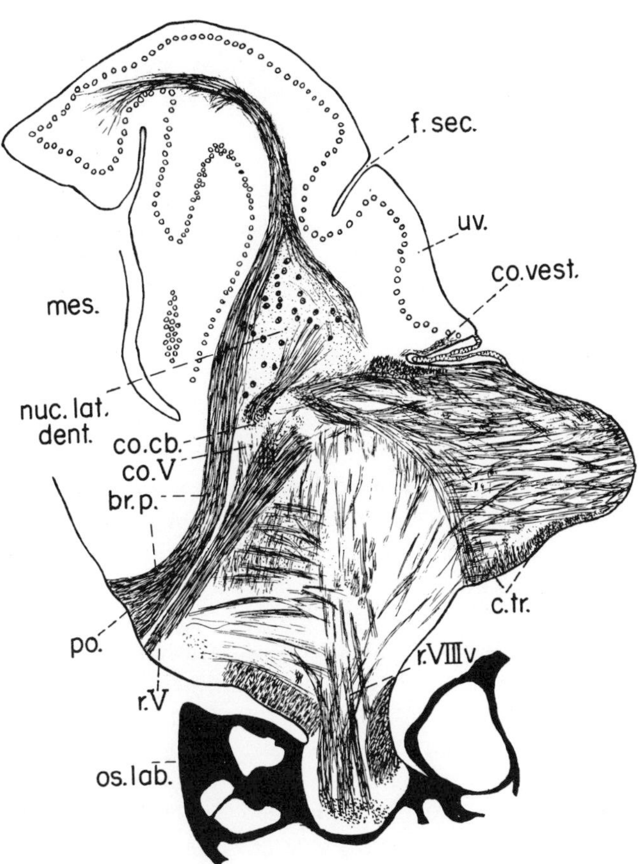

Figure 83. Cerebellum of *Myotis.* Sagittal section through the nucleus lateralis (dentatus) and the entrance of the VIII root into the medulla. Pyridine-silver stain. ×33. (Larsell, 1936b.)

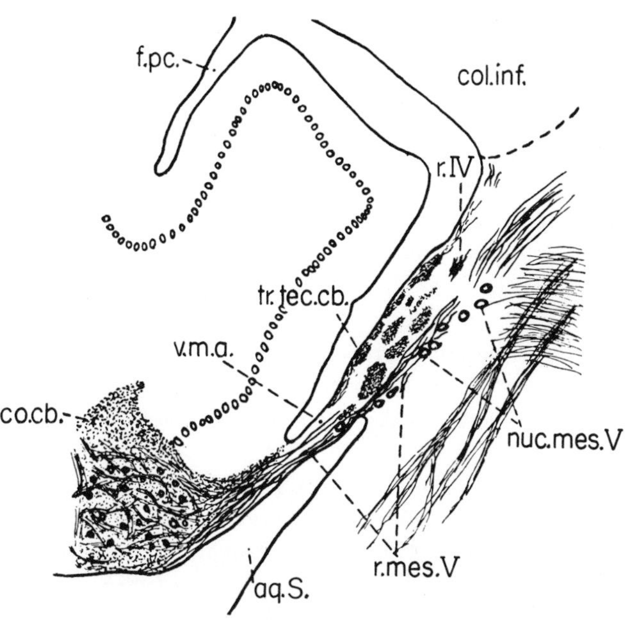

Figure 84. Sagittal section through the anterior part of cerebellum and anterior medullary velum of *Myotis.* Pyridine-silver stain. ×52. (Larsell, 1936b.)

fortunately more specific distribution could not be followed. In the bat, with its reduced optic apparatus, its well-developed acoustic centers and end organs, and its especially large inferior colliculus, the tectocerebellar tract undoubtedly plays an important role in certain acoustic reflexes, as I suggested in my earlier description (Larsell, 1936b) of the bat's cerebellum. Subsequent experimental demonstration in birds (Whitlock, 1952) and in other mammals (Snider and Stowell, 1944) of the relation of the tectocerebellar tract to the activation of folia or lobules VII and VIII by acoustic stimuli appears to confirm the suggested relationship, although the investigations of these authors do not include a study of reflexes.

Direct fibers from the region of the nuclei of the dorsal funiculus reach the cerebellum by way of the inferior peduncle, forming small scattered fascicles that intermingle with those from the vestibular nuclei. They can be followed into the base of the cerebellum in pyridine-silver preparations but are lost among the many other fibers beyond this region. No distinct lateral cuneate nucleus is evident in the bat and the precise origin of these fibers could not be ascertained. Other fibers from the medulla oblongata probably include some from the reticular formation but they were not identified.

Olivocerebellar fibers arise from a group of cells which corresponds in position to the inferior olivary nucleus of other mammals. The fibers take a rostrodorsal course and, after decussating, reach the cerebellum with other fibers from the medulla oblongata that pass through the inferior peduncle.

Pontocerebellar fibers arise from a small pons which is entirely pretrigeminal (fig. 83). The fibers form a compact fascicle which takes a course parallel with the trigeminal root and enters the lateral part of the base of the cerebellum rostral of the cerebellar commissure. Some smaller fascicles, which are distinguishable from trigeminal fibers by their darker color and more compact arrangement, are intermingled with the trigeminal root. The principal pontocerebellar bundle appears to be distributed chiefly to lobules HVII and HVIII, the ansoparamedian lobule of Bolk. Some extend toward the paraflocculus.

Mesencephalic trigeminal root fibers, accompanied by large cells, were found in the anterior medullary velum of the bat (fig. 84). Some of the fibers enter the base of the cerebellum but are lost in the confusion of other fibers. No evidence of the associated large cells, such as has been reported in the opossum (Larsell, 1936a) and in man (Pearson, 1949a, 1949b), was found in the bat.

Direct vestibular fibers pass to the small flocculus, as in reptiles, birds, and other mammals. A larger number enter the vestibular commissure (figs. 80, 81) and are distributed by it to the nodulus, apparently to the fastigial nucleus, and some probably pass into the uvula.

The vestibulocerebellar tract comprises numerous fascicles of fibers from the vestibular nuclei. These continue rostrally and dorsally into the base of the cerebellum, with many passing through the superior vestibular nucleus. These fascicles probably are derived, however, from the medial and inferior vestibular nuclei, as Voris and Hoerr (1932) described in the opossum and as Brodal and Torvik (1957) demonstrated by experimental methods in the cat. Secondary vestibular fibers, included in the vestibular commissure, are distributed to the nodulus, uvula, and flocculi of both sides.

The brachium conjunctivum arises from the nucleus lateralis (dentatus) and the nucleus interpositus. Fibers from the pars parafloccularis of the nucleus lateralis (dentatus) arch dorsally and rostrally before reaching the brachium conjunctivum. The brachium can be followed as a compact mass into the midbrain (figs. 79, 81) and, after decussation, to the red nucleus and the thalamus. No clear evidence of descending fibers from the brachium itself to the tegmentum of the bulb was observed but it was noted that fibers appearing to arise in the nucleus interpositus leave the nucleus as small fascicles, without joining the anteriorly directed bundle, and descend into the tegmentum. Possibly the short base of the cerebellum of *Myotis* accounts for the failure of these apparently descending fibers to first continue forward with the main bundle of the brachium as they do in other mammals. Further analysis of the component elements of the brachium conjunctivum could not be made in pyridine-silver and iron-hematoxylin preparations.

The fasciculus uncinatus is large in the bat and its fibers are somewhat coarser than those of the brachium conjunctivum. It arises from the fastigial nucleus, forming a number of fascicles that arch around part of the lateral (dentate) nucleus and the caudal part of the brachium conjunctivum (fig. 81). The fascicles converge into a fairly compact bundle which takes a course parallel and medial to the fiber tracts of the inferior peduncle and reaches the vestibular nuclei.

The flocculobulbar fascicle or angular bundle of Löwy (1916) is readily visible in the bat (figs. 81, 82) but its connections are difficult to establish. Both pyridine-silver and iron-hematoxylin series clearly show fibers from the flocculus. The fascicle, however, is large in proportion to the small flocculus of the bat; it forms a compact collection of fibers at the angle between the base of the flocculus and the medulla oblongata and then spreads medially and rostrally. Dow (1936) has shown by the Marchi method in the rat that the corresponding bundle arises from the floccular cortex and ends in Bechterew's nucleus, with no fibers reaching the fastigial nucleus. This appears to be true also in the bat.

CORPUS PONTOBULBARE

A thin zone of granule cells extends ventrally from the flocculus toward the entrance of the acoustic nerve and covers the dorsal cochlear nucleus externally. Rostrally this zone continues to the brachium pontis; caudally it reaches the level of entrance of the glossopharnygeal nerve. It is thin rostrally but increases in thickness caudalward and changes from a zone of closely packed granules to one resembling the molecular layer of the flocculus. In addition to scattered small cells it contains large cells which, in Cox-Golgi preparations, somewhat resemble Purkinje cells. The large cell bodies are situated in the inner part of the layer, with their branching dendrites extending toward the surface. Their axons form internal arcuate fibers whose destination was not ascertained. Fine terminals of the cochlear nerve and, apparently, also from the underlying cochlear nuclei end in the cortexlike layer. Some fibers that appear to derive from the vestibular commissure are present in its rostral portion, which is closely related to the flocculus.

Part of this area forms the floor of an anterior diverticulum of the recessus lateralis of the fourth ventricle which is covered laterally by choroid plexus. Much of this area extends beyond the lateral border to the tenial attachment of the plexus so that it is exposed on the dorsolateral external surface of the medulla oblongata. It appears to correspond, on a relatively more expanded scale, to the corpus pontobulbare of Voris and Hoerr (1932) in the opossum but not to the mass of cells and fibers described under the same designation by Essick (1907, 1912) in man, which is related to the dorsal column nuclei. In the bat the relations of the cortexlike layer are with the cochlear and possibly the vestibular systems, so that it corresponds more closely to the tuberculum acusticum of other mammals. This layer appears to represent an elaboration of the inferior fold of the rhombic lip which is continuous in early stages of cerebellar development with the portion of the superior fold which becomes the flocculus. Possibly it represents a specialization of part of the rhombic lip which is functionally related to the ultrasonic equipment of the small bats.

WESTERN POCKET GOPHER

THE Western pocket gopher (*Thomomys* sp.) belongs to the rodent family Geomidae. They spend their lives in extensive burrows and are rarely seen above ground. The legs are short and adapted for digging; the eyes and ears are small. The body is stout and the tail, which is scantily covered with hair, is shorter than the body (Burt and Grossenheider, 1952, p. 82).

The cerebellum described here was obtained from a small and probably young specimen of *Thomomys* (bulbivorus?). The general pattern of the cerebellum resembles that of the rat but it is more flattened and elongated so that in median sagittal section the form of the lobules approaches that of the mole. The hemispheres are relatively smaller than in the rat but larger than those of the mole. The paraflocculus is small.

CORPUS CEREBELLI

The anterior lobe (figs. 85A, 86) presents a pattern intermediate between that of the 5-day-old and the 7-day-old rat. Lobules I and II show no indication of subdivision and lobule III has only a suggestion of a furrow. A slender lobule HIII extends into the hemisphere. Lobules IV and V are differentiated, in median sagittal section, by the intraculminate fissure; but this fissure extends only a short distance on either side of the midline, in contrast with the preculminate fissure, which reaches the anterior ventral cerebellar margin. The hemispheral representations of lobules IV and V, accordingly, form a single lobule which may be designated lobule HIV + V.

The posterior lobe (figs. 85B, 86) was more difficult to describe. In median sagittal section its pattern, with some variations, is intermediate between that of the 7-day-old and the 10-day-old rats. In dorsal view, however, several of the principal fissures depart from those of the rat in their hemispheral relations. The fissura secunda and the prepyramidal fissure are very similar to the corresponding fissures of the rat, both in vermal and lateral relations, and lobules VIII and IX are readily recognizable. Rostral to the prepyramidal fissure a deep furrow, which appears in sagittal section to correspond to the combined posterior superior and intercrural fissures of the adult rat (fig. 25C), is superficially continuous in the gopher with the hemispheral segment of the posterior superior fissure. When this hemispheral segment is spread open one sees that the vermal fissure continues as a furrow on its anterior surface; this furrow evidently represents declival sulcus 1. The medial end of the hemispheral posterior superior fissure of either side turns caudally alongside the vermis and ends opposite a very shallow furrow in the dorsal surface of the vermis, which probably represents the vermal segment of the posterior superior fissure, while the more prominent fissure rostral of it may be regarded as the vermal part of declival sulcus 1. The fissure between the posterior superior fissure, so interpreted, and the prepyramidal fissure is deep and continues without interruption into the hemisphere. Here it forms a deep boundary between a group of two superficially visible folia from a group of three whose anterior boundary is the posterior superior fissure. These two groups of hemispheral folia will be described in greater detail. The vermal segment of the fissure separating them appears in sagittal section to correspond to the combined posterior superior and intercrural fissures of the rat, but its hemispheral relations rule out the posterior superior fissure. Together the continuous vermal and hemispheral segments of the furrow correspond to the ansoparamedian fissure of larger mammals in which sublobule VIIB is well developed, and the prominent segment between it and the prepyramidal fissure in the gopher appears to correspond to this sublobule.

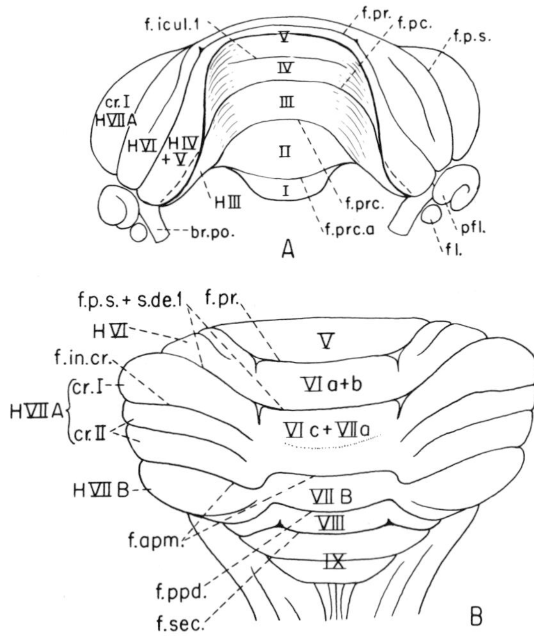

Figure 85. Cerebellum of young pocket gopher (*Thomomys* sp.). A. Anterior view. B. Dorsal view.

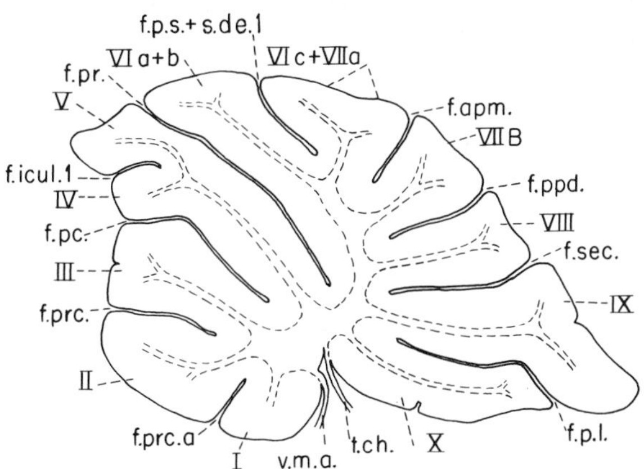

Figure 86. Cerebellum of young pocket gopher (*Thomomys* sp.). Midsagittal section. ×11.

The posterior part of the segment of cortex between the vermal parts of the ansoparamedian fissure and declival sulcus 1 appears to correspond to sublobule VIIA of larger species which have prominent subdivisions of lobule VII. In the gopher it is only faintly delimited from folium VIc. A somewhat similar pattern was seen in early stages of pig embryos in which the vermal part of the ansoparamedian fissure appears earlier than the posterior superior fissure. Sublobule VIIA of the pig, however, although retarded in differentiation from lobule VI, eventually becomes large, whereas folium VIIa of the gopher is small. This variation in the gopher, if not merely individual, is of interest in relation to the probably reduced vision of the gopher.

The vermal segment between the fissura prima and declival sulcus 1 has a terminally branching medullary ray and appears to correspond to folium VIa + VIb. Folium VIc is isolated behind the deep declival sulcus 1, apparently as a part of the segment which also includes VIIa, if my interpretation is correct. Folium VId is merely suggested in the posterior wall of the fissura prima. Lobule VI, so interpreted, conforms with that of the rat and other species except for the greater depth of declival sulcus 1 and the slight differentiation between folia VIc and VIIa.

HEMISPHERAL LOBULES

The hemispheral lobules caudal to the fissura prima are well differentiated. A short caudally directed groove, continuous with the fissura prima, partly separates lobule VI, superficially, from its hemispheral continuation, lobule HVI, but the two are joined beneath and behind this groove (fig. 85B). In addition to the furrow on its hidden posterior surface lobule HVI has a superficial one that divides its broad anterior surface and corresponds to declival sulcus 2. The ansiform lobule (HVIIA) comprises a large undivided crus I and a crus II that consists of two folia. Both crus I and crus II are directly continuous with the granular and medullary layers of the vermian division VIIa (fig. 85B). The intercrural sulcus is deep in the hemisphere but is not represented in the vermis. The paramedian lobule is composed of two broad folia which have a granular layer that is continuous only with sublobule VIIB (fig. 85B). A layer of cortex that is continuous with the deep anterior and lateral part of the pyramis extends lateralward on the dorsal surface of a fibrous peduncle and leads from the pyramis and uvula to the paraflocculus. Before the parafloccular folia are reached this cortex separates from the parafloccular peduncle and continues as a flattened tapering sheet to the underside of the inferior folium of the paramedian lobule. This hidden connection between pyramis and paramedian lobule corresponds to the anterior division of the copula pyramidis of the rat embryo and to the pars copularis of the paramedian lobule of adult cerebella of many species.

FLOCCULONODULAR LOBE

Lobule X, the nodulus, is flattened and extends caudalward beneath the uvula as in other fossorial species (fig. 86). The flocculus is connected with it by a short peduncle. The posterolateral fissure is distinct from the midline to the flocculus so that the flocculonodular lobe is sharply delimited from the corpus cerebelli.

RABBIT

DESCRIPTIONS of the cerebellum of the rabbit (*Oryctolagus cuniculus*) have been published by G. E. Smith (1902, 1903b), Bradley (1903), Bolk (1906), Winkler and Potter (1911), Riley (1929), and Brodal (1940b). These were based on *Lepus cuniculus*, and Bradley included some features of the cerebellum of the European hare, *Lepus timidus*, because they differ from the rabbit's. The present account is based on fetal and adult cerebella of a large albino race of *Oryctolagus cuniculus*. As judged from the published illustrations, the fissures are deeper and the folia more prominent in adults of this race than in the species described by the authors cited. (Presumably these features have a reciprocal relationship with the larger body size of Oryctolagus.)

Development

The development of the lobules and fissures of the rabbit cerebellum, from their earliest appearance in the fetus to the second day after birth, was described by Bradley. The sequence of differentiation and the general pattern of the earlier fissures and subdivisions are similar to those in the rat and pig fetus. Beginning with the 28-day-old fetuses a more detailed account than Bradley's is needed to follow the transitions to the adult pattern of lobules and fissures and to lay the basis for an interpretation of this pattern.

The posterolateral fissure, the vermal segment of which was designated fissure IV by Bradley, was recognizable in the 18-day-old rabbit fetus. The liplike posterior portion of the cerebellum which is delimited by this fissure extends laterally over the recessus lateralis of the fourth ventricle and is continuous with the similar rhombic lip of the medulla oblongata. The lateral part of the lip above the recessus lateralis develops into the flocculus and the medial portion develops into the nodulus. The larger division of the cerebellum, rostral of the posterolateral fissure, is the corpus cerebelli. The flocculonodular lobe and the corpus cerebelli, accordingly, begin to differentiate at about the eighteenth day of gestation in the rabbit fetus (fig. 87).

CORPUS CEREBELLI IN FETUS AND ADULT

The fissura prima (fissure II of Bradley) forms a shallow groove in the 21-day-old fetus. It deepens rapidly so that the anterior and posterior lobes soon are distinctly separated from each other. The anterior lobe becomes divided into dorsal and ventral segments (lobes B and A of Bradley) by fissure I of Bradley. Fissure I in the rabbit corresponds to the preculminate fissure of the developing cerebellum of the rat and other species. In the 23-day-old rabbit fetus, as illustrated by Bradley, it is a short shallow groove, the only one in the anterior lobe; by the twenty-eighth day of gestation it is the most prominent fissure both in depth and lateral extent. At birth fissure I almost reaches the cerebellar margin, whereas the other furrows of the anterior lobe end far from the border (fig. 89B).

Sulcus *c* of Bradley has appeared in the ventral segment of the 24-day-old fetus. From this stage to the 28-day-old fetus it seems to correspond to the precentral fissure of the rat, but when followed in newborn and young rabbits sulcus *c* corresponds, except for its greater relative depth, to the intracentral fissure of fetal and adult rats (cf. figs. 88–90 with figs. 20, 22). A furrow below sulcus *c* is shown in Bradley's figures of 25- to 28-day-old fetuses and in my 28-day-old fetus and young rabbits. Rapid growth of the ventral part of the anterior lobe that begins shortly before birth and continues in the young rabbit brings this furrow into correspondence with sulcus *c* of Bradley's figures of the adult rabbit and rat, along with my precentral fissure *a* of the rat. It seems justifiable to designate sulcus *c* by precentral fissure *a* in the rabbit. In newborn, young, and adult rabbits a second furrow,

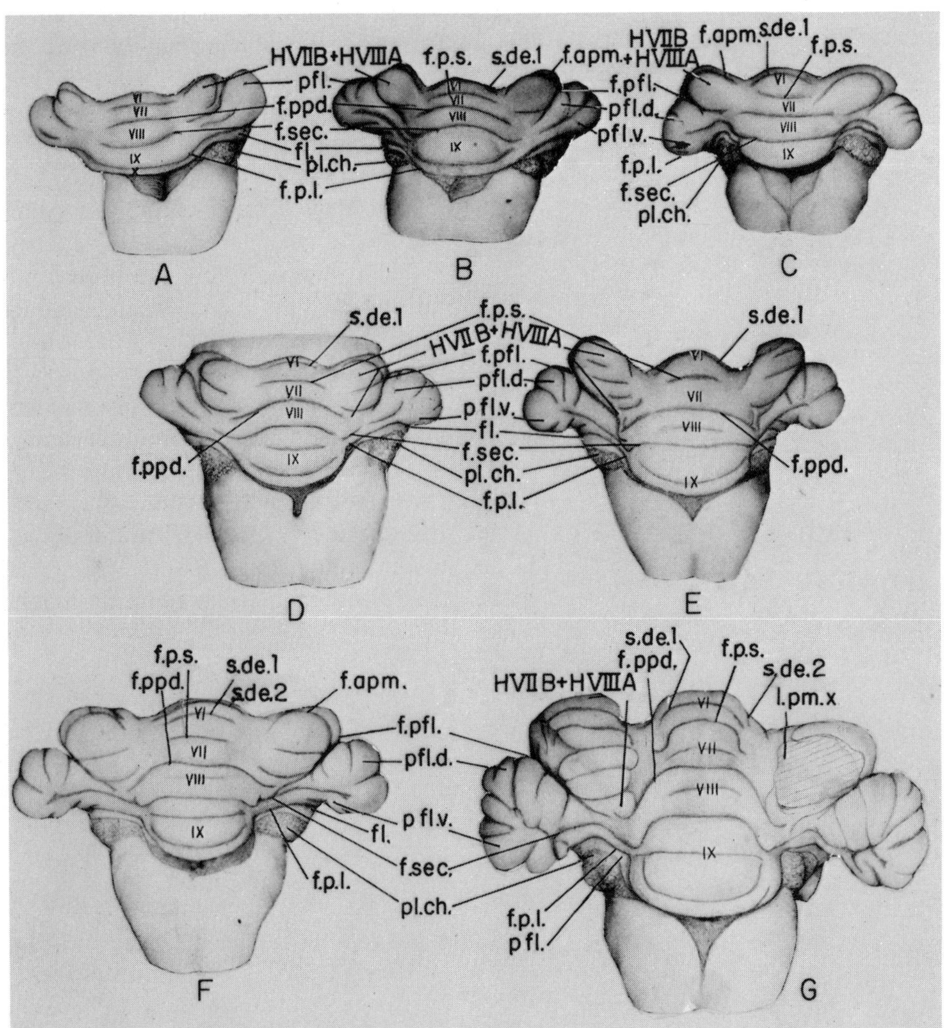

Figure 87. Dorsal view of cerebellum of rabbit (*Oryctolagus cuniculus*) from late fetal stages to newborn. A–E. 48 hours old. F. 3 days old. G. 6 days old. On right side paramedian lobule dissected away.

corresponding to the precentral fissure *a* of the rat and pig, is present beneath the intracentral fissure. The relations of fissures and lobules as seen in median sagittal sections are confirmed by the anterior views of the hemisphere (figs. 88–92).

If the foregoing interpretation of fissures is correct the ventral segment of the anterior lobe is subdivided in the newborn and subsequent stages of the rabbit into a small lobule I, a lobule II of variable size, and a large lobule III which comprises two subdivisions of considerable size that may be designated sublobule IIIA and IIIB. The intracentral fissure, which separates the two sublobules, varies in depth but they conform to lamellae IIIa and IIIb of the rat and to sublobules IIIa and IIIb of the pig, described below.

The dorsal segment of the anterior lobe (lobe B of Bradley) is partially subdivided in the 28-day-old fetus by a short and relatively shallow furrow (fig. 88), which is mentioned but not named by Bradley. This is the intraculminate fissure dividing the dorsal segment into lobules IV and V. In the adult rabbit the dorsal segment extends into the hemisphere where a short gap separates it from a lateral furrow that appears to represent a hemispheral segment of the fissure (fig. 93). Phases of its extension lateralward are shown in the young animals (figs. 89B, 91B).

The above analysis of the anterior lobe of the rabbit is in agreement with the development of this lobe in rat and pig embryos and, through the postnatal stages described, to the adult pattern in the rabbit. The large size and early subdivision of lobule III, as interpreted, appear to be in keeping with the importance of the lower extremity,

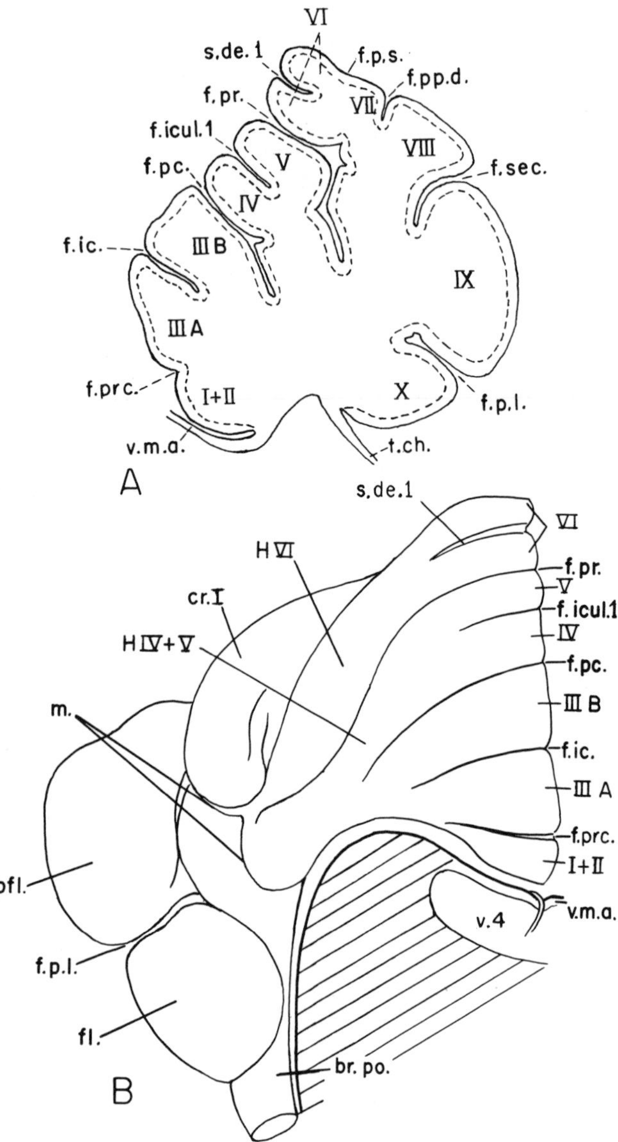

Figure 88. Cerebellum of 28-day-old rabbit fetus. A. Midsagittal section. B. Anterior view.

while the small size and late differentiation of lobule I to be consistent with the relative insignificance of the tail in the rabbit.

The fissura prima ends just short of the rostrolateral margin of the cerebellar cortex in the 28-day-old fetus (fig. 88B). Lobules III, IV, and V are continuous, laterally, with an unfoliated strip of cortex parallel with the anterior margin of the cerebellum. No sharp boundary could be drawn between vermis and hemisphere but lobules IV and V have a common hemispheral representation in the 28-day-old fetus and lobule III is also continuous with it. At 6 days postpartum the preculminate fissure reaches the lateral cerebellar border, dividing the hemispheral extension of the anterior lobe into a ventromedial lobule HIII and a lateral lobule HIV + V (fig. 91B). The lateral representation of sublobule IIIB is carried rostralward with the growth of the hemisphere and also expands, hiding the hemispherical part of sublobule IIIA from surface view. In the adult rabbit lobule HIII lies rostral to the brachium pontis. Lobule HIV + V is incompletely divided by the intraculminate fissure (fig. 93).

The rostral portion of the posterior lobe, corresponding to Bolk's lobulus *c*, expands and differentiates more slowly than the remainder of the vermis. The differentiation of the subdivisions of the posterior lobe, therefore, could be followed more readily by describing the fissures and lobules in order of their appearance.

The furrow designated fissure III by Bradley in the rabbit corresponds to the fissura secunda that differs from Bradley's fissure III in the pig, which corresponds to the prepyramidal fissure. Fissure III appears in the 22-day-old rabbit fetus and delimits lobule IX, the uvula,

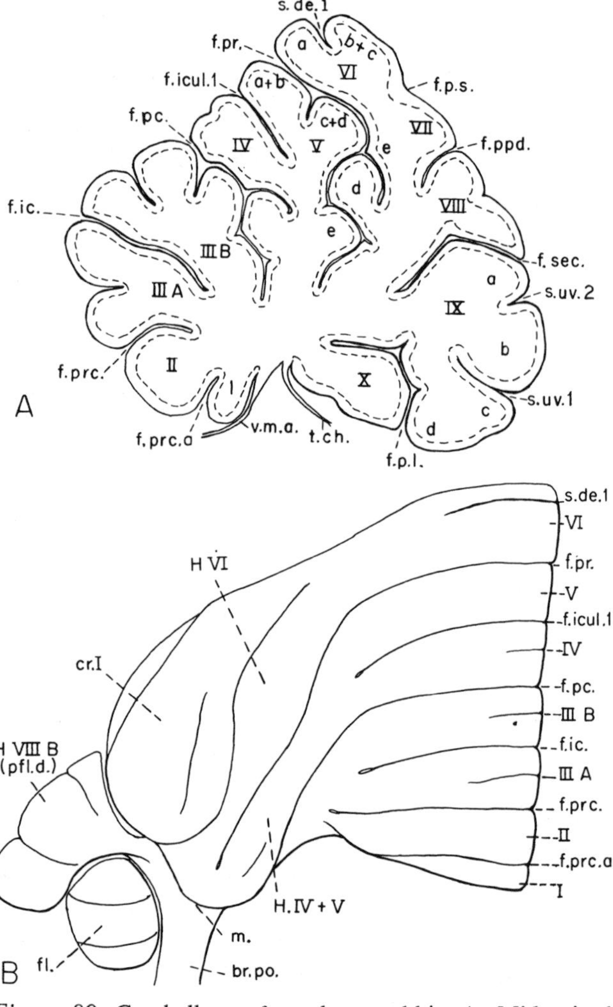

Figure 89. Cerebellum of newborn rabbit. A. Midsagittal section. B. Anterior view.

from the remainder of the posterior lobe. In young and adult rabbits lobule IX shows the superficial subdivisions characteristically found in other mammals and in birds, with four folia being represented in rabbits 48 or more hours old (figs. 90–92). Brodal (1940b), following Bolk's terminology, designated this subdivision lobulus *b* in the adult rabbit and indicated the four folia by the numerals 1, 2, 3, and 4, corresponding respectively to folia IXd, IXc, IXb, and IXa of my terminology. They are separated by uvular sulci 1, 2, and 3, which are deep in the adult cerebellum.

Brodal applied Bolk's term lobulus *c* to the region of the cerebellum between the fissura prima and fissura secunda; this interpretation does not agree with that of Ingvar (1918) who stated that the two caudal folia formed the pyramis. According to Brodal no fissure of the vermis of the adult rabbit can be convincingly homologized with the prepyramidal fissure of other mammals. In our 28-day-old rabbit fetuses a distinct furrow has appeared rostral to the fissura secunda. Bradley also observed this furrow in the 28-day-old fetus, designated it fissure *a*, and regarded it as having considerable morphological significance, although he noted that fissure *a* is relatively shallow in the adult rabbit. Fissure *a* extends lateralward as the rostral boundary of a lateral continuation of the two folia, mentioned above, that could only be interpreted as the copula pyramidis. The copula has connections with the dorsal paraflocculus and the paramedian lobule, as in the rat and other species. The further differentiation of adjacent structures that can be homologized with those of other mammals, together with

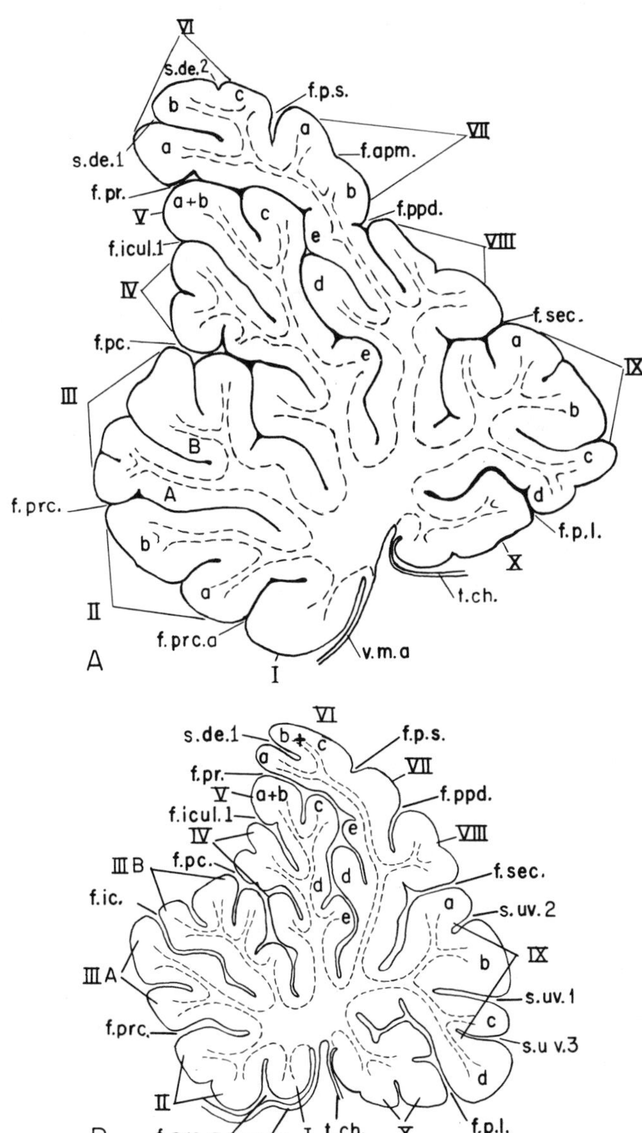

Figure 90. Cerebellum of rabbit. Midsagittal section. A. 48 hours old. B. 3 days old.

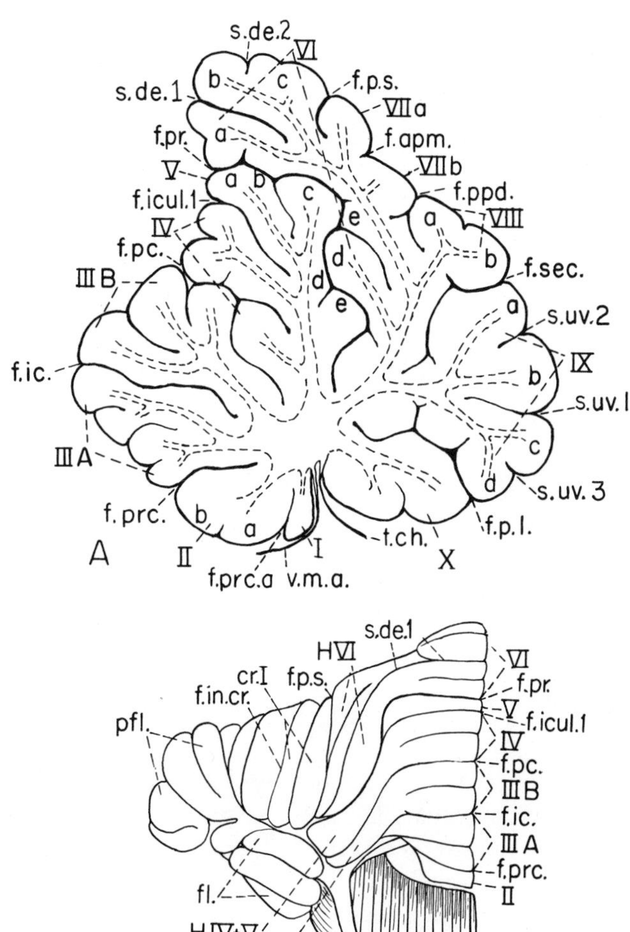

Figure 91. Cerebellum of 6-day-old rabbit. A. Midsagittal section. B. Anterior view.

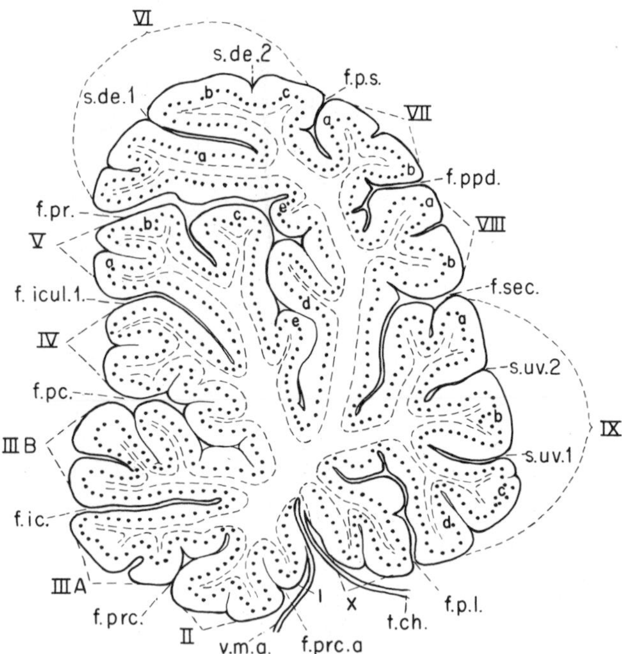

Figure 92. Midsagittal section of cerebellum of adult rabbit (*Oryctolagus* sp.).

the lateral relations of the two folia situated in front of the fissura secunda and of the furrow rostral to these, clearly demonstrates that the folia represent the pyramis and the furrow represents the prepyramidal fissure. The prepyramidal fissure does not open into the parafloccular fissure at any stage of cerebellar development in the rabbit, which is different from its state in bats and in more than 30-day-old opossums. In the rabbit, as in the rat and pig, a cortical connection between the copula pyramidis and the paramedian lobule prevents continuity of the two fissures at all stages of development (figs. 87A–G). In the adult rabbit the prepyramidal fissure terminates laterally beneath the caudal part of the paramedian lobule (fig. 94B). Its vermian segment curves ventralward, in sagittal section, and the walls are formed by small folia in the large rabbits used in our investigations (fig. 92).

Rostral to the prepyramidal fissure a shallow groove is visible in the 28-day-old fetus, which is also shown but not labeled in Bradley's figures of sagittal sections through the cerebellum of fetal and adult rabbits and in Brodal's figures of the adult. The furrow deepens rapidly after birth but remains confined to the vermis. In its development and adult relations the furrow corresponds to the vermal segment of the posterior superior fissure of other species and delimits lobule VII rostrally. Laterally the furrow disappears at the medial border of a medullary area in the floor of the paravermian sulcus. A shallow furrow appears in lobule VII, at about the end of the second day postpartum, which is visible in sagittal sections (figs. 90A, 92) but not always in surface views of two- and three-day-old rabbits (fig. 87E, F). This furrow corresponds to the vermian segment of the ansoparamedian fissure of other species that divides lobule VII into two folia representing small versions of sublobules VIIA and VIIB of many mammals. Because of their resemblance, even in the adult rabbit, to folia rather than lobules they are designated VIIa and VIIb.

The rostrally projecting portion of the posterior lobe is short in the 28-day-old fetus. A deep groove, declival sulcus 2, divides it into two folia. By 48 hours after birth, this segment was recognizable as lobule VI on account of the deepening posterior superior fissure. Declival sulcus 2 has deepened and a shallow declival sulcus 1 has appeared on the dorsal surface in the 28-day-old fetus. Lobule VI is thus divided into the three typical folia, VIa, VIb, and VIc, in the young rabbit; folium VIa by the adult stage has grown into a lamella with two secondary surface folia (fig. 92). In Brodal's figure (modified from Winkler and Potter, 1911) of a median sagittal section of

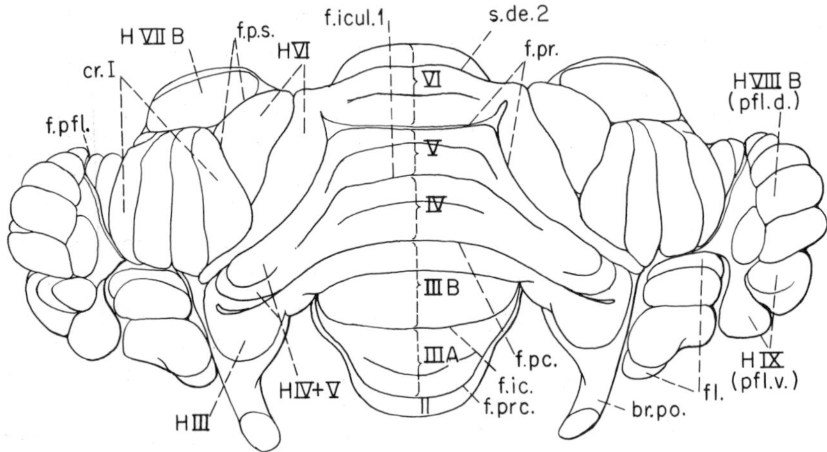

Figure 93. Anterior view of cerebellum of adult rabbit (*Oryctolagus* sp.).

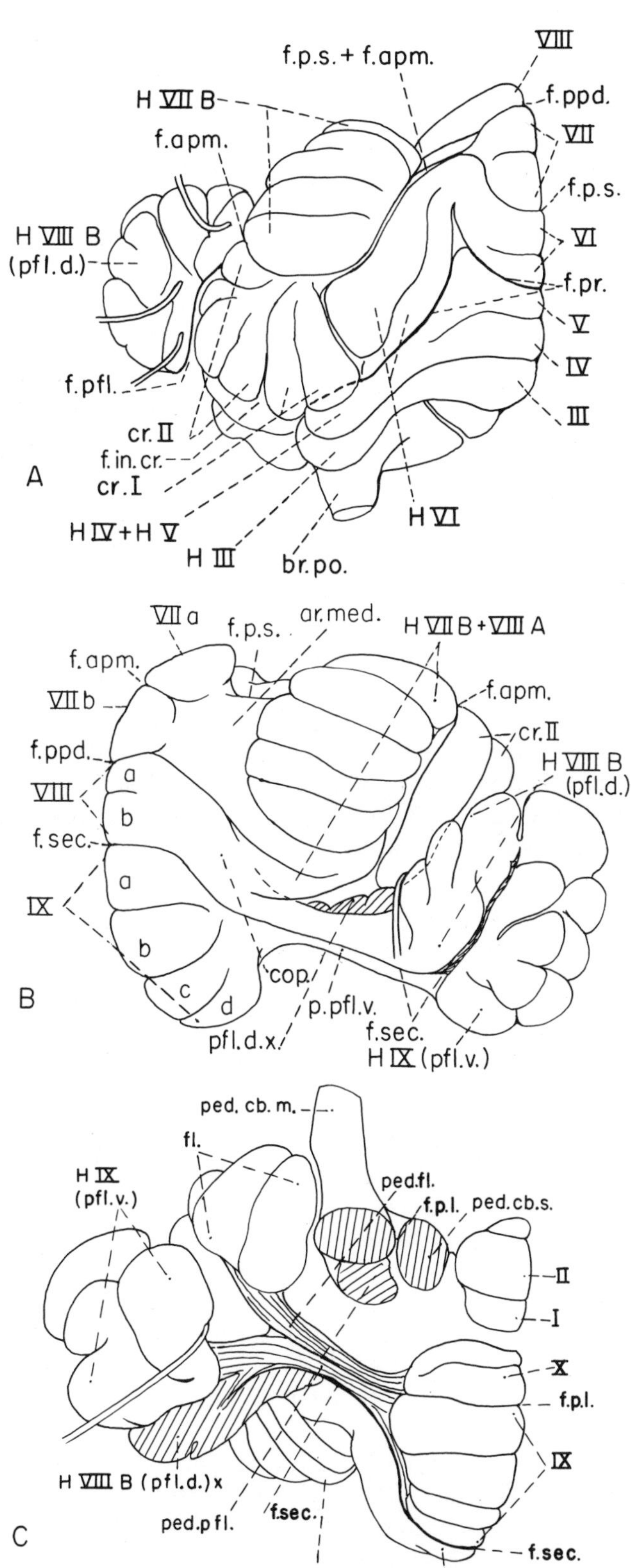

Figure 94. Cerebellum of adult rabbit (*Oryctolagus* sp.). A. Anterodorsal view. B. Posterolateral view. C. Ventral view.

the adult rabbit cerebellum, declival sulcus 2 (not labeled) is deep but only a shallow groove on the dorsal surface is suggestive of declival sulcus 1. Bradley (1903), in the adult rabbit, designated declival sulcus 2 as fissure *b* and described it as being parallel with the fissura prima for some distance in the hemisphere. His figures show declival sulcus 1 and folia VIa, VIb, and VIc but they are unlabeled.

Lobules VI, VII, and VIII, although relatively small and separated by shallower fissures than in most mammals of comparable size, are clearly differentiated in the adult rabbit. The flattening of the lobules and the shallow fissures result from the rostral elongation of much of the posterior lobe above the anterior lobe in the same manner as in many marsupials, shrews, bats, and other rodents. If this elongated region were telescoped together, rostrocaudally, as in other marsupials, shrews, bats, and rodents, in addition to higher mammals, more pronounced lobules and deeper fissures would result.

HEMISPHERAL LOBULES

In the 28-day-old fetus declival sulcus 2 of lobule VI, although deep, extends only to the lateral margin of the vermis. Folia VIa and VIb + c, which it separates, converge laterally into a broad hemispheral fold of cortex, the rudiment of lobule HVI. The hemispheral segment of declival sulcus 2 has extended to the cerebellar margin in the 6-day-old rabbit and completely divided lobule HVI into two folia (fig. 91B). By the adult stage lobule HVI has expanded and lobule VI has projected far rostralward, with a resulting sharp notch between them. Across the floor of this notch, however, the two lobules maintain continuity by a constricted zone in which declival sulcus 2 may be interrupted (fig. 94A). Brodal (1940b) regarded only the first folium behind the hemispheral segment of the fissura prima as part of the lobulus simplex of Bolk. The second folium he assigned to the ansiform lobule because it does not present a smooth transition from vermis to hemisphere owing to the interruption by the paravermian sulcus. The development of lobule VI and its laterally related folia in late fetal and young rabbits, however, demonstrates that both of the hemispheral folia mentioned above are continuous medially with lobule VI and constitute the hemispheral part of Bolk's lobulus simplex, more specifically designated in this volume as lobule HVI.

A similar although less distinct demarcation of the hemispheral from the vermal part of the lobulus simplex was also found in the pig, cat, and man, as described later on. In many mammals of which only the adult cerebellum has been available, lobules VI and HVI are connected by a constricted nexus in the floor of the paravermian sulcus and lobule HVI is as distinct as the hemispheral lobules related to lobules VII and VIII. The conception of a single division of the cerebellum including both vermal and hemispheral folia immediately behind the fissura prima, which Bolk (1906) defined as the lobulus simplex, is not justified on morphological grounds, as its development shows. Except in the smaller primates and some other small species lobules VI and HVI, considered together, have far from a simple pattern. In the interests of morphological clarity as well as descriptive accuracy, in view of the many exceptions, the term lobulus simplex should be discontinued.

The ansiform lobule is differentiated from lobule HVI by the gradual formation of the hemispheral segment of the posterior superior fissure. In the 28-day-old fetus this segment of the fissure is well defined although the vermal segment is still shallow, deepening in later stages as already described. The two segments do not become confluent so that it is difficult to relate them with each other in the distorted cerebellum of the rabbit. The interpretations indicated in figures 87, 93, and 94, however, appear to be justified by the relations of the two segments to the respective vermal and hemispheral lobules which they delimit. The ansoparamedian fissure has appeared in the 28-day-old fetus. The ansiform lobule is undivided except for a slight groove on its anterior surface. In the 6-day-old rabbit five folia show and in the adult there are six; the two medial ones are delimited from the lateral group of four by a furrow that is deeper than the others and which I interpreted as the intercrural sulcus (fig. 94A). The two medial folia constitute crus I and the lateral group crus II. Riley (1929) described an intercrural sulcus in *Lepus* as delimiting a group of two or three lateral folia from the medial group, but Brodal (1940c) was not convinced that this furrow could be distinguished. This author's photographs of the cerebellum of the rabbit, presumably *Lepus cuniculus*, show six folia that appear to be included by him in the ansiform lobule. The one most medially situated, however, resembles lobule HVI, described above, which has only one folium that was assigned by Brodal to the "lobulus simplex." The five folia situated lateral of this one in *Lepus* correspond to the five of the ansiform lobule of young *Oryctolagus*. In adults of the latter species the ansiform lobule partially covers the ventrolateral part of lobule HVI (fig. 94A). It is probable that the four folia of crus II represent more complete foliation in this larger race of rabbits.

The paramedian lobule forms a small knob, in the 28-day-old fetus, which is separated from the paraflocculus by a deep parafloccular fissure and from the ansiform lobule by the ansoparamedian fissure (fig. 94A, B). The paramedian lobule lies opposite lobules VII and VIII at this stage of development but is crowded forward by the rapid growth of the paraflocculus. The vermal relations of the ansiform and paramedian lobules are obscured by the rostral displacement of both. In its early development the paramedian lobule is more directly continuous with lobule VII than with lobule VI by an area of unfoliated cortex. As it expands rostralward the anterior portion of the lobule lies lateral of lobule VI (fig. 87). By the adult stage the area medullaris has appeared, separating the cortex of this region into vermal and hemispheral zones. The absence of fissures across this area makes it difficult to determine the relations of the vermal and hemispheral segments to each other. Association fiber connections between the paramedian lobule and the vermis were demonstrated by Jansen (1933) with the Marchi method. The spread of degenerated fibers, following lesions in the paramedian lobule, included lobules VI, VII, and VIII, but no evidence of fibers from the vermis to the paramedian lobule or other hemispheral division was obtained. In the rat, as already noted, there is continuity of cortex between the paramedian lobule and sublobule VIIb, especially of the vermis. In other species, which will be described, medullary connections were found between the deep part of the paramedian lobule and sublobules VIIA, VIIB, and VIIIA; the most extensive of these appear to be made with sublobule VIIB. In the rabbit the caudal folium of the paramedian lobule is clearly continuous by a narrow cortical band with the copula pyramidis and through the latter with lobule VIII (figs. 87G, 94B).

The dorsal paraflocculus is continuous medially with lobule VIII, whereas the ventral paraflocculus is continuous with lobule IX. The parafloccular peduncle lengthens and becomes relatively more attenuated as the cerebellum grows in volume. In the newborn rabbit the dorsal paraflocculus has begun to foliate (fig. 89B). The ventral paraflocculus begins to foliate at about the end of the third day postpartum (fig. 87). By six days postpartum the paraflocculus has assumed the characteristic form of the lobulus petrosus of the adult rabbit (fig. 87), with both dorsal and ventral paraflocculi taking part in its formation. The parafloccular fissure which separates the paraflocculus, rostromedially, from the remainder of the cerebellar hemisphere gradually extends medially and reduces the width of the zone of cortex situated between it and the lateral end of the prepyramidal fissure. This cortical band connects lobule VIII with the paramedian lobule, as already described (figs. 94B, C).

FLOCCULONODULAR LOBE IN FETUS AND ADULT

Lobule X, the nodulus, was recognized by Bradley (1903) as a distinct cerebellar division, with respect to its vermal as well as its lateral relations, under the designation lobe E. It is well differentiated in the 21-day-old fetus, with the vermal segment of the posterolateral fissure deepening as the lobule increases in size (figs. 88–91). In the adult rabbit lobule X has two superficial folia and one in the depth of the posterolateral fissure (figs. 92, 94C).

The flocculus has been mentioned in connection with the first appearance of the posterolateral fissure. In the 28-day-old fetus it is visible rostrally as a large rounded lobule ventromedial to the paraflocculus. Four folia may be seen in anterior view of the adult cerebellum (fig. 93). A fibrous floccular peduncle, closely associated with the parafloccular peduncle, connects the flocculus and nodulus (fig. 94C). The posterolateral fissure is distinct from one side of the cerebellum to the other in fetuses and young rabbits but in the adult sometimes only traces of it can be seen as a result of the intimate merging of the floccular and parafloccular peduncles. This close association of the medullary bands leading to the flocculus and paraflocculus in the rabbit and many other species led G. E. Smith (1902, 1903c) to regard these two lobules as components of a major lobe of the cerebellum which he designated the floccular lobe. The differences in the vermal relations of flocculus and paraflocculus in the opossum, bat, and mole enabled me (Larsell, 1934) to differentiate the flocculus as part of the flocculonodular lobe and the paraflocculus as an outgrowth of the corpus cerebelli. The developmental history of these subdivisions of the rabbit cerebellum, as in the rat and other mammalian embryos subsequently studied, demonstrated the same fundamental morphological relations. In addition it showed that the two flocculi, the nodulus, and the connecting peduncle constitute a flocculonodular lobe.

ARMADILLO

THE nine-banded armadillo (*Dasyurus novemcinctus*), approximately the size of the domestic cat, attains a total length of 71 cm to 81 cm, about half of which is the tail. The body is rather stout and the animal weighs from 4 kg to 7.7 kg. The long and narrow head, the body, and the tail are covered with armor but the large external ears and the underparts are naked. Vision apparently is limited, since the animal was described as being more sensitive to vibrations in the ground than to visual impressions when approached (Palmer, 1954).

Cerebellum

The cerebellum of the armadillo, as seen from above, is strongly elliptical in outline, with a rostral projection. The vermis is prominent and is sharply delimited from the hemisphere on either side by a narrow but fairly deep paravermian sulcus; in the lower walls and floor of the sulcus the medullary substance is exposed (fig. 95). Although it projects rostrally beyond the anterior surface of the hemispheres the vermis has a considerably longer dorsoventral than anteroposterior axis (fig. 96A). The hemispheres are relatively narrow from the paravermian sulcus to their lateral surfaces and are strongly arched upward. Their folia, except on the anterior cerebellar surface, are nearly transverse and resemble those of the vermis (fig. 95). Continuity of vermal and hemispheral folia and lamellae is interrupted, except on the anterior surface, by the medullary area. The paraflocculus is relatively large, has considerable foliation, and is somewhat flattened against the side of the hemisphere (fig. 97). The cerebellum is typically divided into the corpus cerebelli and the relatively small flocculonodular lobe.

CORPUS CEREBELLI

The fissura prima is unusually deep because the apices of the anterior and posterior lobes adjacent to its mouth are folded into its walls instead of forming superficial folia or lamellae, as in most species. The anterior lobe is large, both in median sagittal section and in anterior view. The superior portion of the posterior lobe is more massive and extends rostralward much less than in the rabbit. The anterior lobe extends to the lateral border of the rostral cerebellar surface and constitutes the greater portion of its area. Both lobes are divided into vermal and hemispheral lobules; the vermal lobules of the posterior lobe differ from those of the anterior lobe by absence of continuity from the hemispheral lobules by a medullary area.

Anterior lobe. The anterior lobe comprises five well-defined lobules (figs. 96A, 97). Lobule I is narrow and projects into the fourth ventricle. Precentral fissure *a*, delimiting it from lobule II, extends to the cerebellar margin. Lobule II includes two folia, IIa and IIb, that converge laterally and continue into the hemisphere as lobule HII and then end against the brachium pontis. Lobule III is divided into three surface and several fissural folia; those of the surface converge laterally into a single broad fold that continues into the hemisphere as lobule HIII (fig. 98). Lobules III and HIII are separated from lobules II and HII by the precentral fissure and from the more dorsal portion of the anterior lobe by the preculminate fissure. Both of these fissures are deep and reach the lateral cerebellar margin. Lobule IV of the armadillo, including the folia of the dorsal wall of the preculminate fissure, is fairly large although the intraculminate fissure, which bounds it from lobule V, is relatively shallow as compared with that in the cat and many other species. The lobule presents two superficial folia but it is probable that the deep sublamella labeled IVa in figure 96A corresponds to sublobule IVA of other species, such as the cat, in which large sublobules IVA and IVB may be represented. The two superficial folia and the fissural folium

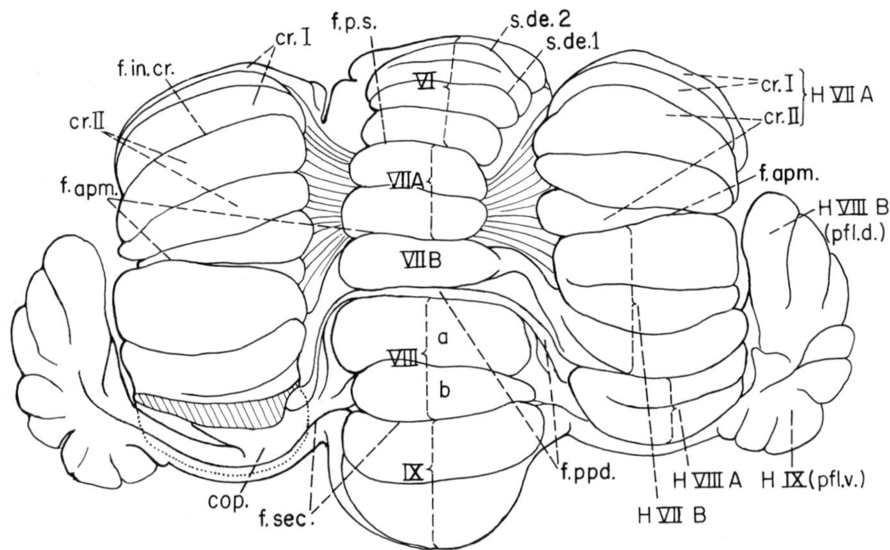

Figure 95. Cerebellum of armadillo. Dorsoposterior view.

immediately below and behind them converge laterally and continue into the hemisphere as lobule HIV (fig. 97). Lobule V presents only two superficial folds, Va and Vb, but the anterior wall of the fissura prima is folded into two large lamellae that appear to correspond to Vd and Ve of other species, described beyond, and a smaller, more superficial fold that corresponds to Vc, except that it forms the outer part of the fissural wall instead of the posterior superficial surface of the lobule (fig. 96A). Variations of position of this lamella are encountered in other species, as will be shown. Two small folia in the deepest part of the anterior wall of the fissura prima probably represent lamella Vf in reduced form. Laterally folia Va and Vb dip into the paravermian sul-

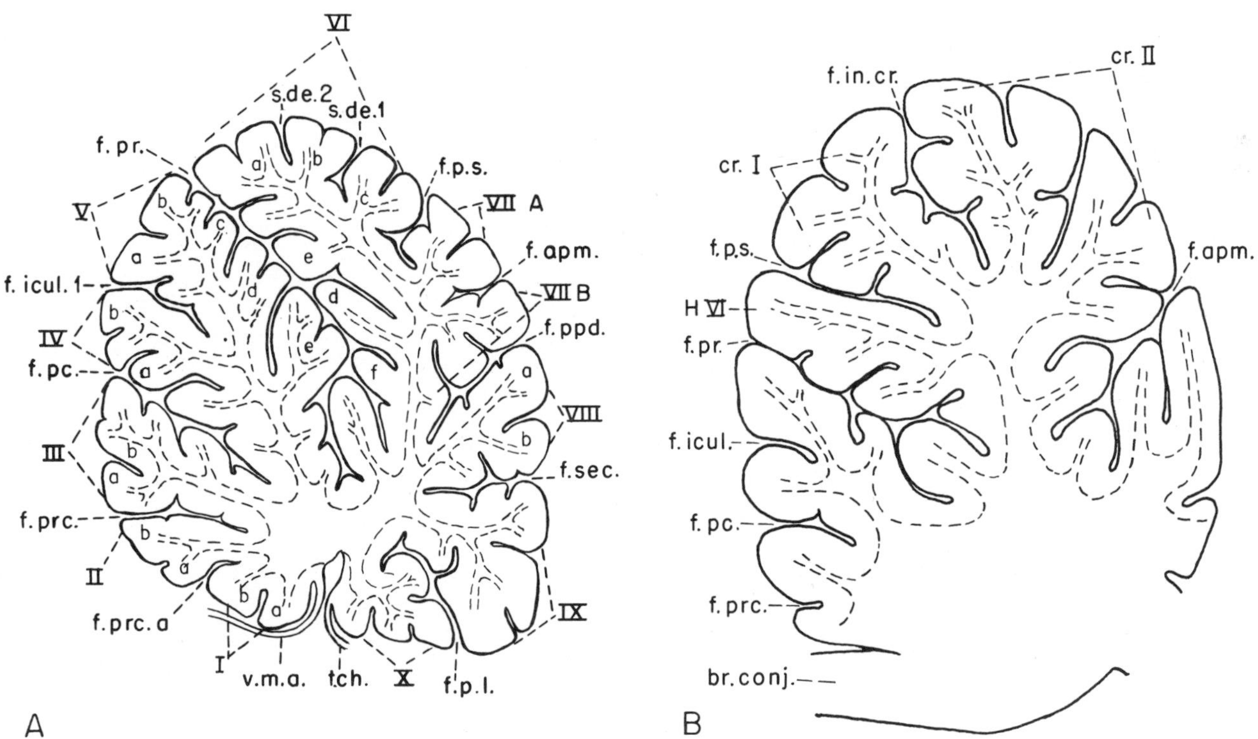

Figure 96. Cerebellum of armadillo. A. Midsagittal section. B. Sagittal section through hemisphere.

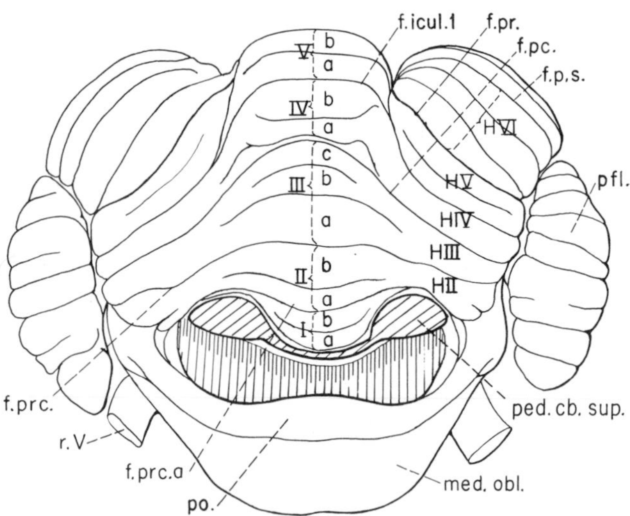

Figure 97. Cerebellum of armadillo. Anterior view, slightly tilted backward.

cus and are continuous with two folia that take a forward direction and emerge on the anterior hemispheral surface as lobule HV. Folium Vc and lamellae Ve and Vd also continue into the hemisphere as laterally diminishing folds of the ventral wall of the fissura prima. Lobule HV, although narrow superficially, has a large cortical surface because of the depth of the hemispheral portion of the fissura prima and the foliation of its ventral wall (fig. 96A).

Posterior lobe. The vermal lobules of the posterior lobe were most conveniently described commencing with lobule IX, the uvula. The posterolateral fissure and the fissura secunda are prominent, with the latter continuing a little way into the parafloccular peduncle (fig. 95). Lobule IX, accordingly, is readily identified. It has three superficial folia which, on the basis of the depth of the intervening furrows and the branching of the intralobular medullary rays, appear to correspond to IXa + IXb, IXc, and IXd of other species. Lobule VIII, the pyramis, is delimited from the remainder of the posterior lobe vermis by a deep prepyramidal fissure. The lobule is relatively small but is superficially divided into two sublamellae, VIIIa and VIIIb, that probably are homologous with sublobules VIIIA and VIIIB of large species. Its fissural walls also are foliated (fig. 96A). A small copula extends caudolaterally on either side; medially it is continuous with the lower folia of the anterior surface of the lobule, with the prepyramidal fissure continuing laterocaudally between it and the paramedian lobule (fig. 95).

The remainder of the posterior lobe vermis, corresponding to lobulus c_2 of Bolk, is relatively very large in the armadillo and has many folds. The most prominent furrow of its dorsal surface appears to represent the posterior superior fissure, although it is not continuous with the hemispheral part of this fissure. It divides lobulus c_2 into two principal segments that correspond to lobules VI and VII of other species (fig. 95). Lobule VII is divided into sublobules VIIA and VIIB by a furrow which I interpreted as the vermal part of the ansoparamedian fissure. A caudolaterally directed band of medullary substance emerges from the base of sublobule VIIB and passes to the deep medullary substance of the paramedian lobule. Although no definite furrow follows the rostrolateral border of this band, the relations of this border to sublobule VIIB and to the paramedian lobule and the hemispheral portion of the ansoparamedian fissure provide the basis for my identification of the vermal segment of the fissure. Lobule VI is large and its relatively prominent lamellae and folia give it a much more extensive cortical surface than lobules VII and VIII (fig. 95). Lobule VI presents three superficial lamellae, VIa, VIb, and VIc; lamella VIa also forms a considerable portion of the dorsoposterior wall of the fissura prima as already noted. Five additional lamellae and folia form the posterior wall of this fissure. Three of these correspond, in relative size and position, so closely to lamellae VId, VIe, and VIf of other species that they were so designated even though they were found to be more deeply situated than usual because of the lengthened outer portion of the fissura prima (fig. 96A).

HEMISPHERAL LOBULES

The fissures and lobules of the posterior lobe were described after being identified by dissection and study of sagittal sections of the lobe, since connections with the

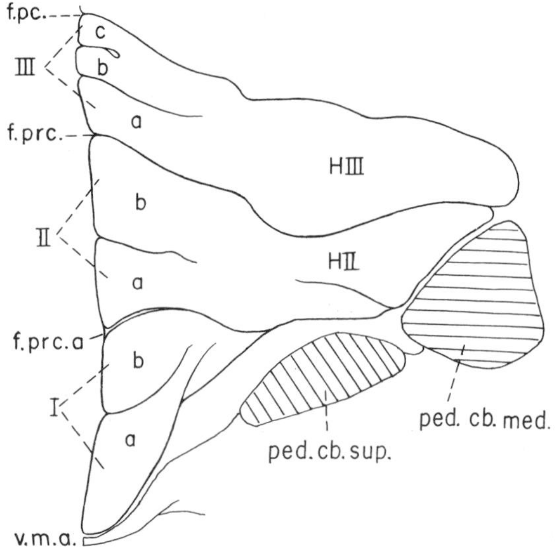

Figure 98. Cerebellum of armadillo. Anterior view showing details of the lower segment of anterior lobe.

vermis were not easy to see superficially. An obliquely sagittal section, beginning dorsally well lateral of the medullary area and passing ventromedially so that the knife emerged through the brachium conjunctivum anteriorly and posteriorly through the proximal part of the parafloccular peduncle, reveals the depth of the fissures and the pattern of the lobules (fig. 96B). The fissura prima is the deepest fissure, as in the vermis, and its walls are greatly folded. The two deep fissures dorsal of it, on the basis of dissection and comparison of their surface relations, are interpreted as the hemispheral segments of declival sulcus 2 and the posterior superior fissure; the latter appears to be quite certain but declival sulcus 2 is not, except as it conforms with the general mammalian pattern. The segment the latter fissure delimits, together with that between it and the posterior superior fissure, forms lobule HVI (fig. 96B).

The ansoparamedian fissure, separating the ansiform and paramedian lobules, is deep and its walls are corrugated. Lobule VIIA, the ansiform lobule, is subdivided into crus I and crus II by a fairly deep intercrural fissure. Crus I presents two broad superficial folia and additional

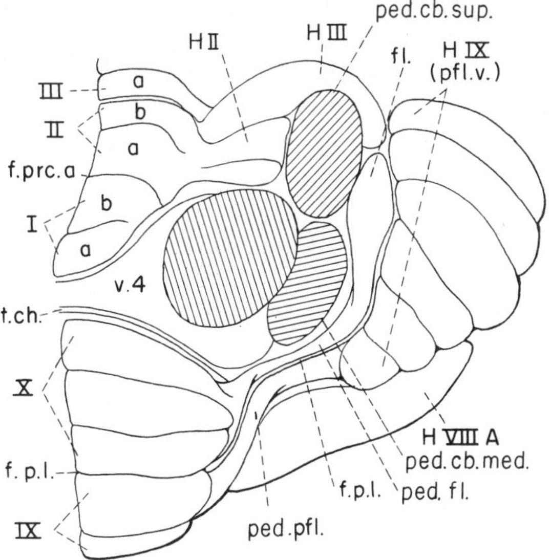

Figure 99. Cerebellum of armadillo. Ventral view.

folds face its delimiting fissures. Crus II also has two superficial folia, as well as two in the anterior wall of the ansoparamedian fissure. The folium nearest the mouth of the fissure is visible externally before shrinking of the specimen by hardening in alcohol.

Lobule HVIIB + HVIIIA, the paramedian lobule, includes five superficial folia and two in the posterior wall of the ansoparamedian fissure (fig. 95). The two most ventrally situated of the superficial folia overlie a layer of cortex and medullary substance, which is separated laterally from the parafloccular peduncle by the medial part of the parafloccular fissure. Rostrolaterally this plate is related to the principal mass of the paramedian lobule; medially it appears more closely related to the small copula than to the ventral part of the common peduncle formed by fusion of the lateral continuation of the copula and the medullary continuation from lamella VIIIb that together constitute the parafloccular peduncle. The plate corresponds to a portion, at least, of the pars copularis of the paramedian lobule of other species. There are indications that the two small inferior lamellae of the paramedian lobule also are related to the pars copularis, but a satisfactory demonstration of such a relationship could not be made; the uvula is the same here as in other species. The fissura secunda extends into the proximal part of the peduncle and a fissure that partially divides the peduncle lengthwise is recognizable laterally and in the proximal portion of the paraflocculus (fig. 95), but it could not be distinguished on the surface of the greater part of the peduncle. Dorsal and ventral paraflocculi also could not be distinctly differentiated.

FLOCCULONODULAR LOBE

Lobule X is small and presents only four folia in median sagittal section. The flocculus is a small club-shaped expansion connected with the nodulus by a slender fibrous peduncle. The posterolateral fissure is deep medially but laterally it is represented only by a faint groove that delimits the floccular from the parafloccular peduncle (fig. 99).

PIG

THE cerebellum of many species of ungulates has been studied by various authors. Reil (1807–8), Leuret and Gratiolet (1839–57), Künnemann (1894), Flatau and Jacobsohn (1899), and Ziehen (1899) described the organ more or less completely in domestic and some wild animals. In his analysis of the cerebellar lobules Bolk (1906) used fourteen species of ungulates ranging in size from the pygmy antelope to the elephant. Riley (1929) described the medullary rays and lobules of the elephant, camel, reindeer, giraffe, and ox in terms of a modification of Bolk's nomenclature, and Scholten (1946), also using Bolk's terms with some modifications, included the ox in his analysis of the paraflocculus. More recently Jansen (1954) described the cerebellum of the elk and the Indian elephant in terms of lobules I–X with respect to the vermis and with the use of Bolk's nomenclature for the hemispheral lobules. Kuithan (1895) studied the development of the organ in the sheep, and Bradley (1903) described cerebellar development in some detail in the pig and sheep and less completely in the ox and horse. Bradley (1903, 1904) also interpreted the adult cerebellum of the pig, sheep, goat, ox, and horse in terms of the patterns of lobules and fissures in fetal material.

The cerebellum of the elephant differs so greatly from that of other ungulates that we will set it aside for the moment. In all other species described or illustrated by various authors, except for the pygmy antelope, the vermis is sinuous to a greater or lesser degree and the hemispheral lobules and fissures have a general similarity of pattern, if one accepts the wide variations. Instead of attempting to make a detailed comparison of this pattern in the numerous species, as interpreted by the authors cited, with my own observations and conclusions, it seems preferable to present the results of a restudy of the development of the cerebellum of the pig (*Sus scrofa*) from early stages to animals who are 3 months old and weigh 40 kg.

The sinuous portion of the vermis, situated between the fissura prima and the prepyramidal fissure, is so complex in the adult cerebellum of larger ungulates that Bolk (1906) designated it lobulus c_2 without further subdivision. Riley (1929) called it c_2 in the reindeer, giraffe, and ox but lobulus *c* in the camel, since he misinterpreted the prepyramidal fissure as the fissura secunda. Scholten (1946) divided his lobulus C_1 (corresponding to Bolk's lobulus c_2) into first, middle, and posterior parts, stating that in the cow and cat the first part, which he homologized (1946) with the declive of the human cerebellum, appears to be connected with the lobulus simplex. A detailed study of the development of the vermian lobules in the pig and of the relations of the sinuous portion of the vermis in late fetuses and young pigs has provided a basis for homologizing all the subdivisions of this species with those of other mammals as well as a basis for understanding their relations to the hemispheral lobules. The homologies established in the pig appear to be valid in the larger ungulates described below.

Thanks to the availability of abundant embryonic material of the pig, the development and differentiation of the fissures and lobules could be followed in closely graded stages both before and after the displacements of some of the lobules that result in the sinuous vermis. The pioneer studies by Bradley (1903) of the fissures and lobules in the pig embryo afford an excellent basis for a restudy of the developing cerebellum in terms of present-day conceptions of its morphology. By comparison with appropriate fetal and postpartum stages of other mammals the homologies of the lobules and fissures could be established with greater certainty than has prevailed before now. The plentiful supply of embryonic material of the pig has allowed for studies comparing the early phases of differentiation of the cerebellum and related parts of the brain with lower vertebrates and with other mammals, especially man, described in a later section. My contribution (Larsell, 1954) is the presentation of the principal features of cerebellar morphology in the pig; these are reviewed here and supplemented by additional details.

Early Development of Cerebellum

The alar lamina of the metencephalon of the 10-mm C.R. length pig embryo is expanded dorsalward on either side and forms the rostrolateral wall of the anterior part of the fourth ventricle, as is also shown in the 12-mm section of the pig (fig. 100). The bilateral expansions constitute the paired rudiment of the cerebellum. They are joined across the median sagittal plane by a thin plate which already is differentiated into ependymal, mantle, and marginal layers. The decussation of the trochlear nerve is prominent at the continuation of this plate with the midbrain. In the anterior part of the plate itself several small groups of nerve fibers indicate the presence of the commissura cerebelli. Fibers corresponding to the vestibular commissure are recognizable at the 12-mm stage of the embryo; it is possible that special neurohistological methods would reveal the fibers of this phylogenetically ancient commissure at an earlier stage.

Fusion of the bilateral halves of the cerebellum has begun along the cerebellar commissure by the 20-mm stage of the embryo. On the external surface of the cerebellum a shallow groove, extending from the lateral wall

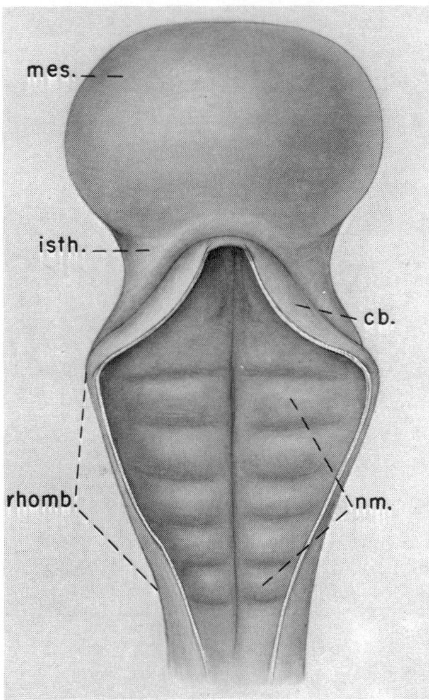

Figure 100. Rhombencephalon and mesencephalon of 12-mm-long pig embryo. Dorsal view showing the bilateral cerebellar rudiment.

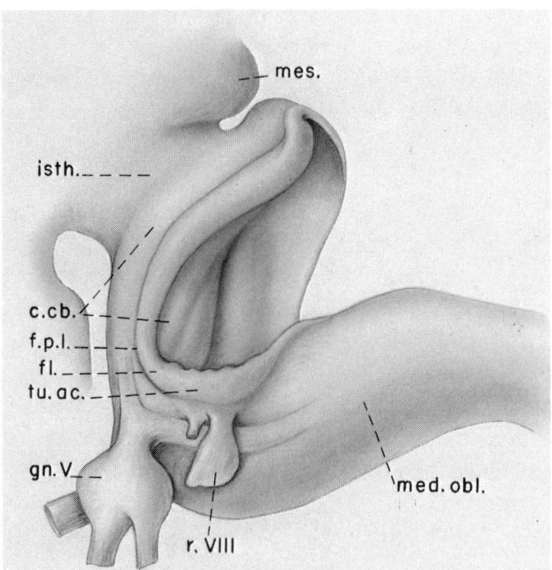

Figure 101. Posterolateral view of cerebellum of 20-mm-long pig embryo. ×14.

of the medulla oblongata to the midline of the fused region, divides the organ into two bilaterally represented portions. The furrow is the incipient posterolateral fissure (fig. 101) which was known as fissure IV of Bradley (1903). Bradley illustrated this fissure as a prominent groove in the 52-mm pig embryo, at which stage no other fissures are present. Bradley also noted that the corresponding furrow is the first to appear in the rabbit fetus and in both species it is associated with the rhombic lip. The incipient posterolateral fissure is continuous with a furrow that delimits the tuberculum acusticum from the lateral surface of the medulla oblongata and apparently is homologous with the external acousticolateral sulcus of urodeles.

The vestibular part of the rhombic lip continues dorsomedially into the cerebellum and forms the rudimentary flocculonodular lobe – the nodular part of which appears much later than the floccular part. The rostral expansion of the remainder of the alar plate becomes the corpus cerebelli. In the pig embryo, as was also shown in urodeles, among the lower vertebrates, the special somatic sensory portion of the alar plate differentiates into the primarily vestibular part of the cerebellum, and the general somatic portion differentiates into the general proprioceptive and exteroceptive division. Along the attachment of the choroid tela of the fourth ventricle to the margin of the incipient flocculonodular lobe proliferating cells soon form a germinal zone. In dissected specimens of later stages lightly stained with carmine, the boundary between this zone and the flocculonodular lobe could be seen because the closely arranged cells of the former produce a band of darker color. In early stages the germinal zone is small, but in subsequent development of the embryo the zone expands, with cells migrating from it into the external granular layer of the developing cortex. By the 62-mm C.R. stage it is much reduced in relative size and it eventually disappears as a well-defined area (fig. 107).

The lateral part of the alar lamina of the myelencephalon proliferates cells which migrate ventrally and rostrally to form the bulbopontine extension and the complex of the inferior olivary nucleus. When the pig embryo reaches the 54-mm C.R. length, the bulbopontine extension is a well-defined band that reaches from the alar lamina of the medulla oblongata to the pons (fig. 102). At this stage the pons has appeared as a small swelling on the ventral surface of the medulla oblongata. It is larger in the 62-mm fetus and the bulbopontine extension is more attenuated although still prominent (fig. 103A). A fibrous strand, representing an early stage of the brachium pontis, extends toward the cerebellum but does not yet reach it. The lateroventral margin of the cerebellar cortex extends from the flocculus to the bottom of the mesencephalocerebellar fissure (fig. 103A). In the 66-mm fetus the pons has enlarged and the bulbopontine extension is much less evident. The brachium pontis has reached the cerebellum and entered it beneath the ventral margin of the cortex. The migrations of cells to the pons and the connections of the pons with the cerebellum appear to be accomplished, so far as external features indicate, in the course of about ten days, if one estimates the time elapsed by correlating the crown-rump (C.R.) measurements I used on fetuses obtained from the commercial abattoir with the measurements, supplemented by age in days, employed by Bradley.

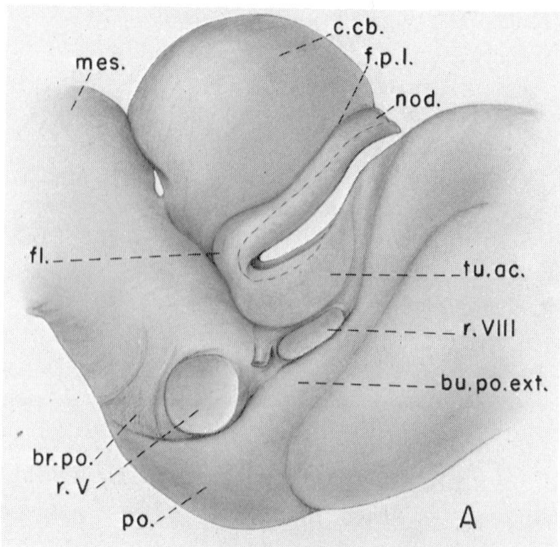

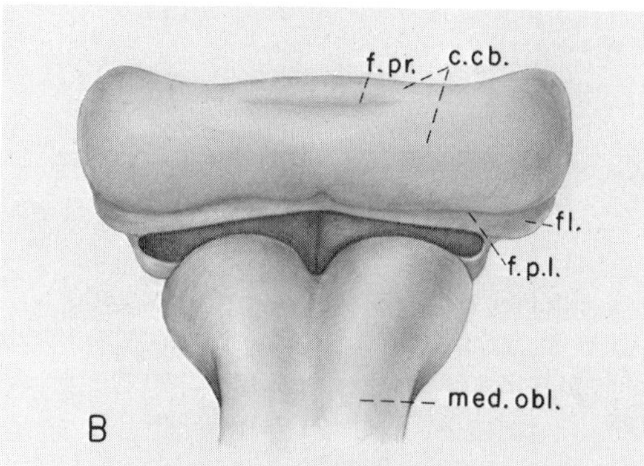

Figure 103. Cerebellum and adjacent structures of 62-mm-long pig embryo. A. Lateral view. ×14. B. Dorsal view.

The corpus cerebelli of the 12-mm pig embryo forms an upward expansion of the remainder of the metencephalic portion of the alar plate. The two sides have begun to fuse rostrally, as already stated, but at this stage the median region, although including cells in addition to commisural fibers, is relatively thin. Lateroventrally the walls thicken and serial sections show that they consist of a mantle layer of loosely arranged cells outside the ependymal layer lining the ventricle. The ventricular surface of the cerebellum shows no boundaries between the corpus cerebelli and the flocculonodular lobe. It forms a rounded dome, continuous caudally with the choroid tela, but the margin of the cerebellum is distinct from the thin tela. The rostral part of the corpus cerebelli has a thicker wall on either side of the median sagittal plane than the more lateral and caudal portions, and it arches upward from the rostral end of the medulla oblongata (fig. 100).

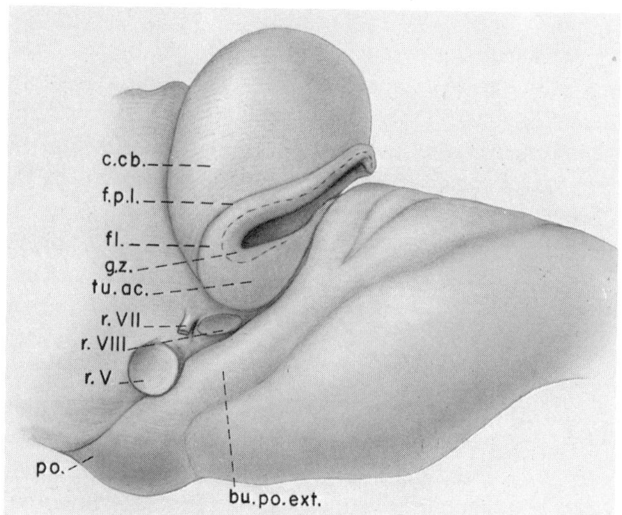

Figure 102. Cerebellum, pons, and bulbopontine extension of 54-mm-long pig embryo. Lateral view. ×14.

By the 20-mm stage the corpus cerebelli has thickened greatly and the medial fusion above the ventricle has extended caudalward (fig. 101). There still remains, however, a deep rostrally directed notch bordered by the dorsomedial continuation of the cerebellar part of the rhombic lip. The posterolateral fissure, the corpus cerebelli, and the incipient flocculonodular lobe are well differentiated at this stage. Rostral to the flocculus a surface elevation, produced by ascending root fibers of the trigeminus, reaches the transition zone between the base of the corpus cerebelli and the upward-turned end of the medulla oblongata. For a considerable period of time, subsequent development consists chiefly of growth in volume of the corpus cerebelli and completion of the arch above

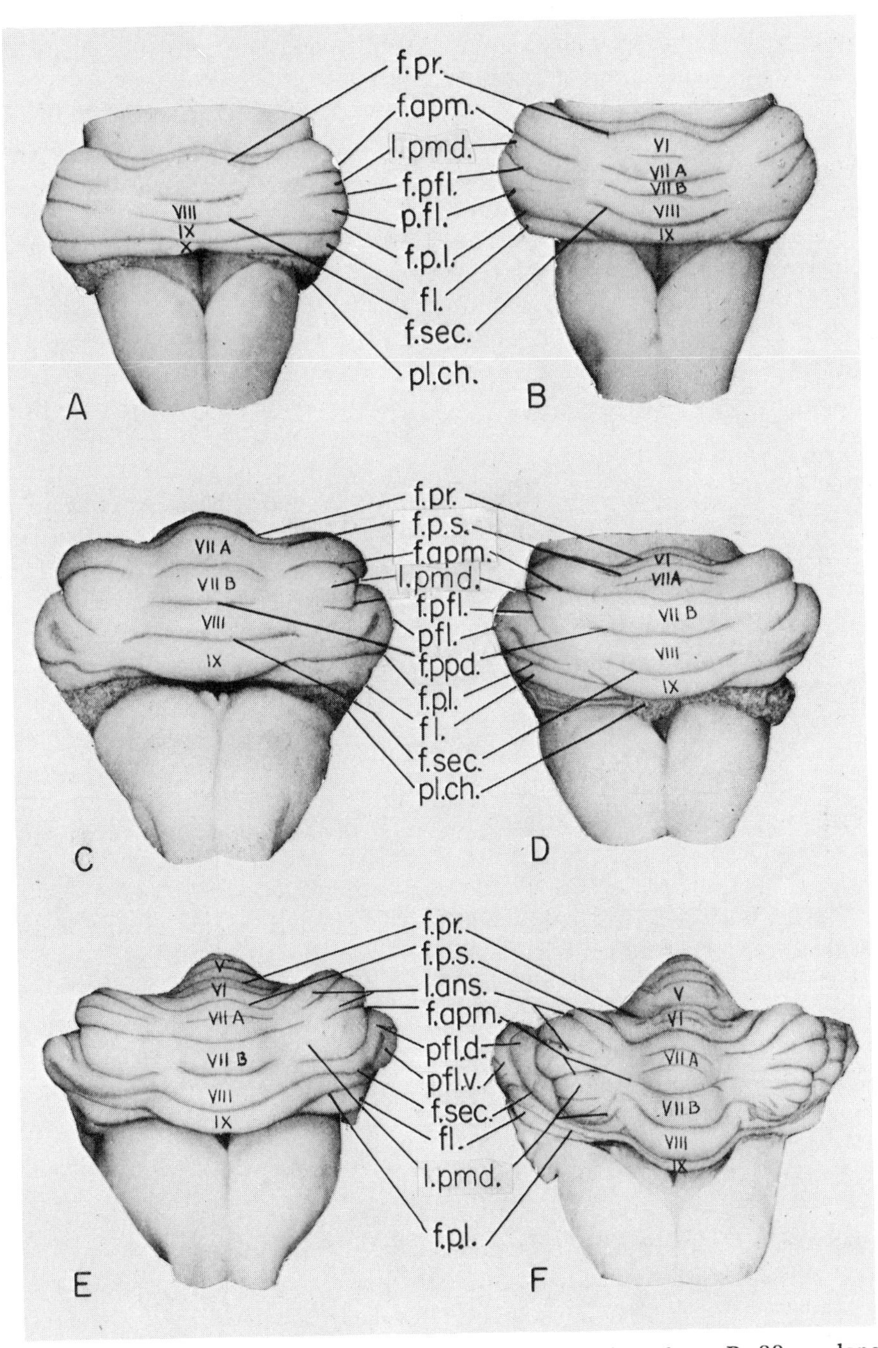

Figure 104. Cerebellum of pig. Dorsal view. A. 80-mm-long fetus. B. 90-mm-long fetus. C. 95-mm-long fetus. D. 110-mm-long fetus. E. 125-mm-long fetus. F. 140-mm-long fetus. Enlarged and retouched photographs.

the fourth ventricle, with the medial region becoming massive (figs. 102, 103). Owing to the sharper pontine flexure the cerebellum tilts posteriorly at this stage. The corpus cerebelli also broadens so that it projects laterally well beyond the margins of the medulla oblongata, with the lateral portions arching downward on each side. In sagittal section the surface forms a semicircle and the ventricular surface tapers to a fastigial peak in the median plane, but it is more rounded beneath the lateral portions of the corpus cerebelli. In surface-stained specimens the margin of the differentiating cortex stands out, in contrast to the lighter staining fibrous surface of the medulla oblongata (fig. 102).

In the 54-mm embryo the medial part of the corpus cerebelli has become massive. The posterolateral fissure is deeper laterally but is still shallow at the midline. The flocculus has begun to expand but there is no indication of the paired rudiment of the nodulus; the incipient flocculonodular lobe consists of the two flocculi and a narrow connecting band that is not definitely fused across the midline.

CORPUS CEREBELLI IN FETAL STAGES AND 3-MONTH-OLD PIG

The fissura prima (fissure II of Bradley) appears in the 62-mm fetus as a short transverse furrow about midway between the anterior and the posterior margins of the corpus cerebelli (fig. 103B). The cortex immediately beneath the fissure is thickened and folds downward. The apical region of the cerebellum of the pig embryo grows slowly but by the 78-mm to 80-mm stage the fissura prima has deepened considerably; it also extends ventrolaterally almost to the rostral margin of the cerebellum on each side. The anterior and posterior lobes of the corpus cerebelli thus are fully delimited from each other (fig. 104).

The anterior lobe of the 66-mm fetus has three short and shallow furrows under which the cortex is thickened and arched inward (fig. 107A). There is so much variation in the folds of the anterior lobe of the pig fetus that it is difficult to establish a consistent pattern of its lobules and fissures. Comparison of the fissures and lobules of later stages (figs. 106, 107B, C, 108) with those of the 66-mm fetus appears to support the interpretations indicated in figure 105A. Lobules III, IV, and V are well defined but lobules I and II are not yet differentiated from each other. The preculminate fissure (Bradley's fissure *c*) subsequently becomes the longest from side to side in the anterior lobe, separating the two lobules of the incipient culmen from lobule III (central lobule). The groove between lobules IV and V is the intraculminate fissure (Bradley's fissure I) and the one between combined lobules I and II, ventrally, and lobule III, dorsally, corresponds to the precentral fissure. This pattern prevails, in general, in later stages although with some variation in individual cerebella. In the 90-mm fetus all the vermal lobules, except I and II, are delimited by relatively deep furrows across the median plane. The fissura prima is now very prominent and is the only furrow of the corpus cerebelli that extends to the cerebellar margin (figs. 105A, B). The preculminate fissure has discontinuous vermal and hemispheral segments in the cerebellum of the 90-mm fetus illustrated in figure 105A. In other fetuses of about the same length this fissure is continuous from near the margin of one side of the anterior lobe to the other, and in still others its hemispheral segment is directed toward the intraculminate fissure. Lobule III sometimes has three folia instead of the two illustrated in figure 107B. In such instances lobule IV is relatively smaller. The cerebella of fetuses 150-mm and 170-mm in C.R. length, as illustrated in figures 107C and 108 respectively, have two lamellae, IIIa and IIIb, that evidently have developed from the two folia of this lobule represented in the cerebellum of the 90-mm fetus selected for the figure.

As the cortex burgeons outward, the fissures become deeper and also extend lateralward toward the cerebellar margin, which gradually is hidden from surface view by the expansion of the cortex. In a fetus of 173 mm in length the preculminate and intraculminate fissures are continuous from the margin of one side to the other (fig. 105B), as is the precentral fissure *a* between lobules I and II. These lobules have differentiated from the earlier common ventrorostral cortical fold by the 140-mm and 150-mm stages (fig. 107C).

In the 150-mm fetus the lobules have foliated into incipient lamellae whose general pattern is unchanged in subsequent fetal stages and in the 3-month-old pig (figs. 108, 109). Both lobules and lamellae, except for increased size and formation of folia, remain very similar in the anterior lobe throughout their subsequent development. Lobule I persists as a simple lamella, lobule II is divided into two surface lamellae, and lobule III is divided by a relatively deep fissure into two large lamellae, IIIa and IIIb, which in the young pig have so increased in size as to merit the designation sublobules IIIA and IIIB. The depth of the intervening furrow in the 3-month-old pig and the close relation of the medullary ray to that of lobule IV could well be indicative of a closer relationship between sublobule IIIb and lobule IV than between sublobule IIIb and sublobule IIIA. Superficially, however, the preculminate fissure, as labeled in figure 105B, extends farther laterally than intracentral sulcus 2. Also the two subdivisions of lobule III are closely related in the

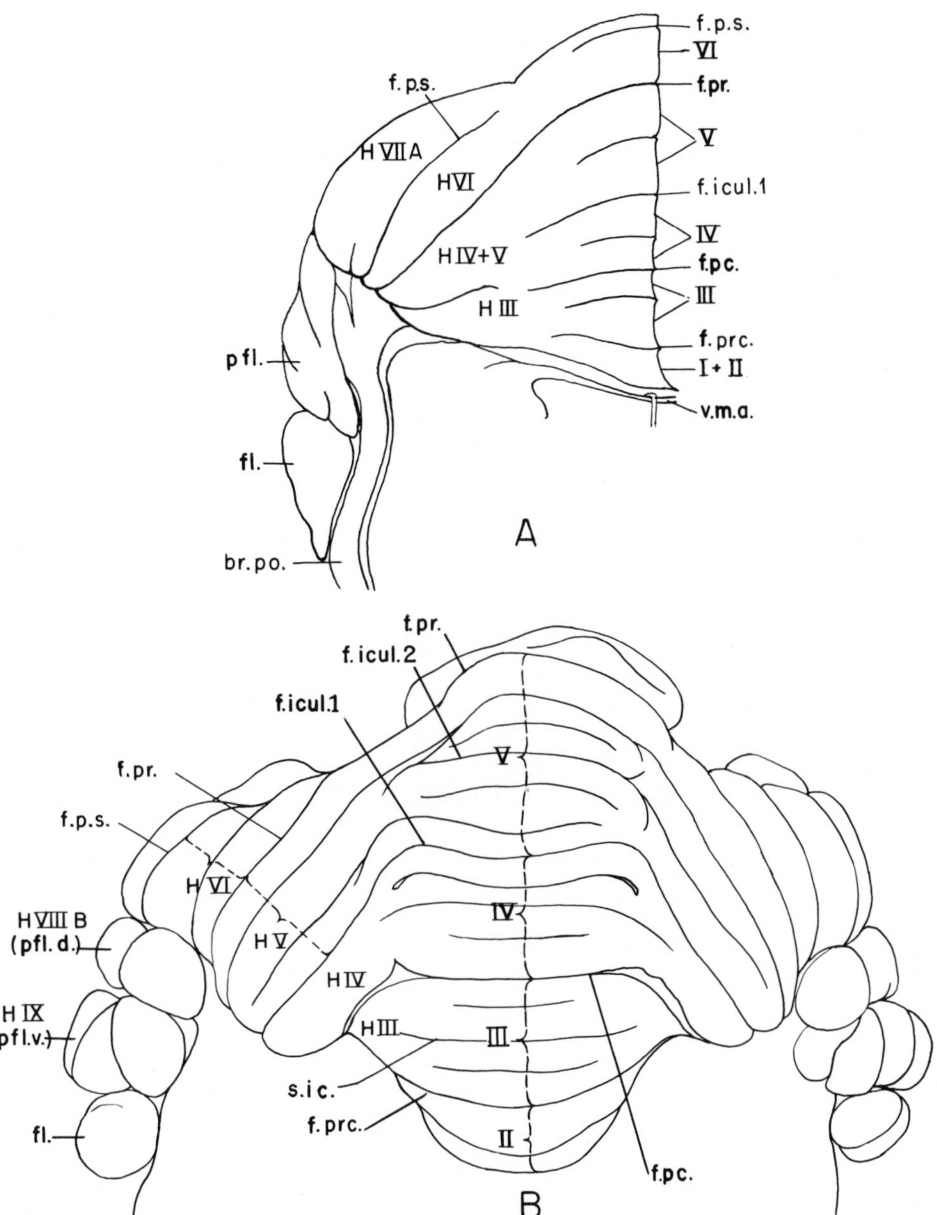

Figure 105. Cerebellum of pig. Anterior view. A. 90-mm-long fetus. B. 173-mm-long fetus. (Larsell, 1954.)

140-mm, 150-mm, and 170-mm fetuses, although the intracentral sulcus 2 is very deep in the fetus last mentioned. Lobule IV is very similar in all the stages, except that in the 170-mm fetus two sublobules are situated between lamella IIIb and lobule V. The more ventral of the two probably corresponds to sublobule IVA of other ungulates; the dorsal one, which resembles lobule IV of the other stages except for its relatively somewhat smaller size, is interpreted as corresponding to sublobule IVB. Lobule V is subdivided into three characteristic superficial lamellae, Va, Vb, and Vc; lamella Va is the largest in all fetal stages and in the young pig. The anterior wall of the fissura prima shows the typical lamellae Vd, Ve, and Vf, of which Ve is characteristically the largest, as in other species.

Bradley (1903) divided the cerebellum rostral of the fissura prima (his fissure *c*) into sublobules A_1 and A_2. He stated that in the 100-mm pig embryo, lobule A_1, the more ventral of the two, is composed of three sublobules, with the uppermost extending into the hemisphere. A single small folium described as adherent to the anterior medullary velum was regarded by this author as a re-

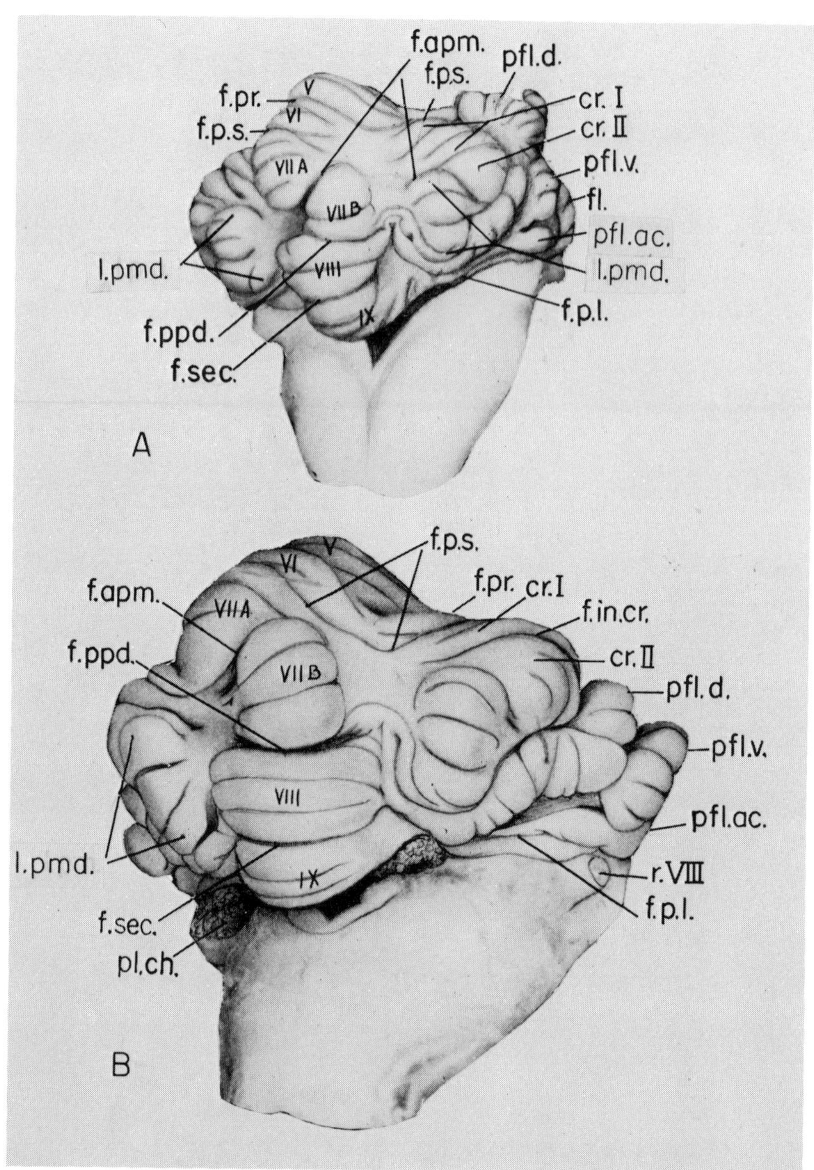

Figure 106. Cerebellum of pig. Dorsolateral view. A. 150-mm-long fetus. B. 170-mm-long fetus. Enlarged and retouched photographs. (Larsell, 1954.)

duced lingula. The three sublobules described and illustrated by Bradley correspond to lobule II and the two subdivisions (IIIa and IIIb) of lobule III, while the lingula corresponds to lobule I of my terminology. Lobule A_2 of Bradley corresponds to lobule IV, and his lobe B to my lobule V. In his figure of a median sagittal section of the adult pig cerebellum, Bradley illustrated three subdivisions ventral to the preculminate fissure, while his lobule A_2 is partially divided into two subdivisions that correspond to sublobules IVA and IVB of other species. Appearing a few years after Bradley's work, Bolk's (1906) illustration of a median sagittal section of the pig's cerebellum shows lobule IV as a single segment which he included with the segment corresponding to my lobule V (Bradley's lobe B) in his lobulus 4.

Lobule I has no hemispheral representation. In the 173-mm fetus lobule II shows a narrow lateral folium that may be regarded as an incipient lobule HII; it is carried ventrally with the keel-like vermal part of lobule II in the young pig. Lobule III extends somewhat beyond the lateral border of lobule II as early as the 90-mm fetus (fig. 105A), forming an incipient lobule HIII which is better represented in the 173-mm fetus (fig. 105B). In the 3-month-old pig it extends considerably onto the hemispheral surface, as shown on the right-hand side of figure 113A. Lobules IV and V are continuous with

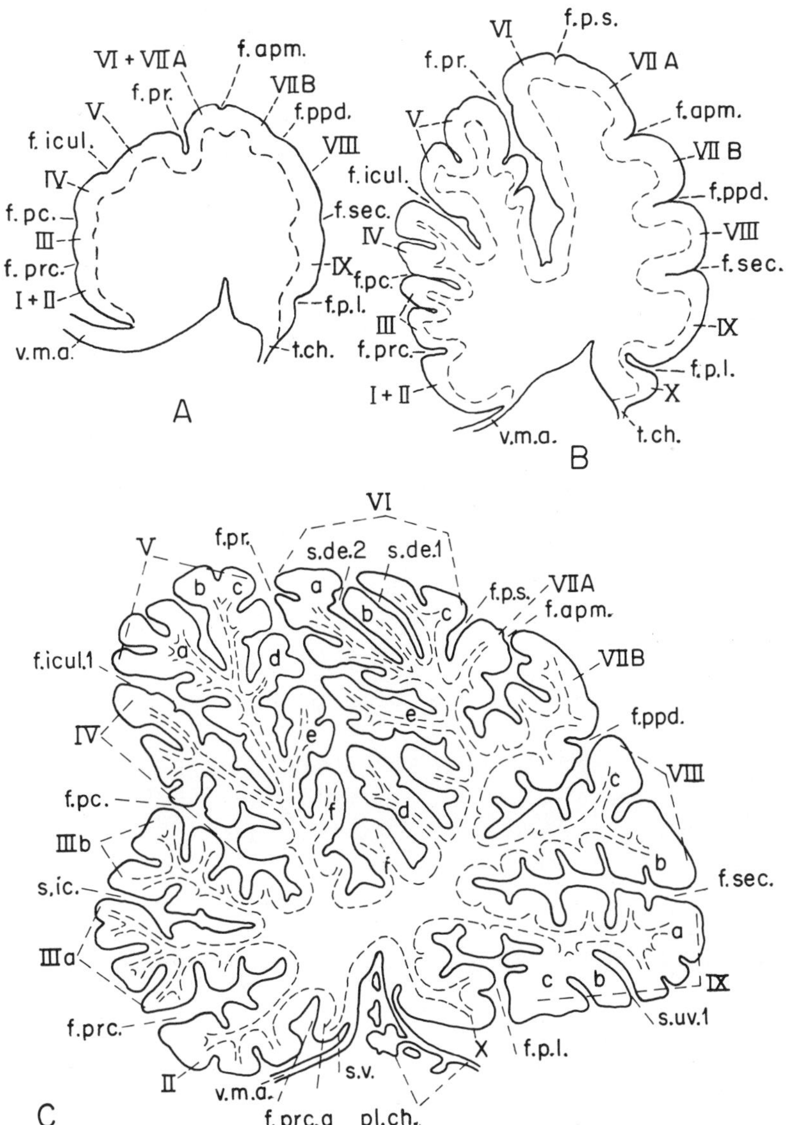

Figure 107. Cerebellum of pig. Midsagittal sections. A. 66-mm-long fetus. B. 90-mm-long fetus. C. 150-mm-long fetus. ×14. (Larsell, 1954.)

broad folia that form distinctly delimited lobules HIV and HV in the 173-mm fetus. In the young pig these lobules constitute a large part of the anterior surface of the hemisphere (fig. 113A). The vermal part of the posterior lobe is subdivided by three shallow furrows in the 66-mm embryo (fig. 107A). These are the fissura secunda, the prepyramidal fissure, and the ansoparamedian fissure, named in the order of their appearance as judged from the thickness of the infolded cortex beneath each one. The ansoparamedian fissure, which corresponds to Bradley's fissure *a* of the pig, sheep, and calf, but not of the rabbit, is situated so far rostrally at this stage that it appears at first sight to correspond to the posterior superior fissure of fetuses of other species. As interpreted from its relations in later stages, however, the posterior superior fissure (fissure *b* of Bradley) is first recognizable on the anterior surface of the hemisphere in the 80-mm embryo and in the vermis in an embryo of 90 mm in length (fig. 105A). Bradley first mentioned the vermal part of the fissure in a 100-mm fetus. The vermal and hemispheral segments of the fissure sometimes join in the 95-mm fetus but more frequently they join at later stages of growth.

Lobule VI, accordingly, is delimited from lobule VII in the 90-mm embryo, but sublobule VIIB has already been differentiated by the ansoparamedian fissure in the 80-mm embryo (fig. 104). The differentiation of lobule VI, therefore, is from sublobule VIIA, rather than from

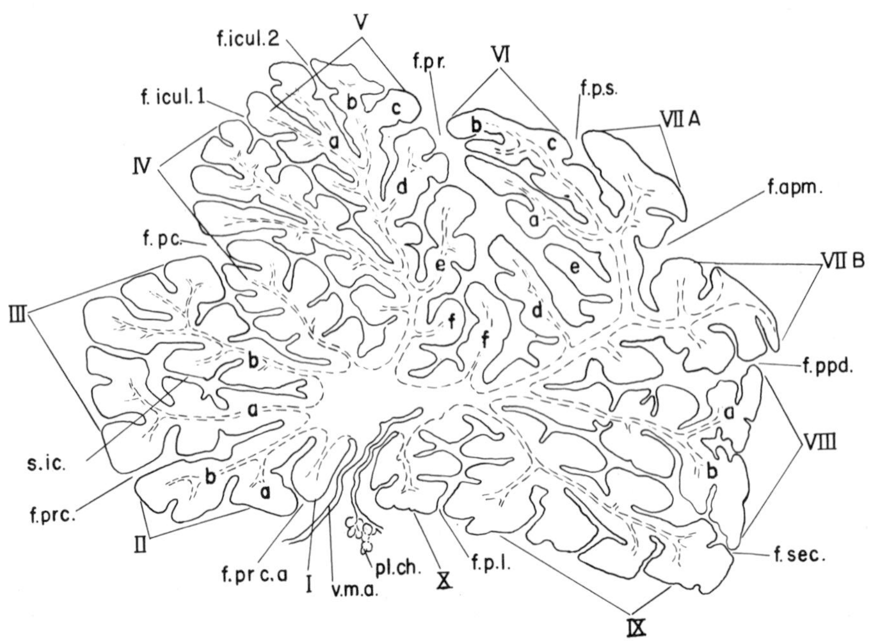

Figure 108. Midsagittal section of cerebellum of 170-mm-long pig fetus. ×12.5. (Larsell, 1954.)

lobule VII as a whole, as in the rat and rabbit in which the vermal segment of the posterior superior fissure appears much earlier than the ansoparamedian fissure. The anomaly in the pig apparently is due to the large size of lobule VII and the ability of the region immediately behind and above the mouth of the fissura prima to yield in a forward direction without early foliation. When first

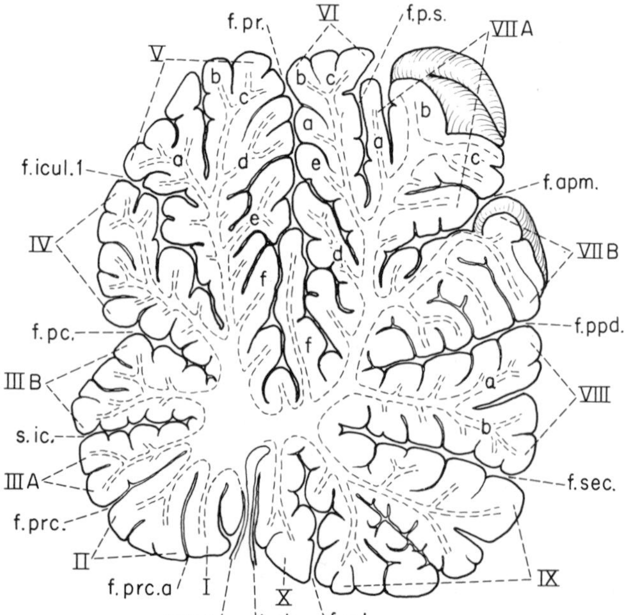

Figure 109. Cerebellum of 3-month-old pig. Midsagittal section.

differentiated the superficial part of lobule VI is small but since the posterior wall of the fissura prima also must be regarded as part of the lobule its total cortical area is extensive (fig. 105A). By the 140-mm stage of the embryo the characteristic lamellae of the lobule have appeared. At this stage lamellae VIa and VIb face the fissura prima, owing to the forward displacement of the superficial part of the lobule by the still medially situated and large sublobule VIIA. As sublobules VIIA and VIIB continue to expand they soon shove the initial stages of displacement to opposite sides of the midline, which provides space behind lobule VI for it to tilt into. Lamellae VIa and VIb are displaced upward and become superficial but VIa also faces the fissura prima as in other species (fig. 107C). These two lamellae and lamella VIc retain their superficial position and their individuality in subsequent developmental stages and in the young pig (figs. 109, 110). Lamellae VId, VIe, and VIf, which are also differentiated in the 140-mm fetus, retain their relative positions and, in general, their relative size in subsequent development.

Lobule VII, in the 90-mm embryo, has a deep ansoparamedian fissure between its two sublobules. In a fetus 143-mm in length, the lobule has become slightly sigmoid, and in the 150-mm and 170-mm fetuses the displacement of sublobules VIIA and VIIB is increasingly pronounced (figs. 106A, B); sublobule VIIA carries with it the superficial posterior part of lobule VI, and sublobule VIIB affects the position of lobule VIII. In the

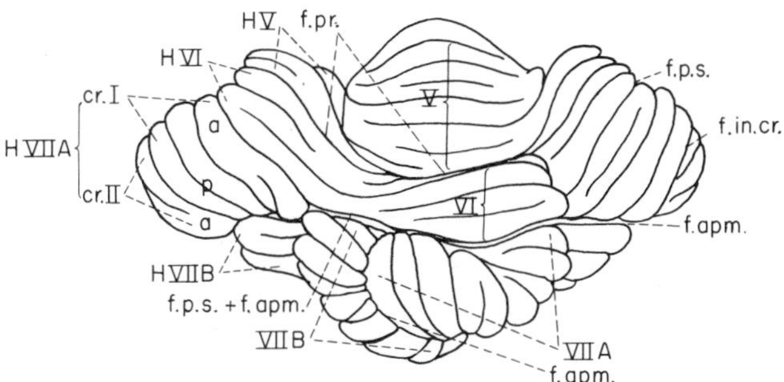

Figure 110. Cerebellum of 3-month-old pig. Dorsal view.

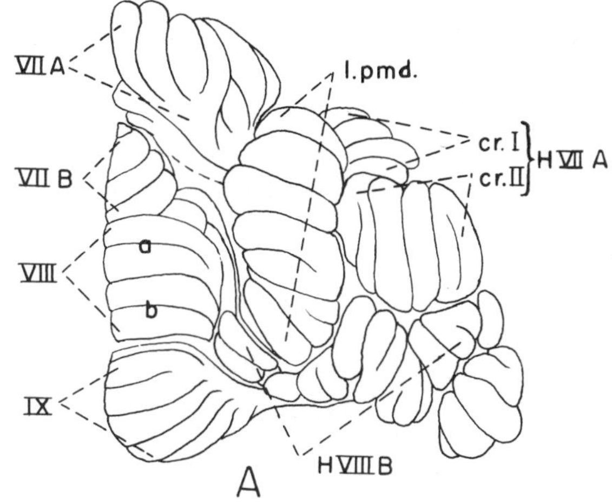

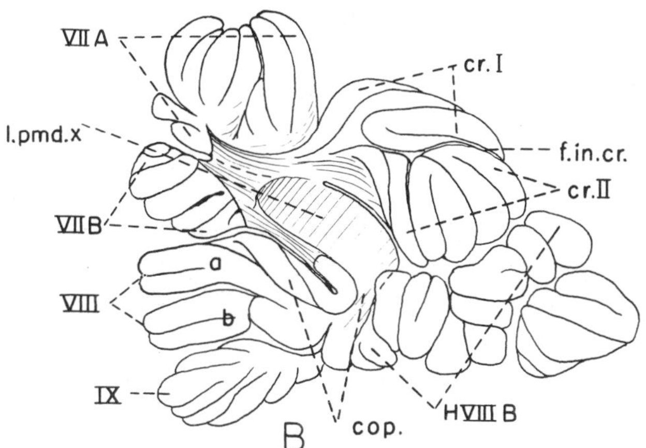

Figure 111. Cerebellum of 3-month-old pig. A. Posterior view. B. Posterior view after paramedian lobule has been dissected away.

3-month-old pig both sublobules have become so large that a median sagittal section of the cerebellum passes through a massive part of each although the principal parts of the two lobules lie on opposite sides of the midline (figs. 109, 110, 111A, 113B). The position and relations of sublobule VIIB in the 140-mm embryo merit special comment. Sublobule VIIB separates the prepyramidal and ansoparamedian fissures; at this stage of development the latter is transverse in the vermis (fig. 104). As sublobules VIIA and VIIB increase in size and are increasingly displaced from their original medial position the vermal part of the ansoparamedian fissure becomes more and more oblique but still remains deep and distinct. In species such as the primates, in which the homolog of sublobule VIIB is reduced to a few folia in the anterior wall of the prepyramidal fissure, the absence of the large segment between the prepyramidal and ansoparamedian fissures brings the two fissures together as a compound cleft, superficially, which separates into its component parts well below the surface (cf. figs. 208, 223).

Lobule VIII, the pyramis, is differentiated by the incipient prepyramidal fissure and the fissura secunda in the 66-mm fetus (fig. 107A). Bradley (1903) mentioned that there were faint indications of fissures in the corresponding region in the 64-mm embryo, but he did not find definite furrows until the 80-mm stage, owing to the lack of intermediate material. In our fetuses of 78 mm to 110 mm in C.R. length both of these fissures are confined to the vermis (fig. 104). Subsequently the fissura secunda extends lateralward and becomes continuous with a furrow that appears in the paraflocculus in the 95-mm fetus (fig. 104C). The united segments form the definitive fissura secunda which is recognizable as a continuous furrow from the paraflocculus of one side to the other in subsequent stages of the fetus and the young pig, as in other species.

The prepyramidal fissure has deepened in the 90-mm embryo (fig. 107B) and is directed on either side toward the rudiment of the paramedian lobule, this relationship becomes more evident as the vermal and hemispheral lobules enlarge (figs. 104D–F). Meanwhile the parafloccular fissure, which delimits the paramedian lobule posterolaterally, extends medialward. In the 125-mm fetus it ends short of, and slightly behind, the prepyramidal fissure, with an oblique bridge of cortex connecting lobule VIII with the caudal part of the paramedian lobule. Behind the paraflocculur fissure lobule VIII is continuous with the dorsal paraflocculus. At the 140-mm stage of the fetus the lateral part of lobule VIII so closely resembles the copula pyramidis of the rat, rabbit, and human fetus that it seems justifiable to regard it as a reduced copula in the pig embryo. It divides into anterior and posterior parts; one connects with the paramedian lobule and the other with the peduncle of the dorsal paraflocculus as in the other embryos investigated (fig. 104F). In the 150-mm and 170-mm pig fetuses the copula is relatively smaller and the portion of the pyramis with which it is continuous has been carried into the floor and the deep anterior wall of the prepyramidal fissure (figs. 106A, B), possibly by the stresses associated with the lateral displacement of sublobule VIIB. The copula and its branches will be considered further in connection with the dorsal paraflocculus and the paramedian lobule.

In median sagittal section lobule VIII remains relatively narrow, dorsoventrally. This is also true in the young pig as compared with the adult pyramis of most other species. At the 150-mm stage of the pig fetus the lobule is divided by a shallow furrow into two superficial lamellae. These subfoliate and the furrow deepens somewhat but the lateral connections of both are with the dorsal paraflocculus as described below. The lateral displacement of sublobule VIIB draws with it the adjacent part of lobule VIII. At first only the rostral folia are involved but gradually the caudal part of the lobule and also the rostral folia of lobule IX are drawn to one side of the midline as sublobule VIIB expands. In the young pig the pyramis has returned to a nearly medial position but it is slightly asymmetrical (fig. 113B).

Lobule IX is delimited dorsorostrally by the fissura secunda. Subject to some variation of position during fetal stages, it has a medial position in the young pig. In the 140-mm embryo, uvular sulci 1 and 2 divide it into folia IXa, IXb, and IXc. Folium IXd has also appeared in the young pig. Laterally the uvula is continuous with the ventral paraflocculus (figs. 111A, 112).

The development of several of the vermal fissures and lobules in the pig strikingly illustrates that the order of appearance of the subdivisions and their delimiting furrows is related to the relative size of the lobules in the fully developed cerebellum of a species, rather than to their significance from the viewpoint of homology. The vermal segment of the ansoparamedian fissure appears very early in the pig, which is in keeping with the precocity and eventual great size of sublobules VIIA and VIIB which it separates. Lobule I, on the other hand, and the precentral fissure do not appear until quite a bit later. The reduced size of lobule I probably could be attributable to its functional insignificance in correlation with the small tail.

HEMISPHERAL LOBULES

Lobule VI is delimited caudally by the hemispheral segment of the posterior superior fissure which, as noted above, appears at about the 80-mm stage of the fetus. The lobule forms the lateral part of the rostral surface of the cerebellum. In the 125-mm fetus it is divided into two broad folia by a furrow which appears to represent the hemispheral part of declival sulcus 2. Some cerebella of this stage and some at earlier stages have a continuous

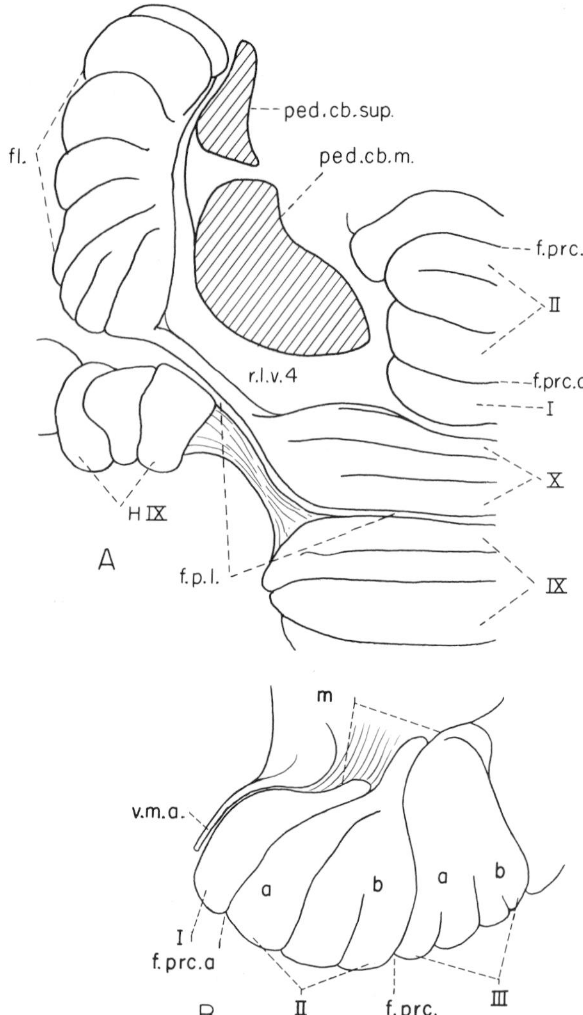

Figure 112. Cerebellum of 3-month-old pig. A. Ventral view. B. Lateral view of lobuli I–III.

posterior superior fissure from the cerebellar margin of one side to the other, which completely delimits lobules VI and HVI from the remainder of the posterior lobe. In others there is a hiatus between the vermal and hemispheral parts of the fissure. The two lobules together correspond to the lobulus simplex of Bolk. In the pig, however, as in other ungulates, the rabbit, and other species, a sharp turn rostralward by the hemispheral portion and a constriction between the latter and the vermal segment that becomes more pronounced in later stages of the fetus and in the young animal (fig. 110) justify differentiation into lobules VI and HVI. Lobule HVI shows three broad surface folia in the 3-month-old pig (fig. 113A). Declival sulcus 1 may continue without interruption from vermis into hemisphere; the vermal and declival parts of declival sulcus 2 usually are discontinuous at the constriction between lobules VI and HVI. In the young pig

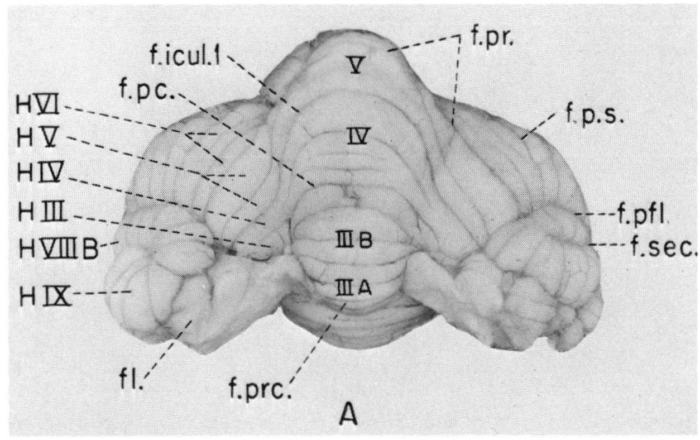

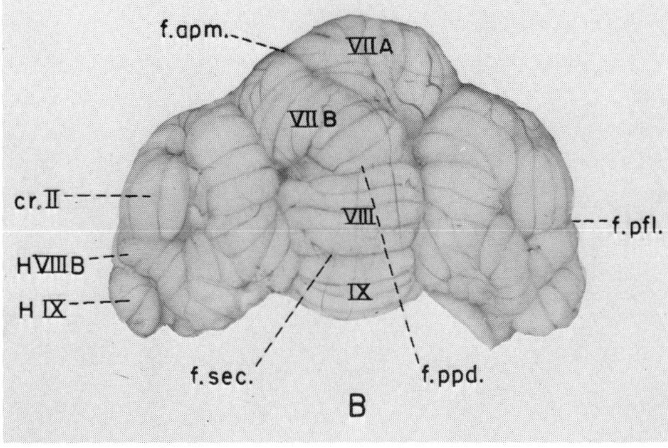

Figure 113. Cerebellum of 3-month-old pig. A. Anterior view. B. Posterior view. Photograph.

there is a sharp dip between the lateral part of lobule VI and lobule HVI on the side toward which displacement of lobule VI and sublobule VIIA has occurred (fig. 113A).

Lobule HVIIA, the ansiform lobule, is clearly continuous with sublobule VIIA in the 110-mm fetus. The vermal part of the ansoparamedian fissure has joined the hemispheral part on either side. In the 125-mm fetus secondary folds have appeared in the lobule (fig. 104E). These are the rudiments of crus I and crus II, with the intercrural fissure being represented by the furrow between the two folia on the right side of the figure and by the furrow between the first and the second folia on the left side (fig. 104). The vermal segment of the intercrural fissure presumably is represented by the furrow in sublobule VIIA of the 110-mm and 115-mm fetuses, and the deeper one in this sublobule of the 140-mm fetus. In the 3-month-old pig crus I comprises three elongated and curved surface folia and others that are hidden in the wall of posterior superior fissure. The surface folia converge toward an isthmus of connection with lobule VIIA (fig. 110). Crus II has five or six shorter and vertically arranged folia that face laterally and posteriorly. Both crura are connected with lobule VIIA by a deep medullary band.

Lobule HVIIB, the anterior part of the paramedian lobule, is delimited rostrally in the 90-mm fetus by the hemispheral part of the ansoparamedian fissure and caudally by the parafloccular fissure. The vermal and hemispheral parts of the ansoparamedian fissure sometimes unite at about the 110-mm stage of the fetus (fig. 104D). They become separated in subsequent stages by stretching and thinning of the cortex incident to displacement of sublobules VIIA and VIIB toward opposite sides and the formation of broad areas between these sublobules and the paramedian lobule on either side (figs. 106A, B). As the lobules increase in size these areas are submerged, forming the floor and lower part of the walls of the paravermian fossae. In the 3-month-old pig the ansoparamedian fissure takes a circuitous course which differs on the two sides. On the side toward which sublobule VIIA is displaced the ansoparamedian fissure begins laterally between crus II and the paramedian lobule and then arches around the dorsal end and upper part of the medial surface of the latter, and then dorsolaterally between sublobules VIIA and VIIB. On the opposite side it continues in front of the paramedian lobule and posteroventrally between this lobule and crus II. The ansoparamedian fissure is deep in the median sagittal plane (figs. 108, 109) because of the large size of sublobules VIIA and VIIB. The prepyramidal fissure continues to elongate in the direction of the posterior part of the paramedian lobule. In the 140-mm fetus this fissure arches in front of the copula and its anterior division onto the paramedian lobule (fig. 104F). At the 170-mm stage the corresponding furrow continues medially into the anterior wall of the prominent vermal segment of the prepyramidal fissure (fig. 106B). In the cerebellum of the 150-mm fetus illustrated in figure 106A the lateral part of the fissure ends medially on the posterolateral surface of sublobule VIIB, and the parafloccular fissure is continuous with the vermal segment of the prepyramidal fissure. Other embryos of the same length, however, show the same relations of the prepyramidal and parafloccular fissures as in the 140-mm and 170-mm stages illustrated in figures 104F and 106B. The extreme lateral part of the prepyramidal fissure delimits a caudomedial crescentic folium of the paramedian lobule which corresponds, except for its deep medial connection, to the pars copularis of other species. The posterior division of the reduced copula (medial in the 170-mm fetus) is continuous behind the parafloccular fissure, with the dorsal paraflocculus.

In the young pig the pars copularis forms a large oblique folium, the most ventral one of the paramedian lobule. It is connected by a distinct medullary band with the medullary substance anterior to and beneath the deep part of the vermal segment of the prepyramidal fissure. The hemispheral part of this fissure has deepened to such an extent that it completely separates the pars copularis from the remainder of the paramedian lobule, except for a deep lateral connection. The prepyramidal fissure also separates the pedunclelike medial continuation of the pars copularis from the medullary connection of the principal mass of the paramedian lobule with the vermis. The posterior division of the copula (medial in the young pig, as in the 170-mm fetus) is connected with the ends of the folia of lobule VIII as it passes caudalward. Its surface expands into two or three caudolaterally directed folia which represent the proximal part of a chain that constitutes the dorsal paraflocculus. The parafloccular fissure continues medially to the lateral part of the vermis between these proximal folia and the pars copularis of the paramedian lobule (fig. 111).

The principal mass of the paramedian lobule is divided into three small folia in the 140-mm fetus. The subsequent foliation and deepening of the first fissure result in two subdivisions that correspond to the pars anterior and pars posterior of the paramedian lobule of other species. In the 3-month-old pig a lateral nearly vertical folium appears to be related to crus II, but dissection shows it to be continuous with the rostral end of the pars anterior (fig. 111B). The pars posterior is connected by a broad medullary band, underlying the floor of the paravermian fossa, with sublobule VIIB. A similar band from the pars anterior merges with the vermal medullary mass beneath sublobule VIIB but some of the connection possibly is with the posterior part of sublobule VIIA.

The paraflocculus, as already noted, is divided into dorsal and ventral parts by a furrow that appears on the lateral surface of the parafloccular rudiment at about the 95-mm stage of the fetus. This furrow lengthens and becomes confluent, medially, with the vermal segment of the fissura secunda which in the meantime has extended lateralward (figs. 104C–F). The completed fissure corresponds to Bradley's sulcus *d* of the pig and other ungulates, but not of the rabbit, and constitutes the definitive fissura secunda. It completely delimits lobule VIII and the dorsal paraflocculus from lobule IX and the ventral paraflocculus except around the end of the fissure where the two limbs of the paraflocculus merge. These features were clearly described by Bradley (1903). In the 125-mm pig fetus each limb of the paraflocculus is continuous with the vermal lobules (VIII and IX, respectively) by a cortex-covered peduncle (fig. 104E). At this stage the distal portion of the dorsal paraflocculus has begun to foliate. In the 140-mm fetus (fig. 104F) foliation has extended caudomedially along both stalks, but in the ventral paraflocculus it extends to the point at which the flocculus begins to expand laterorostrally. Medialward from this point the ventral paraflocculus tapers into a short fibrous peduncle which broadens as it approaches and joins lobule IX (figs. 111A, 112). The most posteriorly situated folium of the ventral paraflocculus enlarges more than the others and probably corresponds to the accessory paraflocculus of Jansen (1950). There are indications that its fibers continue medially into the inferior folia of lobule IX, which suggests that the ventral paraflocculus may also correspond to the avian paraflocculus. The peduncle of the dorsal paraflocculus is surmounted by folia nearly all the way to its attachment with the pyramis in the 170-mm fetus. In the 3-month-old pig the peduncle has lengthened and the dorsal paraflocculus comprises an elongated series of folia that reach the rostral cerebellar surface, which continues there with the ventral paraflocculus. The fissura secunda distinctly separates the dorsal from the ventral paraflocculus as in fetal stages (figs. 113A, B).

FLOCCULONODULAR LOBE IN FETUS AND 3-MONTH-OLD PIG

Although the flocculus is recognizable in the 20-mm embryo (fig. 101), the nodulus is not distinguishable from the tenial margin until approximately the 50-mm stage of the embryo, when a cortical swelling begins to form on either side of the midline immediately ventral of the posterolateral fissure (fig. 102). The germinal zone in the tenial margin enlarges, with its closely packed cells creating a different appearance from that of the incipient nodulus as seen in sagittal sections. The paired rudiments of the nodulus gradually extend toward the midline from either side and fuse to form a single vermal segment (lobule X) as in birds (1948) and the human embryo (1948b).

In the 54-mm fetus the flocculus forms a lateral expansion of the cerebellar continuation of the rhombic lip (fig. 102). At the 62-mm stage a constriction has appeared between it and the tuberculum acusticum, and the band connecting the flocculus and incipient nodulus is somewhat attenuated (fig. 103). The flocculus elongates rostralward beneath the paraflocculus and becomes visible as the most inferior lateral part of the anterior cerebellar surface (figs. 105A, B). It is foliated by the 150-mm stage of the fetus. In the young pig three or four terminal folia appear in the anterior view of the cerebellum while six or seven terminal folia appear on its lateral and ventral surfaces (figs. 112, 113B). The flocculus is attached to the nodulus by a short peduncle that is entirely detached from the parafloccular peduncle; the lateral part of the posterolateral fissure completely separates the two (fig. 112).

The nodulus varies in form, as seen in sagittal sections in early stages of its development, owing to variations in depth of the vermal part of the posterolateral fissure. These variations without doubt result from the stresses of growth that affect the cerebellum and the choroid plexus which is attached to the tenial border of the germinal zone (figs. 107–109). The posterior surface of the nodulus curves forward into the fissure and only this surface is underlaid by developing cortex. By the 78-mm stage of the embryo the posterior surface has expanded so that it bulges caudalward, deepening the posterolateral fissure above it and giving rise to a shallow furrow approximately at the dorsal border of the germinal zone. This furrow appears to correspond to the sulcus taeniae of Hochstetter (1929) in the human embryonic cerebellum, while the posterolateral fissure was called the sulcus anonymus by Hochstetter. Continued expansion of the posterior portion of the nodulus forces its ventricular surface forward; the lobule gradually encroaches on the ventricular space that in earlier stages formed a large-based triangle in sagittal section. The germinal zone assumes first a ventral and then gradually a rostral position with respect to the nodulus. The posterior medullary velum eventually constitutes the greater part of the posterior wall of the fastigial recess of the fourth ventricle (figs. 107–109). By the 150-mm stage of the fetus three folia have formed on the posterior surface of the nodulus; later two additional ones appear on the rostroventral surface (figs. 107, 108). As a result of enlargement and caudal expansion of the corpus cerebelli in subsequent development, lobule X is crowded ventrally and rostrally into the fourth ventricle and is hidden from view in later fetal stages and in the young pig. It remains relatively small in sagittal section but is wide between the floccular peduncle attachments so that a considerable cortical area results (fig. 112).

OX

THE cerebellum of the ox (*Bos taurus*) is characterized by the relatively small size of the hemispheres as compared with the vermis. The anterior part of the vermis projects forward as a prominent vertical ridge well beyond the anterior surfaces of the hemispheres, and the dorsal and posterior portions of the vermis extend beyond the corresponding hemispheral surfaces. The greatest dorsoventral measurement in the median sagittal section is approximately the same as the longest anteroposterior measurement. The dorsal and posterior segment of the vermis, beginning a short distance behind the fissura prima, are so far displaced to one side or the other of the midline in the adult cerebellum that a greatly exaggerated sigmoid pattern results. A deep and wide paravermian fossa separates the dorsal vermal segments from the hemisphere on either side and continues posteriorly as a narrower paravermian sulcus. The displacement of the vermal lobules affects the arrangement of the hemispheral lobules, several of which are not strictly bilaterally symmetrical in position. The anterior lobules of the hemispheres do not overlap the brachium pontis, with the result that the outspread portion of this fiber mass is exposed as it enters the hemisphere. The paraflocculus is relatively small in proportion to the remainder of the organ.

Some of the physical characteristics of the ox that probably have a relationship with the degree of development of various individual lobules may be noted briefly. The body is large and heavy. The legs are short, and the hindlegs are longer than the forelegs. The unilateral independence of both pairs is quite limited. The movements of the ox are generally slow and in running they are quite clumsy. The neck is short and thick; the head is large and heavy. The thick tongue is of unusual importance in gathering food and is aided by the somewhat prehensile lips. The eyes are laterally placed but there is considerable overlap of the visual fields (Riley, 1929, p.83). The tail is long and active.

CORPUS CEREBELLI

The fissura prima, which divides the corpus cerebelli into anterior and posterior lobes, opens on the dorsal surface of the cerebellum (fig. 114B). The anterior lobe is foreshortened anteroposteriorly despite its ridgelike form (fig. 114). It includes approximately one-third of the area of the median sagittal section of the cerebellum, in contrast to the anterior lobe in the horse and camel which comprises about one-half the area of such a section. In the ox, the lobules, accordingly, are relatively smaller and the principal fissures are shorter (fig. 115B).

Lobules I and II together form a keel-like ventral projection. Lobule I is elongated dorsoventrally and is relatively large. The anterior medullary velum is attached near the fastigium so that it constitutes the greater part of the anterior wall of the fastigial recess of the fourth ventricle; all of lobule I is situated rostral of this part of the velum. As seen laterally lobule I comprises seven or eight folia whose intervening furrows end short of the cortical margin. Some of the folia are partially subdivided by shallow furrows that extend but slightly on either side of the midline. The precentral fissure *a* is quite deep and reaches the cortical margin on the lateral surface (fig. 115A). Lobule II has three broad surface lamellae that correspond to lamellae IIa, IIb, and IIc of smaller species. All three lamellae extend farther lateralward than those of lobule I and the rostralmost one appears to have fibrous connections with the brachium pontis.

Lobule III is much larger than lobule II; it comprises two subdivisions, each consisting of several lamellae so that the two may be regarded as sublobules IIIA and IIIB (fig. 114A). The lateral extremities of both are connected with the brachium pontis by fibrous bands.

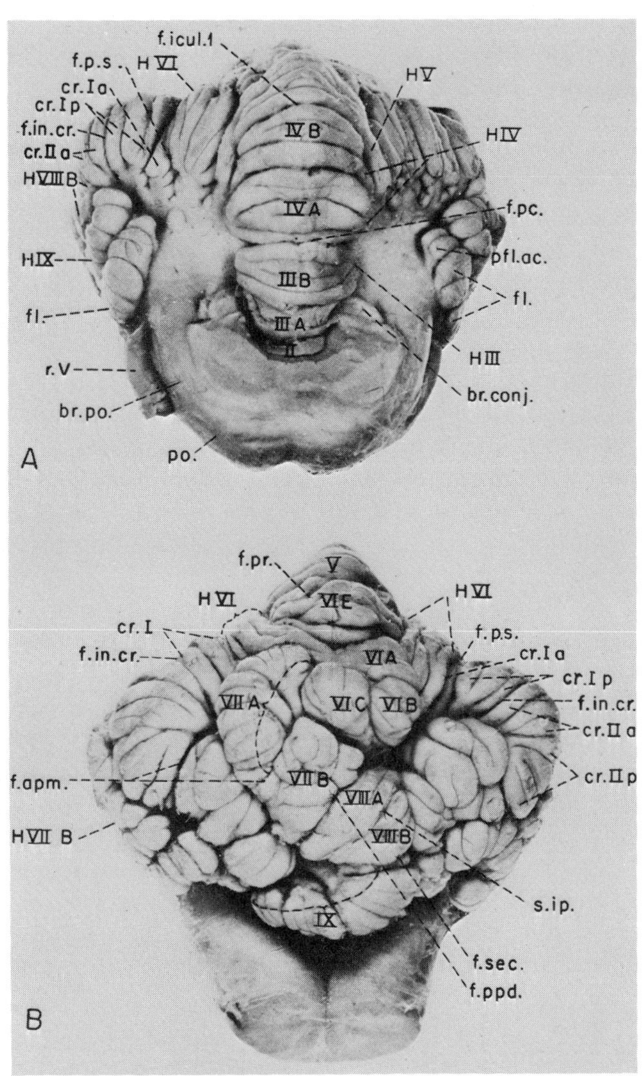

Figure 114. Cerebellum of ox (*Bos taurus*). A. Anterior view. B. Dorsal view.

Whether the lateral parts of the anterior lobe should be regarded as hemispheral or vermal depends on the connections. The preculminate fissure, separating lobule III from lobule IV, is prominent superficially although it is relatively shallow since this part of the anterior lobe is indented (fig. 115B).

Lobule IV is large and distinct owing to the depth of the intraculminate fissure, which delimits it from lobule V. The lobule comprises two subdivisions that because of their large size, as seen in the anterior view of the cerebellum, were designated sublobules IVA and IVB. Both taper toward the brachium pontis and are connected with it by fibrous bands. The lateral part of the lobule extends so far onto the hemisphere that it probably justifies the designation lobule HIV although no superficial boundary is visible between vermal and hemispheral parts.

Lobule V has the typical pattern of three superficial divisions that correspond to lamellae Va, Vb, and Vc and three sagittally elongated lamellae in the anterior wall of the fissura prima that correspond to Vd, Ve, and Vf of other species. The lobule tapers ventrolaterally into an expanded lamella which is joined in the depths of the fissura prima by folia from the anterior wall of the fissure to form lobule HV, most of which is hidden from surface view (fig. 114A).

The vermal lobules of the posterior lobe were more difficult to analyze because of the strongly sinuous form of the remainder of the vermis (fig. 114B). Bradley (1904) illustrated the cerebellum of several stages of the ox embryo before lateral displacement of the vermis has begun. In embryos 150 mm and 175 mm in length the posterior superior, ansoparamedian, prepyramidal, and secunda fissures (fissures *b*, *a*, III, and *d*, respectively, of Bradley) are similar to these fissures in the pig embryo before distortion of the vermis occurs. The lobules which they delimit also correspond quite closely to those of the pig. The median sagittal section of the 175-mm calf embryo shows a large segment which resembles lobule VI of the pig except that the three superficial subdivisions, corresponding to my lamellae VIa, VIb, and VIc, are much larger. Folds in the posterior wall of the fissura prima, corresponding to lamellae VId, VIe, and VIf, also exist in the ox embryo. Lobules C_2 and C_3 of Bradley appear to correspond to my sublobules VIIA and VIIB, and lobules D_1 and D_2 unquestionably correspond to lobules VIII and IX, respectively, both of the pig and of the adult ox described below. In the calf cerebellum the posterior superior fissure is unmistakable in the hemisphere; medially it merges with the ansoparamedian fissure as a result of displacement of sublobule VIIA entirely to one side of the principal vermal axis. Between the vermian part of the fissure and the fissura prima there are four subdivisions of lobule VI whose continuations into the hemisphere are delimited from each other by fissures that extend laterally from the vermis. Whether the most anterior of these subdivisions corresponds to the anterior fold of Bradley's lobule C_1 of the 175-mm embryo or represents a hypertrophied lamella of the posterior wall of the fissura prima could not be determined without examining fetal stages intermediate between those illustrated by Bradley in the calf. The interpretation of my material that conforms most closely with the general pattern of lobule VI is to regard the most anterior of the superficial subdivisions in the ox as a greatly hypertrophied lamella VIe, which becomes sublobule VIE, and the remaining three subdivisions as lamellae VIa, VIb, and VIc (fig. 115B). Sublobule VIE, as a result of its enlargement, has become interposed between the fissura prima and lamella VIa which faces this fissure in most mammals. The two deeper lamellae of the posterior wall of the fissura prima then correspond to lamellae VId and VIf of other species, except that lamella VId is relatively smaller. Lamella VIa has enlarged in the calf so that it may be regarded as sublobule VIA. It and lamella VIb are medially situated but lamella VIc is partially displaced to the right.

Applying the same interpretation to lobule VI of the adult cerebellum, one sees that the caudal part of sublobule VIE has been slightly displaced to the right and sublobule VIA and lamella VIb are strongly displaced in the

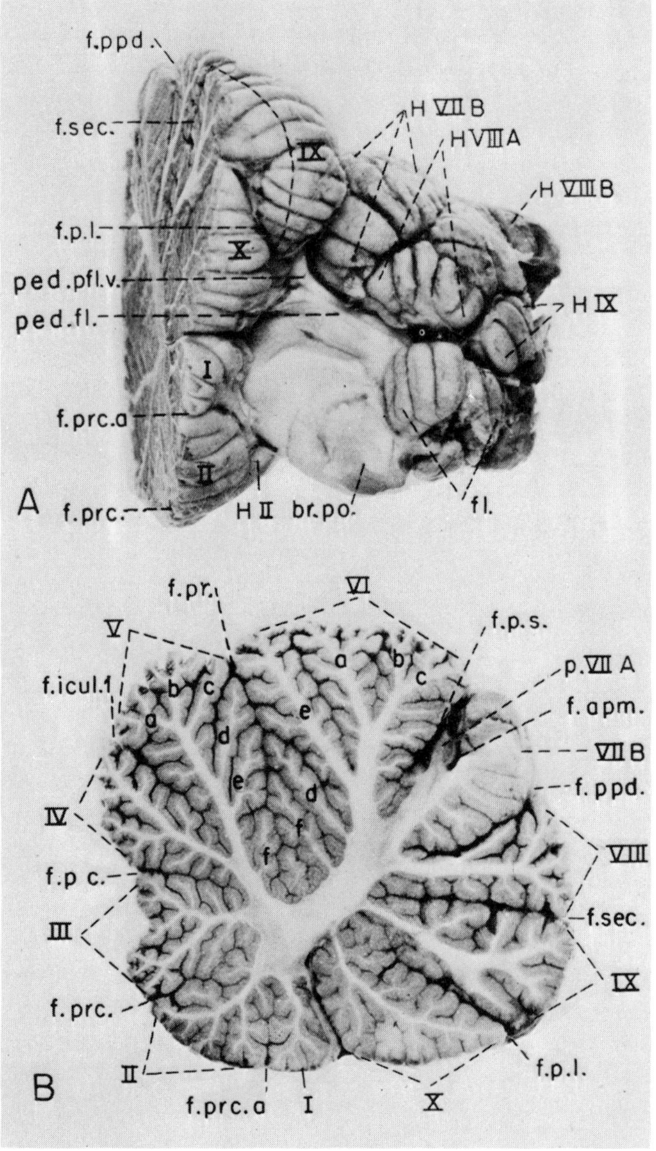

Figure 115. Cerebellum of ox (*Bos taurus*). A. Posteroventral view of right half. B. Midsagittal section of cerebellum of calf.

same direction and toward the paravermian fossa (fig. 114B). Lamella VIc has been carried medially by the displacement to the left of sublobule VIIA. In the calf this sublobule is displaced to the right. The hemispheral continuation of lamella VIc passes into the deep part of the anteromedial wall of the paravermian fossa and continues laterally into the deep part of the posterior superior fissure. On the left side, where the fossa is narrower, the hemispheral relations of lamella VIc are essentially the same.

The median sagittal section of the calf's cerebellum illustrated by Riley (1929, p.80) shows a large subdivision and three smaller ones that correspond to sublobules VIE and VIA, and lamellae VIb and VIc, as described above in the calf, but the deep furrow corresponding to the posterior superior fissure was not labeled. Riley designated as lobulus C_2 all the vermis between the fissura prima and the fissure delimiting his lobule C_1 (the pyramis). A similar emergence to the surface by subdivisions of the posterior wall of the fissura prima was sometimes encountered in other species, especially cetaceans. In the small number of ox cerebella studied or adequately illustrated in the literature, and in the larger number of cetacean cerebella illustrated by Jansen (1950, 1953, 1954) or described on subsequent pages of this book, a sublobule which I interpreted as sublobule VID, or possibly VID + VIE, is always present. Riley's (1929) figures of several cetacean cerebella show a corresponding subdivision. Sublobule VIE seems to be a characteristic feature of the ox cerebellum. In the numerous human cerebella examined either lamella VId or VIe may be enlarged and reach the cerebellar surface, but as a rule both remain hidden in the fissura prima.

The three subdivisions of lobule VI which lie behind sublobule VIE are so large and have so much subfoliation in the adult cerebellum that they could be regarded as sublobules. In the calf, however, only the most anterior of these three divisions is large enough to be considered a sublobule. The remaining two, both in the calf and the adult cerebellum, therefore, were arbitrarily called lamellae VIb and VIc (fig. 114B). The furrow between sublobule VIA and lamella VIb is fairly deep and continues prominently into the hemisphere; it corresponds to declival sulcus 1 of other species. The shallower furrow between lamellae VIb and VIc (declival sulcus 2) dips laterally into the anterior wall of the hemispheral part of the posterior superior fissure. The furrow between sublobules VIE and VIA does not strictly correspond to declival sulcus 3 of other mammals in which lamella VIe is small or lacking; therefore, in the ox I designated it declival sulcus 3′.

Lobule VII comprises two large sublobules, VIIA

and VIIB, which are both displaced to one side or the other of the midline (fig. 114B). The vermal part of the posterior superior fissure in the adult specimen takes a sagittal course between lamella VIc and sublobule VIIA, which is deflected to the left; the fissure then turns lateralward, on the right side, and continues toward the paravermian fossa, separating lamella VIc from sublobule VIIB. From the paravermian fossa the fissure then passes rostrolaterally into the hemisphere, serving in its course as the posterolateral boundary of lamella VIb (fig. 114B). On the left side it separates sublobule VIIA from part of the hemispheral continuation of lobule VI before becoming entirely hemispheral. In the cerebellum of a calf sublobule VIIA is displaced so far to the right that its connection with the medial part of the vermis is by a sheetlike stalk which is interposed between lamella VIc and sublobule VIIB. The posterior superior fissure penetrates deeply in front of this sheet, while the ansoparamedian fissure is less deep behind it; the two fissures merge superficially as a compound fissure (fig. 115B). The ansoparamedian fissure of the large cerebellum is included with the posterior superior fissure as a common fissure between lamella VIc and sublobule VIIB, but it turns laterocaudally to separate sublobules VIIA and VIIB at the left of the midline and then merges with the paravermian sulcus. Finally the ansoparamedian fissure turns sharply laterally and caudally as the boundary between the anterior part of the paramedian lobule and the ansiform lobule (fig. 114B). Sublobules VIIA and VIIB are of unusually large relative size in the ox. Despite the difference of arrangement they conform in morphological relationships with the corresponding sublobules of the pig, camel, and horse, as described elsewhere.

Lobule VIII, the pyramis, is so far displaced to one side of the midline that a median sagittal section passes through its reduced lateral portion (figs. 114B, 115B). The folia of its dorsal and upper posterior surfaces extend laterally as a prominent copula in the smaller cerebellum. In the larger cerebellum a medullary peduncle from the corresponding part of the pyramis gives rise farther laterally to a group of folia continuous with the same parts of the pyramis. In both instances the deep folia of these groups are continuous with the caudal part of the paramedian lobule. The peduncle from pyramis to dorsal paraflocculus is quite distinct from what is connecting the uvula and ventral paraflocculus. The prepyramidal fissure is obliquely directed, disappearing in a deep fossa on either side of the pyramis.

Lobule IX, the uvula, is so strongly deflected to one side that a median sagittal section of the cerebellum gives an entirely inadequate conception of its large size, as is evident from comparison of figures 114B and 115. It is subdivided into four groups of folia that apparently correspond to lamellae IXa, IXb, IXc, and IXd of other species. The fissura secunda is deep and prominent in the vermis and separates the proximal parts of the dorsal and ventral parafloccular peduncles. After the peduncles fuse the fissure is discernible as a shallow groove on the surface of the common peduncle.

HEMISPHERAL LOBULES OF POSTERIOR LOBE

The superficially visible part of the hemispheral continuation of lobule VI comprises three segments which are related to sublobule VIE and lamella VIb. The continuation of lamella VIc is hidden in the anterior wall of the posterior superior fissure. Sublobule VIE tapers lateralward on either side into a superficially visible triangular zone situated between the hemispheral parts of the fissura prima and declival sulcus 3′. The folia of this zone dip sharply ventralward and laterally, forming the posterior wall of the fissura prima, but they do not reach the anterolateral cerebellar surface. The hemispheral continuation of sublobule VIA is different on each side. It is separated from the vermis by a constricted zone and then widens into three large folia that continue onto the anterior cerebellar surface and reach the cerebellar margin, expanding in such a manner as to hide the hemispheral folia of sublobule VIE mentioned above. The displacement of sublobule VIA in the adult cerebellum disturbs the superficial arrangement but the pattern is similar to that in the calf. Declival sulcus 1 extends into the hemisphere as a deep cleft which delimits the extension of sublobule VIA from that of lamella VIb (fig. 114B). The latter is narrow as it leaves the vermis but it spreads laterally as folia hidden in the anterior wall of the posterior superior fissure. The lateral extension of lamella VIc dips deep into the paravermian fossa and continues rostrolaterally as the deep anteromedial wall of the posterior superior fissure. The four groups of hemispheral folia constitute lobule HVI. The great distortion of this lobule in the ox and the differences between the right and left lobules are related to the hypertrophy of sublobule VIE and the increased size of lobule VII, with the resultant crowding of the vermian segment behind the fissura prima.

Lobule HVIIA, the ansiform lobule, is divided into crus I and crus II (fig. 114B). The intercrural fissure is deep in the hemisphere but its identity is lost in the vermis. Crus I comprises five lateroventrally elongated surface folia that are divided by a furrow of intermediate depth into crus Ia and crus Ip, including two and three folia respectively. Crus II is subdivided into crus IIa and crus IIp, with the latter comprising a triangular group of folia on the posterolateral hemispheral surface. Crus I and crus II converge medially into a common deep medullary band which continues into the medullary base of sublobule VIIA.

Lobule HVIIB, the paramedian lobule, comprises two groups of folia that correspond to the pars anterior and the pars posterior of this lobule in other mammals. Both parts are connected with the expanded medullary base of sublobule VIIB by deep medullary bands. They differ in position on the two sides of the posterior cerebellar surface because a large loop of the sinuous vermis forces a different arrangement of the hemispheral lobules of the two sides (fig. 114B). From the deep portion of the pars anterior two superficially visible folia extend caudolaterally, on one side, into a triangular area between crus IIp and the dorsal paraflocculus, but they are not visible on the side toward which sublobule VIIB is deflected. The hemispheral continuation from the copula forms a distinct pars copularis of the paramedial lobule; it is attached to the parafloccular peduncle (fig. 115A).

The dorsal paraflocculus (lobule HVIIIB) comprises a series of loops on the posterior and lateral cerebellar surfaces (figs. 114B, 115A). Its folia are attached to the portion of the parafloccular peduncle that is clearly continuous with sublobule VIIIB. The loops begin as small cortical folds on the peduncle immediately lateral of the copular folia but are separated from the latter by a deep fissure; they increase in size lateralward and form a chain that reaches the anterior cerebellar surface, at which point they turn ventrally and caudally toward the ventral paraflocculus.

The ventral paraflocculus (lobule HIX) is delimited from the dorsal paraflocculus by a well-defined rostrolaterally directed continuation of the fissura secunda. The fissure extends to the rostral tip of the paraflocculus but is hidden farther medially by the loops of the dorsal paraflocculus. The peduncle of the ventral paraflocculus becomes flattened toward the vermis and arches upward as a broad band into the base of lobule IX (fig. 115A), separating itself from the peduncle that connects lobule VIII with the dorsal paraflocculus.

FLOCCULONODULAR LOBE

Lobule X, the nodulus, is unusually long anteroposteriorly and is also wide so that it is relatively larger than in most species (figs. 115A, B). The posterior medullary velum is attached to its base near the fastigium. The vermal part of the posterolateral fissure is unusually deep. The flocculus forms a large group of folia which half encircles the brachium pontis (fig. 114A). It is connected with the nodulus by a floccular peduncle, which is parallel with the parafloccular peduncle but is separated from the latter by a distinctly visible continuation of the posterolateral fissure (fig. 115A). The large flocculus and unusually large nodulus give the flocculonodular lobe of the ox a relatively large size in proportion to the corpus cerebelli.

HORSE

THE cerebellum of the horse (*Equus caballus*) is larger and more rounded than that of the ox and camel. It is irregularly globular in form and somewhat compressed dorsoventrally; the transverse axis is greater than the rostrocaudal axis although the anterior part of the organ is more elongated than in the other ungulates described. The posterior surface is nearly vertical. The vermis is wide and regular on the anterior and dorsal surfaces and becomes narrower and sigmoid on the posterior surface. The hemispheres are relatively large, the paraflocculus is a tortuous series of lamellae flattened against the hemispheres, and the flocculus is relatively smaller than that in the ox and camel. A paravermian sulcus extends from the anterior surface to the posterior inferior surface. It is deep on the caudal, dorsal, and posterior surfaces, where it forms a fossa between the vermis and the hemisphere.

The horse is a perissodactylate ungulate whose physical characteristics are well known. The body is heavy and elongated. The legs are powerful and are capable of independent movement in pawing and kicking. The lips are thick, muscular, and somewhat prehensile, and the tongue is elongated. The eyes are capable of considerable rotation and the movements of the external ears have a wide range. The tail without its long hairy brush is relatively short. The rapid and well-coordinated movements of the horse are in strong contrast with those of the ox and camel.

CORPUS CEREBELLI

The corpus cerebelli as seen in sagittal section is divided into approximately equal anterior and posterior lobes by the fissura prima. This fissure is unusually deep and tilts backward, reaching the posterior dorsal surface. It extends rostrolaterally to the cerebellar margin above the brachium pontis (fig. 116).

The anterior lobe is divided into lobules I–V which apparently correspond to the five segments found by Bradley in an 18-week-old fetal horse. Lobules I and II were included in the lingula of more recent authors. Bolk (1906), however, did not label these or the remaining subdivisions of the anterior lobe of the horse. Lobule I forms a rounded projection extending ventrally and caudally into the fourth ventricle and turning rostralward in a way that gives it the shape of an inverted helmet that more or less completely covers lobule II (fig. 116). As illustrated in the well-executed figures of Leuret and Gratiolet (1839–57) and Sisson and Grossman (1953) and in the more diagrammatic figures of Bolk and others, the corresponding segment has a variety of other patterns. In my specimens the pattern of the lamellae of lobule I differs considerably from that of other large mammals and more nearly resembles the human lingula as most frequently encountered. The lobule comprises a series of transverse folia on the rostral and dorsal surfaces of a medullary sheet that is continuous with the medullary body at the fastigium and covers the lobule laterally as well as posteriorly and ventrally, with a narrow recess of the fourth ventricle extending between the lateral walls and the brachium pontis. The arrangement of the folia suggests that lobule Ia, instead of remaining a single folium as in most species, has developed into a flattened lamella of several folia resting on the medullary sheet with a terminal lamella projecting above it. A single folium with a distinct but small medullary ray appears to represent lamella Ib or Ib + c of other species (figs. 116, 117). Removal of the lateral medullary sheet exposes the lateral surface of this foliated lamella. The lamella was regarded as part of lobule I rather than lobule II because of the depth and relations of the furrow identified as the precentral fissure *a*. Lobule II is relatively small and more or less hidden from view by lobule I, but its folia may reach the ventral cerebellar surface (fig. 117). Lob-

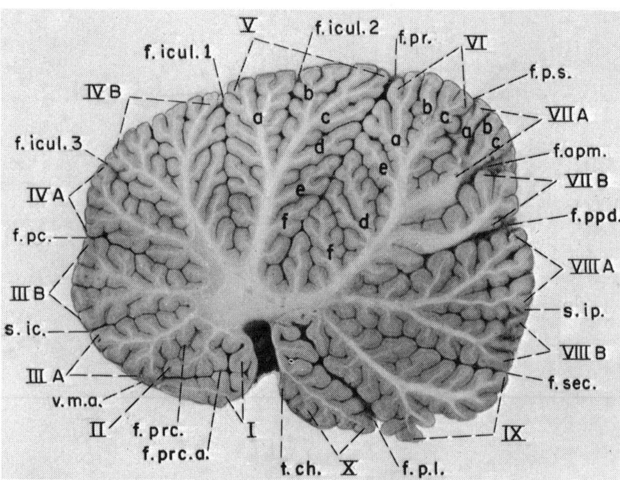

Figure 116. Cerebellum of horse (*Equus caballus*). Midsagittal section.

ule II corresponds to the sublobule centralis anterior of Ziehen in man. A tapering dorsolateral continuation forms a small lobule HII.

Lobule III, the lobus centralis of common usage, comprises two large sublobules, IIIA and IIIB, which are separated by a deep intracentral sulcus 2. Both are continued onto the anterior surface of the hemispheres and the two are connected around the end of the furrow just named. The hemispheral representation of sublobule IIIB is the more prominent; together with that of sublobule IIIA it forms a relatively large lobule HIII. The preculminate fissure is deep and prominent and extends to the cortical margin on either side (fig. 116).

Lobule IV, the pars ascendens monticuli of Flatau and Jacobsohn (1899) and the lobus ascendens of more recent authors, is unusually large in the horse (figs. 116, 118, 119). It comprises three large sublobules which have a constant pattern. In my material and in the illustrations of all authors except Bolk (1906) the most ventral of the three sublobules is the largest and is attached to the deep part of the common medullary ray. In Bolk's figure of a sagittal section of the horse cerebellum the ventral sublobule, although reaching the anterior cerebellar surface, is much smaller than the other two. This suggests that the ventral sublobule corresponds in hypertrophied form to lamella IVd of the camel, pig, and some other species. The two more dorsal subdivisions then would correspond to sublobules IVA and IVB of the ox, camel, and various other mammals. Lobule HIV includes hemispheral continuations of all three vermal sublobules (fig. 119). It forms a rounded eminence which is entirely separated from lobules HIII and HV by the preculminate and intraculminate I fissures. The fissures of lobule HIV itself, however, do not reach the cortical margin, since the folia of the lobule are connected around their ends by a narrow zone of cortex.

Lobule V is greatly elongated dorsoventrally and has a large dorsal surface which is divided by a rather deep furrow, corresponding to intraculminate fissure 2 of the primates and many other species, and several shallower ones (fig. 116). If the segment rostral of the deeper fissure is regarded as homologous with lamella Va, which has become enlarged to form sublobule VA as in the larger primates, then the remaining lamellae, including both the superficial ones and those in the anterior wall of the fissura prima, fall into the pattern characteristic of lobule V generally in all but the smaller species. Lamellae Vb and Vc are superficial but Vd is more deeply submerged than is typical owing to the dorsoventral elongation of the lobule. Lamellae Ve and Vf have their characteristic positions in the deep part of the anterior surface of the fissura prima, and the cortex of the deepest part of this surface has folded into a distinct folium Vg. Lobule HV is formed by lateral expansion of the superficial and fissural folia of lobule V. No distinct boundary between vermal and hemispheral parts of these folia can be drawn but the lateral enlargement into a rounded lobule is noteworthy (fig. 119).

Lobule VI shows the typical pattern of three secondary folds if those, which are lamellae in the horse, are interpreted as indicated in figure 116. The superficial lamellae, VIa, VIb, and VIc, are narrow rostrocaudally but are elongated dorsalward. Lamella VId, characteristically the largest, is subdivided into two secondary la-

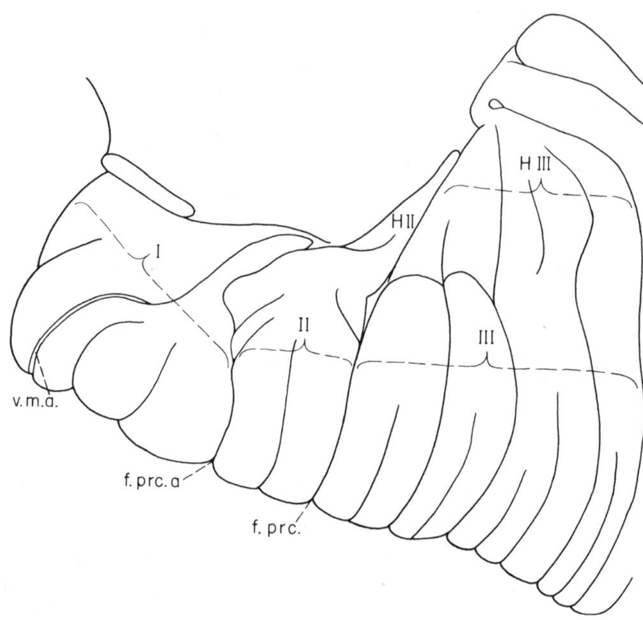

Figure 117. Cerebellum of horse. Left half of the inferior segment of the anterior lobe.

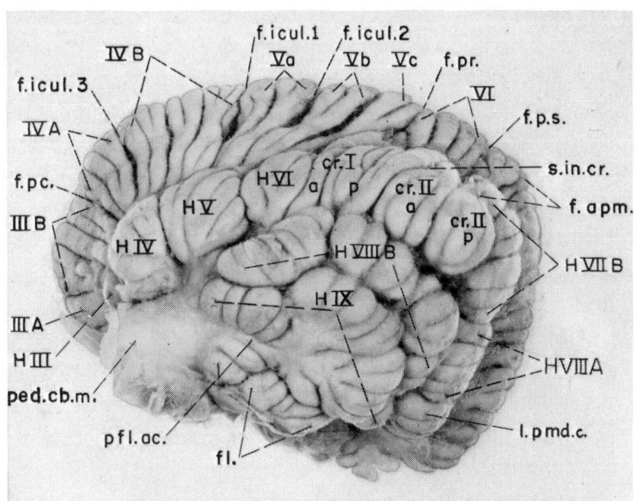

Figure 118. Cerebellum of horse. Lateral view of left half.

HEMISPHERAL LOBULES OF POSTERIOR LOBE

Two superficially visible folia and hidden folia in the posterior wall of the fissura prima and the anterior wall of the posterior superior fissure continue rostrolaterally from lobule VI and expand to form lobule HVI. This has an oval surface area which includes four superficially visible folia (fig. 119). Additional folia, continuous with various vermal lamellae, constitute its fissural surfaces. Declival sulcus 1 passes into the posterior wall of the fissura prima so that the upper part of this wall and part of the superficial surface is a continuation from lamella VIa. Lamella VId is continuous with a hemispheral lamella constituting the majority of the anterior surface of mellae. Lamella VIc is a distinct fold and VIf is relatively large. The deepest cortical fold in the posterior wall of the fissura prima, which in most species is a simple folium, is enlarged in the horse to a lamella that may be designated VIg. The posterior superior fissure is quite deep in the vermis.

Lobule VII is divided by a deep vermal segment of the ansoparamedian fissure into sublobules VIIA and VIIB. The sigmoid curvature of the vermis begins with lobule VII in the horse, with sublobules VIIA and VIIB being displaced to opposite sides of the midline so that only a reduced lateral portion of each appears in a median sagittal section of the cerebellum (fig. 116). Medullary substance is exposed on the ventrocaudal surfaces of each, which represents the medullary bands that lead to the ansiform lobule (HVIIA) and the paramedian lobule (HVIIB) respectively. The prepyramidal fissure is deep and prominent.

In its dorsal portion, lobule VIII includes three surface lamellae that correspond to sublobule VIIIA of many mammals, and a large lamella that corresponds to sublobule VIIIB. The anterior folia of VIIIA turn ventrocaudally on either side, forming a tapering copula pyramidis. The fissura secunda is exceeded in depth in the median plane only by the fissura prima (fig. 116).

Lobule IX is deflected to one side so that its longitudinal axis is oblique to the midline. The lobule is relatively large in the horse but only three elongated lamellae, visible on the lateral surface, represent the characteristic subdivisions of this vermal segment. These appear to correspond to lamellae IXa, IXb, and IXc. Lamella IXd is obscured by the caudal elongation and the oblique axis of the uvula.

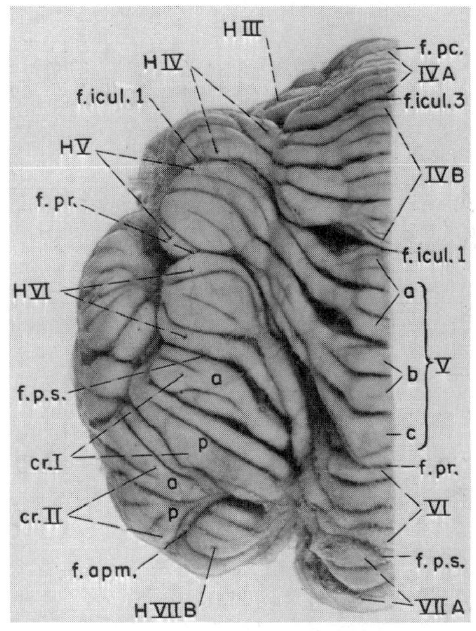

Figure 119. Cerebellum of horse. Dorsal view of left half.

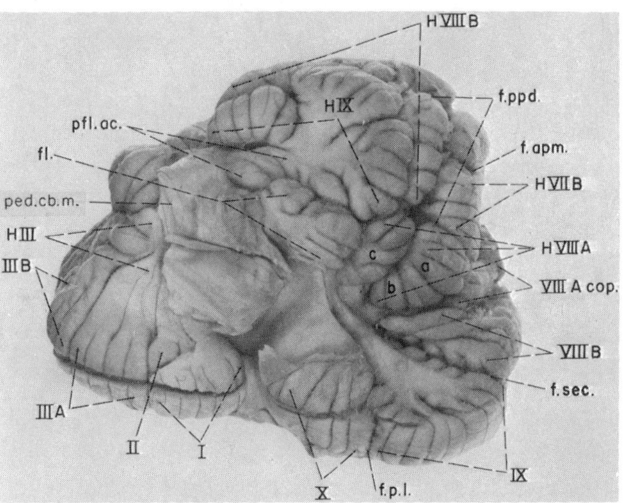

Figure 120. Cerebellum of horse. Ventral view of left half.

lobule HVI and may appear at the lateral surface. Lamellae VIe and VIf have continuations onto the anterior surface. The hemispheral representation of lamella VIb is on the superficial surface of HVI, while that of lamella VIc is largely on its posterior surface, facing the deep hemispheral segment of the posterior superior fissure.

Lobule HVIIA has continuity with lobule VIIA only by a medullary pedunclelike connection beneath the paravermian fossa, which is deep between these two segments. It is divided into crus I and crus II by a deep and corrugated intercrural fissure (figs. 118, 119). Crus I consists of rostrolaterally elongated folia and is subdivisible into Ia and Ip. Save for its lateral tip crus Ia is hidden as the principal part of the posterior wall of the posterior superior fissure. Crus Ip includes the elongated superficially visible folia. Crus II is divided into a lateral group of five elongated folia, which constitute crus IIa, and a posterior group of five or six, which converge medially and are connected with the medullary peduncle of crus IIa by a vertical, flattened medullary band (fig. 119).

Lobule HVIIB, the paramedian lobule, is divided into pars anterior and pars posterior, with the medullary bands of both continuing with the deep medullary layer of sublobule VIIB. The pars anterior and the pars posterior include six and seven folia, respectively, that together form a long chain from the dorsal to the ventral cerebellar surfaces (fig. 118). A group of four or five smaller folia form a pyriform lobule, lateral of the pars posterior, which is connected by an elongated lamella with the copula pyramidis; the lobule therefore corresponds to the pars copularis of the paramedian lobule of other species. The deep ends of its folia are continuous with the deep part of the pars posterior. In the horse the pars copularis covers the distal part of the parafloccular peduncle but is quite distinct from the dorsal paraflocculus. Its cortex-covered peduncle is adherent to the proximal part of the parafloccular peduncle but separates from it before reaching the pyramis and passes into sublobule VIIIA, while the peduncle of the dorsal paraflocculus passes into sublobule VIIIB. The pars copularis of the paramedian lobule therefore may be regarded as lobule HVIIIA (fig. 120).

Lobule HVIIIB, the dorsal paraflocculus, begins as a chain of small folia beneath the pars copularis; the folia increase in size as the series emerges, and the chain ascends parallel with the pars posterior and then turns rostralward, extending as far as lobule HV (fig. 118). A group of folia whose axes are nearly vertical is attached to the brachium pontis immediately ventral of the anterior part of the dorsal paraflocculus; it is not clear whether they should be regarded as part of the dorsal paraflocculus or as belonging to the ventral paraflocculus. The group is separated from the dorsal chain described by a deep fissure which is a direct continuation of the fissure between the remainder of the two paraflocculi. This, in turn, is continuous with the fissura secunda. This fissure bifurcates distally into a forward directed branch and a broader and deeper furrow which is directed ventrally in front of the expanded part of the ventral paraflocculus (fig. 118). The group of folia rostral of the ventrally directed fissure appears to be more closely related to the ventral paraflocculus.

Lobule HIX, the ventral paraflocculus, comprises a series of large lamellae that are somewhat flattened against the principal mass of the posterior lobe. Lobule HIX is attached to a wide medullary band that constricts into a peduncle in its medial course and then expands as it enters the uvula (fig. 120). Rostrolaterally the medullary band is attached to the brachium pontis. Ventral of its attachment two or three folia that apparently belong to the ventral paraflocculus are attached directly to the brachium pontis. They are completely separated from the rostral end of the flocculus by the deep distal part of the posterolateral fissure (figs. 118, 120). The expanded portion of the ventral paraflocculus evidently corresponds to the lobulus petrosus of many species but whether the deeply separated caudomedial part could be regarded as representing the accessory paraflocculus of Jansen in other large mammals must remain an unanswered question. The length of the fibrous parafloccular peduncle, which it shares with the remainder of the ventral paraflocculus, makes it impossible to determine if this group of folia is connected with any specific part of the uvula, as is the accessory paraflocculus.

FLOCCULONODULAR LOBE

Lobule X, the nodulus, is greatly elongated caudalward so that it forms a relatively very large lobule. However, it is attached to the medullary body by only a thin band of medullary substance which forms the posterior wall of the fastigial recess. The posterior medullary velum is attached at the base of a large cluster of folia that constitutes the major part of the nodulus (fig. 118). The flocculus consists of ten or eleven obliquely directed external folia that continue in reduced number onto the hidden surface of the lobule (fig. 120). It is attached to the nodulus by a short peduncle which, as Ingvar (1918) pointed out, is partially covered with cortex. The peduncle spreads medially, forming a broad triangular band that is continuous with the medullary substance of the nodulus. The posterolateral fissure forms a deep furrow between the flocculus and the ventral paraflocculus; this fissure is reduced in depth along the peduncle but forms a prominent fissure in the vermis.

CAMEL

THE one available cerebellum of the camel (*Camelus* sp.) differs somewhat in form from that of *Camelus bactrianus* described by Riley (1929). Presumably my specimen is the cerebellum of the dromedary, *Camelus dromedarius*, but there was no available information regarding its source. The cerebellum is broad and relatively short. The general pattern of lobules and fissures resembles an exaggerated form of the ox. The lobules are larger and overlap the margins of the cerebellar cortex so that the peduncles are well hidden. The hemispheres, paraflocculi, flocculi, and nodulus are relatively large. The vermis is broad anteriorly and projects only slightly beyond the general rostral surface except on the ventral side. Behind the fissura prima the vermis becomes narrow and assumes an exaggerated sigmoid form. On either side of the sigmoid portion a deep fossa penetrates to a series of medullary bands which expand medially and laterally into the bases of the vermal and the hemispheral segments that they interconnect. In the fresh cerebellum this paravermian fossa probably is less open than in the preserved specimen illustrated in the figures. The deeper part of the walls and the floor of the fossa are devoid of cortex; the upper walls are foliated, with the folia increasing in number toward the surface and expanding as the hemispheral and vermal lobules. A deep and narrow paravermian sulcus continues caudalward from the paravermian fossa.

The camel is one of the larger artiodactylate ungulates. The body is heavy and elongated. The tail is relatively small and of little functional significance. The legs are long and, according to Riley (1929), have little or no unilateral independence. The animal walks in a slow, shuffling manner and runs awkwardly. The neck is elongated, the head is relatively large. The upper lip is prehensile, helping the elongated tongue to draw food into the mouth; both lips are large. The external ears are small. The eyes, whose movements are limited, are laterally situated, with the fields of vision overlapping but slightly (Riley, 1929).

CORPUS CEREBELLI

Lobule I is elongated dorsoventrally, forming a keel as in the ox (figs. 121, 123C). It is narrow from side to side and the folia are short, ending on the exposed medullary lateral surface of the lobule. Folium Ia lies against a thin sheet of medullary substance that continues beyond the ventral tip of the folium as the anterior medullary velum. In addition lobule I includes two surface lamellae (Ib and Ic) and a number of small folia on its anterior and posterior surfaces. Precentral fissure *a* is deep and extends to the cerebellar margin on either side of the vermis (fig. 122).

Lobule II comprises two large surface lamellae that are separated by a furrow that penetrates about halfway to the base of the lobule. Lamella IIa expands slightly beyond the lateral surface of lobule I but also has a keel-like form. Lamella IIb extends beyond the lateral border of the keel and expands slightly, forming a suggestion of a hemispheral lobule. The precentral fissure, separating lobule II from lobule III, is deep and extends to the cerebellar margin on either side (fig. 123A).

Lobule III is divisible into sublobules IIIA and IIIB. In comparison with the other subdivisions of the anterior lobe they are relatively small in the camel. They merge laterally around the ends of intracentral fissure and form a small triangular lobule HIII (figs. 122, 123A).

Lobule IV is prominent both in median sagittal section and as seen on the rostral cerebellar surface (figs. 121, 123). Its two subdivisions are so large that they must be designated as sublobules IVA and IVB. The preculminate fissure, delimiting IVA from lobule III, is the most conspicuous furrow on the anterior cerebellar surface,

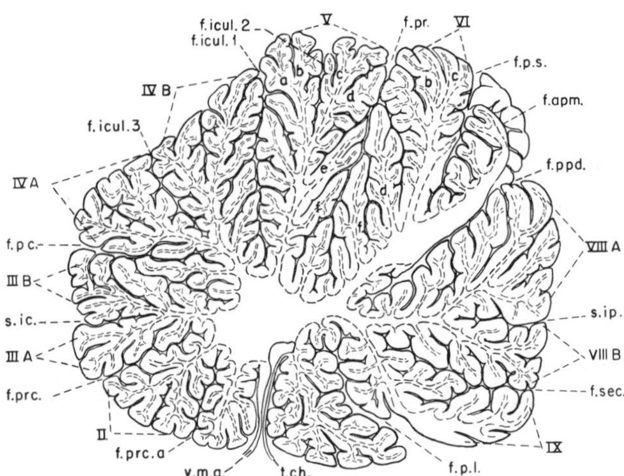

Figure 121. Cerebellum of camel. Sagittal section slightly to the right of the median plane.

and it completely divides the anterior cerebellar surface from margin to margin. An elongated lamella, which forms the greater part of the dorsal wall of this fissure, continues into the lateral part of sublobule IVA but does not reach the surface. The two sublobules are separated by a rather deep intraculminate fissure 3, but they taper laterally and join around the end of this fissure forming lobule HIV. Most of this lobule is hidden in the floor and medial wall of the hemispheral part of intraculminate fissure I, while only two folia that continue from sublobule IVA are visible on the anterior cerebellar surface (fig. 123A).

Lobule V, in sagittal section, presents a dorsoventrally elongated form that tapers gradually from its external surface toward the medullary body (fig. 121). The fissura prima and intraculminate fissure I both are unusually deep in the camel. The surface lamellae, namely, Va, Vb, and Vc, are elongated dorsoventrally, with Vc facing the fissura prima. Lamella Vd is not distinct unless represented by the folium ventral of VIc. The largest fold in the

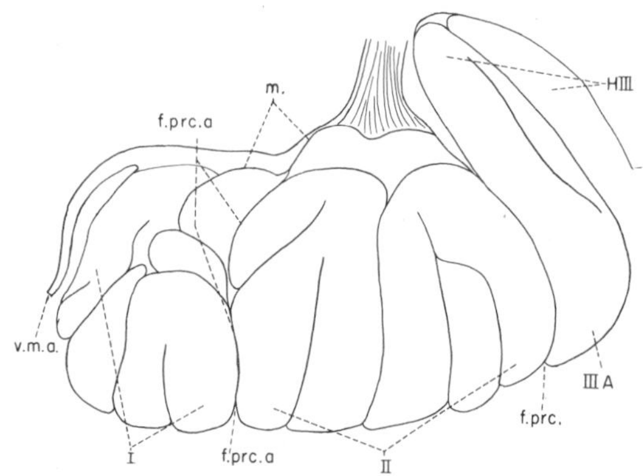

Figure 122. Cerebellum of camel. Lateral view of lobules I and II.

anterior wall of the fissura prima was regarded as lamella Ve, which is typically the most prominent in other species. As in other cerebella having an unusually deep fissura prima there are two lamellae ventral of Ve that were designated Vf and Vg.

The hemispheral representation of lobule V is prominent in the camel (fig. 123A). The vermal lamellae become reduced on each side of the vermis and then expand on the anterior cerebellar surface into a gourd-shaped lobule HV. A deep lamella from sublobule IVB extends across the floor of intraculminate fissure I into lobule HV which also is augmented by a hemispheral continuation of lamella IVf, described below, that crosses the floor of the fissura prima.

Lobule VI includes three surface subdivisions which may be regarded either as large lamellae or small sublobules. I labeled them lamellae VIa, VIb, and VIc. The lobule is deflected diagonally to the right, beginning with VIa, to such an extent that a median sagittal section would miss most of its superficial region. The section illustrated in figure 121, accordingly, had been cut slightly to the right of the midline so that it includes the anterior lamellae of the lobule under consideration. As the figure shows, three additional elongated lamellae constitute the posterior wall of the fissura prima. These correspond to lamellae VId and VIf of other mammals. The posterior superior fissure is identifiable between lobule VI and sublobule VIIA on the left side but merges with the ansoparamedian fissure on the right side, disappearing on both sides in the depths of the fossa. Declival sulci 1 and 2, recognizable in the vermis, also are lost in the fossa. The caudal part of lamella VIc turns slightly toward the midline. Its medullary substance is continuous with that of sublobule VIIA (fig. 123B) beneath the posterior superior fissure.

Lobule VII forms a loop of folia which for the most part lies to the left of the midline (fig. 123C). It is divided into sublobules VIIA and VIIB by the vermal segment of the ansoparamedian fissure. In the sagittal section illustrated, only the medullary peduncle leading to the two sublobules and the cut-off medial tip of VIIA are shown, with sublobule VIIB lying entirely at the left of the plane of section. Owing to the lateral displacement of lobule VII the anterior-superior wall of the prepyramidal fissure is formed, mainly from the medullary band leading to the lobule (fig. 121).

Lobule VIII, the pyramis, must be regarded as comprising two sublobules, VIIIA and VIIIB, separated by a fairly deep intrapyramidal sulcus. The folia of sublobule VIIIA converge on its lateral surface and in the depths of the paravermian sulcus; they expand laterally to form a group of copular folia, the most submerged of which is

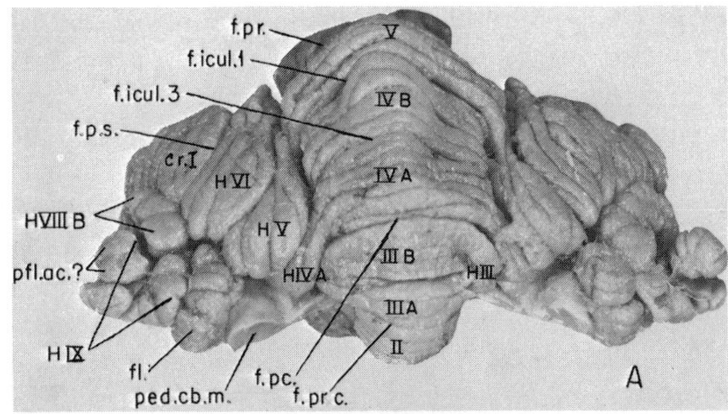

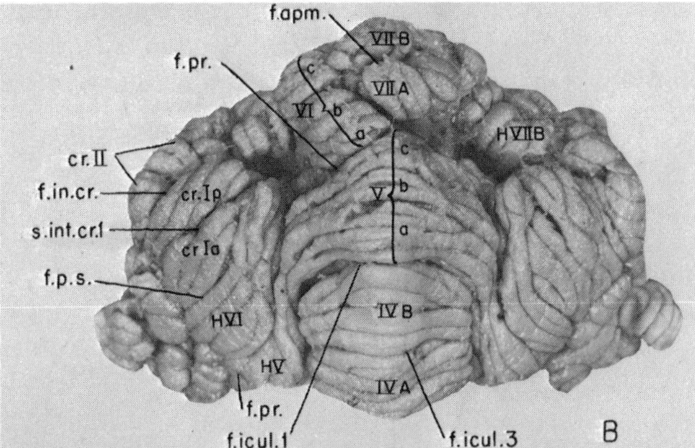

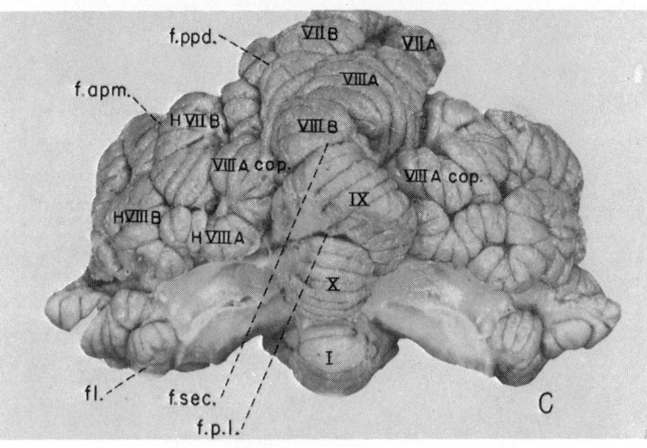

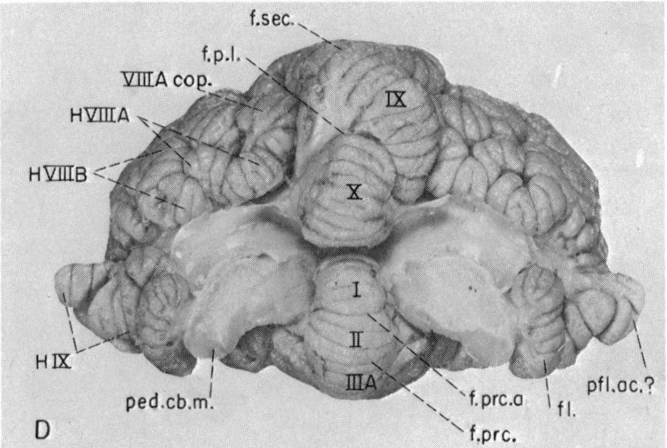

Figure 123. Cerebellum of camel. A. Anterior view. B. Dorsal view. C. Posteroventral view. D. Ventral view.

continuous rostrolaterally with the pars posterior of the paramedian lobule. The group is attached to the rostral part of the medullary peduncle leading to the paraflocculus. The prepyramidal fissure continues laterally in front of the copular group of folia and merges with the parafloccular fissure.

Lobule IX, the uvula, is somewhat flattened and most of it is situated at one side of the midplane. The fissura secunda has an oblique direction. The distortion of the lobule makes it impossible to identify the three to four principal lamellae (or folia) characteristic of the uvula in the cerebellum of most mammals and birds. The medullary peduncle leading to the paraflocculus is broad and distinct for some distance lateral of the uvula but it soon passes into a rounded peduncular band in which there is no sign of the fissura secunda.

HEMISPHERAL LOBULES OF POSTERIOR LOBE

The medullary substance of lobule VI and sublobule VIIA continues laterally as a common medullary band in the floor of the paravermian fossa. In the lateral wall of the fossa folia appear and expand to form lobules HVI and HVII, and the hemispheral segment of the posterior superior fissure forms a deep cleft between them. Lobule HVI has a broad triangular surface including four or five large folia in its widest part (fig. 123A, B) and its surfaces on the delimiting fissures also are formed of large folia. Lamella VIe is confined to the vermis; lamella VId continues uninterruptedly to form part of the posterior wall of the fissura prima; lamella VIf crosses the floor of this fissure and becomes included in the lower part of its anterior wall. The anterior wall of the posterior superior fissure is formed of folia that appear to be lateral representations of lamella VIc, although declival sulcus 1 could not be followed into the hemisphere. The two groups of surface folia of HVI more clearly are medially related with lamellae VIa and VIb.

Lobule HVIIA, the ansiform lobule of Bolk, comprises three or four superficial elongated folia, rostrally, and nine or ten that form the lateral part of the hemisphere (fig. 123B). The rostral group constitutes crus I and the caudal group forms crus II. Three or four folia in the posterior wall of the posterior superior fissure are separated from two which form the dorsal part of this wall by a furrow that is deeper and more prominent than the others and may represent intracrural sulcus 1. The more ventral group of folia may represent crus Ia, and the dorsal and surface group crus Ip, but this is not certain. Two groups of folia in crus II more clearly correspond to crus IIa and crus IIp of other species. The intercrural fissure is deep, disappearing medially in the paravermian fossa.

The paramedian lobule (figs. 123B, C) includes three groups of folia, anterior, intermediate, and posterolateral, which are separated from each other and from neighboring lobules by deep fissures. Each group forms the crown of a stalklike medullary mass which merges with the deep medullary body. So far as connections between the subdivisions of the paramedian lobule and the lobules of the vermis could be determined, the medullary stalk of the anterior subdivision, which corresponds to the pars anterior of the lobule in other species, continues into the medullary mass at the base of sublobule VIIB. The intermediate and posterolateral divisions are less completely divided from each other and apparently correspond to the pars posterior of the lobule in smaller species. They have connections through a common medullary stalk with the medulla beneath sublobule VIIB and in the floor of the prepyramidal fissure. The ansoparamedian fissure takes a tortuous course from one lateral margin of the cerebellum to the other (fig. 123B, C).

The copula pyramidis is prominent in the camel. It comprises six superficial folia on the medullary stalk that continues lateralward from the pyramis. These constrict medially, but their cortex is continuous with that of the anterior folia of sublobule VIIIA. Laterally the copula is continuous with the pars copularis of the paramedian lobule (fig. 123C).

The paraflocculus is a large and convoluted mass of folia that is attached to a broad fibrous band whose vermal connections are with the bases of lobules VIII and IX. The folia of the dorsal paraflocculus begin beneath the copula and continue in an unbroken chain to the inferior rostral surface of the cerebellum (fig. 123A), from which it is separated by the prominent parafloccular fissure. The ventral paraflocculus, as in other species, is continuous rostrally with the dorsal paraflocculus. The ventral paraflocculus expands into a series of laterally projecting folia that form the petrosal lobule; no ventral parafloccular folia were found on the long stretch of the peduncle between this lobule and the vermis. As it approaches the vermis the parafloccular peduncle broadens and then is divided into two parts by the fissura secunda. The anterior part enters the base of sublobule VIIIB and the posterior part enters lobule IX. The lower surface of one side of the latter lobule consists of the entering medullary peduncle. The lobulus petrosus, in all probability, corresponds to the accessory paraflocculus of other species.

FLOCCULONODULAR LOBE

The flocculonodular lobe is large in the camel. The posterolateral fissure could be followed from nodulus to flocculus. It is deep between the nodulus and uvula, becomes a shallow groove between the floccular and parafloccular peduncles, and then becomes a deep and prominent cleft between the flocculus and ventral paraflocculus. The nodulus (lobule X) is larger in proportion to the remainder of the cerebellum than in any other species investigated except the ox. Its anteroposterior axis is slightly oblique as a result of the strong lateral displacement of the inferior part of the uvula. The flocculus also is unusually prominent (figs. 123A, C), since it is composed of twelve nearly transverse folia. Its peduncle arches laterorostrally from the nodulus in the border of the posterior medullary velum.

FUR SEAL

THE cerebellum of the fur seal (*Callorhinus ursinus*) has the form of a broad arch that extends on either side to a level considerably ventral of the under surfaces of the medulla oblongata and pons (fig. 124). The vermis presents a prominent ridge on the dorsal surface but slopes gradually onto the hemispheral surface on either side with no trace of a paravermian sulcus. The posterior and inferior surfaces, however, are deeply indented by a paravermian sulcus on either side of the vermis. The dorsal paraflocculus is a massive lobule that forms the ventral portion of the hemisphere except anteromedially; here the smaller but very large ventral paraflocculus forms the medial part of the ventral surface and extends to the lower anterior surface. These two lobules and the paramedian lobule, which is also of unusually large size in comparison with the species described on the preceding pages, together present a greater surface area than all of the remainder of the hemisphere. The disproportionately large size of these three lobules prevails in other pinnipeds and even more strikingly in cetaceans.

The fur seal has an elongated body and neck, with the latter also being very thick, especially in males. In common with other pinnipeds the thigh and arm and nearly all of the leg and forearm are enclosed by the body integument. The hand and foot are elongated, and the entire extremity constitutes a flipper. The hindlimbs and tail together serve as a propulsive organ in the water. The hindlimbs can be turned forward on land to aid the forelimbs in supporting the body weight; in the Phocidae forward flexion of the thigh is not possible. The fur seal has small external ears. The fields of vision overlap and the eyes probably have well-conjugated movements as in *Phoca*. The male fur seal attains a head-body length of 2 meters or more and a weight of 180 kg to approximately 320 kg (Palmer, 1954).

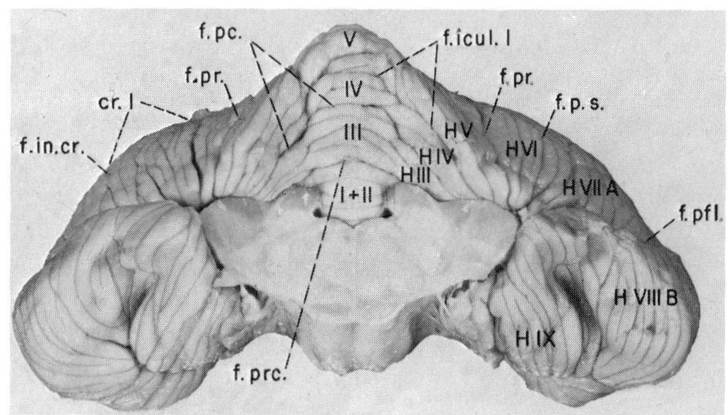

Figure 124. Cerebellum of fur seal (*Callorhinus ursinus*). Anterior view. ×1.3. Photograph.

CORPUS CEREBELLI

The exposed surface of the anterior lobe is relatively small in proportion to the entire cerebellum, owing to the large paraflocculi and the paramedian lobule. As compared with the remainder of the corpus cerebelli the anterior lobe is fairly large superficially. In median sagittal section of the cerebellum it constitutes nearly one-half of the area (fig. 127). Lobules I and II together form a large segment whose two components are not easily differentiated from each other. In sagittal section this segment is very similar in outline, number of lamellae, and distribution of medullary rays to lobules I and II of the dog and some other species. The illustrations of Bolk (1906) and Riley (1929) of median sagittal sections of the cerebellum of the harbor seal, *Phoca vitulina*, show the corresponding part of the anterior lobe as being divided by a fissure into two distinct segments which Bolk designated lobuli 1 and 2. Riley, who based his lobuli entirely on the pattern of the medullary rays, included in his lobulus 1 only the lamella corresponding to that labeled lobule I in figure 127; the remainder of the anterior lobe

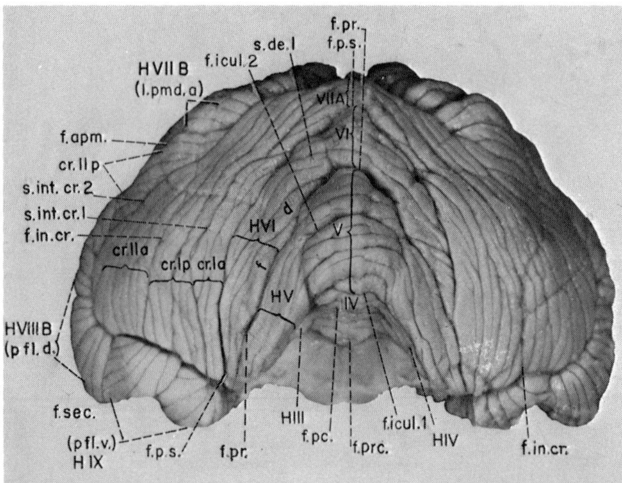

Figure 125. Cerebellum of fur seal. Anterodorsal view. ×1.3. Photograph.

ventral of the preculminate fissure was designated lobulus 2 by him. Jansen (1954, fig. 21) interpreted as lobule I, using my terminology, the corresponding lobule of *Phoca groenlandica*. The furrow designated precentral fissure in figure 127 corresponds to the precentral fissure of the dog and other species and to the deeper furrow, mentioned above, of the harbor seal. This fissure was interpreted by Jansen as the preculminate in the Greenland seal. On the lateral surface of the fur seal it fails to reach the cerebellar margin, although the fissure delimiting lobule I almost does so. Whether or not these are constant patterns in *Callorhinus* is unknown but the information at hand indicates that lobules I and II are incompletely differentiated from each other. The rostralmost lamella of the combined lobules has a small hemispheral representation corresponding to lobule HII of other species.

Lobule III is well defined by the precentral and preculminate fissures. It is divided into two large surface lamellae and is very similar in sagittal section to Bolk's lobulus 3 in *Phoca vitulina* and Jansen's lobule III in *P. groenlandica*, although Jansen labeled its ventral furrow the preculminate fissure. A ventrolateral extension on either side forms a small lobule HIII on the anterior cerebellar surface (fig. 124).

Lobule IV is narrow in median sagittal section but the intraculminate fissure, delimiting it from lobule V, is deep and continues ventrolaterally to the cerebellar margin (fig. 125). A corresponding lobule, designated 4b by Bolk and IV by Jansen, was found in the two species of *Phoca*. Riley included it, together with Bolk's lobulus 4a (my lobule V), in his lobulus 4 and did not differentiate a lobulus 3. Jansen included the anterior subdivision of lobule V, as I regarded it, with lobule IV of the Greenland seal. In this species the fissure corresponding to that labeled intraculminate fissure 2 in figure 125 apparently is much deeper than in the fur seal. The fissure corresponding to the intraculminate fissure, however, is shown as still deeper in Jansen's figure. The differences of interpretation require fetal material for reconciliation. A single broad surface lamella and a number of folia hidden in the delimiting fissures constitute lobule HIV.

Lobule V comprises surface lamellae Va, Vb, and Vc and lamellae Vd, Ve, and Vf on the anterior wall of the fissura prima. The undesignated folds in the posterior wall of the intraculminate fissure are also included. Lamella Va is so large that it could almost be regarded as a sublobule; it corresponds to the dorsal subdivision of Jansen's lobule IV of the Greenland seal. Lamella Vf is unusually large in the fur seal as well as in Riley's figure of the harbor seal. Three elongated superficial lamellae and folds hidden in the fissura prima and intraculminate fissure constitute lobule HV (fig. 125). The fissura prima, as in most mammals, is the deepest of the fissures shown in median sagittal section. As seen on the anterior cerebellar surface it dips rather sharply to the ventral margin (fig. 125).

The vermal lobules of the posterior lobe were readily recognized both in sagittal section and superficially (figs. 125, 126, 127). Lobule VI has three surface lamellae (VIa, VIb, and VIc) and the typical folia and lamellae (VId, VIe, VIf, and VIg) that form the posterior wall of the fissura prima. The posterior superior fissure is deep and distinct on the dorsal and rostral cerebellar surfaces. Lobule VI of Jansen's figure of *Phoca groenlandica* is relatively much smaller superficially and is divided by a deep fissure that corresponds in position to declival sulcus 2. In Riley's figure of the harbor seal the corresponding lobule, labeled c_3, also is larger than in *Callorhinus*, but the deeper of the two principal furrows corresponds to declival sulcus 2.

Lobule VII includes only one obvious segment but the connections of the cortical folds in the anterior wall and floor of the prepyramidal fissure are with the paramedian lobule. The ansoparamedian fissure continues from the hemisphere into the upper part of the anterior wall of the prepyramidal fissure (fig. 127). The greater part of lobule VII, which is situated above and rostral to the vermal continuation of the ansoparamedian fissure, accordingly corresponds to sublobule VIIA of other carnivores and ungulates. Its cortical folds are continuous either directly or by medullary sheets with the ansiform lobule. The intercrural fissures of the two sides, however, do not meet in the vermis. The cortical folds of the greater part of the anterior wall of the prepyramidal fissure and its floor correspond to sublobule VIIB.

Lobule VIII is narrow, with its lateral surfaces dipping

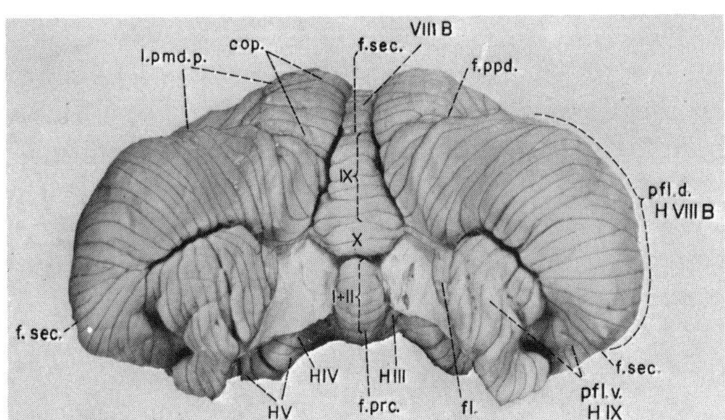

Figure 126. Cerebellum of fur seal. Posteroventral view. ×1.3. Photograph.

deep into the paravermian sulcus on either side. It is divided into sublobules VIIIA and VIIIB, both of which are extensive in sagittal section (fig. 127). Cortical folds from the anterior surface of sublobule VIIIA extend lateralward into the pars copularis of the paramedian lobule, as do those of its superficial and posterior surfaces. There is no distinct copular group of folia. Sublobule VIIIB is continuous with the dorsal paraflocculus with respect to both its cortical folds and its medullary substance. The latter forms a short massive peduncle which is covered by the folial connections.

Superficially lobule IX, the uvula (figs. 126, 127), has the form of a truncated pyramid, with its base resting on the nodulus. Its area in median sagittal section is extensive. The four lamellae typical of this lobule when it is large, namely IXa, IXb, IXc, and IXd, are well differentiated in other species. The fissura secunda is deep.

HEMISPHERAL LOBULES OF POSTERIOR LOBE

The hemispheral lobules of the posterior lobe, except the paramedian lobule and the paraflocculus, form relatively simple elongated surface areas, which are narrow as they approach the vermis but expand toward the cerebellar margin. In lobule HVI vermal lamellae VIb and VIc extend lateroventrally onto the anterior wall of the hemispheral segment of the posterior superior fissure. Lamella VIa and lateral continuations of VId and VIe that emerge from the posterior wall of the fissura prima form the surface of the lobule. Declival sulci 1 and 2 both disappear into the anterior wall of the posterior superior fissure.

Lobule HVIIA is narrow medially but expands widely on the rostrolateral surface of the hemisphere and divides into crus I and crus II (fig. 125). Three folia that emerge to the surface from the posterior wall of the posterior superior fissure form crus Ia; this subdivision is delimited from crus Ip by intracrural sulcus 1, which is deeper than the adjacent furrows. Crus Ip consists of three to four elongated superficial folia that continue medially with the superficial lamellae of sublobule VIIA. The intercrural fissure is deep and has strongly foliated walls. Crus II is composed of elongated folia that are continuous with the superficial lamellae of sublobule VIIIA. These are augmented by folia that emerge from the various fissures, giving rise to a broad expanse of hemispheral surface. A deep furrow, known as intracrural sulcus 2, divides this expanse into an anterior elongated region (crus IIa) and a posterior crus IIp of semilunar forms.

The paramedian lobule comprises three groups of folia separated by deep fissures. The rostrolaterally situated group is connected with sublobule VIIB; it corresponds to the pars anterior of other species. The caudomedial group of folia is connected with the base of sublobule VIIB and forms the pars posterior. A triangular group of transversely directed folia is connected with sublobule VIIIA, as already described, and appears to combine the copular folia and the pars copularis of the paramedian lobule. It covers the lower posterior folia of the pars posterior, and its tapering lateral part continues both into this part of the paramedian lobule and the dorsal paraflocculus.

The dorsal paraflocculus (lobule HVIIIB) is the largest lobule of the cerebellum in *Callorhinus*. It is composed of a series of lamellae attached to a massive peduncle from the base of lobule VIII, the most medial of which are continuous with those of sublobule VIIIB. The dorsal paraflocculus expands to the point where it forms the larger part of the ventral and posterior cerebellar surfaces, and then it arches around and beneath the hemisphere to the anterior cerebellar surface where it is sepa-

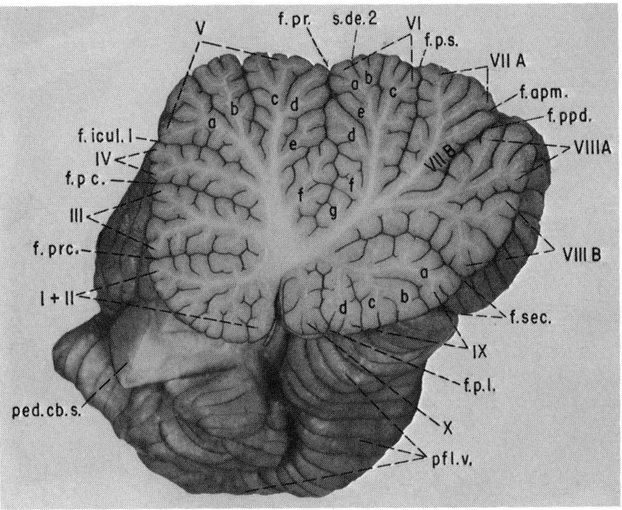

Figure 127. Cerebellum of fur seal. Midsagittal section.

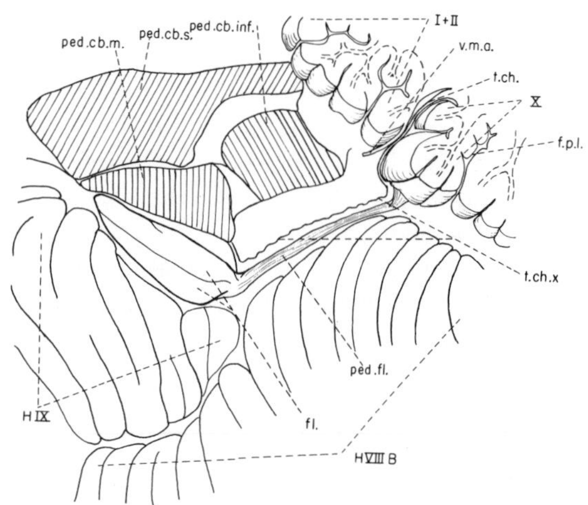

Figure 128. Cerebellum of fur seal. Ventral view, showing right half of flocculonodular lobe with surroundings.

rated from the ventral paraflocculus by a deep continuation of the fissura secunda (fig. 126).

The ventral paraflocculus (lobule HIX) comprises a series of folia that extend medially on the ventral cerebellar surface but do not reach the vermis. They are connected, however, with lobule IX by a prominent medullary band. A proximal group of folia that is separated from the main mass of the ventral paraflocculus by a deep and prominent fissure appears to represent the accessory paraflocculus.

FLOCCULONODULAR LOBE

Lobule X, the nodulus (figs. 126, 127), is small and has but two superficial cortical folds. The posterior medullary velum is attached at the fastigial base of the lobule. The folia converge laterally toward a slender and short floccular peduncle (fig. 128). The flocculus is relatively small and most of it is hidden in the cleft between the brachium pontis and the ventral paraflocculus; its lateral surface comprises five short folia. The posterolateral fissure is deep between the flocculus and ventral paraflocculus and can be followed to the vermis.

CALIFORNIA SEA LION

THE cerebellum of the sea lion (*Żalophus californianus*) is larger than that of the fur seal. The general pattern is the same but there are striking differences in the relative size of many of the lobules which are of interest considering the similarity between the two species in body type and habitat. These differences are pointed out in the description of the individual lobules. The entire cerebellum is more flattened in the sea lion, forming a relatively thin arch from one side to the other (fig. 129). The surface area of the hemispheres is large (fig. 130) and, as in the fur seal, the dorsal and ventral paraflocculi are very large (fig. 131). The flocculus is smaller than in *Callorhinus*.

The sea lion is a large seal whose hindlimbs bend forward and help support the body when the animal is on land. These limbs and the tail are incompletely incorporated in order to serve as a propulsive organ in water. The forelimbs are well adapted for support of the body on land and have considerable unilateral independence of movement. The distal portions of both forelimbs and hindlimbs are flippers but the sea lion is capable of fairly rapid movements on land; in the water its activities are agile and remarkably well coordinated. The animal is capable of being trained to perform activities requiring a high degree of skill. The body and very mobile neck are elongated and the head is small. The tongue is of moderate size and can be protruded. The eyes are large, frontally situated, and their movements are well conjugated. Adult males attain a head-body length of more than 2.4 meters and a weight of 227 kg to 281 kg (Riley, 1929; Palmer, 1954).

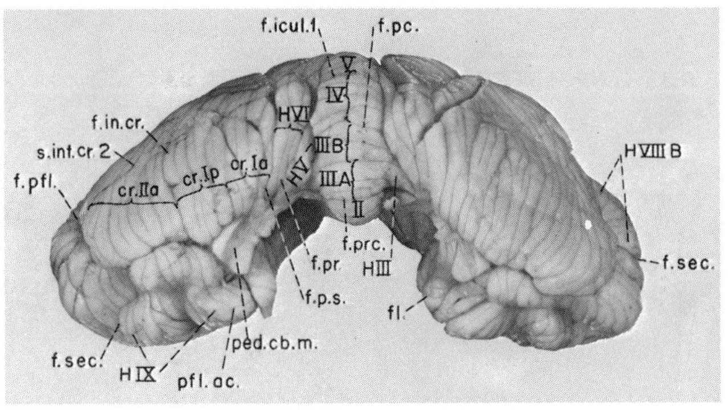

Figure 129. Cerebellum of California sea lion (*Zalophus californianus*). Anterior view. Photograph.

CORPUS CEREBELLI

The ventralmost subdivision of the anterior lobe appears, as in the fur seal, to constitute a single vermal lobule (figs. 132, 133). The cortical folds are short and those of the dorsal surface are not continuous with the ventral folds. The latter end on the medullary substance which projects forward and forms part of the lateral surfaces of the segment. A furrow that is deeper and more prominent both on the lateral surface and in median sagittal section delimits the two caudal lamellae from an anterior group of four (figs. 132, 133). The corresponding region of the anterior lobe of the sea lion was described by Riley (1929) as consisting of two distinct segments, designated lobuli 1 and 2, and a deep fissure is illustrated between them in median sagittal section of the cerebellum. The lobuli of Riley correspond to the two groups of lamellae described above, and the fissure corresponds to the precentral fissure *a* of other species. It appears justifiable to interpret the two groups of cortical folds as lobules I and II; the latter is separated from lobule III by the precentral fissure. Riley's descriptions and illustration of this and other parts of the vermis of this species as compared with my own observations and photographs indicate that the cerebellum available to me came from a smaller and probably much younger animal.

Lobule III (figs. 129, 132), which corresponds to lob-

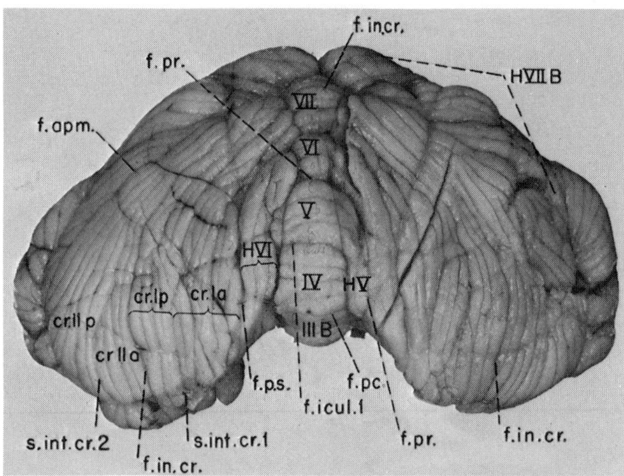

Figure 130. Cerebellum of California sea lion. Dorsoanterior view. Photograph.

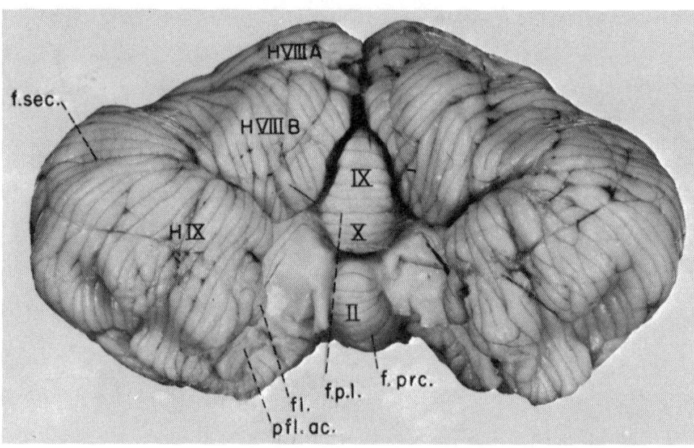

Figure 131. Cerebellum of California sea lion. Ventroposterior view. Photograph.

ulus 3 of Riley, is larger in the sea lion than in the fur seal. (The two surface lamellae of the latter are represented by small sublobules.) Lobule HIII, however, is relatively small in the sea lion. The preculminate fissure is deep and prominent.

Lobule IV is large, with its surface being subdivided into two large lamellae (fig. 130, 132). In Riley's description and illustration the corresponding segment, included with my lobule V in his lobulus 4, consists of two much larger subdivisions that correspond to sublobules IVA and IVB of many species. Lobule HIV includes the lateral continuation of the vermal lamellae, which constitutes the medial wall of a deep cleft whose lateral and posterior walls are formed by lobule HV.

Lobule V is relatively smaller than in the fur seal both in my material and in Riley's illustration. Lamellae Va, Vb, and Vc are reduced, but lamellae Vd, Ve, and Vf are unusually large (fig. 132). Riley called attention to the extensive development of the folial groups on the anterior wall of the fissura prima but he did not specifically designate them. Lobule HV turns sharply rostralward in the paravermian sulcus and comprises a nearly vertically directed sheet of lamellae that are hidden for the most part in the hemispheral part of the fissura prima. On the right side of figure 129 two of the folia appear at the surface.

Lobule VI is very similar to that of the fur seal. Lamellae VIa, VIb, and VIc are represented in simple form on the surface, while VIe, VId, VIf, and VIg are represented in the posterior wall of the fissura prima, with VId usually being the largest (fig. 132).

Lobule VII is not obviously divided into sublobules. The three large surface lamellae (fig. 132) are connected laterally with the ansiform lobule. The deep part of the anterior wall of the prepyramidal fissure, however, is continuous with the pars anterior of the paramedian lobule. The furrow labeled ansoparamedian fissure in figure 132 represents the vermal boundary between folia passing laterally into the ansiform lobule and those to the paramedian lobule. The portion of lobule VII ventral of this fissure must therefore be regarded as homologous with sublobule VIIB, and the larger part, including the three superficial lamellae, as corresponding to sublobule VIIA. In Riley's figure of the median sagittal section of the sea lion cerebellum a much deeper fissure, apparently corresponding to the ansoparamedian fissure, is shown and the portion of the vermis which it delimits anteriorly reaches the surface. This subdivision, however, cannot correspond to sublobule VIIB if Riley's interpretation of the pyramis (his lobulus C_1) is correct, but if one regards the pyramis as including two sublobules, as I found to be

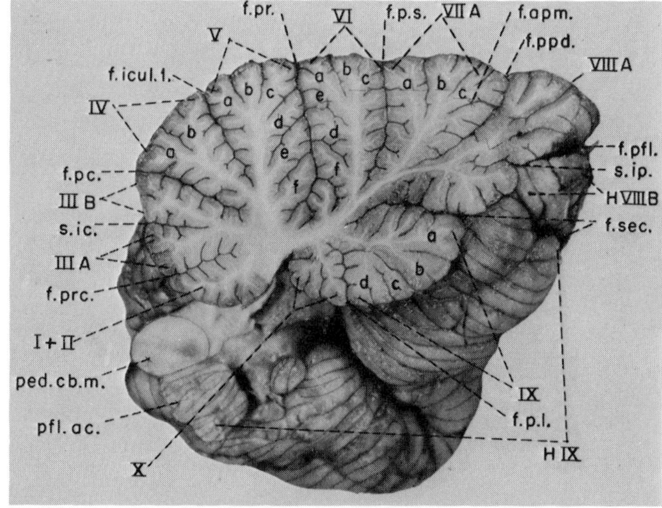

Figure 132. Cerebellum of California sea lion. Midsagittal section. Photograph.

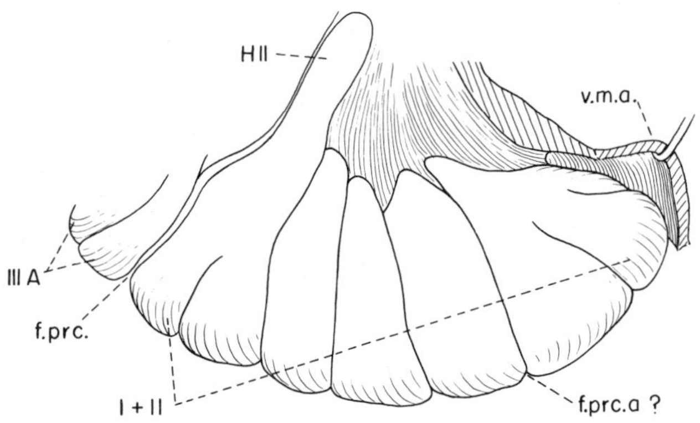

Figure 133. Cerebellum of California sea lion. Drawing shows details of ventral part of anterior lobe.

the case, then the pattern is the same in the two cerebella although the subdivisions of my lobules VII and VIII were much larger in Riley's specimen.

The three superficial lamellae of sublobule VIIA are much larger than in the fur seal and the anterior one is delimited from the others by a much deeper fissure. Riley's more schematic figure shows the corresponding part of the vermis of the sea lion as relatively much larger but similarly subdivided, except that the furrow between the first and second lamellae is shallower. The anterior lamella in my specimen appears to represent a combination of the rostral surface lamella of Riley's illustration and the fur seal, with the upper folia of the posterior wall of the superior posterior fissure of the latter usually being found in other species. There are similar variations in other species, but they may possibly be individual differences as in the sea lion. In three cerebella of the adult fin whale, however, Jansen (1953) found a similarly situated but larger subdivision which he attributed to the declive (my lobule VI); this raised the question of the identity of the posterior superior fissure. In the sea lion the lamella in question clearly is part of sublobule VIIA and the posterior superior fissure is not in doubt.

Lobules VIII and IX are connected by a common medullary ray with the ray from the medullary body which also leads to lobule VII. Lobule VIII comprises an elongated sublobule VIIIA and a smaller sublobule VIIIB. Lobule IX is very similar to that of the fur seal and is subdivided into the four characteristic superficial lamellae, namely, IXa, IXb, IXc, and IXd. The fissura secunda is deep and prominent (fig. 132).

HEMISPHERAL LOBULES OF POSTERIOR LOBE

Lobule HVI turns rostralward and is represented on the dorsal and anterior cerebellar surfaces by three elongated folia. The hemispheral segments of the fissura prima and posterior superior fissure are deep, with lobule HVI forming a vertical plate between them (fig. 130). Lamellae VIa and VIb dip into the lateral wall of the fissura prima, subfoliate, and form the upper part of this wall. Lamellae VIe, VId, and VIf extend lateralward, forming the deep part of the wall. The medial wall of the posterior superior fissure is formed by lateral continuations of lamella VIc and the undesignated folia lining the anterior wall of the vermal segment of the fissure. The deepest of these folia cross the floor of the lateral part of the fissure to its posterior surface.

Lobule HVIIA forms most of the dorsal and anterior surface of the hemisphere (fig. 130). The intercrural fissure is deep and its walls are corrugated by numerous folia. Both crus I and crus II are subdivided by furrows which correspond to intracrural sulci 1 and 2, respectively, of other species. These also have corrugated walls but are shallower than the intercrural fissure. In the sea lion crus Ia is relatively broader on the surface than in most other species. On the right-hand side of the specimen its folia all continue medially with the large anterior lamella of sublobule VIIA; on the left side, however, only the deep folia of the lateral wall of the posterior superior fissure continue with this lamella and its medullary base, while the superficial and posterior folia end on a medullary band in common with those of crus Ip. This band dips beneath the paravermian sulcus into the common base of the remainder of sublobule VIIA. Crus IIa spreads widely on the lateral hemispheral surface. Crus IIp has a crescent-shaped group of surface folia on its caudolateral border, is directed obliquely forward beneath crus IIa, and has extensive surfaces which face intracrural sulcus 2 and the ansoparamedian fissure (figs. 129, 130).

The paramedian lobule (HVIIB + HVIIIA) comprises the pars anterior, pars posterior, and pars copularis (figs. 130, 131). The vermal segment of the ansoparamedian fissure and the folia ventral of it continue into the floor of the larger and deeper fissure between crus IIp and the pars anterior. The actual boundary line between the two hemispheral sublobules occurs in the lower rostral wall of the more obvious fissure. The pars anterior of the paramedian lobule includes folia in this floor and a plate which continues upward from those in the posterior wall of the hemispheral part of the ansoparamedian fissure. The folia of this plate converge medially into a medullary band that joins the medullary ray leading to lobule VII. Laterally, deep folia of the plate cross the floor of the ansoparamedian fissure to its anterior (crus IIp) wall. The pars posterior of the paramedian lobule likewise tapers medially, with the folia terminating deep on the medullary ray common to lobules VII and VIII. The pars copularis is continuous with the folia on the anterior and dorsal surfaces of sublobule VIIIA. The dorsal folia of sublobule VIIIA continue beneath the deep cleft of the paravermian sulcus into the dorsal and most prominent part of the pars copularis. This may represent a combined copula and pars copularis but there is no distinct group of copula folia. The paramedian lobule of the sea lion accordingly may be considered as principally lobule HVIIB, but the connections with lobule VIIIA make its caudal part lobulus HVIIIA (fig. 131).

The dorsal paraflocculus (figs. 130, 131) begins beneath the pars copularis and immediately lateral to sublobule VIIIB as a series of oblique folia which quickly become increasingly elongated and continue as a series on the ventrolateral surface of the cerebellum that forms the largest subdivision of the organ as already mentioned.

The ventral paraflocculus also is large but does not reach the uvula except by a medullary band. The fissura secunda can be followed along this band, in which it makes a shallow groove, to the deep lateral fissure that completely separates the dorsal from the ventral paraflocculus down to their medullary base.

It is clear in dissections that both lobules receive pontine fibers, except possibly the most medial group of five folia of the ventral paraflocculus. There are inconclusive indications that this group corresponds to the accessory paraflocculus of Jansen. The group is attached to the proximal part of the ventral parafloccular peduncle and also is divided by a deep fissure from the remainder of the ventral paraflocculus (fig. 131).

FLOCCULONODULAR LOBE

The flocculus forms a small spindle-shaped group of folia between the ventral paraflocculus and the brachium pontis. The rounded ventral surface is exposed and the lateral surface is pressed against the ventral paraflocculus (fig. 131). A slender, arched peduncle connects flocculus and nodulus. Lobule X, the nodulus, is relatively small, as in the fur seal. The choroid tela is attached near the fastigium. The posterolateral fissure can be followed along the slender peduncle between its vermal and floccular parts. As in the fur seal the flocculonodular lobe of the sea lion is very small (figs. 131, 132). In the Greenland seal Jansen (1954) described the flocculus as being composed of a series of 12 to 13 short but well-developed folia and a large nodulus, which is illustrated.

CETACEA

THE cetaceans include species ranging in length from about 1.2 meters to the 33 meters attained by the blue whale, *Balaenoptera musculus*, the largest of all animals. The fin whale, *Balaenoptera physalus*, may reach a length of approximately 25 meters, while the porpoise, *Tursiops truncatus*, ranges from 3 meters to 3.4 meters. The head of cetaceans varies in form and in relative size, with reference to the body, in different species. The neck is not distinguishable. The forelimbs are paddlelike flippers which were said to be used chiefly for maintaining the balance of the body and for steering; external hindlimbs are lacking. Swimming is accomplished chiefly by the tail which has two horizontal flukes. A dorsal fin is present in some species. The eyes are small but well developed and vision is reportedly good. External ears are lacking and the outer opening of the ear is by a minute aperture not far behind the eye on either side. In the *Mystacoceti* the external auditory passage was said to be blocked by a mass of wax a number of centimeters in length. Their hearing is dull in the air but very acute in the water.

Cerebellum

The cerebellum of cetaceans is large. Jansen (1953) found an average breadth of 20.4 cm in five cerebella of the fin whale, the largest having a breadth of 21.6 cm. In twelve cerebella of the sei whale (*Balaenoptera borealis*) the average breadth was 18.9 cm (Pilleri, 1966). The weight of formalin-hardened specimens, after the membranes were removed, ranged from 1170 gm to 1330 gm. The largest of three porpoise cerebella that I measured was 10.8 cm in breadth. The weight, unfortunately, was not recorded. The entire brain of the fin whale, after formalin hardening, weighed 5.95 kg in one specimen and 7.98 kg in another, according to Ries and Langworthy (1937). The cerebellum of this species, according to Jansen (1953), accounts on the average for 20 percent of the total brain weight.

In another species of *Mysticeti*, *Balaenoptera borealis*, Pilleri (1966) found a figure of the same order of magnitude; the cerebellum of eleven specimens averaged 19.6 percent of the total brain weight. A definitely lower ratio is encountered in *Odontoceti* where the cerebellum accounts for approximately 15 percent of the total brain weight (Putnam, 1928; Pilleri, 1966; Jansen and Jansen, 1968).

The cerebellar hemispheres are unusually large in Cetacea, owing to great hypertrophy of the dorsal and ventral paraflocculi and the paramedian lobule. The vermis of the fin whale comprises a series of lobules whose superficial folia are transverse, in general, and are continuous, beneath an anteroposteriorly directed shallow and incomplete paravermian sulcus, with obliquely directed folia of the hemispheres. Some of the more posterior vermal lobules are partially displaced to one side of the midline. In *Tursiops* the paravermian sulcus is deep and narrow on either side of the vermis, which forms a prominent ridge between the hemispheres. The hemispheres of both species are divided into lobes, homologous with the hemispheral subdivisions of smaller mammals, each of which is represented superficially by groups of elongated folia. The vermal lobules are separated by deep fissures that are continuous with hemispheral fissures.

The cerebellum of various species of cetaceans has been described to a greater or lesser extent by Beauregard (1883), Guldberg (1885), Flatau and Jacobsohn (1899), Bolk (1906), Riley (1929), Langworthy (1932), Wilson (1933), Jelgersma (1934), Scholten (1946), and Pilleri (1963, 1964, 1966). The divergent interpretations of lobules and fissures by these authors confused matters. The illuminating studies of Jansen (1950, 1953, 1954) on the development of the organ in fin whale embryos and his descriptions of the adult cerebellum of the bottle-nosed whale, *Hyperoodon rostratus*, and the fin whale clarified the situation. Jansen stated that the pattern of the cerebellum in these two species is very much alike and conforms with the fundamental plan of its morphology in mammals generally.

I was able to compare my observations on the cerebellum of the porpoise (also called bottle-nosed dolphin), *Tursiops truncatus*, with Jansen's whale cerebella at Oslo. *Tursiops* has a fishlike body with no external differentiation between the head and the trunk. The forelimbs are reduced to a pair of fins which reportedly have very little unilateral independence. Porpoises show great agility in swimming, and can move with great speed and leap out of the water. The fields of vision of the laterally situated eyes do not overlap. The lower jaw projects somewhat beyond the upper one but the head is relatively small. The tongue is short and not protrusible (Riley, 1929).

The cerebellum of the porpoise is large in comparison with that of most mammals but, as noted above, is only about one-half as wide as the cerebellum of the fin whale. The dorsal surface is less arched, anteroposteriorly, so that the organ is relatively longer than that of the whales described by Jansen. As compared with other mammals, the porpoise cerebellum shares with the whales striking differences in the relative size of many of the lobules and their subdivisions. Lesser differences between the lobules and fissures of the whales and the porpoise are described below.

Interpretation of the subdivisions of the large and complex cetacean cerebellum is so dependent on following its developmental history that since I lacked embryonic material of the porpoise I made close comparison of the lobules and fissures of the organ in *Tursiops* with those of the fin whale, described both embryologically and in the adult by Jansen (1950, 1953, 1954). Semidiagrammatic figures of the cerebellum of a 102-cm C.R. length embryo of the porpoise were given to me by Jansen for further comparison with the adult organ.

Development of Cerebellum in Fin Whale

The posterolateral fissure antedates all others, as in other mammals, and divides the cerebellum into the flocculonodular lobe and the corpus cerebelli (Jansen, 1950, 1954). The next fissure in sequence of appearance in the fin whale embryo is the prepyramidal rather than the fissura prima, according to Jansen. This order is anomalous since in all other species, with the possible exception of the rat in which the sequence of fissure development has been closely followed, the fissura prima is the first to appear in the corpus cerebelli. Usually it is followed by the fissura secunda which, in the posterior lobe, is followed in turn by the prepyramidal fissure. In the human embryo, however, the prepyramidalis precedes the secunda although it follows the fissura prima. Similar departures from the more common sequences of other fissures occur in species that have unusually large or small lobules adjacent to individual fissures, e.g., the vermal segment of the ansoparamedian fissure of the pig. The prepyramidal fissure, as interpreted by Jansen in the fin whale embryo, appears in the median part of the corpus cerebelli in an embryo of 14.5 cm in length. Between this stage and the 24-cm C.R. length embryo a number of fissures have appeared; the deepest, next to the prepyramidal fissure, in the 24-cm stage, was regarded by Jansen as the fissura prima. A furrow right behind the prima is tentatively identified as the posterior superior fissure, while behind the prepyramidalis the fissura secunda is faintly shown. In the 26-cm C.R. length embryo (fig. 134) the fissura prima is the deepest of the vermal fissures and, as in embryos of other species at approximately corresponding stages of cerebellar development, it is the most prominent, dividing the corpus cerebelli into anterior and posterior lobes.

CORPUS CEREBELLI

Anterior lobe. The anterior lobe of the 26-cm embryo (fig. 134) has two shallow furrows: the deeper one Jansen called the intraculminate fissure and the shallower and more ventral one, the preculminate fissure. They appear to correspond, respectively, to the preculminate and precentral fissures of the rat, pig, and other embryos already described. Jansen (1954) regarded his intraculminate fissure as identical with what I called the preculminate fissure in other species. These fissures deepen and others appear (figs. 134–137), dividing the anterior lobe into five segments called lobules I–V by Jansen in the 160-cm C.R. length and later embryos and in the adult whale (figs. 135, 136). Except for the difference in interpretation of the preculminate fissure, which Jansen regarded as separating lobules II and III rather than lobules III and IV, and the resulting inclusion by him of lobule III in the culmen, the lobules and fissures of the anterior lobe appear to be identical with those of other species. Lobules I, II, and III are relatively large in median sagittal section of the later fetal and the adult cerebellum, but their hemispheral continuations are greatly reduced. Lobule IV, by the 160-cm stage, has two large subdivisions that correspond to sublobules IVA and IVB of many other species. Lobule V of the 220-cm C.R. length (fig. 135E) and later stages, including the adult whale,

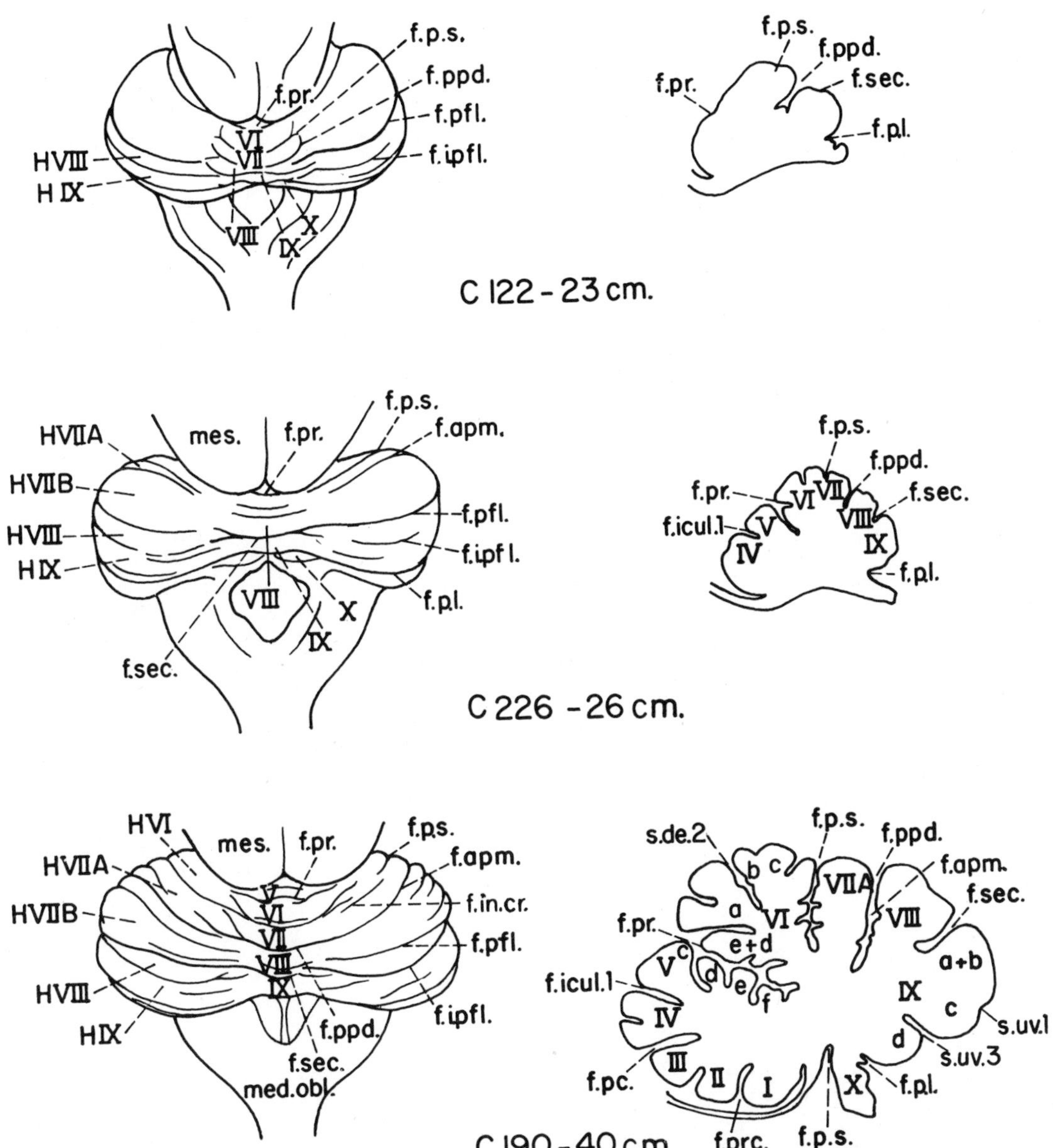

Figure 134. Cerebellum of fin whale (*Balaenoptera physalus*). C122. Dorsal view (×4) and midsagittal section (×6) of 23-cm-long fetus. C226. Dorsal view (×4) and midsagittal section (×6) of 26-cm-long fetus. C190. Dorsal view (×4) and midsagittal section (×6) of 40-cm-long fetus. (Modified from Jansen, 1950, 1954.)

presents an arrangement of lamellae which is similar to that of other large mammals in pattern.

In the adult porpoise (figs. 139–142) the anterior lobe comprises about one-third of the area of the median sagittal section of the cerebellum (fig. 138). Lobule I includes five small surface lamellae and a number of folia on its fissural surfaces. The lobule is narrow transversely, forming a keel-like projection into the anterior part of the fourth ventricle (fig. 141), but it is separated from the ventricle by the anterior medullary velum (fig. 143). The velum is attached to a triangular projection of medullary substance behind the lobule. Lobule II, separated from lobule I by a deep precentral fissure *a*, comprises two large surface lamellae that correspond to IIa and IIb of other mammals. The lobule is narrow, forming an anterior continuation of the keel, but the folia of lamella IIb continue rostrolaterally as small lobule HII (fig. 141). Lobule III comprises two surface lamellae and smaller deep lamellae or folia. The precentral fissure, delimiting it from lobule II, extends nearly to the lateral border of the anterior lobe. The preculminate fissure, separating lobule III from lobule IV, is deeper and continues to the

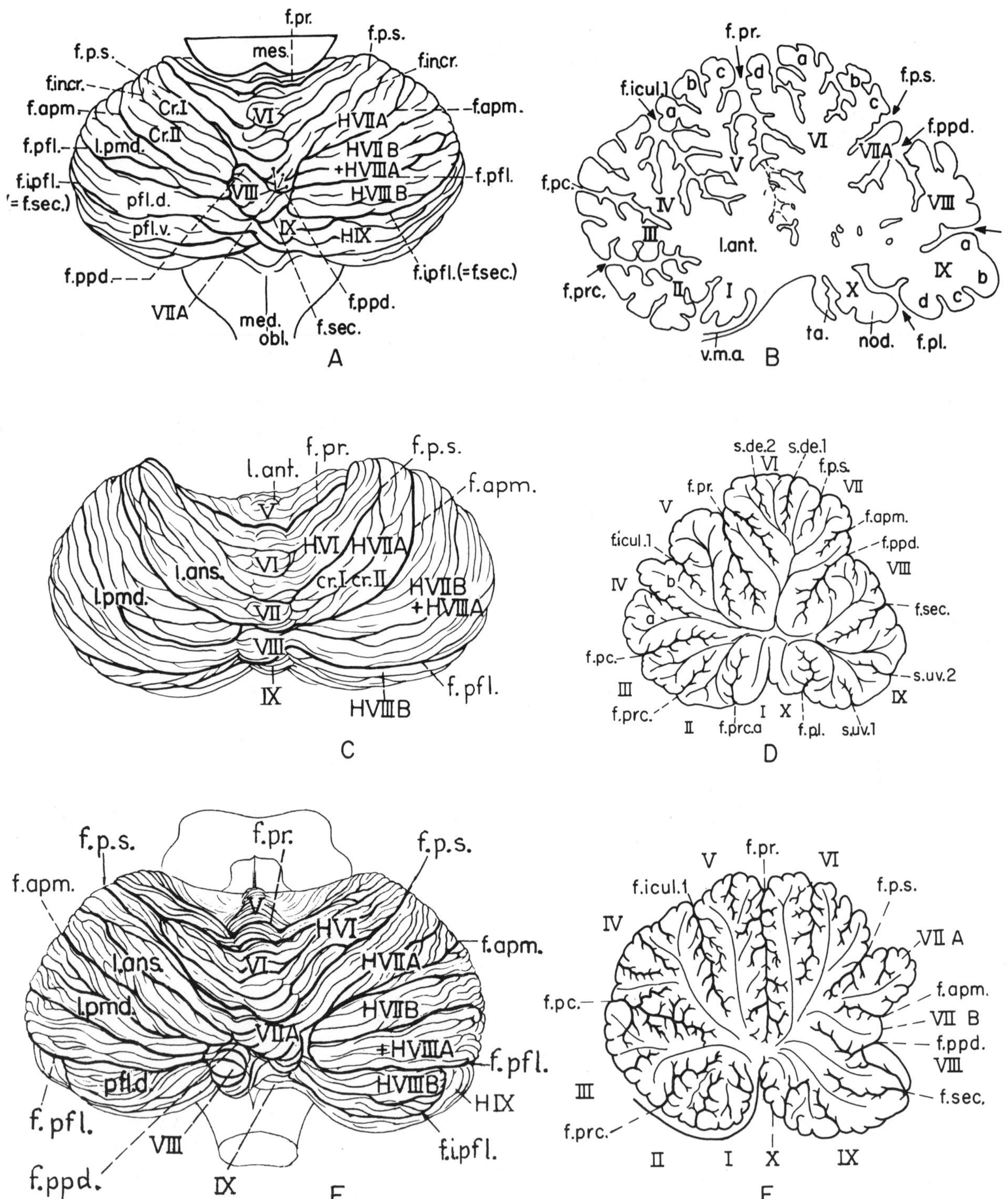

Figure 135. Cerebellum of fin whale (*Balaenoptera physalus*). A, B. Dorsal view and midsagittal section of 123-cm-long fetus. C, D. Dorsal view and midsagittal section of 160-cm-long fetus. E, F. Dorsal view and midsagittal section of 220-cm-long fetus. (Modified from Jansen, 1950, 1954.)

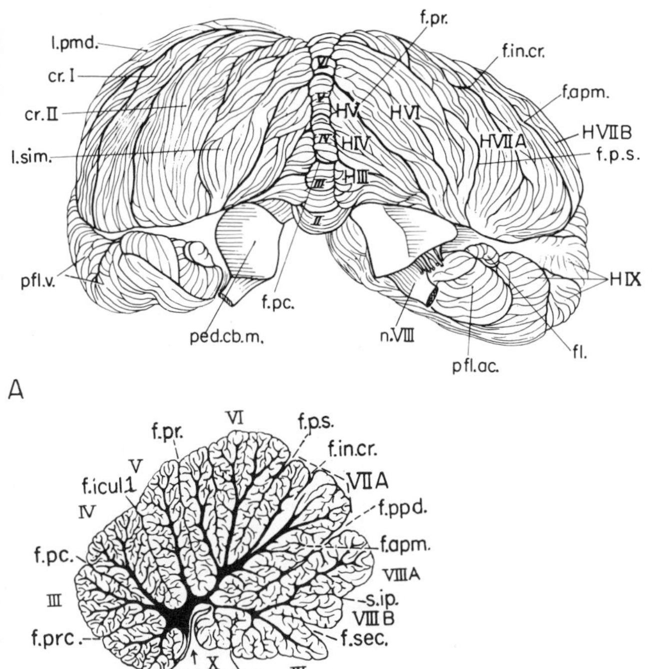

Figure 136. Cerebellum of adult fin whale (*Balaenoptera physalus*). A. Anterior view. B. Midsagittal section. (Modified from Jansen, 1954.)

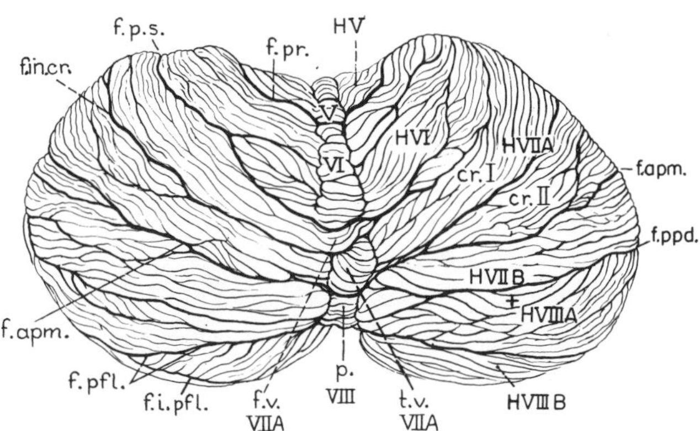

Figure 137. Cerebellum of adult fin whale (*Balaenoptera physalus*). Dorsal view. Same specimen as figure 136. (Jansen, 1953.)

cortical margin of the lobe. Lobule IV is divided into relatively large sublobules IVA and IVB (fig. 138), as also noted in the whale embryo by Jansen. Intraculminate fissure 3 ends short of the anterior ventral margin of the cerebellum; the hemispheral representation of sublobule IVA is continuous around its tip with that of sublobule IVB. Together the two hemispheral parts form a small triangular lobule HIV (fig. 139). Lobule V presents three small surface lamellae (Va, Vb, and Vc) and more prominent ones in the anterior wall of the fissura prima (fig. 138). Intraculminate fissure 1 is so deep in the porpoise that the folia and small lamellae of its posterior wall add considerably to the cortical surface of lobule V. The fissura prima turns sharply ventralward on either side of the vermis and forms the lateral boundary of a small lobule HV (figs. 139, 140). The surface folia of this lobule are continuous, beneath the paravermian sulcus, with those of lobule V, but the deeper part of lobule HV, forming the medial wall of the hemispheral segment of the fissura prima, is continuous with the folia of the anterior wall of the vermal segment of the fissure. Lobule HV is relatively smaller in the porpoise than in the fin whale as illustrated by Jansen (1954).

Because of the small size of the hemispheral lobules of the anterior lobe and the relative narrowness of its vermal lobules (figs. 139, 140, 141), the anterior lobe as a whole is smaller in proportion to the entire cerebellum in cetaceans than in any other group of mammals. It is noteworthy that in median sagittal section of the cerebellum (figs. 138, 144B) its vermal lobules together represent approximately as large a share of the total area as in many other species in which some of the vermal lobules of the posterior lobe are unusually large, as they are in the cetaceans. Lobule I is relatively larger than in most mammals but, as Jansen (1953) commented, it is surprising that it is not a great deal larger in cetaceans which have such enormous development of the tail. In view of the experimental evidence that the "lingula" is the principal lobule functionally related to the tail (Chang and Ruch, 1949; Hampson, Harrison, and Woolsey, 1952), one would expect to find this part of the cetacean cerebellum to be hypertrophic. The lingula of classical terminology includes

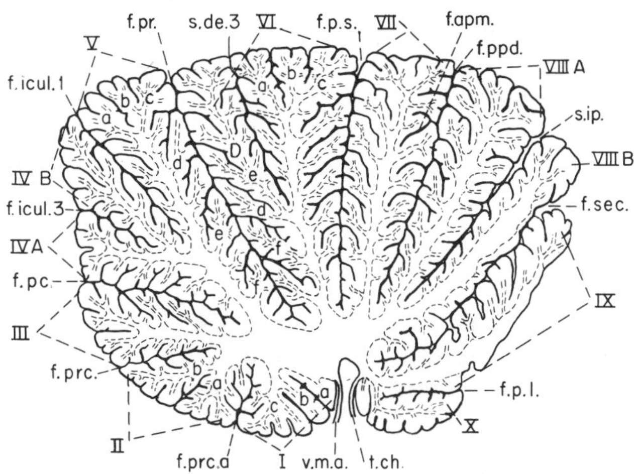

Figure 138. Cerebellum of porpoise (*Tursiops truncatus*). Midsagittal section. (Redrawn and reinterpreted from Langworthy, 1932.)

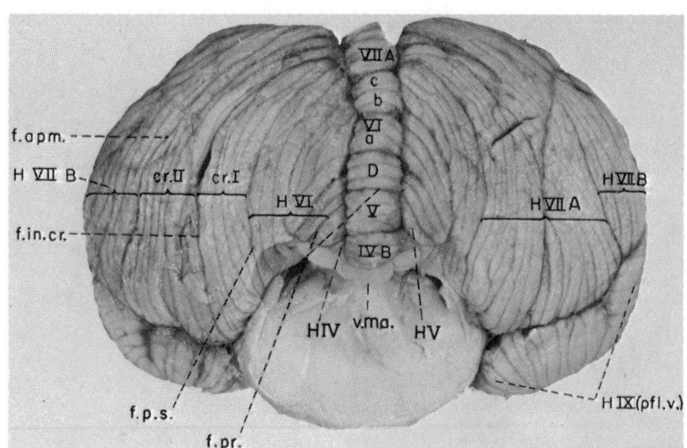

Figure 139. Cerebellum of porpoise (*Tursiops tursio*). Anterior view.

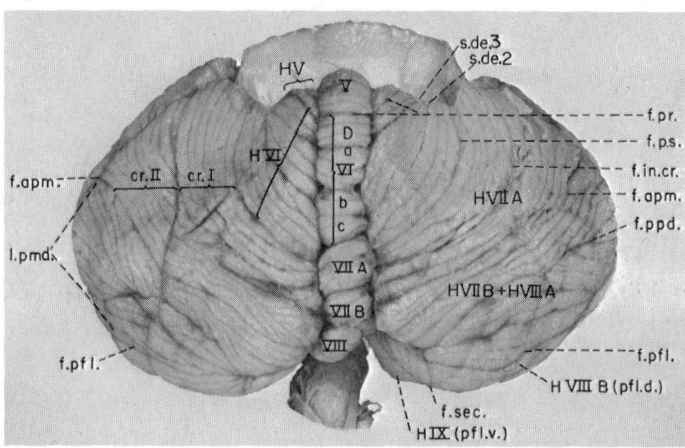

Figure 140. Cerebellum of porpoise (*Tursiops tursio*). Dorsal view.

both lobules I and II, as already noted. In Cetacea, which lack hindlimbs, lobule III probably is also related to the base of the tail or the transitional part of the trunk.

Without considering any modifications of musculature that were involved in the formation of the powerful tail of cetaceans, but remembering that in the spider monkey (Chang and Ruch, 1949) the subdivision of the anterior lobe corresponding to lobule II also is functionally related to the tail, one may assume that the tail-related functional significance of lobule II is increased in cetaceans and what is related to the nonexistent hindlimb has become modified or has disappeared. The relatively large size of lobules I, II, and III which, as a group, constitute a large proportion of the anterior lobe would then have a plausible explanation. The two sublobules of lobule IV are in keeping with the two corresponding divisions in other mammals, such as the horse, that have elongated and powerful trunks. The small superficial area of lobule V appears to be compensated for by the increasing length of the lobule and the area of its cortex which results from the great depth of the fissura prima.

Posterior lobe. The posterior lobe of Jansen's 26-cm C.R. length fin whale embryo is divided into four segments by the posterior superior and prepyramidal fissures and the fissura secunda (fig. 134). These segments were called lobules VI, VII, VIII, and IX by Jansen

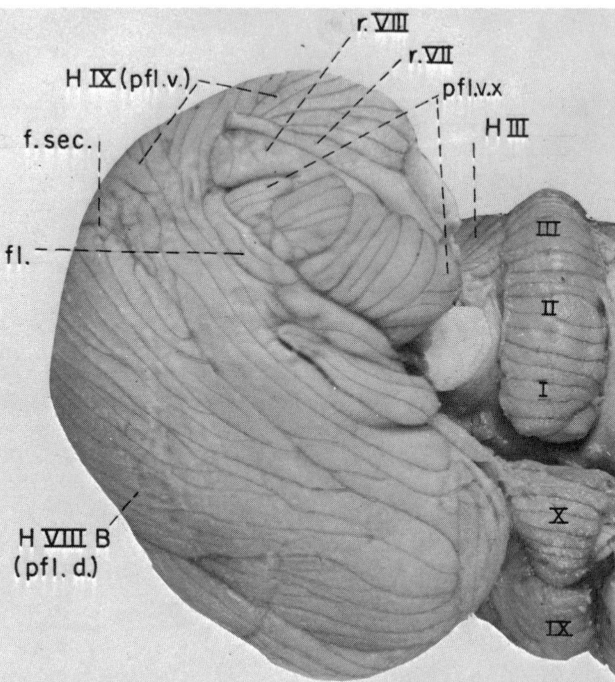

Figure 141. Cerebellum of porpoise (*Tursiops tursio*). Ventral view.

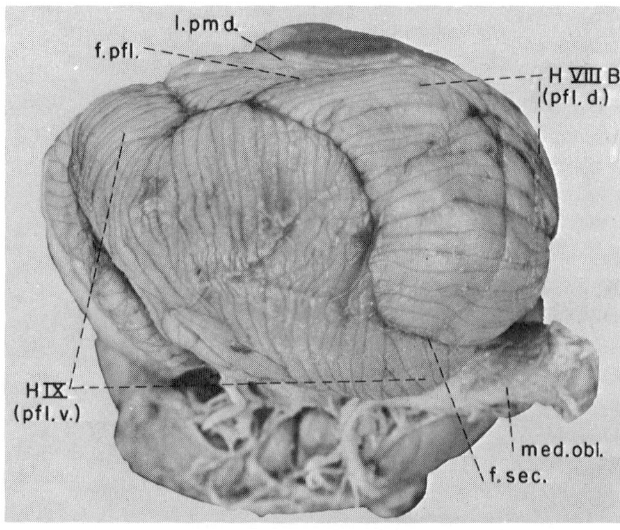

Figure 142. Cerebellum of porpoise (*Tursiops tursio*). Lateral view.

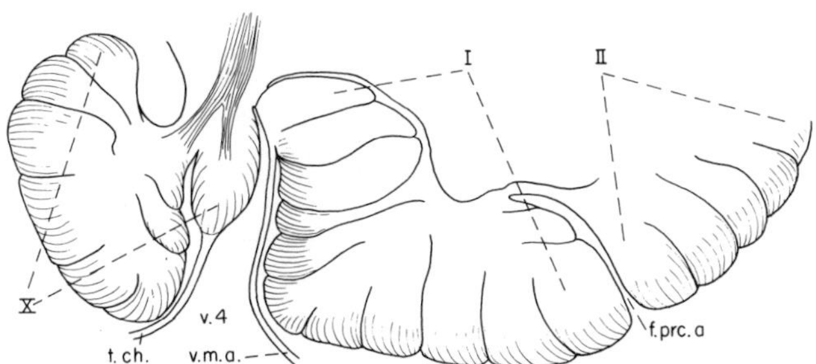

Figure 143. Cerebellum of porpoise showing details of lobules I, II, and X in lateral view.

(1954) in the 160-cm and larger embryos and in the adult. Lobule VI, in the 160-cm embryo (fig. 135C, D), is divided into three superficial lamellae by declival sulci 1 and 2, and a much larger section facing the fissura prima is divided by a deeper fissure which corresponds to declival sulcus 3 of the rat. The superficial lamellae are homologous with VIa, VIb, and VIc of the rat and other species. The large division in the posterior wall of the fissura prima, the end of which reaches the external surface, corresponds to folium VId of the rat and possibly to VId + VIe of many larger species. As illustrated by Jansen (1950, 1953, 1954a) in the 220-cm and larger embryos of the fin whale and also in the adult, this division has expanded so much that it equals some of the primary divisions of the posterior lobe in size (fig. 135F). In the adult cerebellum illustrated by Jansen (1954a) its medullary ray is a direct branch of the posterior medullary limb instead of branching from the ray to the remainder of lobule VI, as it usually does. The developmental history of the division, however, shows that it is a subdivision of lobule VI and Jansen (1954) called it division *a* of this lobule in the adult whale; a corresponding large division in the elephant was similarly named. Since it corresponds in position to folium VId in the rat and to a similar folium or lamella in all other mammals, the term sublobule VID appears appropriate in species in which it attains an unusually large size (figs. 138, 144).

Lobule VI of the porpoise (figs. 138, 139, 140) is similar to the corresponding lobule of the whale but its subdivisions, especially sublobule VID, are relatively smaller. This difference in sublobule VID probably can be correlated with differences in specific areas and muscles of the head to which the trigeminal and other cranial nerves are distributed. The tongue, which is very large in the fin whale and, relatively, very much larger than in the porpoise, suggests itself as one such sensory area and group of muscles.

Lobule VII, situated between the posterior superior and prepyramidal fissures, was regarded by Jansen as the homolog of the folium and tuber vermis of classical terminology. In the whale embryos, according to Jansen, it can be divided into VIIa and VIIb, as in the rat. Dorsal views of the cerebellum of his 50-cm, 160-cm, and 430-cm C.R. length embryos and also of the adult fin whale cerebellum give the appearance of continuity of the ansoparamedian fissure from each hemisphere with a vermal fissure (fig. 137). In the 160-cm embryo and in the adult fin whale a fairly deep fissure, as seen in sagittal section of the cerebellum, appears to correspond to the vermal part of the ansoparamedian fissure as seen in dorsal view (figs. 135D, 136). A correspondingly situated but shallower furrow is shown in Jansen's figures of the cerebellum of younger embryos in sagittal section. In the younger embryos one, and in some, two furrows indent the anterior wall of the prepyramidal fissure; such furrows are more numerous in the 160-cm embryo and in the adult, with one appearing to be deeper than the others. Neither the more dorsal furrow nor those in the fissural surface of lobule VII were labeled by Jansen, but he stated that there are indications that the ansoparamedian as well as the intercrural fissures are continuous with sulci on the oral bank of the prepyramidal fissure.

Comparison between lobule VII in the monkey and human fetuses and lobule VII in the adult monkey, chimpanzee, and human is illuminating. The fairly deep furrow that opens onto the posterodorsal surface of lobule VII in the 160-cm whale embryo appears to correspond to the vermal part of the ansoparamedian fissure of one hemisphere in the embryonic cerebellum of monkey and man and also in the adult cerebellum of the monkey, chimpanzee, and man. As is most clearly evident in the developing human cerebellum the ansoparamedian fissure of the contralateral hemisphere continues onto the anterior surface of the prepyramidal fissure, i.e., into the posterior part of lobule VIII below the first one mentioned, with the two rarely, if ever, becoming directly confluent. Also in the macaque the ansoparamedian fissure of one hemisphere ends below the other on the posterior surface of lobule VII. Various modifications were found in species, such as the cat, that have a strongly sigmoid vermis. In Jansen's (1950) figures of the cerebellum of a 220-cm C.R. length fin whale embryo the posterior vermis is quite sigmoid in form and sublobules VIIA and VIIB are separated by what appears to be a single deep vermal segment of the ansoparamedian fissure (fig. 135). In other whale embryos illustrated by Jansen the unnamed furrows seem to be similar in their relations to the vermal continuations of the ansoparamedian fissures of the primates and the posterior surface of lobule VII below the more dorsal of these furrows could be regarded as sublobule VIIB, as in primates.

Lobule VII of the porpoise is relatively large and its fissural surfaces have a great deal of foliation (figs. 138, 144). There is no obvious division into sublobules VIIA and VIIB. A somewhat deeper furrow on its posterior surface may represent the vermal continuation of the ansoparamedian fissure of one hemisphere although attempts to demonstrate the vermal relations of this fissure were inconclusive. The posterior surface of lobule VII which faces the prepyramidal fissure below the presumptive ansoparamedian fissure would then correspond to sublobule VIIB of the fin whale. The remainder of lobule VII in the porpoise has little resemblance to sublobule VIIA of the whale. In the 160-cm fin whale embryo and in some of the younger stages illustrated by Jansen (1950, 1954) a furrow in the dorsal surface of the lobule, situated between the vermal part of the ansoparamedian fissure and the posterior superior fissure, appears to represent the incipient vermal segment of the intercrural fissure. In Jansen's (1954) figure of the adult fin whale cerebellum in median sagittal section a deep intercrural fissure divides what I regarded as sublobule VIIA into folium vermis and tuber vermis. Neither the vermal segment of the intercrural fissure nor the two subdivisions that it separates could be identified in the adult porpoise.

Lobule VIII, as identified by Jansen in the 160-cm fin whale embryo, is already well defined in his 26-cm-long embryo (fig. 134). Some of the later stages have a furrow in the posterodorsal surface of the lobule which Jansen called the parafloccular fissure. In the cerebellum of one 40-cm embryo, the parafloccular fissure is shown in the posterior surface of the lobule, slightly above the fissura secunda; its position corresponds approximately to that of the intrapyramidal sulcus of the adult rat. Although the position of the furrow is more dorsal in the

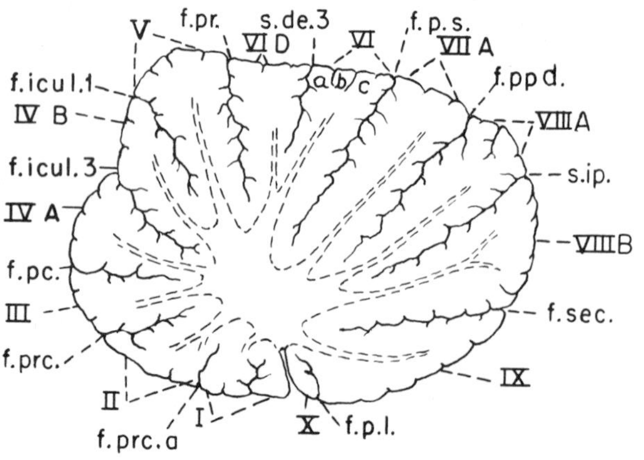

Figure 144. Cerebellum of newborn *Phocaena phocaena* of 102-cm C.R. length. Midsagittal section. (Oslo collection.)

other embryos illustrated by Jansen, here it corresponds to my intrapyramidal sulcus of the monkey and other embryos, including the human. As it deepens in the fin whale embryo lobule VIII becomes divided into two sublobules that are comparable, as Jansen noted, to sublobules VIIIA and VIIIB which I described (Larsell, (1953a) in the adult cat and monkey and subsequently identified in many other species including man (1953b). In the adult fin whale, sublobule VIIIA is considerably larger than VIIIB, as also is true in man and many other species.

The hemispheral segment of the parafloccular fissure is shown in Jansen's figure of the cerebellum of a 21-cm C.R. length whale embryo. It extends medialward into the pyramis, dividing the cortex which is continuous from the latter to the hemisphere into a rostral part, connecting sublobule VIIIA with the paramedian lobule of Bolk, and a caudal part, connecting sublobule VIIIB with the dorsal paraflocculus. Evidently the medially extending hemispheral segment of the fissure, by the 40-cm stage of the embryo, is represented in the pyramis by the indentation already described. This was not specifically stated by Jansen but his figures of dorsal views of the cerebellum of 50-cm-long or longer whale embryos show the parafloccular fissure as being continuous across the vermis, in close relation with the fissura secunda. In no instance, according to Jansen, did it join the prepyramidal fissure.

In the rat the sulcus copularis, which is the medial continuation of the parafloccular fissure as already noted, divides the copula pyramidis: one branch continues from it to the paramedian lobule and another continues with the dorsal paraflocculus. The sulcus copularis extends toward, but does not reach, the ventrally situated intrapyramidal sulcus. The parafloccular fissure of the 90-day-old monkey embryo also extends toward the more dorsally situated and deeper intrapyramidal fissure of this species, and a suggestion of a shallow furrow connects the two. In human infants the parafloccular fissure appears to be continuous with the intrapyramidal fissure, and this also is true in many adult cerebella. It is very probable that Jansen's vermal segment of the parafloccular fissure in the whale embryo and my intrapyramidal sulcus in embryonic and/or adult cerebella of a variety of species are one and the same. Sublobule VIIIA is continuous laterally with the posterior part of the ansoparamedian lobule of Bolk and sublobule VIIIB with the dorsal paraflocculus; the two are separated by the hemispheral part of the parafloccular fissure. The pattern is the same in the whale embryo but it is obscured in the adult by the great hypertrophy of the paramedian lobule and the dorsal paraflocculus.

Lobule VIII of the porpoise is divided into sublobules VIIIA and VIIIB, with the two sharing a short ray of attachment to the medullary body (figs. 138, 144). In the adult fin whale the corresponding medullary ray is much longer before it divides into branches to the individual sublobules, but the two sublobules in the porpoise are relatively much more elongated than in the fin whale. Sublobule VIIIB, as in the whale, is smaller than VIIIA and is more or less displaced to one side of the midline. The two sublobules correspond to those similarly named in the cat and rhesus monkey (Larsell, 1953a), as Jansen noted with reference to the subdivisions of the pyramis in the fin whale.

In the electrophysiological studies of Snider and Stowell (1942, 1944), auditory stimulation induced action potentials in lobule VIII and also in lobule VII of the cat. The differentiation of lobule VIII, alone, in the small bats whose auditory sense is highly developed but whose vision is greatly reduced points to this lobule as the principal "auditory" segment of the vermis. The hypertrophy of this lobule in Cetacea, which is especially pronounced in the porpoise, appears to be correlated with the extraordinary development of the auditory mechanism and the centers in the brainstem that are related to hearing in cetaceans.

According to Langworthy (1932) in regard to *Tursiops*, and Ogawa and Arifuku (1948) and Osen and Jansen (1965) in regard to *Odontoceti* and *Mysticeti* the cochlear nerve and acoustic center of the brainstem are very large. The acoustic sense in *Odontoceti* was said by the Japanese authors to have reached a degree of development which is unique among mammals. Kellogg, Kohler, and Morris (1953), in experimental studies on *Tursiops*, observed reactions to vibrations in water as high as 80,000 c.p.s. and Kellogg (1959) ascertained that such reactions included avoidance of obstacles, discrimination of sounds, and others. Reysenbach de Haan (1958) emphasized the great importance of hearing in *Odontoceti*, stating that in *Mystacoceti* it is somewhat less important. According to this author (1960) Cetacea are sensitive to ultrasonic frequencies much higher than 100,000 c.p.s. and are capable of producing very high tones. In *Odontoceti* the nuclei and the reflex and coordination centers that are especially significant for interpretation of ultrasonic frequencies were said to be particularly well developed, which suggests a parallelism with the central acoustic system of bats.

With reference to the cerebellum, the morphological homology of lobule VIII of cetaceans, as defined above, with the pyramis of the bat, cat, monkey, and other mammals together with the relatively larger lobule VIII of the porpoise, an odontocete, as compared with the fin whale, a mystacocete, indicate that this lobule is the auditory segment of the organ. Whether the two sublobules in Cetacea and other mammals are further differentiated functionally remains to be determined by further experimental research.

Lobule IX, the uvula, becomes foliated during development in the fin whale into three or four folia, according to Jansen (1954). However, he was uncertain of their correspondence, respectively, to the subdivisions of lobule IX in other species. In the porpoise lobule IX is relatively larger than in the fin whale. It is elongated dorsalward behind sublobule VIIIB (figs. 138, 144), and also is partly displaced to one side, with the lateral part of the lobule expanding posterolaterally. Two principal fissures divide it into three but these cannot be homologized with any certainty with those of other mammals. The two most ventrally situated, however, probably represent lamellae IXc and IXd.

HEMISPHERAL LOBULES AND FISSURES

The first furrows that appear in the hemispheres, according to Jansen (1954), are the parafloccular and intraparafloccular, which are both present in the 21-cm C.R. length fin whale embryo. The parafloccular fissure extends medialward so that in the 23-cm embryo it ends between the lateral extremity of the prepyramidal fissure and the medial end of the intraparafloccular fissure of Jansen (fig. 134). The latter appears to correspond morphologically to the furrow which in the rat and other embryos I called the lateral segment of the fissura secunda. In the fin whale embryo, according to Jansen, it usually but not always joins the vermal segment of the fissura secunda, as does the lateral segment of the fissura secunda in other embryos. The parafloccular fissure of the whale appears to be the more precocious of the two, as it is in other embryos. According to Jansen its medial end sometimes joins the fissura secunda but never the prepyramidalis. As noted above, the vermal part of the fissure, when established, corresponds to my intrapyramidal sulcus. Two additional fissures, tentatively identified as the posterior superior and the ansoparamedian by Jansen, have appeared in the 24-cm embryo and are distinct in the 26-cm embryo (fig. 134).

The rudiments of the dorsal and the ventral paraflocculus and the paramedian lobule are quite distinct in the 26-cm embryo (fig. 134). A narrow zone between the posterior superior and ansoparamedian fissures represent the rudiment of lobule HVIIA, the ansiform lobule of Bolk. In the 50-cm embryo it has increased in size and the intercrural fissure has appeared, dividing this lobule into crus I and crus II (fig. 134). A narrow zone between the posterior superior fissure and the faint lateral continuation of the fissura prima of the 23-cm embryo evidently is the rudiment of lobule HVI, the hemispheral part of Bolk's lobulus simplex.

The hemispheral lobules and fissures of the adult porpoise are similar in general to those of the adult fin whale, as described and illustrated by Jansen, but with some differences. Lobule HVI is more distinctly demarcated from lobule VI in the porpoise than in the fin whale (fig. 139). This is because of the pronounced paravermian sulcus in this part of the porpoise cerebellum (fig. 140). The hemispheral lobule is relatively smaller in the porpoise than in the fin whale and does not spread so far laterally; it is quite similar, however, to Jansen's illustration of the corresponding lobule of the bottle-nosed whale. This fact and the greater size of lobule VI in the fin whale (the head including the lower jaw of which is relatively much larger than in the other two species) permit the suggestion that the greater development of lobules VI and HVI in the fin whale possibly is correlated with the larger area of distribution of the trigeminus. In the porpoise lobule HVI comprises three distinct groups of folia, the most posterior of which is less clearly subdivided into a small anterior group and a larger and more elongated posterior group (figs. 139, 140). The most rostral segment of the lobule is separated from the remainder by a lateral continuation of declival sulcus 3; the vermal connection of the folia is with sublobule VID. Emerging from the lateral wall of the paravermian sulcus the folia form the lower medial surface of lobule HVI. The second folial group is delimited posteriorly and laterally by a fissure which probably represents the hemispheral segment of declival sulcus 1, although the dorsal folia of the group are related to lamella VIb rather than lamella VIa, as are the more ventral folia. The third and largest folial group is related to lamellae VIb and VIc and those in the anterior wall of the posterior superior fissure.

Lobule HVIIA, the ansiform lobule, is narrow medially but wider on the anterior and anterolateral surfaces of the hemisphere (figs. 139, 140). Its posterior and lateral boundary, the ansoparamedian fissure, forms a deep cleft which reaches the anterolateral cerebellar surface. The anteromedial wall of its deepest portion is formed by eight folia of the ansiform lobule. The intercrural fissure, which divides the lobule into crus I and crus II, also is deep and prominent. Both of its walls have six to seven folia. The posterior wall of the posterior superior fissure includes five folia. Crus I is narrow medially but widens on the rostral surface of the hemisphere. No distinct subdivision into crus Ia and crus Ip is recognizable. A relatively deep fissure divides crus II into two parts that probably correspond to crus IIa and crus IIp. Although the superficial surfaces of both crus I and crus II are relatively small the depth of the delimiting fissures and the many folia of their walls give to each a considerable cortical surface. The relative reduction of the exposed surfaces, as compared with many other large mammals, appears to represent, in part at least, a rostrocaudal compression that results in deep rather than broad sublobules. Both crus I and crus II are quite similar in surface view to the corresponding subdivisions of the fin whale as illustrated by Jansen (1954).

The paramedian lobule, as defined by Jansen (1950) in the fin whale, is very similar in the porpoise although Wilson (1933) stated that it cannot be delimited satisfactorily in *Phocaena* or *Tursiops*. In *Balaenoptera sulfurea*, however, Wilson differentiated it as a distinct lobule expanding laterally between the ansoparamedian and parafloccular fissures as a large hemispheral subdivision. Scholten (1946) included both the paramedian lobule and the dorsal paraflocculus of Jansen in his crus II, as Jansen pointed out. In late embryos of the fin whale the paramedian lobule comprises three subdivisions connected medially with the rostral part of the pyramis, according to Jansen (1950); the rostral subdivision also has a small connection with the caudal part of the posterior tuber facing the prepyramidal fissure. The adult fin whale has three or four groups of folia that taper medially and have similar vermal connections (Jansen, 1954). If the ansoparamedian fissure ends in the anterior wall of the prepyramidal fissure, as suggested above and as Jansen (1954) confirmed by his statement that this fissure is continuous with sulci in the oral bank of the prepyramidal fissure, then the anterior subdivision must be continuous with the posterior tuber or lobule VIIB. This does not rule out possible continuity of part of this hemispheral division with part of lobule VIIIA. In some cerebella of the monkey and man the floor of the prepyramidal fissure and its lower posterior wall also are continuous with the anterior division of the paramedian lobule. This division corresponds to lobule HVIIB of other species; two divisions behind it, which are continuous medially with lobule VIIIA, represent lobule HVIIIA which in some species I found to be subdivided into two parts, one continuous with the greater part of the sublobule and the smaller caudal part continuous with the copula pyramidis. Similar relations are suggested in Jansen's figures of the fin whale. The porpoise has three subdivisions of the lobule (fig. 140), but owing to the depth of the paravermian sulcus and the uncertain vermal part of the ansoparamedian fissure, I was unable to satisfactorily establish their vermal relations. As in the fin whale the paramedian lobule is the second largest division of the cerebellum and forms a large portion of the hemisphere.

Chambers and Sprague (1955a) considered the para-

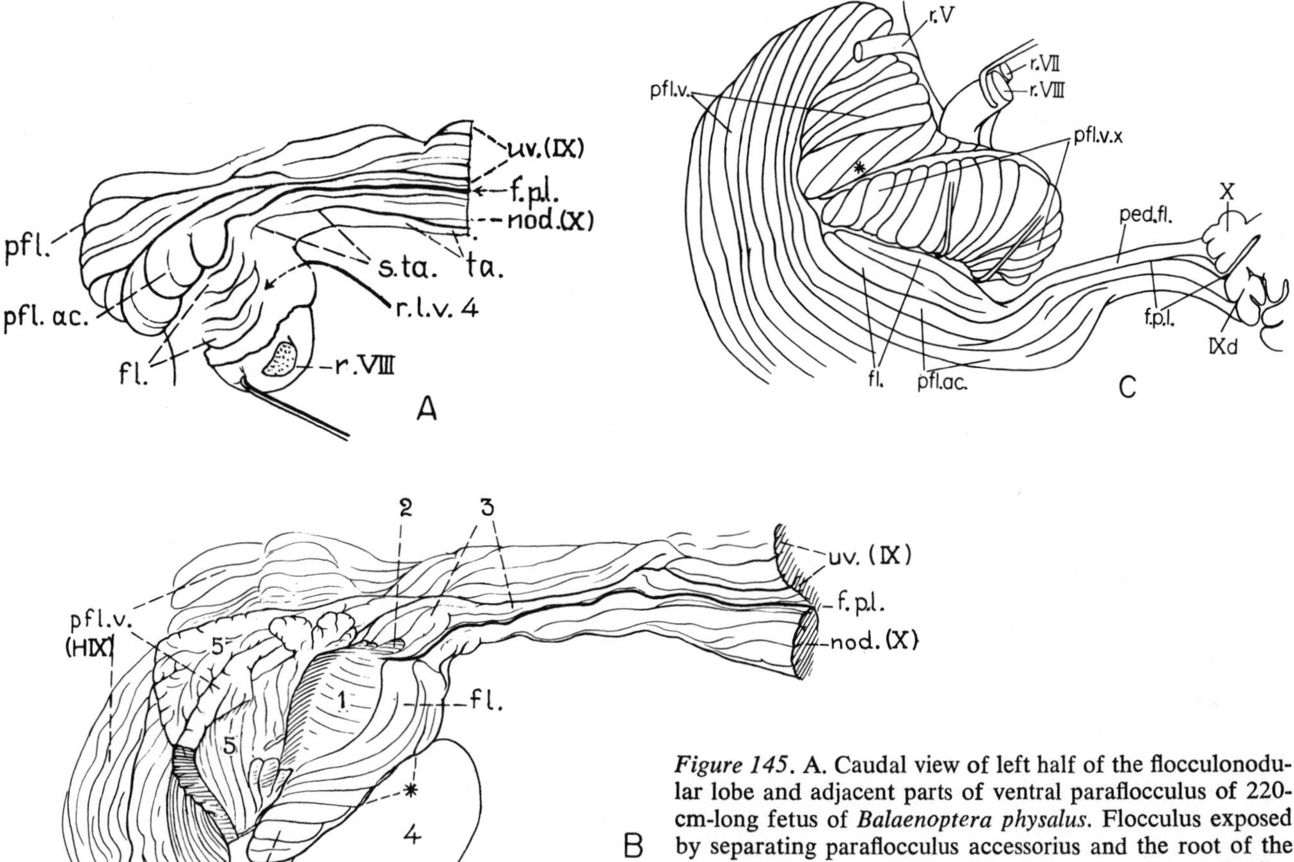

Figure 145. A. Caudal view of left half of the flocculonodular lobe and adjacent parts of ventral paraflocculus of 220-cm-long fetus of *Balaenoptera physalus.* Flocculus exposed by separating paraflocculus accessorius and the root of the statoacoustic nerve. Dissection. (Jansen, 1950.) B. Similar view of flocculonodular lobe in adult *Balaenoptera physalus.* 1. "Bed" of paraflocculus accessorius. 2. Cut surface of paraflocculus accessorius. 3. Folia connecting paraflocculus accessorius with caudalmost folia of uvula (IXd). 4. Brachium pontis. 5. Cut surface of ventral paraflocculus. Asterisk marks a slight marginal defect of the flocculus. Dissection. (Jansen, 1953.) C. Cerebellum of porpoise (*Tursiops truncatus*). Ventral view showing the relations of the flocculonodular lobe. Ventral paraflocculus arches around VII and VIII nerve roots and forms a spindle-shaped terminal hook which is pulled rostralward by retractors in figure; it is completely separated from the remainder of the paraflocculus ventralis by a deep cleft but is continuous rostrally with the paraflocculus ventralis by folia in the depth of this cleft and around its lateral end. Dissection.

median lobule in the cat and monkey as the posterior part of the intermediate zone of Hayashi and of Jansen and Brodal. They presented evidence that the intermediate zone serves the pyramidal system control of the extremities. Since the paramedian lobule of cetaceans is by far the largest lobule, both relatively and actually, found in any mammal and the distal part of the forelimb (the flipper) is greatly modified and the hindlimb is absent, except for buried rudiments in the whales, their interpretation of the paramedian lobule does not seem applicable to the whale and porpoise or to the pinnipeds described above. The large size of the lobule in cetaceans is more consistent with a representation of the entire body, as Jansen (1953) suggested, such as Snider and Stowell (1944), and Hampson, Harrison, and Woolsey (1952) found with reference to the paramedian lobule of the cat and monkey in electrophysiological studies. If the ansoparamedian fissure ends in the posterior surface of lobule VII, as indicated above, the anterior division of the lobule is separated from the anterior one by a fissure which I regarded as the hemispheral continuation of the prepyramidalis. This division, continuous medially with sublobule VIIIA, becomes lobule HVIIIA. The posterior division is small and appears to correspond to the pars copularis of lobule HVIIIA of other species.

The paraflocculus of cetaceans has been variously interpreted but until Jansen elucidated its morphology by his embryological studies there was no clear recognition of the dorsal and ventral paraflocculus. Flatau and Jacobsohn (1899) interpreted the dorsal paraflocculus of *Phocaena* as corresponding to the inferior semilunar lobule of the human cerebellum, i.e., the homolog of crus II.

Riley (1929) described the paraflocculus of *Phocaena* as forming fully one-third of the hemisphere, but neither in this species nor in the narwhal, *Monodon,* did he differentiate the two subdivisions. In *Balaenoptera sulfurea* Wilson (1933) described the paraflocculus as being extremely large, comprising nine lobules, but he did not mention the dorsal and ventral parafloccular divisions. According to this author the paraflocculus receives probably 60 percent of the pontine fibers, with the remaining 40 percent passing into the rest of the hemisphere. Scholten (1946) regarded the subdivision which other authors described as the homolog of the paraflocculus as including the paraflocculus and paramedian lobule – the latter was said to be much the larger of the two. The paraflocculus, according to Scholten, is relatively small.

The dorsal paraflocculus, as defined by Jansen primarily on the basis of his studies of embryonic and adult material of the fin whale, extends lateralward from the side of the pyramis almost to the lateral cerebellar surface. It is separated from the superficial part of the pyramis by the paravermian sulcus, from the paramedian lobule by the parafloccular fissure, and from the ventral paraflocculus by the intraparafloccular fissure (fig. 142). In the porpoise the dorsal paraflocculus is relatively more expanded laterally, forming a pyriform lobule whose small end is continuous beneath the paravermian sulcus with the medullary substance leading into sublobule VIIIB. It probably can be regarded as lobule HVIIIB, as in other mammals. The parafloccular fissure is deep and prominent.

The ventral paraflocculus, as interpreted by Jansen in the fin whale and bottle-nosed whale and by myself in the porpoise, is the largest of the cerebellar subdivisions (figs. 141, 142). It forms the entire ventral surface and part of the lateral surface of the cerebellum and constitutes about one-half of the volume of the organ in the fin whale (Jansen) and a somewhat smaller proportion in the porpoise. Medially the ventral paraflocculus is continuous with lobule IX, the uvula; some of the folia were found by Jansen in the fin whale to be continuous occasionally with folia of the pyramis at the bottom of the fissura secunda.

The accessory paraflocculus was described by Jansen (1950) in the embryonic fin whale and the adult bottle-nosed whale; later he described (1953, 1954) it in the adult fin whale, Greenland seal, and Indian elephant. Pilleri (1963, 1964, 1966) identified the accessory paraflocculus in *Delphinapterus leucas, Eubalaena australis,* and *Balaenoptera borealis.* The accessory paraflocculus represents the hemispheral continuation of the caudalmost folia of the uvula (IXd). Figure 145A, B illustrates the relations of the lobule in the fetal and adult fin whale. In the porpoise it comprises a series of fourteen or fifteen short obliquely arranged folia that form a lobule whose medial connections, as in the whales, are with the most caudal folia of lobule IX (figs. 141, 145). It was incorrectly designated the flocculus by Langworthy (1932) in the porpoise. Jansen regarded it as the homolog of the Nebenflocke of Henle in the human cerebellum, an interpretation which I concurred with.

FLOCCULONODULAR LOBE

The flocculonodular lobe is small in cetaceans. The nodulus appears to be bilateral in origin (Jansen, 1954) as in other mammalian embryos. It attains a rather small to moderate degree of development relative to the remainder of the vermis. In the porpoise it has a triangular form, as seen from beneath, and a small floccular peduncle extends laterally from the base of the triangle on either side (fig. 145C). The peduncle expands into four or five flattened and atrophic folia that constitute a rudimentary flocculus hidden by the accessory paraflocculus. The posterolateral fissure is fairly deep in the vermis. Along the floccular peduncle it is a shallow groove which delimits the peduncle from medially directed folia of the accessory paraflocculus (fig. 145).

CAT

THE cerebellum of the cat (*Felis domestica*) is wide and relatively short (fig. 146). The vermis, like that in ungulates, is broad rostrally but is narrower and sinuous on the dorsal and posterior cerebellar surfaces. The hemispheres, not including the paraflocculus, are small; the paraflocculus is large and arches forward around the cerebellar base to form a prominent feature of the anterior surface of the organ (fig. 146A). The flocculus is elongated beneath the paraflocculus and also is visible in an anterior view (fig. 149A). The paravermian sulcus is narrow and deep on the posterior cerebellar surface and on the side of the dorsal surface toward which the lateral deflection of the corresponding part of the vermis is directed. On the rostral surface a deep cleft, the floor of which is formed by the outspreading of the brachium pontis before it enters the cerebellum, separates the ventral part of the anterior lobe from the paraflocculus and part of the remainder of the hemisphere. This cleft is formed by the forward bulge of the anterior lobe and the rostralward displacement of the hemisphere during growth, rather than by the relatively retarded expansion of the cortex between the vermis and the hemisphere that results in the paravermian sulcus of the posterior lobe. The question of hemispheral representation of the lobules of the anterior lobe is discussed below; at this point it should be stated that no furrow strictly comparable with the paravermian sulcus is present on the anterior cerebellar surface. For descriptive purposes the cleft between the medial and lateral parts of the anterior surface was designated the anterior sulcus.

The physical characteristics of the domestic cat are so well known that little description is necessary. The body is elongated and rather heavy. The legs are relatively short and have considerable unilateral independence of action, especially the forelimbs. The tail is long and probably serves an equilibratory function in some of the animal's movements. The muscular activities are agile, rapid, precise, and extremely well coordinated. Locomotion can be rapid but a fast pace cannot be maintained for long. The eyes are directed forward and are conjugated in their movements. The external ears are of medium size and have considerable latitude of movement. The auditory range is extensive. The tongue is large and projectable as in lapping fluids, but it is not prehensile.

CORPUS CEREBELLI

The fissura prima divides the corpus cerebelli into two parts whose relative areas in median sagittal section depend on variations in lateral displacement of the vermis in individual cerebella. The anterior lobe, however, is smaller than the posterior lobe. In the adult cat the anterior lobe bulges forward prominently since its surface is convex in the horizontal as well as the sagittal plane (figs. 146, 147). The lateral margin of the anterior lobe lies against the spread of the brachium pontis deep in the anterior sulcus. In the 140-mm fetus the anterior lobe is less rounded from side to side and the lateral extremities of its segments are generally similar to those of other species (fig. 149). Interpretation of these segments in terms of vermal and hemispheral subdivisions must take into account the experimental results of Brodal and Jansen (1946) on the distribution of pontocerebellar fibers. According to these authors the lateral parts of the anterior lobe of the cat probably are connected predominantly with the rostral paramedian gray of the pons. The vermis, including the medial part of the anterior lobe, receives pontine fibers from the dorsolateral paramedian and part of the ventral pontine gray substance and the ventral half of the nucleus reticularis tegmenti pontis. In the rabbit, in which the hemispheral lobules of the anterior lobe are more evident superficially, these lobules receive fibers from the rostral one third of the paramedian gray, with

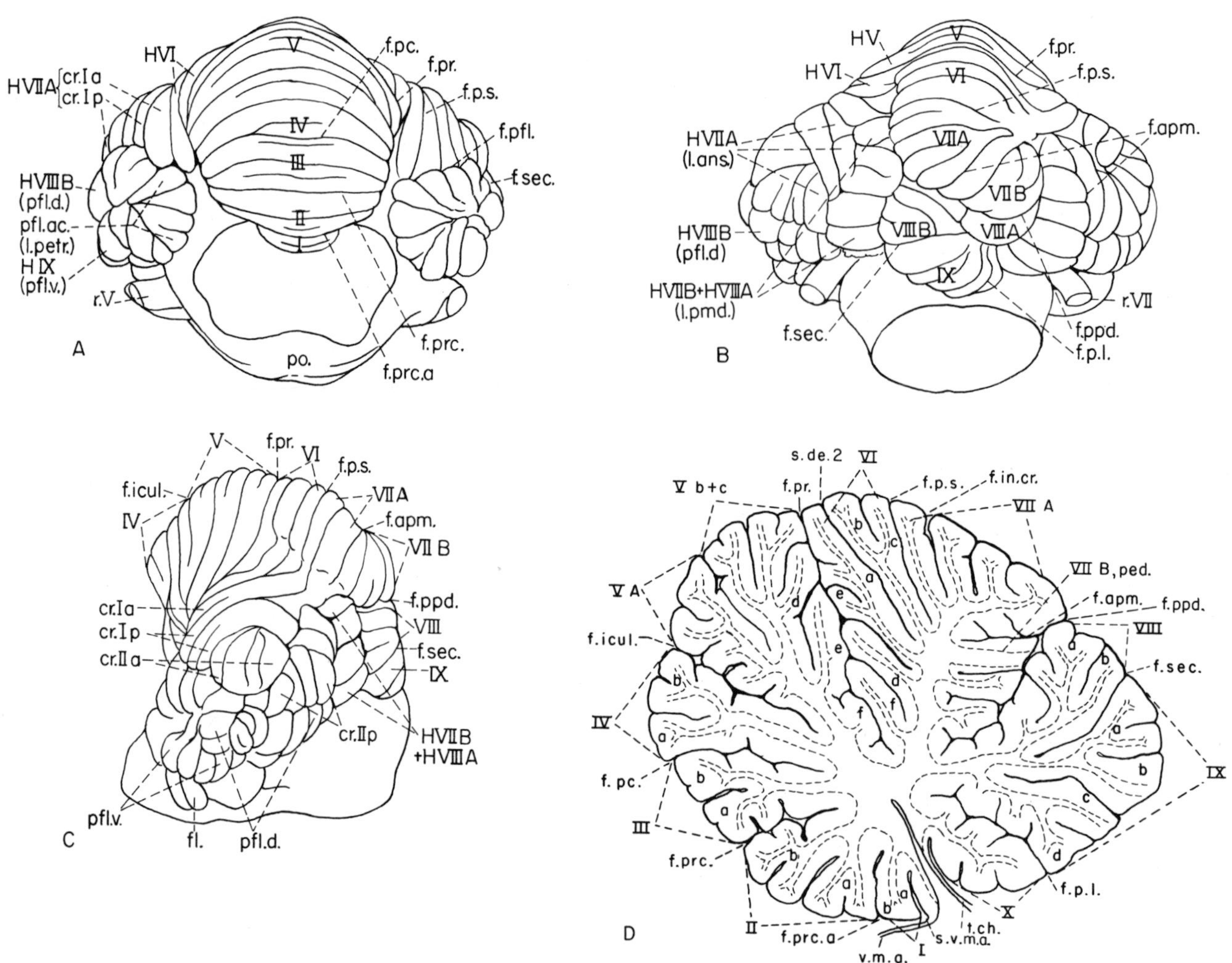

Figure 146. Cerebellum of adult cat. A. Anterior view. B. Posterodorsal view. C. Lateral view. Outlines of photographs after removal of pia mater and surface-staining with carmine. D. Midsagittal section. (Larsell, 1953a.)

the source of those to the vermis being the same as in the cat. Chambers and Sprague (1955a, 1955b) demonstrated that the anterior lobe in the cat is functionally divided into a medial zone of vermal cortex related to the fastigial nuclei and an intermediate zone of paravermal cortex related to the interpositus nuclei. On the basis of the experimental results of Brodal and Jansen and Chambers and Sprague it appears justifiable to differentiate vermal and hemispheral lobules in the anterior lobe of the cat despite the absence of any pronounced surface indications of boundaries. Such indications are subject to modifications related to the form of the cerebellum and the relative size of the lobules involved in individual species. In the anterior lobe of the cat five vermal lobules, with all but the most ventral one having hemispheral representation, are recognizable if the keel-like projection below the general ventral cerebellar surface is recognized as lobule I.

Lobule I is relatively small in the cat as compared with the rat. It is delimited rostrally by a furrow which extends from the anterior ventral cerebellar margin of one side to the other, corresponding to the precentral fissure *a* of other species (fig. 149A). In a cat fetus of 140 mm it has two folia, Ia and Ib; the anterior medullary velum is attached to the posterior surface of folium Ia which forms the lower anterior wall of the fastigial recess (fig. 148). In a 1-hour-old kitten the lobule shows the same general outline and relations (fig. 150). A 3-week-old kitten shows a compact medullary ray branching rostroventrally from the white substance that forms the anterior wall of the fourth ventricle. This ray passes into folium Ib which represents the principal part of the lobule; folium Ia receives a direct continuation from the medullary body. In the adult cerebellum represented in figure 146D, lobule I is composed of a narrow but tall folium and a

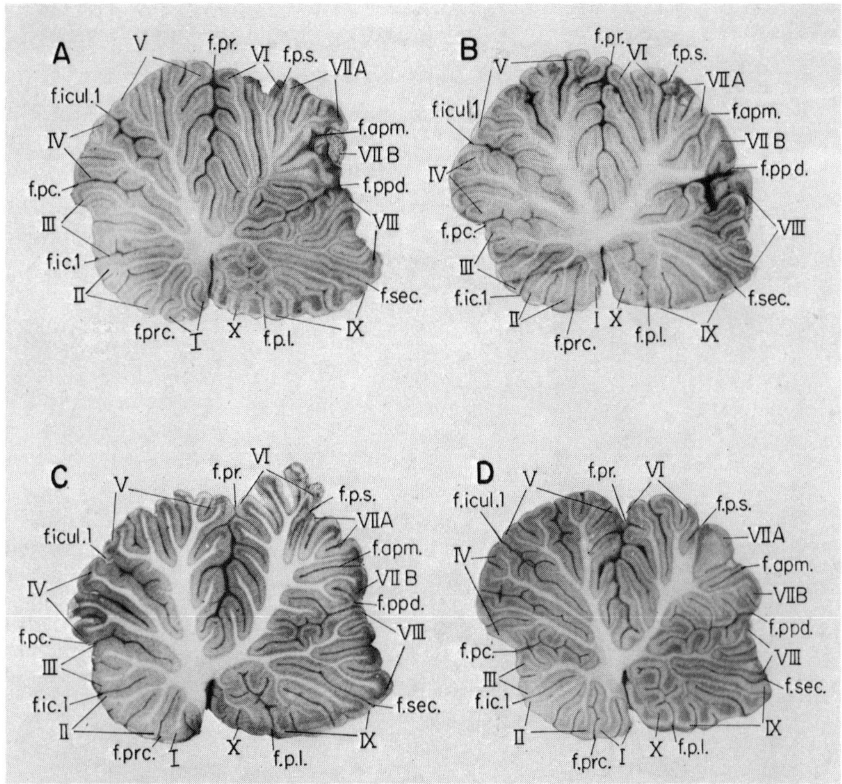

Figure 147. A–D. Midsagittal sections of cerebella of four adult cats, showing the principal variations of vermal lobules I–X. Photographs after surface-staining with carmine. ca. ×2. (Larsell, 1953a.)

plate of cortex and medullary substance which forms the ventral part of the anterior wall of the fourth ventricle. Folium Ia is elongated ventrally and the anterior medullary velum, in this and other adult cerebella, is attached to its tip. The lobule in the adult cat thus consists of two characteristic folia. The lobule is, relatively speaking, much smaller than in fetal and neonatal stages on account of the great increase in size of the remaining lobules of the anterior lobe during postnatal development. No hemispheral representation is evident.

Lobule II presents two folia in the 140-mm fetus and the newborn kitten. In this respect, as well as in outline, it closely resembles lobule II of the adult rat. The two folia have become lamellae in the 3-week-old kitten, each of which has two surface folia. In the adult cat the pattern varies from two folia, as in the fetus, to two lamellae (figs. 146D, 147). The rostral lamella, IIb, tapers onto the lateral surface of the anterior lobe (fig. 146A), forming lobule HII. This lobule has pontine connections corresponding to those of the remainder of the lateral part of the anterior lobe, according to the diagrams of Brodal and Jansen (1946).

Lobule III is subdivided by the intracentral sulcus into lamellae IIIa and IIIb in the fetal and kitten cerebella illustrated (figs. 148, 150). In the adult cerebellum the intracentral sulcus, as a rule, is relatively shallow but sometimes it is deep (fig. 147); in such instances, lobule III consists of two lamellae as in the kitten cerebellum illustrated in figure 150. In the 140-mm fetus only two folia of lamella IIIa reach the surface, but in the newborn kitten both IIIa and IIIb present two surface folia. In adult cats there is much variation of this lobule (figs. 147A–D). It tapers onto the lateral surface of the anterior lobe and forms a small lobule HIII which has connections with the rostral paramedian gray of the pons.

Lobule IV, in the 140-mm fetus, already is divided by a deep furrow into sublobules IVA and IVB (fig. 148). These are also visible in the 3-week-old kitten (fig. 153). In the newborn kitten (fig. 150) and in adult cerebella (figs. 147A–D) lobule IV shows different degrees of subdivision, apparently varying with the relative size of the adjacent parts of lobules III and V. When these lobules are large lobule IV is only partly divided; when they are small lobule IV usually consists of two sublobules, more or less distinct from each other, which may be designated IVA and IVB. The preculminate fissure pene-

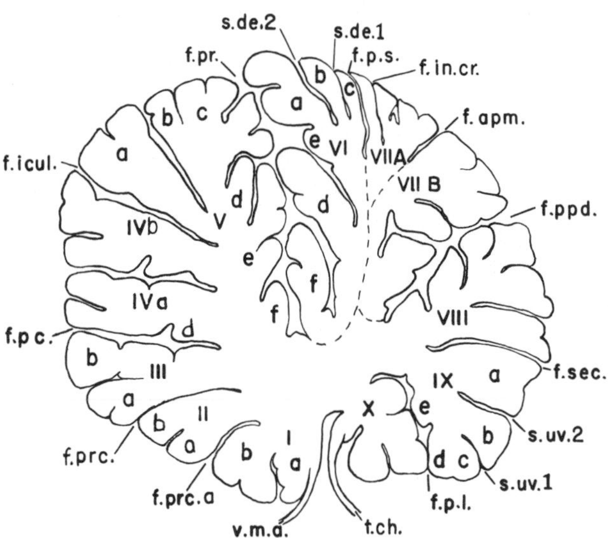

Figure 148. Cerebellum of 140-mm-long cat fetus. Midsagittal section. ×8. (Larsell, 1953a.)

trates so deeply that it almost reaches the medullary body in the 3-week-old kitten and the adult; it completely divides lobule IV from lobule III. Laterally lobule IV continues onto the medial wall of the anterior sulcus. Because of its pontine connections the lateral part may be regarded as lobule HIV. Intraculminate fissure 1, delimiting lobules IV and HIV from lobules V and HV, reaches the cortical margin.

Lobule V comprises a large anterior division that corresponds to sublobule VA of many species and two superficial lamellae, Vb and Vc, in addition to the characteristic lamellae Vd, Ve, and Vf that occur in the anterior wall of the fissura prima. All are recognizable in the 140-mm fetus and undergo little change except increase in size and secondary foliation. The interlobular and intralobular fissures also deepen. It is noteworthy that despite the greatly increased depth of the fissura prima in the adult cat the foliation of its anterior surface involves only the lamellae already present in the 140-mm fetus, principally lamella Va, which usually is the largest as in other species (figs. 148, 149A, 150). The lateral continuation of lobule V turns sharply ventralward, ending against the brachium pontis, which forms the floor of the anterior sulcus. The lateral portion was regarded as lobule HV.

Lobule VI comprises two usually elongated lamellae that reach the dorsal cerebellar surface and two or three smaller lamellae in the inferior part of the posterior wall of the fissura prima (figs. 146D, 154). The two principal folds of this wall correspond in position, general form, and size to lamellae VId and VIf of other species and were so identified. Both are differentiated in the 140-mm cat fetus and lamella VId is much the larger of the two. Presumably lamella VId is the first deep fold of the lobule to appear, as in other species. Sometimes lamella VIf is the larger in the adult cerebellum (figs. 147A, D). Both of the lamellae that reach the external cerebellar surface are subfoliated and the two are separated by a relatively deep fissure. This furrow and the folia of the two lamellae are difficult to homologize with the fissures and folds of lobule VI as found in most other mammals. In my earlier description of the cat cerebellum I (Larsell, (1953a) interpreted the deeper furrow as declival sulcus 2 of the rat and the cortical folds that it separates as folia VIa and VIb. The posterior fold of the lobule was re-

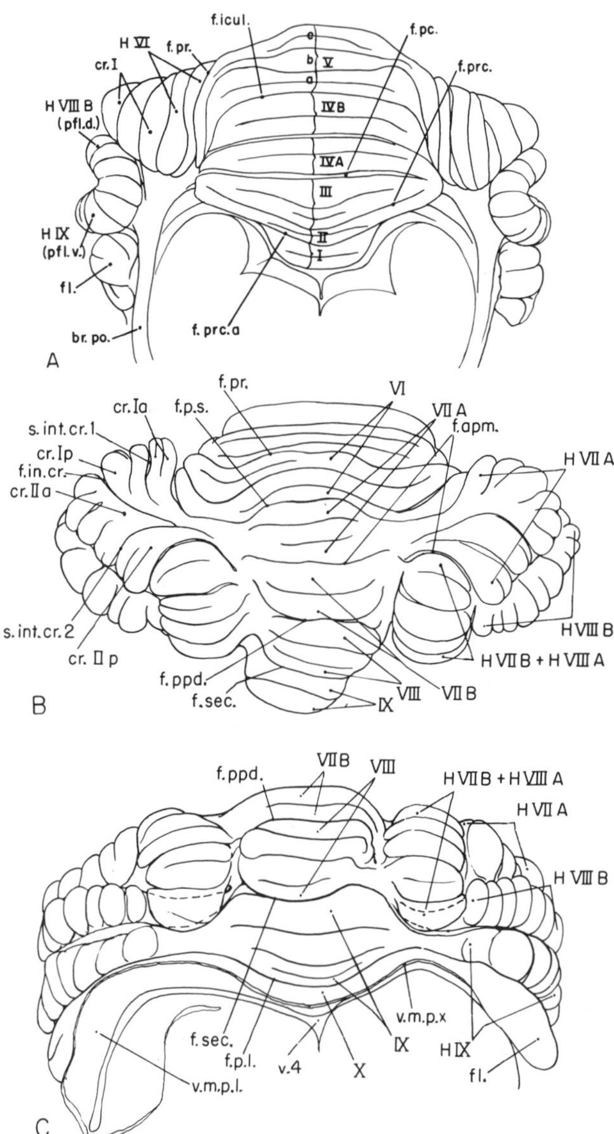

Figure 149. Cerebellum of 140-mm-long cat fetus. A. Anterior view. ×7. B. Dorsal view. ×6. C. Posterior view. ×6. (Larsell, 1953a.)

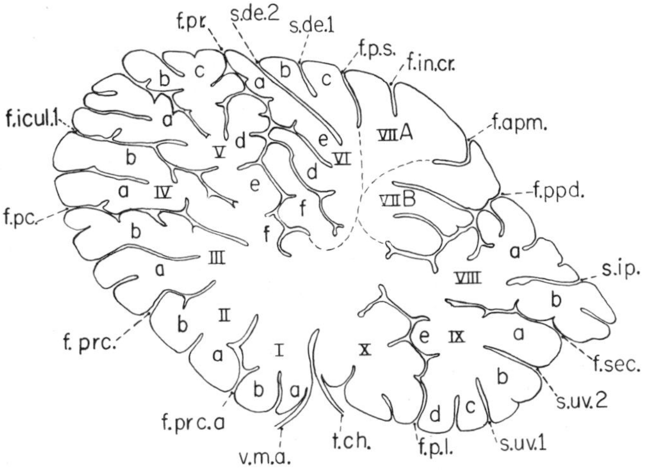

Figure 150. Cerebellum of newly born kitten. Midsagittal section. ×10. (Larsell, 1953a.)

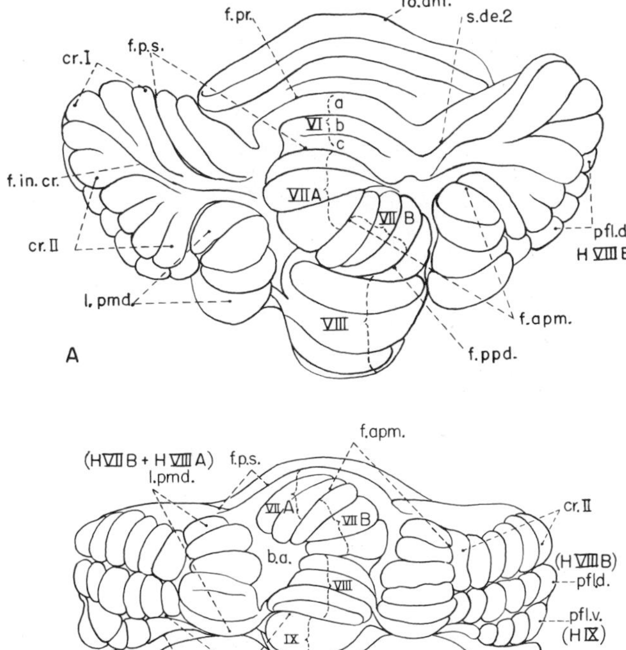

Figure 151. Cerebellum of newly born kitten. A. Dorsal view. B. Posterior view. ×6. (Larsell, 1953a.)

garded as lamella VIc. Study of lobule VI in many additional cat brains and its relations to lobule HVI and comparison with numerous other species made it seem probable that the deeper fissure is declival sulcus 1 and that folia VIa and VIb are represented by the subdivisions of the lamella anterior of it. The cortical folds that were interpreted earlier as VIb and VIc probably only represent lamella VIc, subdivided into folia VIc[1] and VIc[2] by a furrow of variable depth which ends blindly on one side of the vermis but usually is continuous, contralaterally, with a fissure of lobule HVI (figs. 151A, 153). Sometimes lamella VIIAa shares a medullary ray in common with lamella VIc which makes lamella VIIAa appear as a subdivision of lobule VI.

Lobule VII is expanded rostrocaudally in the 140-mm cat fetus so that it presents the largest surface outline, in the median sagittal plane, of any of the vermal lobules (fig. 148). A medial continuation of the ansoparamedian fissure divides it into sublobules VIIA and VIIB. The latter already is crowding into the prepyramidal fissure and, as shown in figure 149B, C, its caudal part is slightly

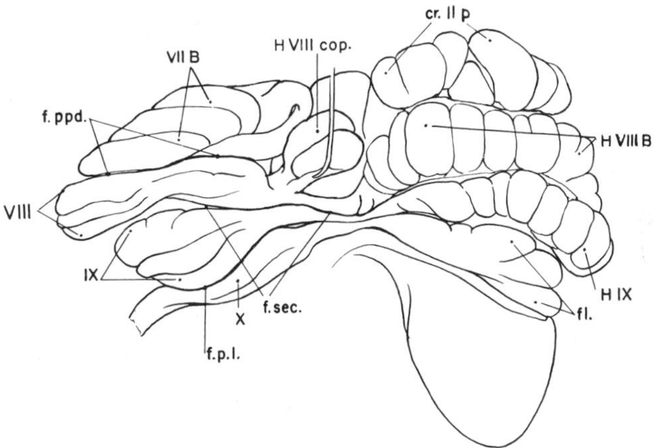

Figure 152. Cerebellum of full-term cat fetus. Posterolateral view of right half showing the relations of the copula part of the paramedian lobule, the paraflocculus, and the flocculus to the caudal vermal lobules. ×6. (Larsell, 1953a.)

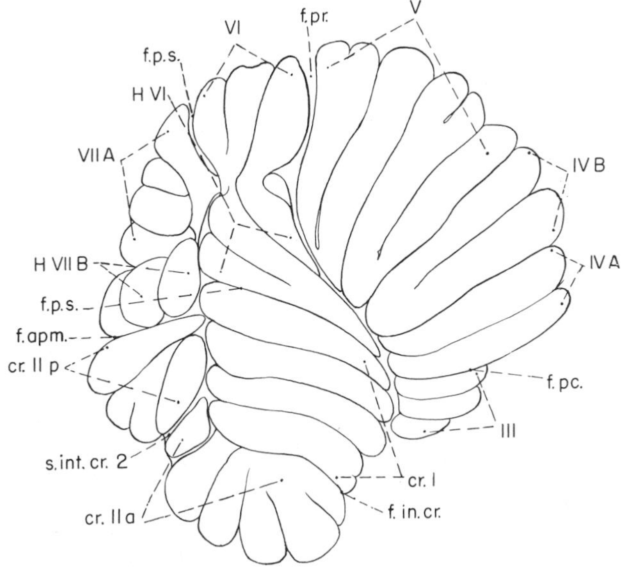

Figure 153. Cerebellum of 3-week-old kitten. Dorsolateral view, tilted posteriorly. ×7. (Larsell, 1953a.)

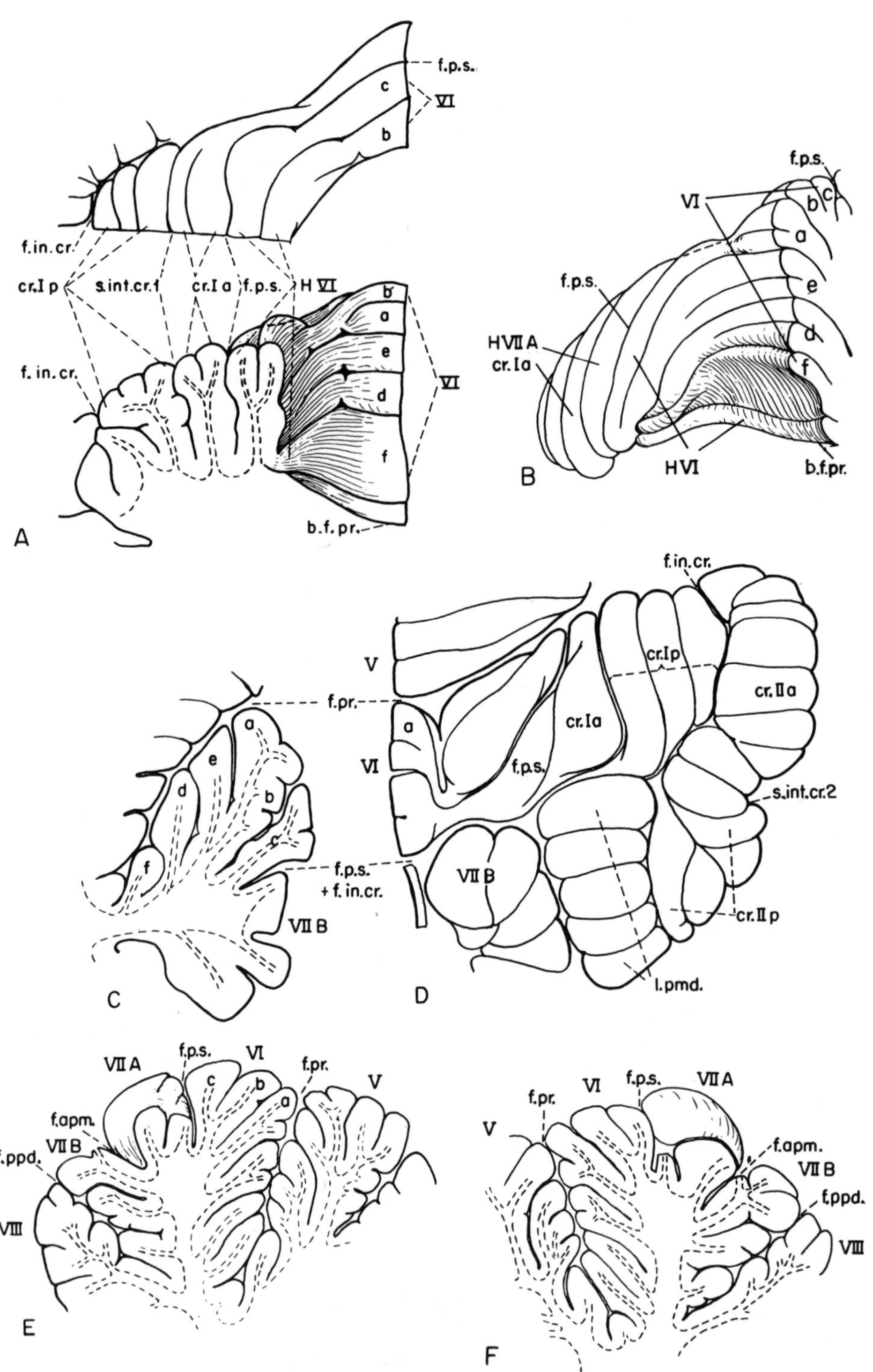

Figure 154. Cerebellum of cat. Dissections showing details of folia and relations between vermis and hemispheres in various specimens. A. Upper half of the figure, dorsal view of lobulus VI; lower half of the figure, rostral view of lobulus VI after removal of anterior lobe. B. Rostromedial view of right half of lobulus VI. C. Sagittal section of lobules VI and VII. D. Dorsal view of right half of hemisphere. E. Left side. F. Right side of sagittal section through lobules V–VII.

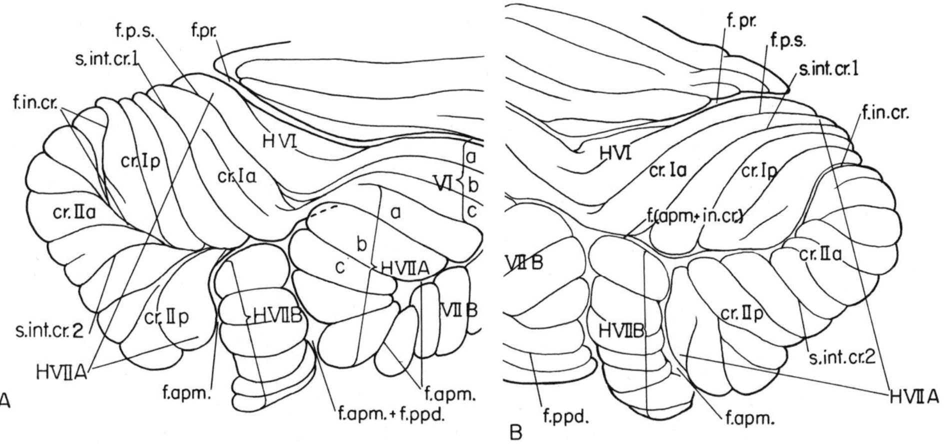

Figure 155. Cerebellum of cat. Dorsal view of left (A) and right (B) hemisphere.

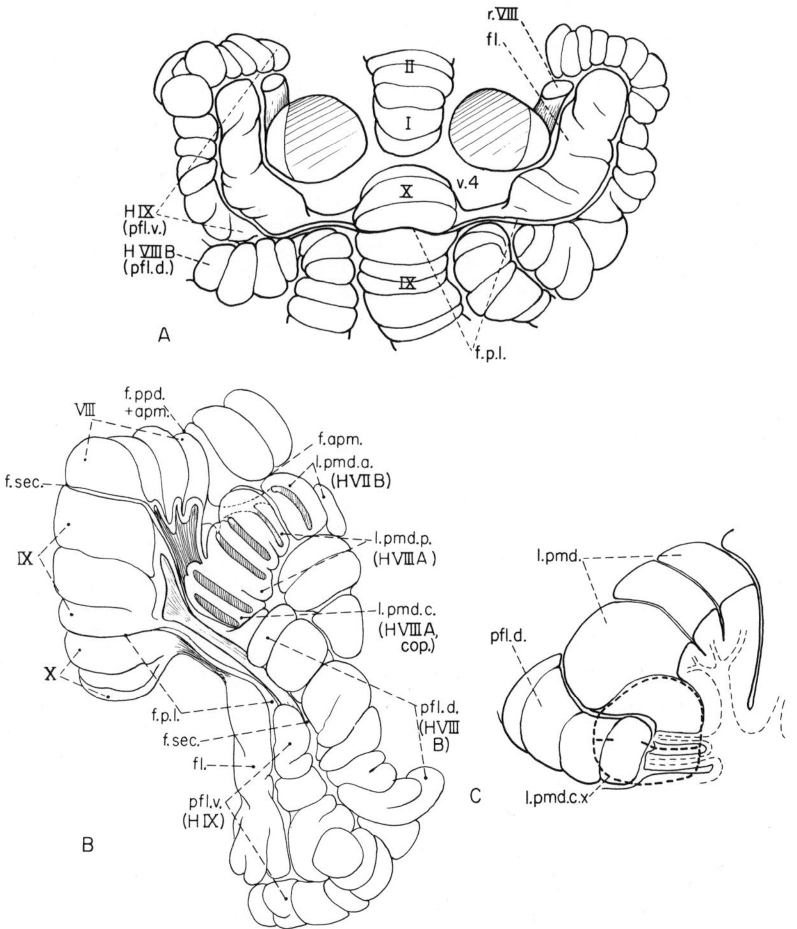

Figure 156. Cerebellum of adult cat. A. Ventral view. B. Posterior region. The areas ruled with short parallel lines represent cut medullary rays to the dissected away folia of the paramedian lobule. The parts of the lateral surfaces of lobules VIII and IX not covered by cortex are represented by larger parallel lines, those of lobule IX continue into the stalk of the ventral paraflocculus. The portion of the stalk of the dorsal paraflocculus visible in the dissection was covered with cortex. ×3. C. Details of paramedian lobule. Pars copularis of the lobule dissected away (bounded by broken lines).

displaced to the right. This lateral displacement is greatly accentuated in the newborn kitten (fig. 151A, B) and is accompanied by a displacement to the left of the caudal part of sublobule VIIA. In the adult cat VIIA is nearly medial, rostrally, but its caudal lamellae are pulled laterally with sublobule VIIB, which lies entirely at one side of the midline. The original left side of sublobule VIIA, as present in the fetal stage, has been drawn into the lateral continuation of the prepyramidal fissure in the cerebellum illustrated (figs. 146, 155). It forms the greater part of the anterior wall of this fissure on the right-hand side of this cerebellum. In the median sagittal plane, however, it is evident from figure 147 that the laterally displaced lobule is continuous with the base of lobule VII by a large medullary band. Stages of transition from the original medial position of sublobule VIIB to its adult relations are illustrated in figures 146B, 149C, 151, and 155. The displacement of the lobules may be either to the right or to the left.

Three divisions of sublobule VIIA are apparent in the 140-mm fetus and in some median sagittal sections of the adult cerebellum (figs. 149B, 147A, C). They represent lamellae VIIAa, VIIAb, and VIIAc; the first corresponds to the folium vermis and the last two correspond to the superficial part of the tuber vermis of the human cerebellum. After displacement of sublobule VIIA has begun the number of lamellae seen in median sagittal section varies with the angle formed between the sagittal plane and the deflected portion of the sublobule. The three lamellae may be seen, however, in dorsal view of the cerebellum. Sublobule VIIB has a variable number of lamellae facing the prepyramidal fissure and four or five reaching the cerebellar surface either as broad lamellae or subdivided into folia.

Lobule VIII, the pyramis, is relatively small in the 140-mm fetus (figs. 148, 149C) and the fissura secunda is rather shallow in the median sagittal section. Both these features result from the displacement of the lobule by the growth of sublobule VIIB (figs. 151, 152). By the adult stage the rostral part of lobule VIII has been drawn to one side and the caudal part has been displaced so far to the other side that the lobule is a horizontally widened segment whose folia are greatly distorted (figs. 146B, 155). In median sagittal sections two subdivisions are visible (figs. 146D, 147). These appear to correspond to sublobules VIIIA and VIIIB of many other species but in the cat their size, as seen in sagittal section, not only is reduced but varies in individual animals because of differences in the amount of deflection of the sinuous portion of the vermis.

Lobule IX, the uvula, also is affected by the crowding of sublobule VIIB. As shown in figure 151B, its rostral part is displaced in company with the ventral part of lobule VIII. In the 3-week-old kitten the deflection is so pronounced that the entire lobule is involved and even lobule X is somewhat affected. By the adult stage the exaggerated sinuous form of the vermis, presented in the kitten, has been reduced by readjustments accompanying the increase in size of the entire cerebellum (fig. 146B).

HEMISPHERAL LOBULES OF POSTERIOR LOBE

Lobule HVI in the 140-mm fetus comprises three superficially visible folia immediately lateral of the vermis, which converge into two on the anterior cerebellar surface. Hemispheral continuations of part of lamella VIa and of lamellae VIe, VId, and VIf constitute the greater part of the lateral wall of the fissura prima. In addition the folia of the anterior wall of the posterior superior fissure are included in the lobule. The developmental changes from the simple relations in the 140-mm fetus to those of the adult are illustrated in figures 149B, 151A, 153, and 154A. There is considerable variation in the dorsal surface area of lobule HVI in the adult (fig. 154) as a result of the differences in the breadth and the forward crowding of the hemisphere.

Lobules VI and HVI, which together correspond to the lobulus simplex of Bolk, in addition to the sharp superficial differentiation from each other, also receive fibers from different parts of the pontine gray substance as demonstrated by Brodal and Jansen (1946). Lobule VI is connected with the same gray masses of the pons as the remainder of the vermis, whereas lobule HVI receives fibers from those that also are connected with the ansiform lobule.

The hemispheral continuations of folia VIa and VIb are separated for a variable distance lateralward by a furrow but they eventually merge into a single superficial folium of lobule HVI. The deep surface of the lobule which faces the fissura prima is formed of lateral continuations of folia and lamellae VIe and VId (fig. 154A). In some cerebella these hemispheral folia are partially visible in dorsal view (fig. 154B). The posterolateral folium of lobule HVI is continuous with lamella VIc, with an extension of declival sulcus 1 separating it from the anterior group.

In the 140-mm fetus (fig. 149B), the posterior superior fissure forms a continuous furrow between lobules VI and HVI, on the one hand, and lobule VII and the ansiform lobule (HVIIA), on the other hand. In subsequent development the continuity is obscured at the paravermian sulcus, but in the adult the posterior superior fissure is recognizable by its depth in the hemisphere. Followed medialward it frequently is joined by the intercrural and ansoparamedian fissures, with the three forming a compound furrow as far as the margin of the vermis (fig. 154D). The posterior superior fissure, however, usually is traceable as a shallow groove in the upper anterior wall of the common furrow, which disappears at the lateral margin of the paramedian sulcus. In the vermis the three fissures are desegregated. When lamella VIIAa is attached to the medullary ray of folium VIc, the vermal segment of the posterior superior fissure is shallower than that of the intercrural fissure. The continuity between the vermal and hemispheral segments in such instances is by a shallow groove across the floor of the paravermian fissure.

Lobule HVIIA already is divided in the 140-mm fetus into crus I and crus II (fig. 149B). In the fully developed cerebellum crus I includes four or five elongated superficial folia that extend rostrally and ventrally (fig. 146). The most rostral of these folia, which becomes the most medial part of crus I on the anterior surface of the cerebellum, terminates as an expansion which extends beyond the ventral border of the others. It is continuous with them, however, by an arch of cortex around the end of the intervening fissure. This folium, which is partly subfoliated medially, is separated from the more lateral group of three or four by a rather deep fissure; it also is directly continuous with lamella VIIIAa of the vermis, whereas the lateral group is continuous by a medially tapering band of medullary substance with the white substance beneath this lamella. The anteromedial lamella of crus I appears to correspond to crus Ia of other species and the posterolateral group to crus Ip (figs. 154C, D, 155). Crus Ia, in part, appears to be included in the middle portion of the cerebellar autonomic eye field as illustrated in Hampson's (1949) diagram of the cat cerebellum. Hampson, Harrison, and Woolsey (1952, p. 309) described the cerebellar area wherein evoked potentials are obtained upon stimulation of the medial wall of the autonomic eye field of the cerebral cortex of the cat which included contralateral crus I, crus II, and the lateral part of the lobulus simplex (lobule HVI). The largest responses occur in crus I and crus II. The rostral folia of the paramedian lobule also are activated. Lam and Ogura (1952) localized evoked potentials from stimulation of the superior laryngeal nerve of the cat in a small area which was described as being situated at the inferomedial angle in the medial adjacent lips of folia 3 and 4 of the paramedian lobule. The crus I area involved corresponds to the enlarged medial part of crus Ia before this folium begins to taper toward the vermis. Judging from the photograph reproduced by these authors the adjacent region of lobule HVI also is involved.

Crus II in the 140-mm fetus comprises six lamellae, some of which are beginning to subfoliate (fig. 149B). By the adult stage a chain of eight to thirteen superficial folia is differentiated; the number varies with the subfoliation of the original six. A group of four to eight folia adjacent to the paramedian lobule is delimited from the more lateral group of six or seven folia by a relatively deep fissure which may be regarded as intracrural sulcus 2 (figs. 146C, 160). The medial group arches caudoventrally; the arching is more pronounced and the group is bigger in large cats. It appears to correspond to the ansula of the lion, seal, and bear, illustrated and briefly described by Bolk (1906), who included it as part of crus II. The group appears to be homologous with crus IIp of the ox, horse, and other species already described. The six or seven folia between crus IIp and crus Ip differ in form from those of both crus Ip and crus IIp; it seems justifiable to designate this group as crus IIa.

The extreme sinuous form of the posterior part of the vermis in the adult cat not only displaces sublobule VIIA to one side but it also displaces it posteriorly, so that it largely overhangs the deep portion of sublobule VIIB. The vermal segment of the ansoparamedian fissure, as a result, is distorted in such a manner that it opens into the prepyramidal fissure instead of on the dorsal cerebellar surface as in the fetal cerebellum (figs. 146B, 160). Successive stages of the shift in position of the fissure, brought about by the rostrocaudal expansion of lobules VII and VIII, are illustrated in figures 146B, 149C, and 151.

Lobule HVIIB comprises six folia in the 140-mm fetus (fig. 149C). Variable subfoliation may increase the number to seven or eight in the adult, in addition to two or three superficially invisible folia, described below, which are attached to the parafloccular peduncle but were regarded as part of the paramedian lobule. The three anterior folia of the lobule are continuous medially with sublobule VIIB, and the caudoventral group of three or four, as a rule, are continuous with the folia of the floor of the prepyramidal fissure and on the lower part of its posterior wall. These two groups, which are separated by a fairly deep fissure, appear to correspond to the pars anterior and pars posterior, respectively, of the paramedian lobule of other species. The two or three small postero-inferior folia, mentioned above, which are attached by medullary rays to the white substance leading to lobule VIII (figs. 156B, 157), correspond to the pars copularis of the paramedian lobule of other species. Although no distinct copula pyramidis can be differentiated from the pyramis in the cat the relations of these folia are entirely similar in other respects to the pars copularis. The paramedian lobule of the cat thus comprises three subdivisions as in many other species described in this volume and as noted by Jansen (1950) in the

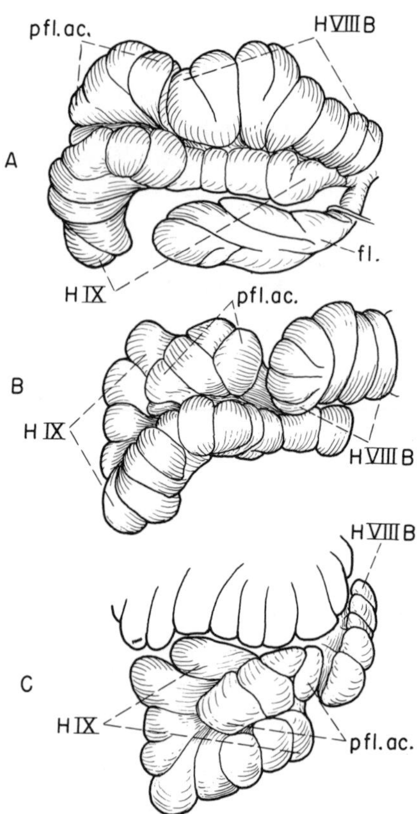

Figure 157. Paraflocculus and flocculus of cat. A. Lateral view. B. Dorsolateral view. C. Anterior view.

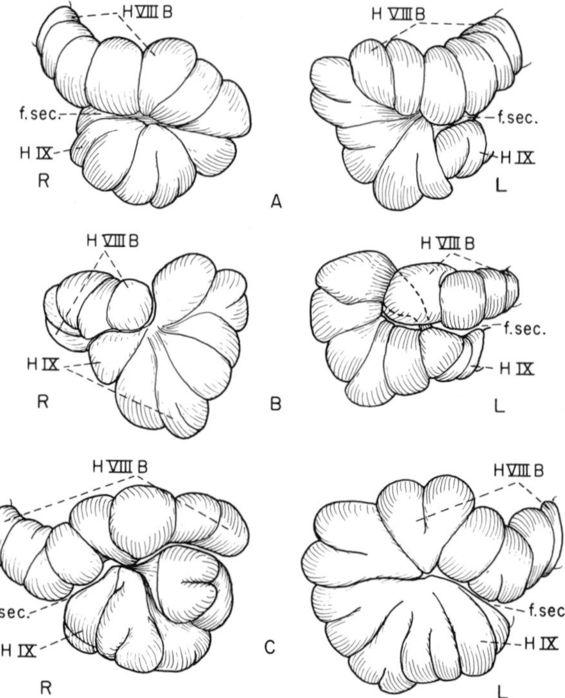

Figure 158. A–C. Right and left paraflocculus in three adult cats, illustrating individual variations.

whales. On the basis of its relations to the subdivisions of the vermis in the cat it may be designated lobule HVIIB + HVIIIA.

The paraflocculus of the cat is distinctly separated into a dorsal and a ventral paraflocculus by lateral continuity of the fissura secunda; the two divisions merge around the laterorostral end of the fissure (figs. 146C, 157, 158). The dorsal paraflocculus is continuous medially by its peduncle with the base of the posterior part of lobule VIII, corresponding to sublobule VIIIB of many species, as is especially clear in the 140-mm fetus and the newborn kitten when the pars copularis of the paramedian lobule is elevated (figs. 152, 156B). The foliation of the dorsal paraflocculus begins as small folia beneath the pars copularis, with increase in size laterorostrally.

The ventral paraflocculus, which is readily visible in the fetus, is continuous with lobule IX by a short peduncle, with foliation beginning at about the same lateral level as in the dorsal paraflocculus. In the newborn cat the peduncle has elongated while in the adult it is obscured by inclusion in a sheet of medullary substance although it can be demonstrated by dissection (fig. 156B, 158, 159). The proximal folia of the adult cat are large and are covered by the flocculus. The more distal ones form a chain parallel with the dorsal paraflocculus. A group of larger folia at the transition from ventral to dorsal paraflocculus appears to represent the accessory paraflocculus (fig. 157).

FLOCCULONODULAR LOBE

Lobule X, the nodulus, has a triangular form in sagittal section of the cerebellum of the 140-mm fetus but elongates in subsequent development so that folia characteristic of the adult nodulus appear. The choroid tela is attached at the base of the lobule behind the fastigium.

The flocculus (figs. 156A, B, 159) is a flattened, foli-

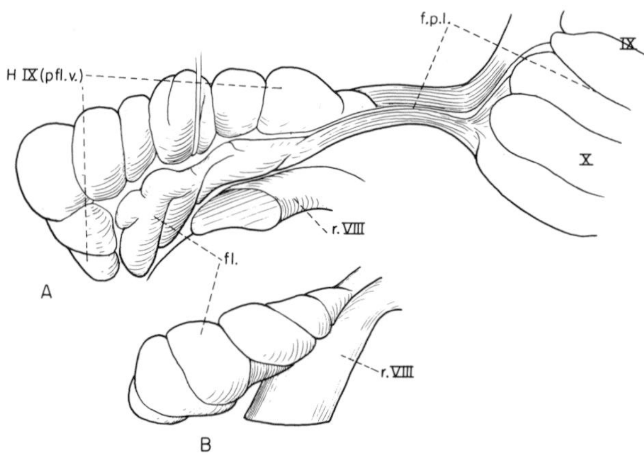

Figure 159. Cerebellum of cat. A. Lateral view of flocculus and ventral paraflocculus. B. Dorsal view of flocculus after dissecting away paraflocculus.

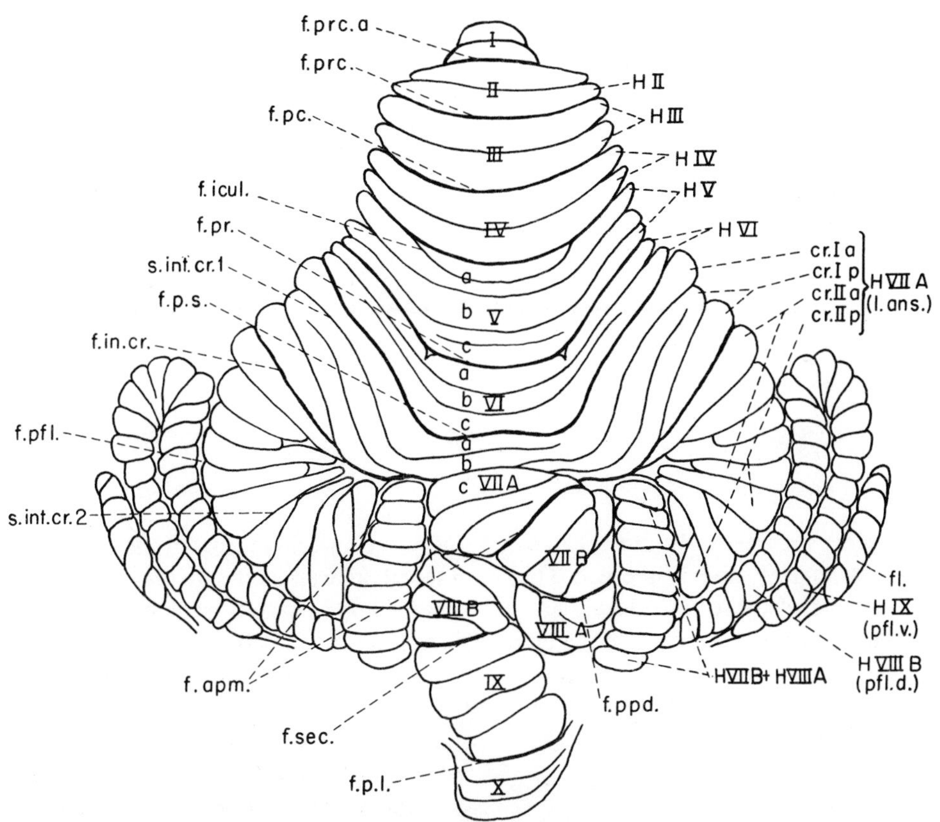

Figure 160. Diagram of cerebellum of cat. The cerebellar surface is folded out in one plane.

ated, and elongated lobule in the adult cat. Its continuity with the nodulus is clearly evident in the fetus and young kittens. In the adult the floccular peduncle, although somewhat buried in the posterior medullary velum lateral to the nodulus, is still demonstrable as a short fibrous band.

The nodulus, the two flocculi, and the connecting peduncles form a distinct flocculonodular lobe (figs. 156, 159). As in other mammals the posterolateral fissure completely delimits it from the corpus cerebelli. In the fetus this fissure can readily be followed from one side of the cerebellum to the other. As the posterior medullary velum increases in thickness, in later development, the fissure is more difficult to follow medially on account of the embedding of the peduncles in the medullary velum. At the lateral border of the nodulus, however, the fissure widens and deepens, penetrating almost to the medullary body.

Figure 160 illustrates diagrammatically the cerebellar subdivisions of the cat and their mutual relations as they appear when the cerebellar cortex is unfolded in one plane. It should be emphasized that peduncles connect the ventral paraflocculus and flocculus with the uvula (IX) and nodulus (X), respectively.

DOG

THE cerebellar hemispheres are relatively more extensive in the dog (*Canis familiaris*) than in the cat. The vermis forms a prominent ridge whose rostral part projects forward but is a less conspicuous feature of the anterior cerebellar surface owing to the greater lateral extent of the hemispheres. A paired broad groove on the anterior surface separates vermis and hemispheres, but unlike the anterior sulcus of the cat, its floor and low lateral wall as well as the medial wall are formed by hemispheral continuations of lobules of the anterior lobe. Therefore, in hemispheral and vermal relations this groove resembles the paravermian sulcus of the posterior lobe, with which it is continuous by a shallower groove (fig. 161A). The vermal part of the posterior lobe is narrower and more or less sigmoid. In very small breeds of dogs there may be little or no deflection to either side of the midline but even in puppies of larger breeds there is some displacement. The paraflocculus is large, extending onto the lower anterior surface of the cerebellum. The flocculus is elongated and relatively large but most of it is hidden beneath the paraflocculus (fig. 161B).

Body size and form, length of legs and tail, and other physical features vary so greatly in the numerous breeds of dogs that no general statements could be made concerning them. The extremities of most breeds are strong. The forelimbs, especially, have considerable unilateral independence of movement. The frontally directed eyes have well-conjugated movements and overlapping fields

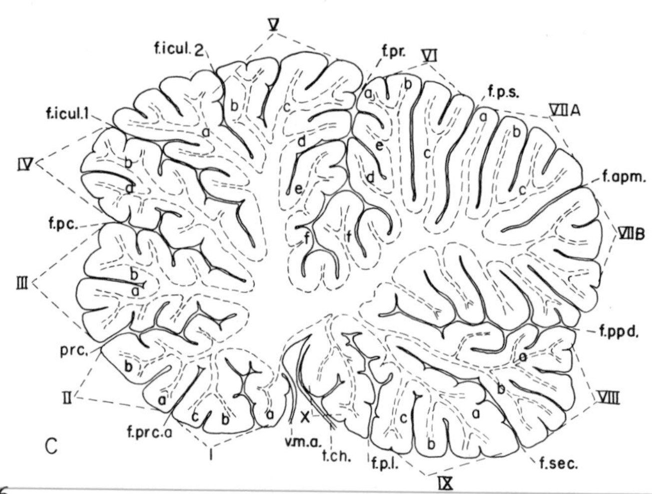

Figure 161. Cerebellum of dog (*Canis familiaris*). A. Antero-dorsal view. B. Ventral view. ×2. C. Midsagittal section of cerebellum of small dog. ×4.

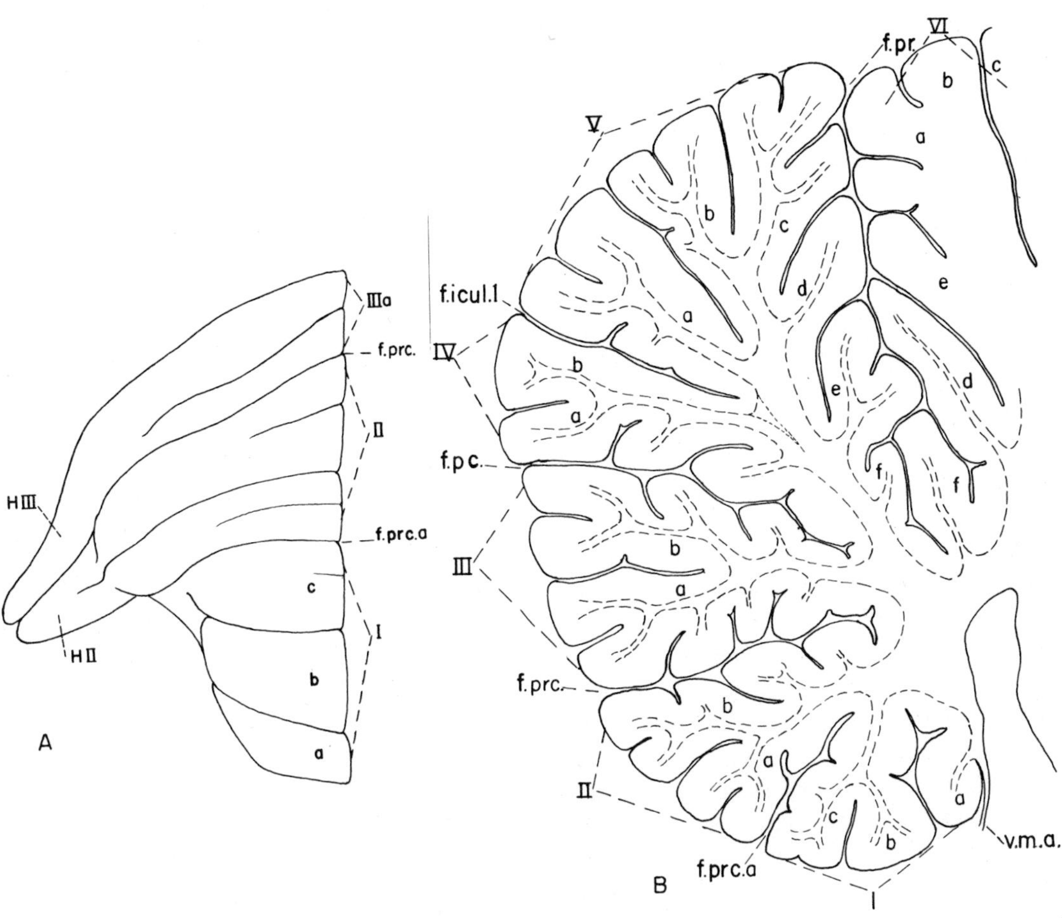

Figure 162. Cerebellum of medium-sized dog. A. Lower segment of anterior lobe. B. Midsagittal section of anterior lobe. ×6.

of vision. Distant vision is poor in dogs but hearing is acute and covers a wide range.

CORPUS CEREBELLI

The vermal portion of the anterior lobe (figs. 161, 162) is large and crowds the posterior lobe caudalward to such a degree that the fissura prima opens onto the dorsal cerebellar surface approximately midway between the anterior and posterior cerebellar surfaces. Lobule I comprises three principal folia that project into the fourth ventricle, pushing the anterior medullary velum beneath them (fig. 161A). Folium Ia is separated from Ib by a comparatively much deeper furrow than in the cat and many other species. Folia Ib and Ic extend laterally, forming a small triangular area on either side of the keel-like body of the lobule. Precentral fissure *a* varies in depth in different specimens; sometimes it is shallower than the furrow between folia Ia and Ib, but laterally it clearly constitutes the boundary between lobules I and II (figs. 161C, 162).

Lobule II has only two surface folia in the puppy and the small adult cerebellum illustrated in figure 161C. In larger dogs the corresponding folds are subfoliated medially (fig. 162) but laterally there are only two folia, as in the small cerebellum; these two converge to form a single fold of cortex which extends onto the anterior hemispheral surface as lobule HII. Lobules I and II sometimes are so indistinctly differentiated from each other, so far as the depth of the precentral fissure *a* is concerned, that they can well be regarded as subdivisions of one lobule. Comparison with the puppy, cat, and fetal stages of other species, however, indicates that the interpretation of the two lobules described is justifiable. The lateral continuation of lobule II onto the ventral surface of the hemisphere also distinguishes the two lobules (fig. 162A). The precentral fissure separates lobule II from lobule III.

Lobule III is divided into two large surface lamellae, IIIa and IIIb, each with two superficial folia. The lobule extends laterally onto the rostral surface of the hemisphere as a triangular continuation of the merged lamellae, forming lobule HIII (figs. 161C, 162).

Lobule IV is separated from lobule III by a deep preculminate fissure. Intraculminate fissure 1, which delimits it from lobule V, varies in depth. In some specimens it is nearly as deep as the preculminate fissure, in others the intraculminate fissure 1 is much shallower (figs. 161C, 162B). In sagittal section lobule IV presents two surface lamellae, designated *a* and *b*, and a characteristic deep lamella *d* at its base. The latter may correspond in an incipient way to sublobule IVA of the cat, but this is so uncertain that the designation used seems preferable. In none of the dog cerebella examined was there any indication of sublobules IVA and IVB in the form frequently found in the cat. Lamellae IVa and IVb converge laterally to form a narrow lobule HIV on the rostral surface of the hemisphere (fig. 161A). Sometimes intraculminate fissure 1 ends so far short of the lateral cerebellar margin that lobule HIV merges with lobule HV.

Lobule V includes three lamellae, namely, Va, Vb, and Vc, that reach the dorsal cerebellar surface (figs. 161C, 162B); two or three folia face intraculminate fissure 1; and the three characteristic lamellae Vd, Ve, and Vf form the anterior wall of the fissura prima. Lamella Va varies in size and secondary foliation more than Vb or Vc. Frequently it is so large that the furrow separating it from Vb is deep enough to merit specific designation, namely, intraculminate fissure 2. The surface lamellae converge laterally with lamellae Ve and Vf, forming a compressed lobule HV. Only one or two folia of HV appear on the anterior surface of the hemisphere; the others form the walls of the fissura prima and intraculminate fissure 1. Lamella Vd extends but slightly into lobule HV.

Lobule VI is relatively small in the dog. It comprises two major subdivisions, the terminal folia of which reach the dorsal cerebellar surface and two lamellae and some smaller folds that face the deep part of the fissura prima (figs. 161C, 163). Lamella VId of the posterior wall of the fissura prima corresponds to lamellae VId and VIf of the cat and other species. Close comparison of the secondary folds of the anterior lamella-like subdivision which lies dorsal of lamella VId, with corresponding folds in the cat and other species, reveals a pattern entirely similar to that formed by folia or lamellae VIa, VIb, and VIe, but on a relatively smaller scale in the dog. The three lamellae are reduced to folia in the small cerebellum illustrated in figure 161C. In the larger specimen (fig. 163) lamella VIa is subfoliated. The posterior major subdivision of the lobule corresponds to lamella VIc of the cat, as interpreted above, and other species. Superficially it is divided into two folia (VIc[1] and VIc[2]) by a

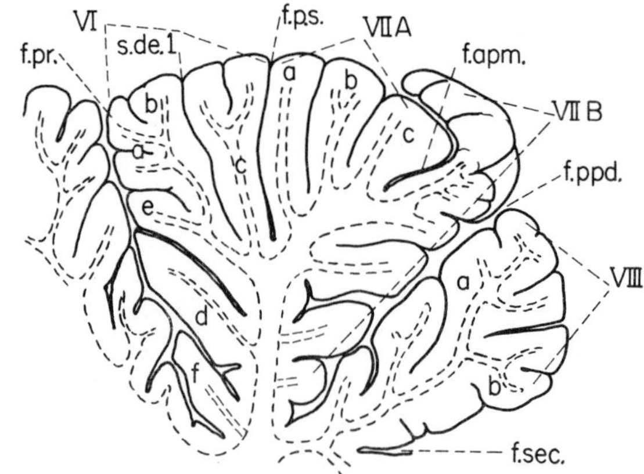

Figure 163. Cerebellum of large dog. Midsagittal section of lobules VI–VIII. Upper folia of VIIB lie immediately lateral to plane of section, continuous laterally with pars anterior and pars posterior of the paramedian lobule.

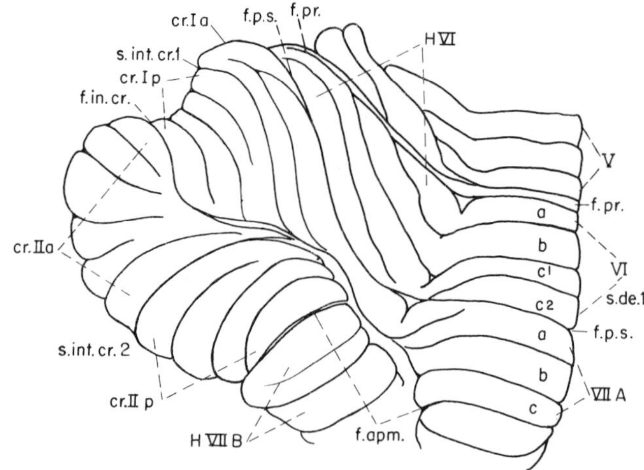

Figure 164. Cerebellum of large dog. Dorsal aspect of left half.

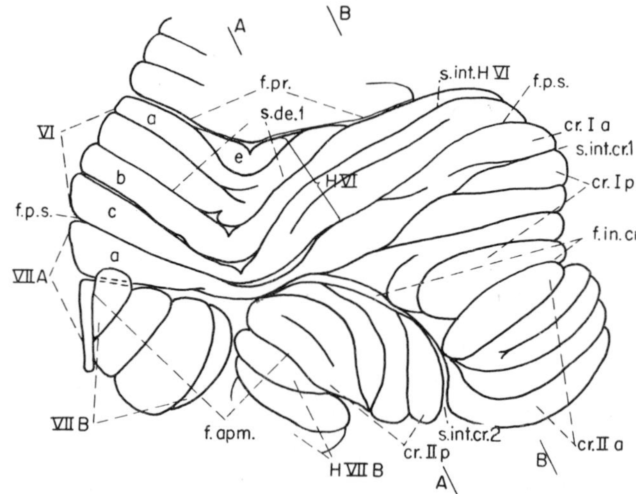

Figure 165. Cerebellum of large dog. Dorsal aspect of right half.

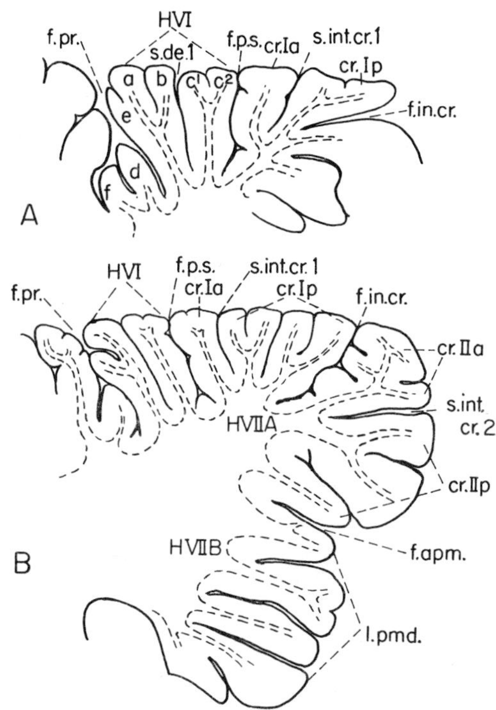

Figure 166. Cerebellum of large dog. A. (Medial) and B. (Lateral) vertical sections of hemisphere. Planes of sections indicated in figure 165.

furrow which, on one side, ends blindly or may appear to reach the posterior superior fissure when it really continues for a short distance in the anterior wall (fig. 164). Contralaterally this furrow is continuous with the intralobular fissure of lobule HVI, described below. Declival sulcus 2 between lamella VIc and the part including folia VIa and VIb is deep but its continuation into lobule HVI is shallow on one side, although deep contralaterally.

Lobule VII is large in the dog and is divided into sublobules VIIA and VIIB by the ansoparamedian fissure, which penetrates into the posterior part of the dorsal surface of the vermis (fig. 161C). In the floor of the paravermian sulcus this fissure is directly continuous with its hemispheral segment. Sublobule VIIA comprises three characteristic superficial lamellae, namely, VIIAa, VIIAb, and VIIAc, the hemispheral connections of which are with the ansiform lobule of Bolk (figs. 165, 166). Sublobule VIIB forms the upper posterior surface of the vermis and the roof of the prepyramidal fissure. Sublobule VIIB assumes a slightly sinuous form: its deflection from the midline also affects sublobule VIIIA and to a slight degree the dorsal folia of lobule VIII (fig. 163).

Lobule VIII comprises two relatively small superficial lamellae which probably correspond, on a reduced scale, to sublobules VIIIA and VIIIB of many other species, but in the dog the term sublobule does not appear warranted by their size (fig. 163). The lobule shares with lobule IX a short ray of attachment to the medullary body (fig. 161C). The fissura secunda, accordingly, is shallow but the prepyramidal fissure is nearly as deep as the fissura prima. From either side of the base of lobule VIII emerges a fibrous band that leads to the dorsal paraflocculus and also affords attachment to the two inferior folia of the paramedian lobule (fig. 167A).

Lobule IX is relatively small and entirely median in position. The three superficial lamellae shown in figure 161B appear to correspond to IXa, IXb, and IXc of other species. A short peduncle leads to the ventral paraflocculus, with a lateral continuation of the fissura secunda separating the ventral paraflocculus from the peduncle of the dorsal paraflocculus (fig. 168).

HEMISPHERAL LOBULES OF POSTERIOR LOBE

Lobule HVI is superficially delimited from lobule VI by a shallow rostral continuation of the paravermian sulcus (fig. 161A). The lobule comprises four superficial folia which arch ventrolaterally onto the medial part of the anterior surface of the hemisphere and hemispheral continuations of lamellae VId, VIe, and VIf in the posterolateral wall of the fissura prima (figs. 164, 165). More clearly than in the cat and other subprimates the folia are divided into two groups that correspond to the pars anterior and pars posterior of lobule HVI of primates, described below. The delimiting fissure is designated the intralobular sulcus. The intralobular sulcus of one side is continuous with declival sulcus 2 of the vermis, while contralaterally it is continuous with the shallow furrow that separates the two folia of lamella VIc.

Lobule HVIIA is divided into crus I and crus II by a deep intercrural fissure. Crus I is subdivided into crus Ia and crus Ip by a shallower intracrural sulcus 1. Crus II likewise is subdivided into crus IIa and crus IIp by intracrural sulcus 2 (fig. 166). The hemispheral segment of the posterior superior fissure, which separates lobule HVIIA from lobule HVI, is deep and may continue to be so until it reaches the vermis on one side or both. It may, however, be interrupted short of the vermis on one side by the medial merging of crus Ia and folium HVIc^{2}, which then continues to lamella VIIAa. Folium HVIc^{2} in such instances is continuous with the anterior surface of lamella VIIAa and this portion of the cortex of the lamella may be separated from the remainder by a shallow furrow (fig. 164). The vermal segment of the posterior superior fissure appears to be continuous with the intralobular sulcus of lobule HVI. Evidently such variations from the more common pattern are due to differences in

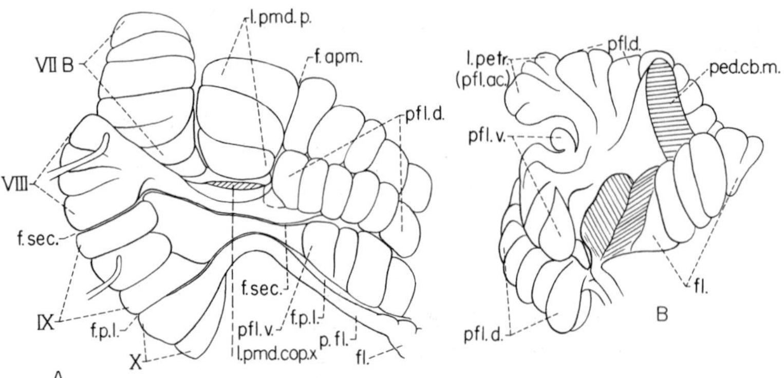

Figure 167. Cerebellum of dog. Ventral aspect. A. Floccular and parafloccular peduncles exposed by dissecting away copular part of paramedian lobule. B. Dorsal hidden surface of flocculus which lies against under surface of ventral paraflocculus exposed by turning back the flocculus.

the folding of this region of the cortex during fetal development.

Crus Ia is an elongated lamella that may have one or two superficial folia. Medially it is directly continuous with lamella VIIAa (figs. 164, 165). Crus Ip presents four or five shorter superficial folia which converge medially into a medullary sheet that is connected with sublobule VIIA. Crus IIa forms the most lateral portion of the hemisphere and crus IIp constitutes the posterolateral portion. The folia of both converge into a medullary band which merges with that of crus Ip and continues into sublobule VIIA. As it approaches the vermis this band forms the floor of a compound fissure produced by the junction of the intercrural and ansoparamedian fissures.

The paramedian lobule (figs. 161B, 168) is connected principally with sublobule VIIB and the folia in the lower anterior wall and floor of the prepyramidal fissure. The lobule comprises six obliquely to transversely arranged folds which, because they are subdivided by shallow furrows in larger dogs, were designated lamellae. The dorsorostral group of three lamellae is delimited from the caudoventral group by a deeper furrow, thus differentiating a pars anterior and a pars posterior. In addition two or three short folia at the lower margin of the pars posterior superficially appear to form a continuation of the lobule. These folia, however, are attached to the anterior part of the medullary band leading medially to the portion of the pyramis from which the copula, when present, extends lateralward in other species. I did not observe a distinct copula in the dog but the folia in question correspond to the pars copularis of the paramedian lobule of other mammals and therefore were so designated in the canine cerebellum. With the exception of this connection with lobule VIII and the possible connection with sublobule VIIA the paramedian lobule is continuous with sublobule VIIB, as stated above, and may be considered primarily as lobule HVIIB; the pars copularis, however, constitutes a small lamella HVIIIA.

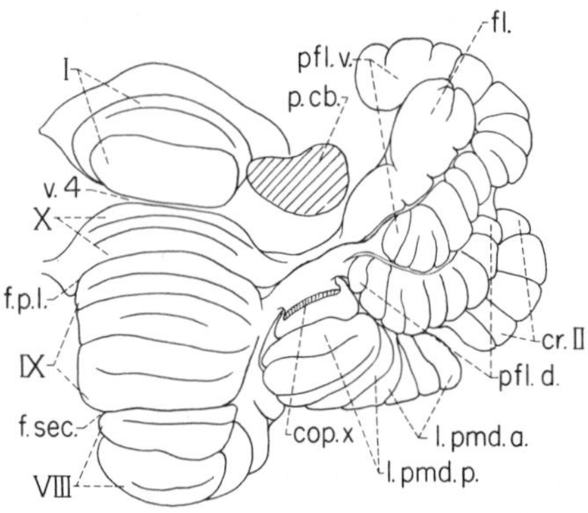

Figure 168. Cerebellum of 5-day-old dog. Ventral aspect. Copular part of paramedian lobule dissected away.

The paraflocculus (figs. 161A, 167, 168) consists of two chains of nearly vertical folia that extend from the lower lateral border of the paramedian lobule almost to the ventromedial margin of the rostral surface of the hemisphere. The more dorsal chain constitutes the dorsal paraflocculus, which is continuous with the deep portion of lobule VIII by a medullary stalk partly covered by the copular part of the paramedian lobule. Lateral of the copular folia the parafloccular peduncle proper becomes surmounted by the folia of the dorsal paraflocculus.

The ventral paraflocculus has a longer medullary peduncle which connects it with the uvula. A continuation of the fissura secunda forms a shallow groove in the unfoliated segment of the common parafloccular peduncle delimiting the ventral from the dorsal parafloccular portion of the peduncle (fig. 167A). Between the two chains of folia the fissura secunda widens into a prominent furrow that separates the two limbs of the paraflocculus as far as their distal loop of junction. A group of large ventral parafloccular folia forms a prominent lateral lobule some distance behind the junction of the dorsal and the ventral limbs. This lobule projects into a recess of the petrous bone and appears to correspond to the accessory paraflocculus of many other species. In the dog this lobule is clearly an enlargement of the ventral paraflocculus.

FLOCCULONODULAR LOBE

Lobule X, the nodulus (figs. 160, 167, 168), is rather small in median sagittal section but is elongated from side to side. The choroid tela has its attachment near the fastigium. The floccular peduncles are short and small in the puppy; in the adult dog they form prominent elongated medullary bands that flatten laterally as they enter the flocculus.

The flocculus (figs. 161B, 168) arches around the brachium pontis parallel to and beneath the ventral paraflocculus. It comprises seven or eight transverse folia that are visible posteriorly on its dorsal and largely hidden surface. Its ventral surface is largely medullary and nearly smooth. The posterolateral fissure is prominent laterally and medially but is reduced to a groove between the floccular and parafloccular peduncles. It can be followed, however, without difficulty (fig. 168).

PRIMATES

The cerebellum of various primates has been described and illustrated by a number of investigators beginning with Treviranus (1822), who studied the organ in *Ateles paniscus*. Illustrations of monkey cerebella made by Serres (1824–27) and Swan (1835) were considered unsatisfactory by Ziehen (1899). Tiedemann (1837) gave an account of the cerebellum of the orangutan and chimpanzee; the atlas of Leuret and Gratiolet (1839–57) contains beautiful and accurate figures of the organ in *Macacus radiatus*, a species of *Ateles* and a baboon. The cerebellum of the baboon also was described by Huschke (1854), the gibbon by Waldeyer (1891), *Semnopithecus* by Künnemann (1894), and the orangutan by Fick (1895). Employing the terminology of human anatomy, as did earlier authors to a more limited extent, Flatau and Jacobsohn (1899) included the cerebellum of the chimpanzee in their comparative studies. Ziehen (1899) briefly reviewed these contributions and added a carefully executed figure of a median sagittal section of the cerebellum of *Macacus speciosus* labeled in terms of the human cerebellum.

Using the nomenclature of his earlier studies on developmental and adult stages of subprimates, Bradley (1905) described the lobules and fissures of five species of primates. After preliminary studies (1902, 1904, 1906) Bolk (1906) selected the cerebellum of a primitive primate, *Lemur albifrons*, for detailed description as representing the structural pattern for mammals generally and compared various modifications of pattern in 23 other species of primates, as well as in subprimates. As already mentioned this author's terminology is based on the cerebellum of the lemur. In his extensive comparative study of the arbor vitae and the relations of the lateral lobules to those of the vermis, Riley (1929) included the cerebellum of nine species of primates ranging from the marmoset, *Hapale jacchus*, to the gorilla and chimpanzee. The monograph of G. Retzius, *Das Affenhirn* (1906), contains superb photographs of the brain, including the cerebellum, of fifty-one species of primates from the lowest to the anthropoid apes. From the photographs superficial features of the cerebellum were briefly described only in a few of the more primitive species and no attempt was made to define its subdivisions in any of the primates. However, the pictures are invaluable despite the absence of labels with reference to the cerebellum because they accurately depict the lobules and fissures of species illustrated more or less diagrammatically by Bradley, Bolk, and Riley. The number of species with which comparisons could profitably be made also is greatly increased by the photographic figures.

The primate cerebellum obviously has been well explored but there has been little agreement regarding the lobules and their subdivisions and little information concerning the lamellae and folia. In an earlier contribution (Larsell, 1953a) I presented an analysis of the cerebellum of the rhesus monkey and a partial one of the spider monkey. Bolk's terminology was used for the hemispheral lobules and my terminology for the vermis of subprimates in connection with this part of the monkey cerebellum. In the following pages the cerebellum of the rhesus and spider monkeys is described more fully and the analysis included the mangabey, capuchin monkey, baboon, chimpanzee, and gorilla. The terminology employed in the preceding pages for subprimates is applied to homologous features in all the primates studied.

The external form of the cerebellum varies considerably in different species. The posterior part of the vermis is slightly sinuous in some species. The greater development of the cerebral cortex in the anthropoid apes is reflected by the relatively much larger cerebellar hemispheres in this group. The paraflocculus undergoes a gradual change of position, modification of form, and relative shortening of its fibrous connections with the vermis and the medullary body. This made it possible to follow the principal stages in the transformation of dorsal and ventral paraflocculus, respectively, into part of the biventral lobule and the tonsilla of the gorilla, chimpanzee, and man. The flocculonodular lobe is clearly recognizable as a unit in all. The flocculus undergoes changes in relative position as a result of modifications of the subdivisions of the paraflocculus and part of the hemisphere as well as an increase in hemispheral size. The dorsal paraflocculus and certain other lobules of the two New World monkeys described (*Ateles* and *Cebus*) resemble their homologs in anthropoid apes and man more closely than do these lobules in the Old World monkeys and baboons. The order of presentation of the seven species described is based on the relative approach to the human cerebellum of these and other cerebellar features, rather than on the usual criteria of systematic position.

Variations in size, habitat, methods of progression, and other factors that involve the physical characteristics of body parts known to have a somatotopical relation to certain lobules of the cerebellum make it desirable to have brief descriptions of the physical characteristics of the groups of primates whose cerebella have been available for study. All the primates have frontally directed eyes whose movements are well conjugated. Vision is excellent and stereoscopic. The external ears vary in size but hearing seems to be acute in all species. The monkeys, baboons, and apes are quadrumanal primarily, but the chimpanzee, gorilla, and some others can stand and walk in erect posture. The macaques (genus *Macacus*) are more stoutly built than the mangabeys, langurs, guenons, and New World monkeys and their muzzles are more prolongated. As between the various species, however, they differ considerably in physical characteristics. The body and legs vary in size and proportions. The tail exceeds the length of the body in some species; in others it is shorter or even may be reduced to a mere stump; in the Barbary ape (*M. inuus*) the tail is entirely absent and is represented by a mere fold of skin that has no connection with the end of the vertebral column (Lydekker, 1901).

A few species, whose vermis is compared below, may be described a little more fully. *M. nemestrinus* may attain the size and strength of a full-sized mastiff dog. Its somewhat piglike slender tail is about one-third the length of the body, which is comparatively stout and broad-chested. The limbs are long and powerful. *M. cynomolgus* has a large and massive body which with the head measures about 55 cm in length. The legs are short and stout and the tail is nearly as long as the head and body. In *M. speciosus* the head and body are about 60 cm long, while the tail is a stump of 5 cm to 7.5 cm; *M. maurus* has a tail length of about 2.5 cm. *M. rhesus* is of moderate size, with long arms and shorter legs; its tapering tail is about one-half the length of the body which measures about 25 cm in the male and from 18 cm to 20 cm in the female. The head is large, the jaws are heavy, and the thick neck is freely movable. The hands and feet have great manual dexterity. This species, although predominantly arboreal, is also at home on the ground. The more strongly built *M. erythaeus* has a body length of nearly 68 cm and a tail length of about 22 cm.

The mangabeys (genus *Cercocebus*) are fairly large monkeys of arboreal habitat. They are closely related to the macaques but the body is more slender and the limbs are proportionately longer (Forbes, 1894). The tail is as long as the body and, at least in some species, is carried over the back. However, it is not prehensile, a characteristic shared by all other Old World monkeys and the baboons.

The baboons (genus *Cynocephalus*) are entirely terrestrial, with their anatomy being modified accordingly. The body is heavy, the neck is long and mobile, and the head is large with an elongated muzzle and jaws. The animals are powerful; their muscular development is second only to that of the great apes among the primates. The forelimbs and hindlimbs are well developed and nearly equal in length. The limbs have unilateral independence of movement, although this is so to a much greater degree in the forelimbs. The forepaws serve as efficient hands and the hindfeet are long. The baboons progress rather awkwardly on all fours, without the capacity for great speed. The tail varies in length relative to the body in different species. In *Cynocephalus sphinx*, one of the smallest of the genus, the body length of a young male is about 67 cm and the tail length is about 50 cm.

The two New World monkeys, *Ateles* and *Cebus*, are arboreal in habit and have long tails. The spider monkey has a long and slender body, a short, freely movable neck, and a small head with a projecting muzzle. The limbs are long and slender, and the forelimbs are especially flexible. The tail, which exceeds the combined length of body and head, is exquisitely adapted as a fifth limb. It is used in climbing, maintaining position, and as an aid in keeping equilibrium during erect progression. The distal part of the tail is hairless on the underside and is ridged like a finger; it is used in picking up objects and exploring the ground, fissures, and other features of the environment. Frequently the distal part of the tail is carried over the head, projecting beyond it in exploratory fashion. The forelimbs and hindlimbs have great unilateral independence, with all four limbs and the tail being able to perform separate activities simultaneously. The fingers are hooked and the thumb is rudimentary or absent. The spider monkeys are among the best adapted of the primates for an arboreal habitat. The brain of *Ateles* is exceptionally large and complex among the monkeys.

The capuchin monkeys (genus *Cebus*) are arboreal in habitat and quick and agile in action. The body is robust; all four limbs are moderately long, slender, and bilaterally independent, but the forelimbs are more so than the hindlimbs. The forelimbs are so well coordinated that *Cebus* was said to be able to catch insects with the hands. Forbes (1894) described the thumb as the most manlike among the apes. In walking this species, unlike the Old World monkeys, places the palms of the hands on the ground (Riley, 1929). The head is relatively large, with a long and freely movable neck. The tail is long and prehensile; it is used as a fifth extremity in climbing and maintaining position, as well as for other purposes, but it does not serve as an additional hand to the same extent as in *Ateles*.

The chimpanzee (genus *Pan*) is heavily built but the body is shorter and less robust than that of the gorilla. Males attain a weight of about 55 kg. The shoulders and chest are broad, which is indicative of great muscular strength. The neck is short, thick, and freely movable, and the head is large. The arms are long but shorter than those of the gorilla, and the legs are short. The hands and feet are long, with the toes being about as long as the fingers. The thumb and great toe are opposable and both hands and feet are capable of great dexterity. The chimpanzee is more agile than the gorilla and more completely arboreal. It can stand and walk erect but the gluteal and calf muscles are weak. It has only two coccygeal vertebrae and no external tail.

The gorilla (genus *Gorilla*) is noted for its great strength and its size, being the largest of the primates. Males may exceed 180 kg in weight and some have been reported to approach 275 kg. The massive body and the wide chest and shoulders are suggestive of great muscular power. The neck is short, very thick, and freely movable; the head is large with heavy jaws. The forelimbs are long, reaching to the middle of the leg when the animal stands erect. The hands are thick and clumsy, with short but functional thumbs. The great toe is thumblike. The forelimbs are used in walking. Although the gorilla can walk in an erect posture, habitual erect progression is prevented by relatively weak gluteal and calf muscles. Even so, the gorilla's muscles are stronger than the chimpanzee's. The habitat is largely terrestrial but tree-climbing is practiced, except perhaps by the heavy males. There is no external tail.

Fetal stages of *M. rhesus* have provided a firm foundation for the interpretation of the lobules and fissures of this species. The pattern established in these fetuses was found in all the species studied in the adult stage, including the New World *Cebus* and *Ateles*. Comparison with the monkeys, on the one hand, and with the fetal and adult human cerebellum on the other hand, has afforded insights into the functioning of the cerebellum of the great apes, whose fetal stages were not available.

RHESUS MONKEY

Development of Cerebellum

THE cerebellum of the 90-day-old monkey (*Macacus rhesus*) fetus shows the vermal and hemispheral lobules and their delimiting fissures with diagrammatic simplicity (figs. 169, 170A). The posterolateral fissure is continuous from side to side between the corpus cerebelli and the flocculonodular lobe. The fissura prima subdividing the corpus cerebelli into anterior and posterior lobes is deep and its walls already have prominent folds. The hemispheres are large. Posteriorly they project as rounded masses on either side of the posterior part of the vermis, which forms a ridge separated from the hemispheres by a narrow and relatively deep paravermian sulcus on either side. This sulcus, however, does not continue onto the superior cerebellar surface, where there is no boundary between vermis and hemispheres.

The anterior lobe is divided into five segments by four interlobular fissures, which correspond to the precentral *a* and precentral, preculminate, and intraculminate fissures of subprimates (fig. 169). The segments that they delimit are homologous with lobules I–V, medially, and lobules HI–HV, laterally. The vermal part of lobules I–IV is divided by a shallow furrow into two superficial folds that represent the earliest lamellae of each lobule. Lobule V has two superficial furrows and two in the anterior wall of the fissura prima, the latter already differentiating lamellae Ve and Vf. An anteroposteriorly directed line connecting the ends of the superficial secondary furrows and continuing to the lateral wall of the posterior part of the vermis indicates the approximate lateral boundary of the vermal parts of the larger transverse segments. The secondary furrows extend into the hemispheres in subsequent development.

As seen in median sagittal section (fig. 169) lobules I and II are relatively large. Precentral fissure *a*, which separates them, is quite deep but extends only a short distance lateroventrally on either side before reaching the cortical margin. Lobule HI, accordingly, is very small. The precentral fissure, between lobules II and III, is longer, which results in a larger lobule HII. The preculminate fissure, between lobules III and IV, is the deepest in the anterior lobe. Preculminate fissure 1 does not reach the cerebellar margin of the left hemisphere in this specimen, although it does so on both sides at later stages. The relatively shallow vermal segment of this fissure (fig. 169) and the later completion of the separation of lobules HIV and HV indicate a closer morphogenetic relationship between lobules IV and V and their hemispheral extensions than appears to be true of other adjoining lobules of the anterior lobe. A closer relationship such as this also is apparent in many of the subprimates, especially among the smaller species.

The vermal portion of the posterior lobe, which is situated between the fissura prima and the prepyramidal fissure, is so small, as seen in median sagittal section, and the two superficial divisions which it presents are so reduced in comparison with other vermal lobules, that the segment appears to represent a single lobule. It corresponds to lobulus c^2 of Bolk (1906) in animals and lobulus X of Hochstetter (1929) in the human embryo. On the grounds of their further development in the monkey and their comparative anatomy, however, the anterior superficial subdivision and the cortical folds of the posterior wall of the fissura prima together represent lobule VI, while the posterior superficial fold and the anterior wall of the prepyramidal fissure constitute lobule VII (fig. 169). The furrow between the two superficial folds, although shallow, is continuous on either side with the hemispheral segment of the posterior superior fissure and represents the vermal segment of this fissure. Both lobules remain narrow in the sagittal plane in the adult stage of the several species of monkeys investigated as well as

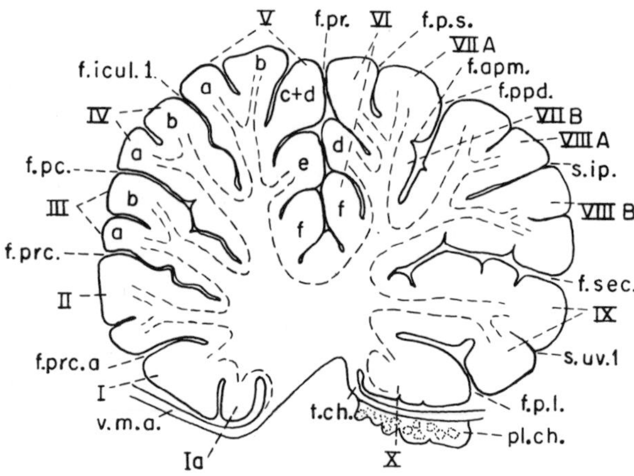

Figure 169. Midsagittal section of cerebellum of *Macacus rhesus,* 90-day-old fetus.

in the additional species illustrated in median sagittal section by Retzius (1906).

Lobule VI already is characterized in the 90-day-old fetus by two prominent lamellae, VId and VIf, in the posterior wall of the fissura prima. The superficial part of the lobule, however, is not differentiated into lamellae VIa, VIb, and VIc, which are characteristic of the adult, until later stages of fetal development (fig. 169).

Lobule VII is divided only by a shallow furrow situated in the anterior wall of the prepyramidal fissure in the usual conception of this cleft between the folium-tuber lobule and the pyramis. The furrow dividing lobule VII is continuous on both sides with the ansoparamedian fissure of the hemispheres and must be regarded as the vermal segment of this fissure (figs. 169, 170D). Presumably the vermal and hemispheral segments arise separately, as in subprimates and the human fetus, but by the 90-day stage of the monkey fetus they have become confluent. In ungulates, carnivores, and some other subprimates the vermal segment of the ansoparamedian fissure opens on the dorsal cerebellar surface. Sublobule VIIB, which is located between the ansoparamedian and prepyramidal fissures, forms a large segment of the sinuous posterior part of the vermis. The corresponding segment of cortex, together with the floor and part of the posterior wall of the prepyramidal fissure described below, must be recognized as homologous with sublobule VIIB, even though it is greatly reduced in the monkey. The remainder of lobule VII, above and anterior to the ansoparamedian fissure, is sublobule VIIA, as its hemispheral relations confirm (fig. 170A, D).

In the 90-day-old monkey fetus the deep part of the posterior surface of lobule HVIIB of the left hemisphere crosses the floor of the junction of the vermal and hemispheral segments of the prepyramidal fissure obliquely and continues with the deep part of the posterior wall of the vermal segment of this fissure. This deep part of the wall is delimited from the more external part by a slight indentation which represents a shallow furrow that extends a short distance in the floor of the hemispheral segment of the prepyramidal fissure. The deep posterior wall then is continuous lateralward with the floor of this furrow which crosses obliquely to the deep part of the posterior surface of lobule HVIIB of the right hemisphere. In later stages of development the anterior and posterior walls of the vermal and hemispheral prepyramidal fissure become foliated, as does its floor. The vermal segment of the ansoparamedian fissure becomes deeper than the other furrows in the anterior wall and is shown in sagittal section as a rostroventrally arching fissure. The early single groove in the posterior wall of the prepyramidal fissure is not recognizable as a distinctive furrow in later stages but it appears justifiable to regard it as the posterior boundary of a portion of sublobule VIIB that folds back onto the base of the pyramis. Considered as such, the furrow also is the ventral limit of sublobule VIIIA, defined below, and can be regarded as the bottom of the prepyramidal fissure proper. The downward continuation of the vermal segment of the prepyramidal fissure, as usually defined, between the two parts of sublobule VIIB, may be differentiated by designating it prepyramidal sulcus 1. The vermal segment or prepyramidal sulcus 1 extends laterally a little way on either side and, above the oblique folia, merges with the hemispheral segment of the prepyramidal fissure. The reduced size of sublobule VIIB in the monkey fetus is generally characteristic in the adult stage of primates, especially when compared with ungulates and carnivores. Undoubtedly this reflects relatively reduced functional significance. The submerged position and impingement of sublobule VIIB on the base of the pyramis in the fetus, which is also characteristic of the adult, probably have resulted from adjustments related to the accommodation of the greatly expanded cortex of the primate cerebellum.

Since the vermal segment of the ansoparamedian fissure reaches the external cerebellar surface in many subprimates, its relations in the monkey and other primates might be better understood by regarding the vermal segment as reaching the surface in these species in company with the vermal part of the prepyramidal fissure; the two then form a compound cleft between sublobules VIIA and VIIIA. Immediately lateral of the vermis, however, the two furrows separate into individual hemispheral fissures.

The vermal lobules behind and below the compound ansoparamedian-prepyramidal fissure could be described briefly in the 90-day-old fetus. Lobule VIII already is divided by the intrapyramidal sulcus into two large sublobules, VIIIA and VIIIB, which each have two superficial lamellae (fig. 169). Lobule IX has two superficial divisions and several folds facing the fissura secunda, which is exceeded in depth only by the fissura prima (fig. 169).

Posterior to the fissura prima the lateral part of the corpus cerebelli is divided into the hemispheral portion of the posterior lobe and the paraflocculus by the parafloccular fissure. This fissure, beginning laterally as a deep cleft, gradually is reduced in depth as it approaches the vermis. The parafloccular fissure probably is the first to appear in the lateral part of the corpus cerebelli and it separates the paraflocculus from the hemisphere in a pattern different from that of the interlobular fissures of the hemisphere proper.

The hemispheral lobules of the posterior lobe are completely delimited in the 90-day-old fetus by fissures that are continuous with those separating the corresponding lobules of the vermis. Only those posterior and ventral of the hemispheral segment of the ansoparamedian fissure, however, are delimited from the vermal lobules by a paravermian sulcus; lobules HVI and HVIIA have unbroken continuity with lobule VI and sublobule VIIA respectively (fig. 170B).

Lobule HVI expands laterally but is undivided. Lobule HVIIA expands into a large segment that is divided by two lateral furrows into the rudiments of three sublobules (fig. 170C). Subsequent development shows that the more posterior furrow is the intercrural fissure, dividing the lobule into crus I and crus II of Bolk. The anteriorly situated furrow is intracrural sulcus 1, subdividing crus I into crus Ia and crus Ip. Crus II is undivided in the 90-day-old fetus. The hemispheral segment situated between the ansoparamedian and prepyramidal fissures, already mentioned as lobule HVIIB, tapers rapidly as it approaches the vermis and is continuous with the sub-

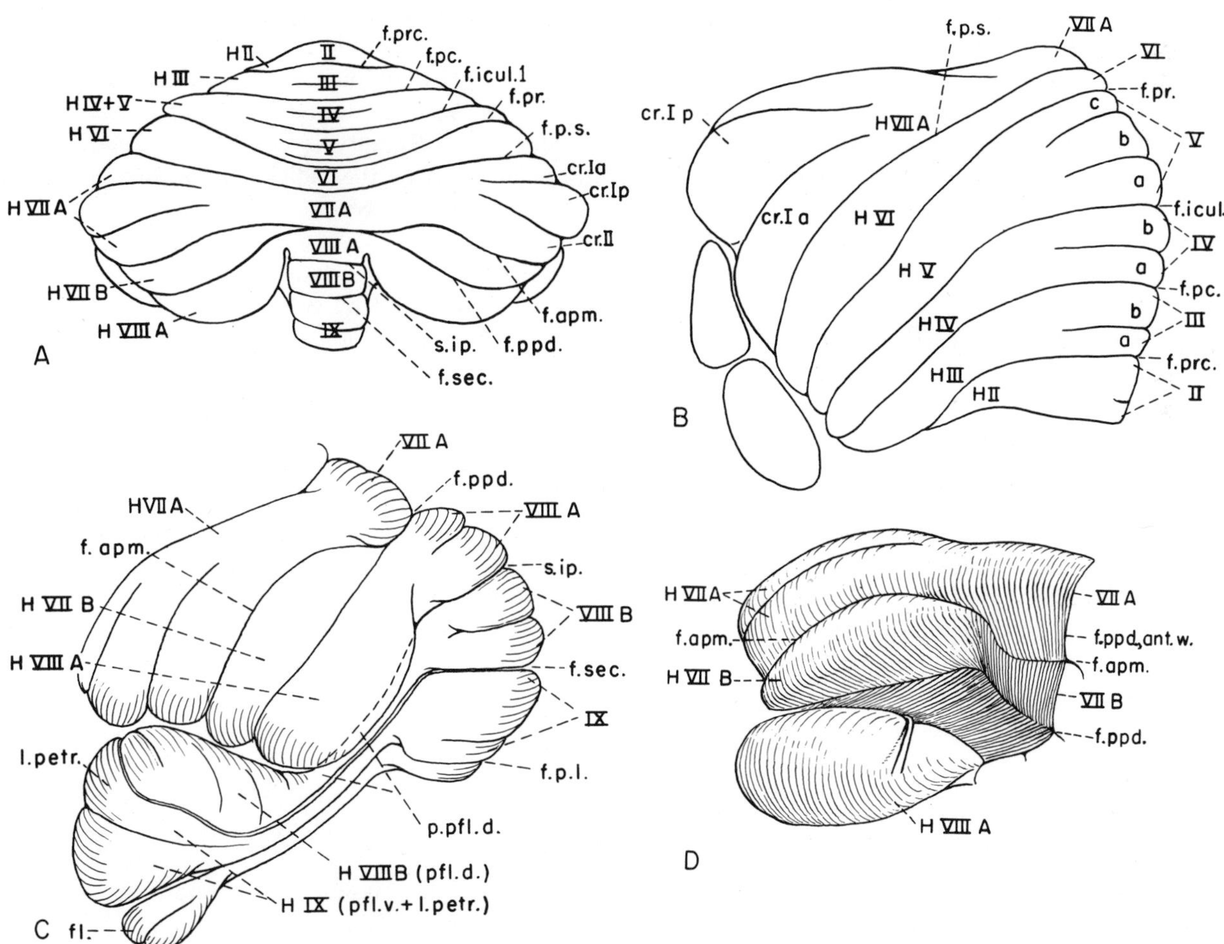

Figure 170. Cerebellum of *Macacus rhesus*, 90-day-old fetus. A. Dorsal aspect. B. Anterolateral view of right half. C. Posterolateral view of caudal part of left hemisphere. D. Anterior wall of the prepyramidal fissure, showing the ansoparamedian fissure and relations between the vermal and hemispheral lobules VII and HVII, respectively.

merged sublobule VIIB as described above. For consistency of terminology one would have to apply the term sublobule to the hemispheral segments related to sublobules VIIA and VIIB, but the large size of the hemispheral segments makes the term lobule, applied to them in the fully developed cerebellum, also more suitable in the fetus. Behind lobule HVIIB is situated a crescentic area that is continuous with sublobule VIIIA; a rostrally directed notch partly separates the two as viewed dorsally (fig. 170B). This is lobule HVIIIA. Its posteromedial border partially overlaps a narrow band that extends from sublobule VIIIB to the paraflocculus (fig. 170C).

The subdivisions of the paraflocculus are poorly defined in the 90-day-old fetus. Comparison with the 115-day-old specimen in which the dorsal paraflocculus, lobulus petrosus, and ventral paraflocculus are unmistakable, however, appears to provide justification for the recognition of the rudiments of these lobules also in the 90-day stage, as labeled in figures 170C and 172A, B. They are connected with the vermis by a fibrous sheet that appears to form a common parafloccular peduncle posteriorly, but which also is continuous beneath lobule HVIIIA with the fibrous substance of the hemisphere. On approaching the vermis the posterior part of this sheet divides into individual attachments to sublobules VIIIA and VIIIB and lobule IX (figs. 172A, 173C, 174C). The fibrous connection with sublobule VIIIA appears to continue into lobule HVIIIA, while the connections with sublobule VIIIB and lobule IX continue ventrolaterally into the paraflocculus. The parafloccular portion of the sheets separates on dissection into a sheet passing into the dorsal paraflocculus and another having the ventral paraflocculus and, apparently, the lobulus petrosus attached to it (fig. 172A). The ventral paraflocculus and petrosal lobule separate by a shorter arc of cleavage that begins beneath a furrow dividing them superficially and ends in the ventral parafloccular portion of the common peduncle (fig. 172B). This description requires confirmation from additional material and, especially, from stages intermediate between the 90-day- and 115-day-old fetuses, but it presents the apparent relations in the 90-day-old specimen.

The dorsal paraflocculus (lobule HVIIIB) is directed ventrolaterally and rostrally as a pyriform lobule situated beneath the posterolateral margin of the hemisphere, from which it is separated by the distally deep but medially shallower parafloccular fissure. Beneath the posteromedial margin of lobule HVIIIA the shallow segment of the parafloccular fissure, indicated by the broken line in figure 170E, separates lobule HVIIIA from the narrow band, mentioned above, which connects the dorsal paraflocculus with sublobule VIIIB. Medially the parafloccular fissure continues as a slight groove that approaches the intrapyramidal fissure and a short shallow furrow that extends toward sublobule VIIIA but ends superficially on the isthmus between this sublobule and lobule HVIIIA. This short furrow appears to correspond to the copular sulcus of the rat (figs. 12B, 16B, 21). As it emerges from beneath the posterolateral margin of lobule HVIIIA, the dorsal paraflocculus has a cortical surface and, as it expands distally, faint furrows indicate incipient foliation. In addition to the connections with the fibrous layer of the hemisphere already mentioned, the lobule receives a strand of fibers from the brachium pontis, as Scholten (1946) found in subprimates.

The rudiments of the lobulus petrosus and ventral paraflocculus, as interpreted above, present laterorostrally rounded surfaces that taper caudomedially to the attachments of the lobules with the parafloccular peduncle. Both lobules form wedges between the distal part of the dorsal paraflocculus and the flocculus (fig. 172A).

The cerebellum of the 115-day-old fetus (fig. 171) has attained the pattern found in the adult monkey. The vermal lobules have the form and foliation of later stages up to the adult. Except for smaller size and shallower secondary furrows the individual lamellae and most of the folia of later stages are recognizable by position and relationships (fig. 171A).

The vermis of later fetuses acquires an increasingly more mature aspect by enlargement of the lobules and their lamellae and by foliation of some of the latter. The interlobular fissures and the furrows between the lamellae deepen and in the 165-day-old fetus there is little difference, save in size, from the vermis of the adult monkey. The greatest variations in the individual lobules are found in the superficial lamellae of lobule VI and sublobule VIIA, which is also true of the adult cerebellum. These lamellae vary so greatly in size and in their relations to the cerebellar surface and the interlobular fissures delimiting the two lobules that some question regarding their individual identities is raised. In the following description these lamellae are interpreted on the basis of their individual continuity with hemispheral lamellae.

Lobule VI, in all the fetuses, is characterized by the two large lamellae, VId and VIf, in the posterior wall of the fissura prima (figs. 169, 171A). These increase in length and VId is foliated in the 115-day and later stages. The more superficial lamellae are shown in early differentiation in the 115-day-old fetus (fig. 171). Lamella VIa faces the fissura prima in this and succeeding stages. In the adult it sometimes reaches the surface (fig. 176). A closely related fold between lamellae VIa and VId is designated VIe because of its apparent homology with a

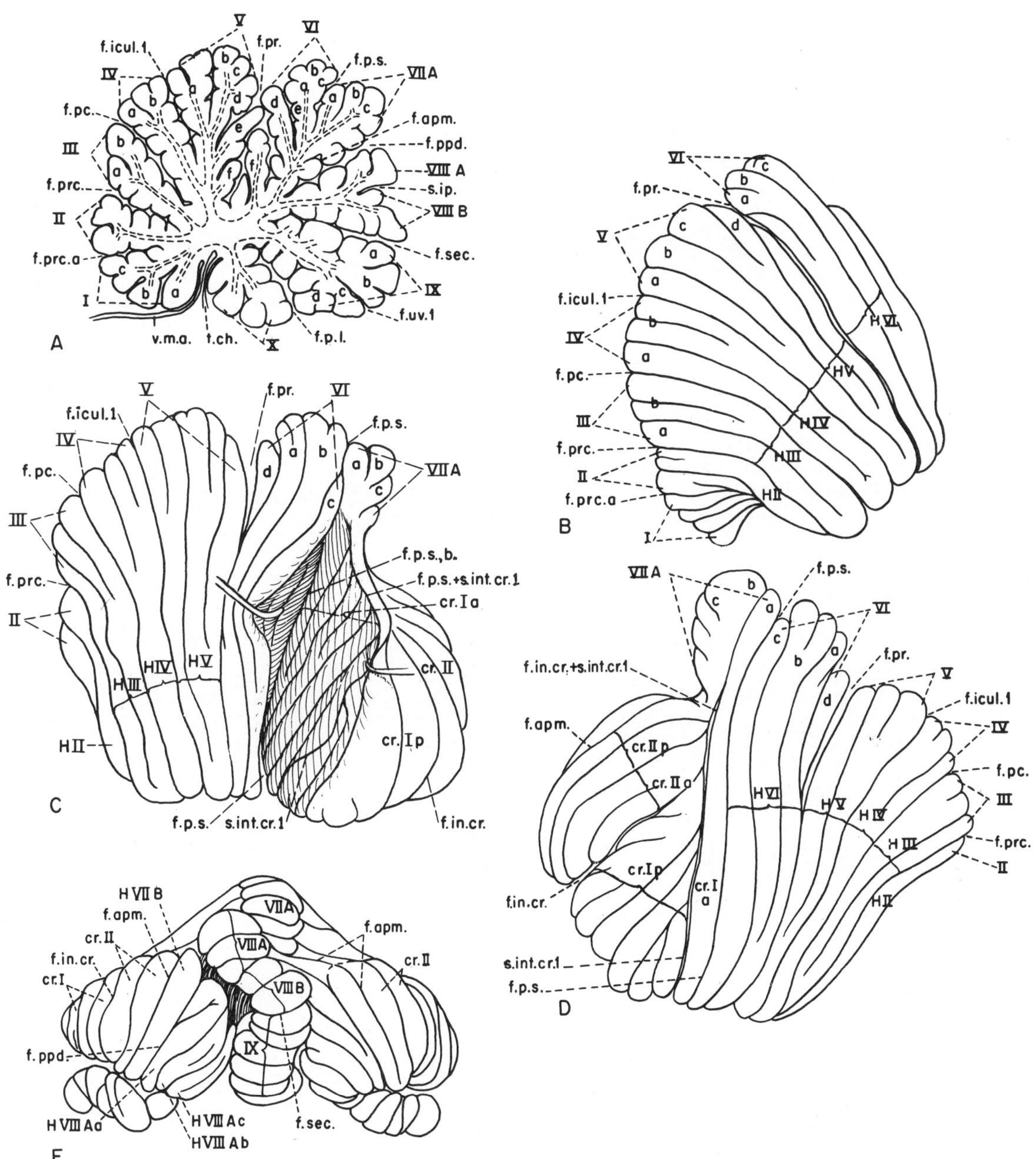

Figure 171. Cerebellum of *Macacus rhesus*, 115-day-old fetus. A. Midsagittal section. B. Lateral view of left half of anterior lobe. C. Lateral view of left hemisphere. Walls of posterior superior fissure spread apart. D. Lateral view of right hemisphere. E. Posterior view.

large lamella in some species of mammals. In the monkeys this fold rarely is large enough to merit individual recognition, but in the 158-day-old fetus and sometimes in the adult it forms an elongated lamellalike fold (figs. 174A, 176). Lamella VIb is superficial in all instances and is divided into two short folia (fig. 173A). Lamella VIc faces the posterior superior fissure in the 115-day- and 158-day-old fetuses, but in the 147-day- and 165-day-old specimens (fig. 173A) it forms an elongated fold that reaches the surface and resembles lamella VIIAa of many adult cerebella in both the form and branching of its medullary ray from the one leading to sublobule VIIA. Its hemispheral continuation, however, is rostral of the hemispheral segment of the posterior superior fissure, which also continues into the vermal segment behind the lamella.

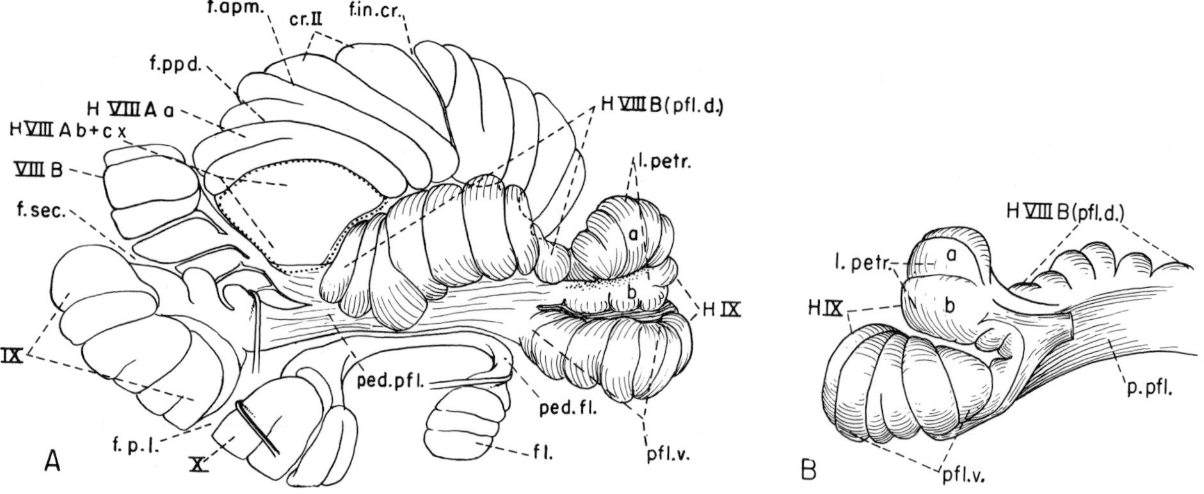

Figure 172. Cerebellum of *Macacus rhesus*, 115-day-old fetus. A. Posterolateral view of right half, showing the flocculus and paraflocculus. Part of paramedian lobule (HVIII Ab–c) dissected away to show the medial relations of the floccular and parafloccular peduncles. B. Medial surface of right paraflocculus.

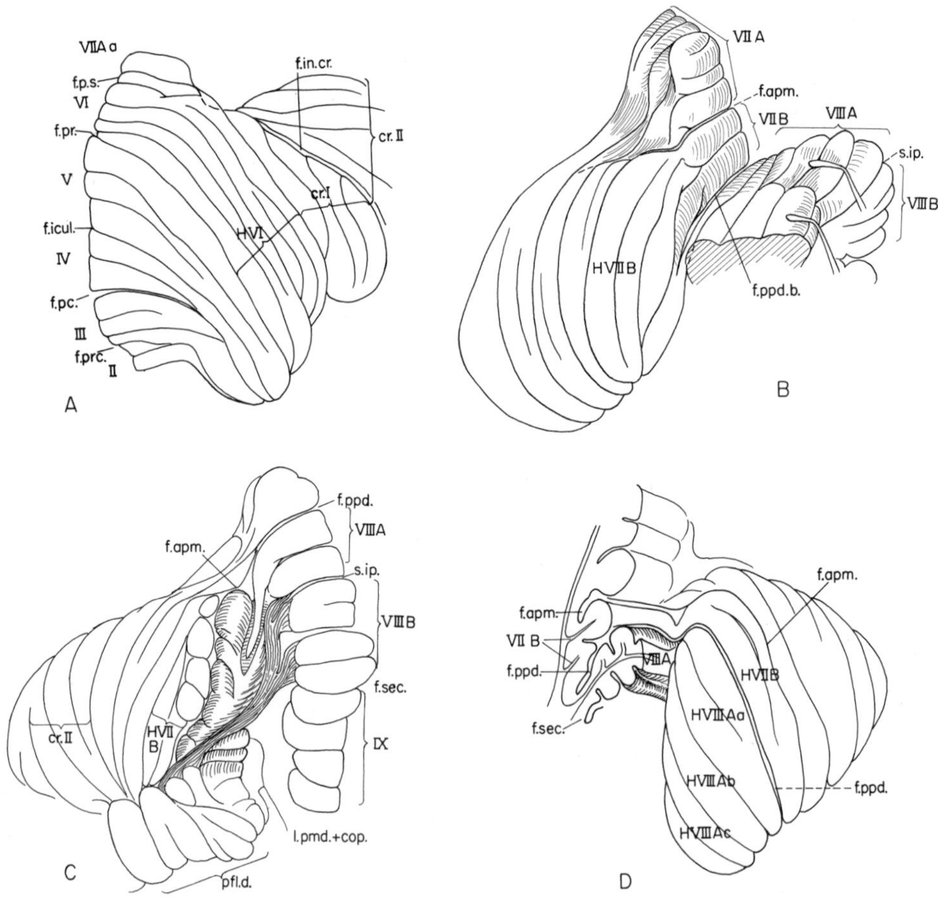

Figure 173. Cerebellum of *Macacus rhesus*, 147-day-old fetus. A. Anterior view of left half of anterior lobe. B. Dorsolateral view of part of left half of posterior lobe. The hidden surface of the prepyramidal fissure exposed by retraction of lobule VIII to show the relation between the vermal and hemispheral folia. C. Posterior view of left hemisphere after removal of paramedian lobule to expose connections of the paramedian and dorsal parafloccular lobules with the vermis. D. Posteromedial view of right hemisphere with related parts of the vermis.

Sublobule VIIA is divided into small superficial lamellae VIIAa, VIIAb, and VIIAc by shallow furrows that extend but a short distance on the lateral surfaces of the segment in the 115-day-old fetus and later. One or two additional folds, lamellae VIIAd and VIIAe, in the 115-day-old fetus, are constant features of the posterior surface of the sublobule above the ansoparamedian fissure of later stages. Sublobule VIIB is submerged and has the same relations to the deep part of the prepyramidal fissure (prepyramidal sulcus 1) as in the 90-day-old fetus. Its surfaces, however, are foliated in the later stages (fig. 173B).

Lobule VIII has expanded greatly in the 115-day-old fetus and its fissural surfaces are foliated. Sublobules VIIIA and VIIIB are separated by a relatively deep intrapyramidal sulcus; they also are displaced, one on either side of the midline, as in the cat and some other species. The median sagittal section of the cerebellum (fig. 171A), accordingly, shows only the reduced lateral part of the base of sublobule VIIIA and the basal portion of VIIIB. The sublobules resume a median position in later fetuses, but frequently some degree of displacement of VIIIA to one side or the other remains in the adult.

The folia of the posterior wall of the prepyramidal fissure, except the deep folia lining prepyramidal sulcus 1, continue as the posteromedial wall of the hemispheral segment of the fissure. The uppermost vermal folia are continuous with the anterior superficial folia of lobule HVIIIA, while the superficial sublamella of VIIIA continue, beneath the paravermian sulcus, with the remaining exposed portion of lobule HVIIIA (fig. 173D).

Sublobule VIIIB comprises three superficial sublamellae and four or five folds in the superior wall of the fissura secunda. Its continuation with the parafloccular complex is overlapped proximally by a short inferior lamella of lobule HVIIIA, lateral to and partly beneath which the parafloccular peduncle is surmounted by the folia of the dorsal paraflocculus (lobule HVIIIB) (figs. 171, 172A).

Lobule IX of the 115-day-old fetus shows the two superficial divisions of the 90-day-old specimen subdivided into lamellae IXa, IXb, IXc, and IXd (fig. 171A). In the 158-day-old fetus (fig. 174A) the lobule is relatively smaller but the lamellae just mentioned are recognizable if the posterior fold in the floor of the fissura secunda is interpreted as lamella IXa. In the earlier stage this lamella is only partly exposed superficially. If the deeper furrow of the 158-day-old fetus is considered to be uvular sulcus 2, instead of uvular sulcus 1, then the superficial lamella above it becomes IXa and the three below are IXb, IXc, and IXd. The second interpretation appears to correspond with the adult pattern in *M. rhesus* and some other species of monkeys, although uvular sulcus 1 is the deeper in some species, as is generally true in subprimates.

All the hemispheral lobules of the anterior lobe are completely delimited on both sides by the interlobular fissures in the 115-day-old and later fetuses (figs. 171B, C, D, 173A). The interlamellar furrows have deepened and extend variable distances toward the margin. They lengthen in subsequent development but end short of the cerebellar margin; some pass into the walls of the interlobular fissures as the latter deepen in the course of expansion and rolling adjustment of the cortex. The lamellae of the individual vermal lobules are continued as hemispheral lamellae between these furrows.

The hemispheral lobules of the posterior lobe have developed greatly by the 115-day stage of the fetus (fig. 171). Lobule HVI has differentiated superficially into three elongated lamellae, HVIa, HVIb, and HVIc, by extension of declival sulci 1 and 2. The furrows in the posterior wall of the fissura prima also have extended from the vermis into the hemisphere, differentiating a deep but short hemispheral continuation of lamella VIf and a longer one of lamella VId — the latter is visible superficially for some distance (fig. 171C, D) when the walls of the fissura prima are spread slightly apart. In the right hemisphere the lobule appears to include four superficial lamellae but the most caudal one is separated from the others by a deep fissure and also is continuous with lamella VIIAa. Comparison with later fetuses indicates that the deep furrow is the posterior superior fissure and the lamella is the superficially emerging border of crus Ia. In the left hemisphere of the 115-day-old fetus crus Ia is almost entirely submerged; intracrural sulcus 1 which delimits it from the remainder of crus I is hidden in the posterior wall of the posterior superior fissure (fig. 173A), except for a short distance where the sulcus reaches the surface. Intracrural sulcus 1 does not reach the furrow between lamellae VIIAa and VIIAb on the left side but crus Ia evidently has fibrous continuity with the base of lamella VIIAa. Lobule HVI shows the same pattern of three superficial lamellae, some of which subdivide into folia, in subsequent stages of development. There are variations, however, in the lamellae that constitute the superficially visible anterior and posterior parts of the lobule; we will return to this point in connection with the adult cerebellum.

Lobule HVIIA in the 115-day-old fetus (fig. 171C, D) shows crus Ia as a thin sublobule facing the posterior superior fissure, with its deep surface folded into elongated folia. The relations of the sublobule to the superficial surface of the right and left hemispheres already have been described. Similar differences in the two hemi-

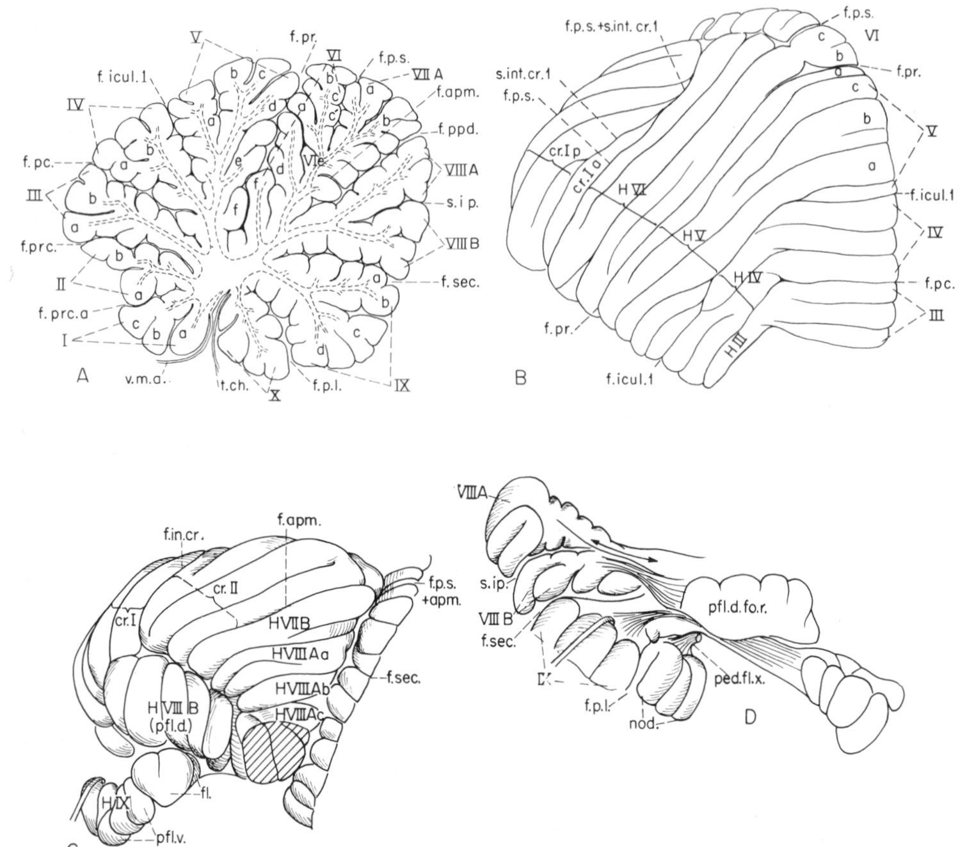

Figure 174. Cerebellum of *Macacus rhesus*, 158-day-old fetus. A. Midsagittal section. B. Anterolateral view of right half. C. Posterior view of left hemisphere. D. Dissection showing relations of right paraflocculus to vermal lobules VIIIB and IX. Flocculus removed.

spheres prevail in later stages of development. In the 147-day-old fetus the margin of crus Ia does not reach the surface in the left hemisphere (fig. 173A, B), but on the right side it is superficial throughout its extent, except for a short stretch just before it reaches lamella VIIAa; here the margin of crus Ia is constricted and also is overlapped by a caudal swelling of lamella HVIc. In later stages the sublobule tends to become more submerged on both sides, with the medial part dipping toward the base of lamella VIIAa and becoming elongated into a fibrous band. This band is delimited from the larger fibrous mass connecting the remainder of crus I with the vermis by a medial continuation of intracrural sulcus 1 which disappears on the medullary band. Crus Ip forms a rounded folial group that tapers toward the vermis and continues to the base of sublobule VIIA as a fibrous band. This is submerged in a compound furrow formed by convergence of the intercrural fissure and intracrural sulcus 1. In subsequent development the folia of crus Ip become grouped as two principal lamellae with broad lateral surfaces that taper medially (fig. 171D).

Crus II becomes divided by intracrural sulcus 2 into crus IIa and crus IIp, both of which are expanded on the rounded posterolateral surface of the hemisphere. Medially both subdivisions reach the posterior part of the base of sublobule VIIA. Crus II largely remains exposed and the more caudal folia of crus IIp are continuous with the posterior folia of sublobule VIIA (fig. 173B).

Lobule HVIIB has become compressed by the 115-day stage of the fetus into a curved plate with a relatively narrow superficial surface but with more extensive surfaces facing the ansoparamedian and hemispheral prepyramidal fissures. Its anterolateral and superficial surfaces blend, as the lobule tapers sharply toward the vermis, and continue into the floor of the hooked (in sagittal section) vermal segment of the ansoparamedian fissure (fig. 171A). The posteromedial surface, facing the hemispheral segment of the prepyramidal fissure, is continuous with the surfaces of the prepyramidal fissure by the folia that cross the floor of the prepyramidal fissure obliquely and continue into the posterior wall of this fissure. These folia represent the connections having similar relations in the 90-day-old fetus.

As a result of my failure to clearly recognize the relations of lobule HVIIB to the floor of the vermal part of the ansoparamedian fissure, whose mouth appears continuous with one of the furrows of the posterior surface of the lobule, I (Larsell, 1953a) misinterpreted the pars anterior of the paramedian lobule as being a submerged segment in the adult cerebellum of the rhesus monkey. In the earlier fetal cerebella a fibrous sheet intervenes between the ends of the folia of lobule HVIIB and those of sublobule VIIB; the continuity of the superficially visible hemispheral segment of the ansoparamedian fissure with the vermal segment is clear at the upper border of this sheet (fig. 173B). Subsequently this sheet is covered by an extension of foliated cortex, with the hemispheral and vermal folia meeting, as some of their intervening furrows also appear to do. In the fetal cerebellum, however, the continuation of the hemispheral ansoparamedian fissure with the deep part of the vermal segment is clear. The hemispheral segment does not always meet the vermal segment (represented by the deeper hooked furrow) on both sides in the simple pattern seen in the 90-day-old fetus (fig. 170). In some of the later fetuses and in many adult cerebella the hemispheral segment of one side becomes continuous with the next furrow above the more prominent one in the posterior surface of lobule VII, so that an offset of the vermal connection of lobule HVIIB of one side results.

Lobule HVIIIA in the 115-day-old fetus is divided by a deep fissure into an obliquely directed elongated lamella which is broad and partially divided medially and into two or three short and smaller lamellae that overlap the proximal part of the parafloccular peduncle (figs. 171E, 172A). These lamellae enlarge and their furrows elongate, more completely dividing them into folia, but further foliation does not occur. As seen in later stages the anterior lamella (HVIIIAa) is continuous with the upper posterior wall of the vermal segment of the prepyramidal fissure. The smaller lamellae (HVIIIAb and HVIIIAe) are attached to a medullary sheet that derives from roots coming from the lateral base of sublobule VIIIA (fig. 173D); the posterior border of the sheet fuses with the paraflocculor peduncle. I found no lateral expansions of sublobule VIIIA, in fetal or adult monkeys, corresponding to the alae pyramidis already mentioned in some subprimates and described further on in the great apes and man. The common fibrous sheet to which the lamellae of HVIIIA are attached and whose posterior border is continuous with the dorsal paraflocculor part of the paraflocculor peduncle appears to correspond to the fibrous part of the copula pyramidis of subprimates (cf. fig. 156B).

The component parts of the paraflocculor complex of the monkeys have been subject to a variety of interpretations. Bradley (1905) thought that the dorsal paraflocculus, as represented in the majority of mammals, is replaced in the adult rhesus and other monkeys by "the enlarged hemispheral segment of lobule D_1," corresponding to lobule HVIIIA which has been described before in the fetus and will be considered in adult monkeys further on in the text. Bradley tended to regard the row of transverse folia "which turns downwards a little in front" as corresponding to the ventral paraflocculus of most mammals. Riley (1929), however, included lobule HVIIIA, although without specific mention, with the "lobulus paramedianus" in his diagrams of several species of monkeys and many subprimates. The paraflocculus was not divided by Riley into dorsal and ventral paraflocculus but "the uncus terminalis" appears to represent the ventral paraflocculus, as I defined it, not only in the monkeys but in a number of subprimates, including the cat and two species of *Canis*. The term uncus terminalis was introduced by Bolk (1906), who regarded the series of folia so designated as corresponding to the human flocculus. Riley, however, differentiated a distinct flocculus in monkeys as well as subprimates and Bradley had pointed out that it is distinct. The confusion resulting from crowded relations of the lobules in this region is apparent from the descriptions of the authors cited and from some misinterpretations in my own (Larsell, 1953a) earlier study of the rhesus monkey. The arrangement of the lobules was clarified by an intensive study of the fetal stages of this species and of these lobules in the adult cerebellum of several other species of monkeys.

In the 115-day-old and later fetuses of *M. rhesus* a fibrous band leading from the base of lobule IX to the paraflocculus is separated from one leading from sublobule VIIIB by a lateral continuation of the fissura secunda, as in other mammalian fetuses. Along the paraflocculor peduncle, however, the fissure disappears but a plane of cleavage extends a short distance medialward from the small hiatus shown in figure 172, between the end of the dorsal series of folia and the rostrolaterally projecting lateral group of the 115-day-old fetus. This plane appears to correspond to the cleavage zone between the rudiments of the dorsal paraflocculus and the petrosal lobule in the 90-day-old fetus (fig. 170C), but the fibrous attachments of the fibrous bands of the two subdivisions merge medially without external evidence of a furrow. In the later fetuses extension of the fissura secunda along the peduncle is doubtful, although a groove that I once (Larsell, 1953a) interpreted as such is visible in the adult. The three series of folia in the 115-day-old and later fetuses (figs. 172, 175) are so distinctly differentiated from the remainder of the hemisphere and from each other that there could be no question about their

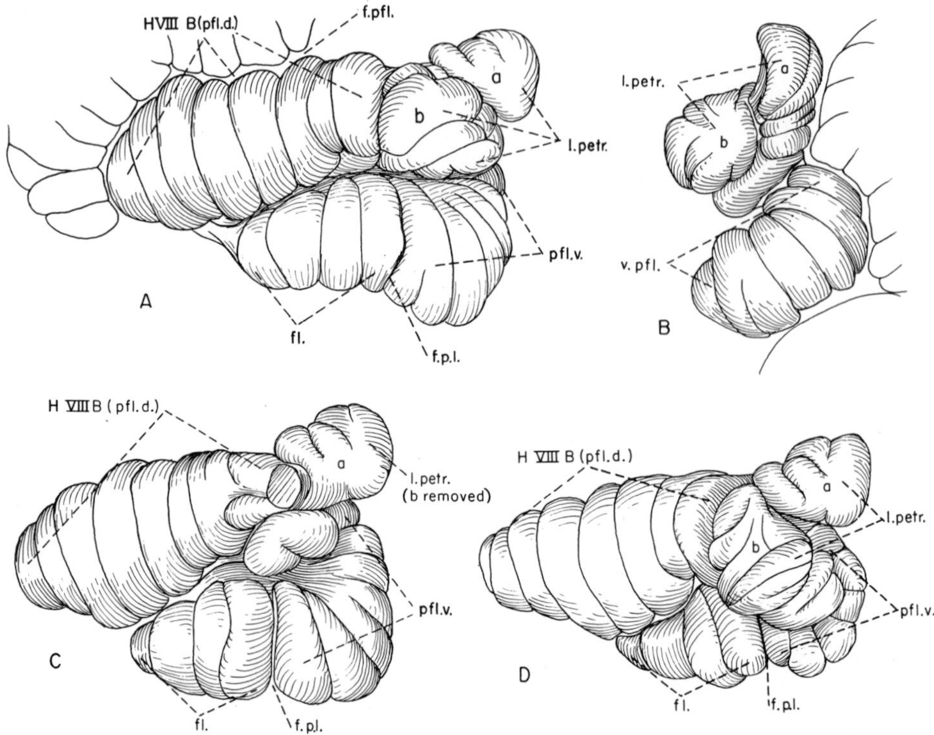

Figure 175. **Cerebellum of *Macacus rhesus*, 165-day-old fetus. A. Flocculus and paraflocculus, lateral view. B. Lobulus petrosus and ventral paraflocculus, anterior view. C. Flocculus and paraflocculus. Lobulus petrosus partly removed to expose deep folia. D. Dorsolateral view of paraflocculus and flocculus.**

correspondence to the three subdivisions of the paraflocculus, namely the dorsal and ventral paraflocculus and the lobulus petrosus. Jansen and Brodal (1942, 1954) made excellent diagrammatic illustrations of the adult rhesus monkey, except that the topographical relations could not be adequately shown in an outspread diagram.

The dorsal paraflocculus is composed of a series of folia that begin under cover of the caudal margin of lobule HVIIIA as small folds attached to a fibrous band leading medially to sublobule VIIIB (figs. 172, 175). Each succeeding folium in a lateral sequence increases in size and also continues onto the posterolateral surface of the parafloccular fissure. The folia end laterally as a small folium at the hiatus, which has already been mentioned; this is apparent in the 115-day-old fetus but in older stages the enlarged adjacent folia cover it up, to a lesser or greater extent.

The lobulus petrosus of the 115-day-old fetus extends laterorostrally as a compact series of folia attached above, below and around the end of a dorsal branch of the parafloccular peduncle (fig. 172B). As seen from the dorsomedial angle the two groups merge into a rounded knob, a medullary band which also branches to the ventral paraflocculus ending in it. From the posteroventral aspect the attachment of the petrosal lobule appears more closely related to the dorsal parafloccular part of the peduncle. In the 165-day-old fetus the petrosal lobule differs somewhat on the two sides. On the right side it comprises two groups of folia, which are designated *a* and *b* in figure 175. Group *a* obviously corresponds to the dorsal folia of the 115-day-old fetus and group *b* appears to represent an expansion of part of the ventral group of the younger fetus, accompanied by a rotation of the lobule and a deepening of the furrow into a cleft. After removal of group *b*, more deeply situated folia are visible which apparently represent the remainder of the earlier ventral group. The fibrous connections of the petrosal lobule with the vermis are lost in the parafloccular peduncle, but there are suggestions of connections with the brachium pontis.

Except for its rostromedial surface, which appears to be connected with the ventral parafloccular part of the parafloccular peduncle, the petrosal lobule of the 115-day-old and later fetuses seems to be more closely related externally with the dorsal than with the ventral paraflocculus. Its relations must be determined by its peduncular connections. I was unable to determine whether these are with the ventral parafloccular part of the parafloccular peduncle alone, as appears true in the 90-day-old fetus (fig. 172B), or if it also has connections with the dorsal parafloccular part of the peduncle. The peduncle separates by cleavage for a short distance medialward, beneath the distal end of the dorsal paraflocculus, but no satisfactory demonstration of the relations in the common peduncle of the fibers leading to the lobulus petrosus and to the two other subdivisions of the paraflocculus could be made.

The ventral paraflocculus comprises a series of folia around the end of a ventral terminal branch of the parafloccular peduncle. Proximally the series begins under cover of the distal part of the flocculus. The series arches medially and then upward beneath and medial of the petrosal lobule. In the 115-day-old fetus the series extends well beyond the distal end of the dorsal paraflocculus (fig. 172), but in the 165-day-old fetus (fig. 175), owing to adjustments of growth, the distal end of the dorsal paraflocculus partly overlies the ventral paraflocculus and is separated from it by a space that continues to the surface as a cleft between the lobulus petrosus and the ventral paraflocculus. Viewed from the dorsolateral angle in the later stages, after removal of the petrosal lobule and part of the dorsal paraflocculus, the ventral paraflocculus is a rounded concavo-convex plate of folia arranged around the end of the parafloccular peduncle. The convex surface abuts on the brachium pontis.

FLOCCULONODULAR LOBE

Compared with the corpus cerebelli the flocculonodular lobe is small in the fetal as well as in the adult monkey. In the 90-day-old fetus (fig. 169), only the ventral surface of the nodulus (lobule X) is slightly foliated. The floccular peduncle is elongated and ends in two small cortical folds that constitute the flocculus. The posterolateral fissure is distinct from the vermis to the ventrolateral cerebellar surface. It is worth noticing that the choroid tela is attached to the anterior surface of the nodulus, immediately behind the fastigium. In subsequent stages (figs. 171, 174A) the surface of the nodulus facing the posterolateral fissure also becomes foliated. The attachment of the choroid tela in the 165-day-old fetus is lower on the ventricular surface of the nodulus and continues onto the lateral surface and then along the margin of the floccular peduncle to the flocculus. The floccular peduncle becomes arched sharply forward on either side of the nodulus, with caudalward growth of the lobule, before continuing to the flocculus. About midway in its course the floccular peduncle receives a band of fibers (not illustrated) from the floor of the fourth ventricle which, together with the portion of the peduncle described here, apparently corresponds to the floccular peduncle of Burdach in man. The flocculus in the 165-day-old fetus shows six folia; the most lateral one overlaps and conceals the proximal folia of the ventral paraflocculus. The two lobules are separated by a narrow cleft representing the posterolateral fissure (fig. 175).

Adult Cerebellum

The adult monkey has relatively much larger cerebellar hemispheres than the subprimates, except for cetaceans and the elephant. The rostral and dorsal parts of the vermis form a ridge above the general cerebellar surface but the folia are continuous from vermis to hemispheres beneath a slight concavity on either side of the vermis. On the posterior surface, the paravermian sulcus is deep and narrow, with the vermis being distinctly delimited from the hemispheres. As a rule the vermal lobules occupy a medial position but a slight deflection may occur as already mentioned. The photographs of Retzius (1906) show a greater displacement of part of the vermis in some other species of macaques. The paraflocculus is situated beneath the hemisphere. The following description is based on the study of many cerebella of various sizes; the smaller ones presumably are from young animals. No records of age or sex, however, were supplied with the brains from various sources. Median sagittal sections of three cerebella are illustrated to present more clearly certain variations of the vermis as well as the more constant features.

CORPUS CEREBELLI

The general pattern of the lobules of the anterior lobe of adult macaques conforms with that of subprimates. A figure of Ziehen (1899, p. 485) illustrating a median sagittal section of the cerebellum of *Macacus speciosus* and the median sagittal sections of six species of *Macacus*, included in the photographs of Retzius, present a pattern which is generally similar to that of *M. rhesus*, as described below; however, there are differences in the size of several of the lobules and the relative depth of some of the fissures. In *M. maurus*, Bolk (1906) designated as lobuli 1, 2, and 3 the segments that correspond to lobules I, II, and III of the terminology employed here. However, Bolk's lobulus 4, which is composed of three large subdivisions, corresponds to lobules IV and V. Lobule V is subdivided into a large anterior division similar to sublobule VA of some cerebella and a posterior division in which lamellae Vb to Vf may be identified. So interpreted, lobule IV and V correspond to lobuli 4a and 4b of *Cercopithecus*, as designated by Bolk. In *M. rhesus*, Riley (1929) designated as lobulus 1 only the caudal folium *a* of lobule I, as I defined it, and included the remainder of this lobule, together with lobules II

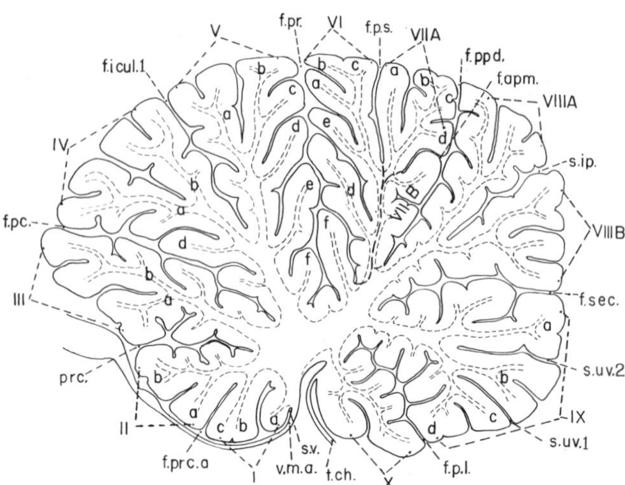

Figure 176. Midsagittal section of a small macaque cerebellum. ca. ×3. (Larsell, 1953a.)

and III, in his lobulus 2. No lobulus 3 was indicated by Riley in *M. rhesus* but he subdivided Bolk's lobulus 4 into sublobuli 4A and 4B, corresponding respectively to lobules IV and V, as defined in this volume. The different interpretations of the lobules are due chiefly to the reliance by Bolk and Riley on the varying medullary rays as the basis of the lobules. In Riley's figure of the vermis of the rhesus monkey the medullary rays to the two dorsal subdivisions of his lobulus 2 are derived from a common stalk of connection with the medullary body. Bolk's figure of the vermis of *M. maurus* shows that the corresponding subdivisions, namely, lobuli 2 and 3 of this author, have separate connections with the medullary body, similar to lobules II and III in several of my specimens of *M. rhesus* (figs. 176, 177). In the cerebellum illustrated in figure 176 lobule II is connected with the medullary body by a ray which also gives off a branch to folium Ib.

Lobule I of *M. rhesus* is variable in size and form. In the cerebellum illustrated in figure 177A it is elongated rostralward and has three surface folia. A smaller cerebellum (fig. 177B) shows two distinct folds; the more rostral one has a slight indentation so that three folia are indicated, presumably corresponding to Ia, Ib, and Ic of lobule I of the larger cerebellum. The latter has three large surface folia, and folium Ic is partially subdivided by a shallow furrow. The anterior medullary velum is attached, at the base of folium Ia, to the rostral surface of the fastigial recess of the fourth ventricle. The lateral surfaces of folia Ia and Ib are nearly vertical, but folium Ic extends laterally as a narrow band of cortex (fig. 180). Precentral fissure *a* is deep in the cerebella illustrated in figure 177A, C, but shallower in figure 176. It extends in all three cerebella to the margin of the cerebellar cortex (fig. 178C). Bradley's (1905) illustration of a median sagittal section of *M. rhesus* shows the corresponding segment elongated rostralward but deeply separated from the segment immediately dorsal. The photograph of Retzius from this species shows an unusually large segment which apparently corresponds to lobule I of figures 178C, 180, and 191.

Lobule II comprises two small superficial lamellae and folia in the delimiting fissures, in the large cerebellum illustrated in figure 177A, but it had three superficial sublamellae in one of the smaller specimens and a slight furrow in the more anterior lamella of another small cerebellum (figs. 176, 177B). It is relatively larger and its furrows are deeper, as a rule, in the cerebella that have a small lobule I. The rostral lamella is similar to the corresponding part of lobule II in the dog and many other species. Bradley's (1905) depiction of the subdivision related to lobule II in the rhesus monkey shows an elongated, lamellalike structure which is included with the segment corresponding to lobule I in his lobule A_1. Furthermore, it is delimited from his lobule A_2 by his fissure *c*, which corresponds to the precentral fissure of figures 176, 177, and 179. In the *M. rhesus* photograph of Retzius the corresponding segment is relatively larger than in most of my specimens. Lobule II extends into the hemisphere as a fairly prominent lobule HII (fig. 180). The precentral fissure reaches the cortical margin but the furrow between the lamellae ends short of the margin.

Lobule III of the small cerebellum illustrated in figure 176 is very similar to Bradley's lobule A_2. Retzius illustrated an entirely similar segment. It is separated from lobule IV by a deep fissure, designated fissure I by Bradley, which according to my interpretation in subprimates corresponds to the preculminate fissure. Riley included lobule III in his lobulus 2 of the rhesus and spider monkeys, but in *Cebus* and *Cynocephalus* he designated as lobulus 3 the segment corresponding to my lobule III. Comparison with lobule III of the rat, rabbit, and pig in embryonic and adult stages and with the dog and other subprimates shows a similarity of position and of division into terminal lamellae IIIa and IIIb by a characteristic fissure. These lamellae and the entire lobule are relatively smaller in the large cerebellum illustrated in figure 177A. In position, general form, and hemispheral relations the segment resembles lobule III of subprimates. In the rhesus monkey it apparently corresponds to the so-called central lobule which has been shown to be functionally related to the antigravity muscles of the lower limb (Nulsen, Black, and Drake, 1948). Adrian (1943) obtained responses in the "central lobule" of macaques when he stimulated the lower extremity. It is not clear whether or not lobule II was involved in the experiments of these in-

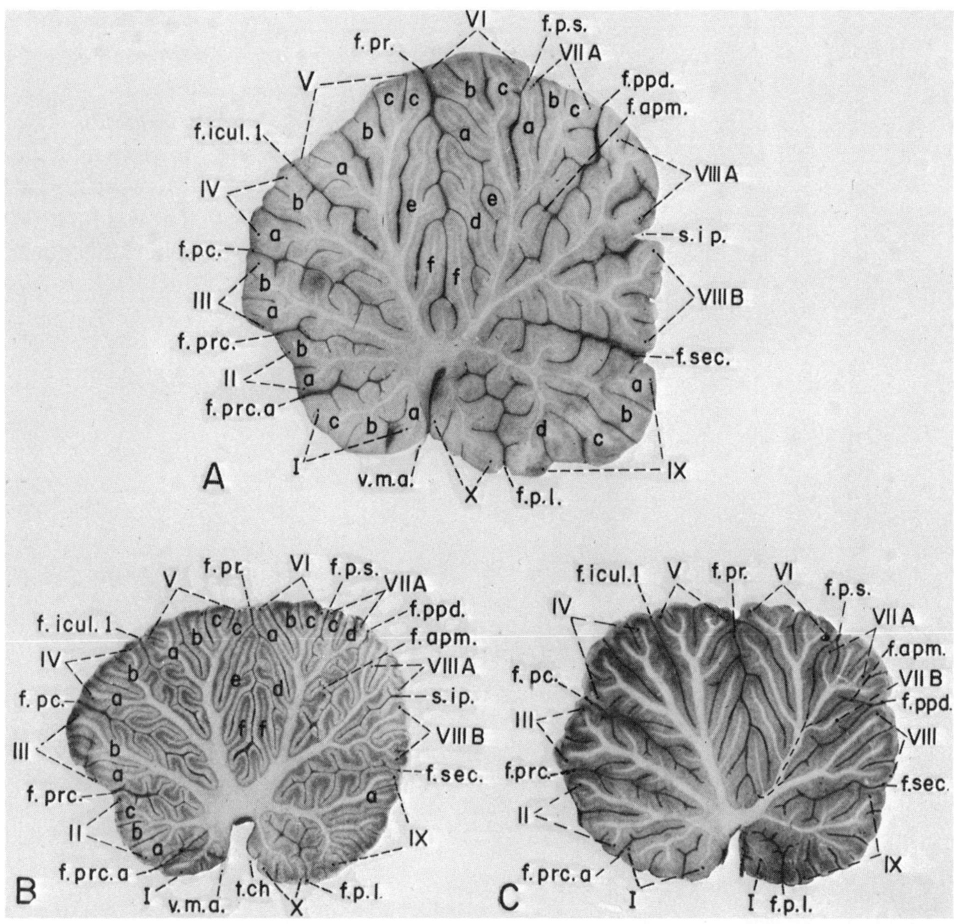

Figure 177. A. Midsagittal section of large cerebellum of *Macacus rhesus*. B. Midsagittal section of medium-sized cerebellum of *Macacus rhesus*. C. Midsagittal section of cerebellum of spider monkey (*Ateles*). Retouched photographs of hemisected cerebella which were surface-stained with carmine. ×2. (Larsell, 1953a.)

vestigators, but probably it was not. The preculminate fissure, forming the dorsal boundary of lobule III and the dorsolateral boundary of lobule HIII, is the deepest fissure of the anterior lobe. As already mentioned, it has reached the cerebellar margin in the 90-day-old fetus. Lobule HIII tapers lateroventrally and nearly reaches the ventral paraflocculus.

Lobule IV varies in size in different specimens (figs. 176, 177). In some it includes two superficial lamellae that are so large and distinct that they almost could be called sublobules. In others the corresponding lamellae are much smaller and the intervening fissure is shallower. In comparison with Bradley's figures, lobule IV corresponds to the rostral division of his lobule B in *Nyctipithecus*, *Cebus*, *Macacus*, and *Cercocebus*. Bolk (1906, fig. 31) labeled as lobulus 4a the corresponding division in *Cercopithecus* but did not differentiate it from the remainder of his lobulus 4 in *M. maurus*, although it is nearly as distinct in his figures of this species as in *Cercopithecus*. In some of the other primate cerebella illustrated by this author the segment corresponding to my lobule IV is designated lobulus 3. The photographs in the Retzius series show the segment deeply separated from lobule V in *M. rhesus*, but the two lobules share a short medullary attachment to the medullary body. In several other species intraculminate fissure 1 is nearly as deep as the preculminate fissure and the medullary rays to lobules IV and V arise separately from the medullary body. The hemispheral relations of lobule IV in the adult do not differ from those already described in the fetus. Two broad superficial folia which continue as lobule HIV reach the rostrolateral border of the cerebellum (figs. 179, 180). Folia in the walls of the delimiting fissures also extend from the vermis into the hemisphere.

Lobule V comprises the three characteristic surface lamellae (Va, Vb, and Vc), three lamellae (Vd, Ve, and Vf) which form the anterior wall of the fissura prima, and several sublamellae in the posterior wall of intracul-

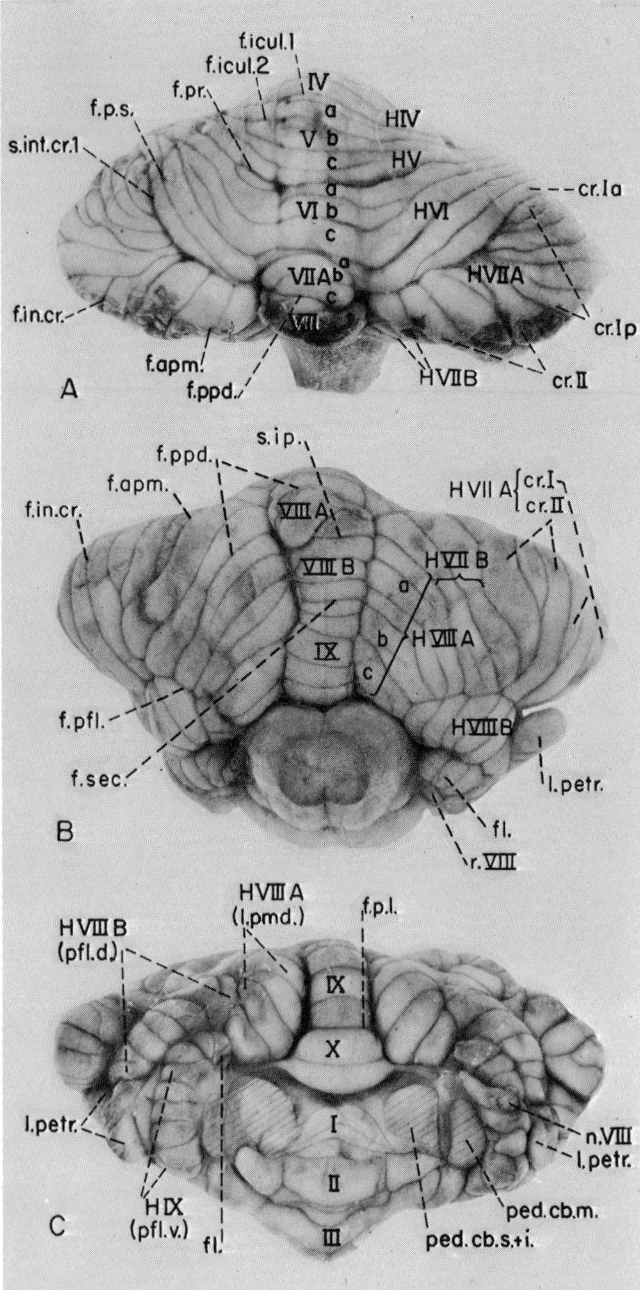

Figure 178. Cerebellum of *Macacus rhesus*, large specimen. A. Dorsal view. B. Posterior view. C. Ventral view. Retouched photographs after removal of pia mater and surface-staining with carmine. ×2. (Larsell, 1953a.)

minate fissure 1 as in the later fetal stages described. Lamella Va is larger than Vb and Vc, and lamella Ve frequently is greatly elongated but is divided into two folia that give it a characteristic appearance (fig. 177A, B). Lamella Vd in such instances is a reduced fold of cortex at the mouth of the fissura prima. Aside from variations of this type lobule V is similar in all the rhesus cerebella examined. It also resembles the posterior part of Bradley's lobule B, the posterior division of Bolk's lobulus 4 in *Macacus maurus*, *Semnopithecus*, *Hylobates*, and the orangutan, as well as Bolk's lobulus 4b of *Cercopithecus*. In Bolk's illustrations the segment corresponding to lamella Va is larger than in my specimens of *M. rhesus* or in the photograph of this species in the Retzius series; it is delimited from the remainder of lobule V by a furrow that corresponds to intraculminate fissure 2 of figures

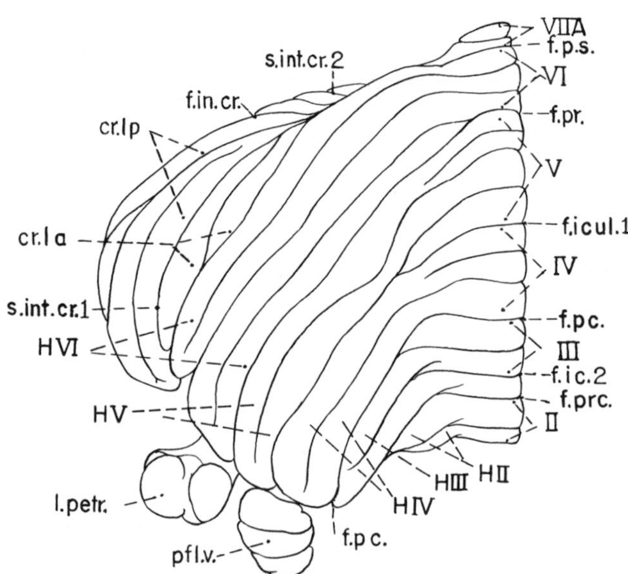

Figure 179. Cerebellum of macaque. Anterior aspect of right half. ×3. (Larsell, 1953a.)

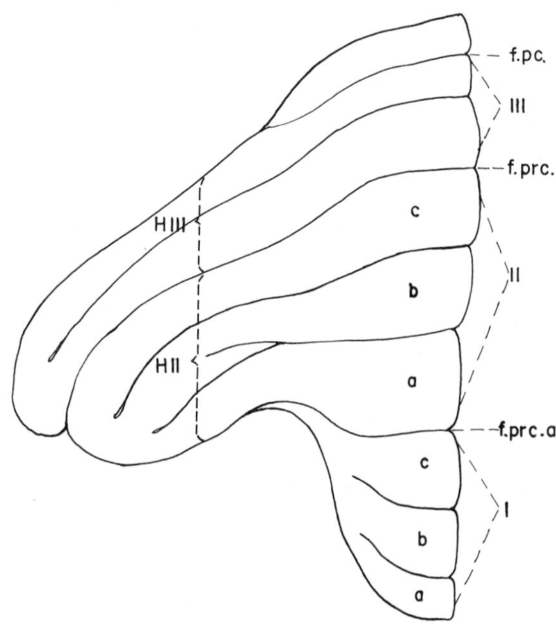

Figure 180. Cerebellum of macaque. Lower segment of right half of anterior lobe.

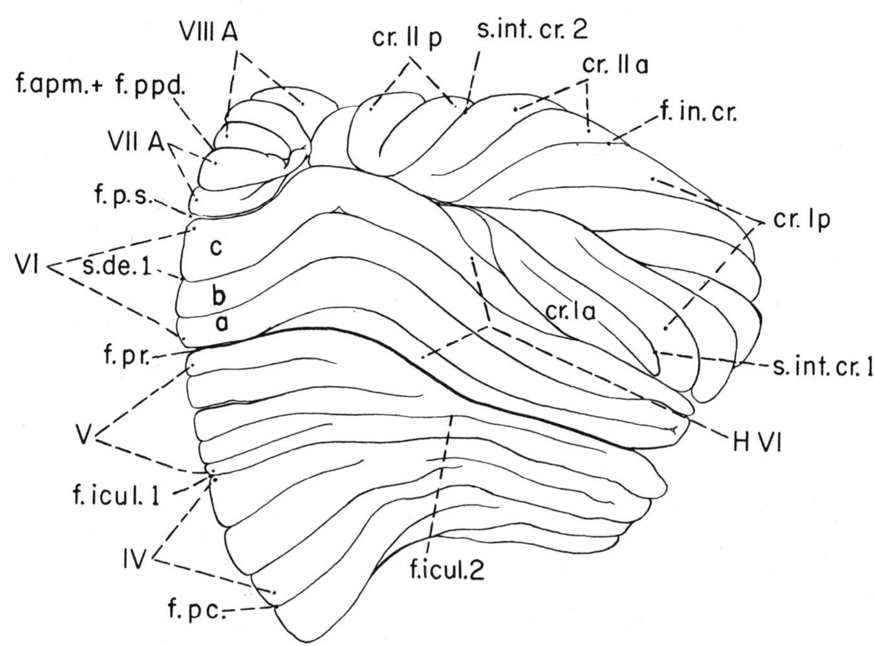

Figure 181. Cerebellum of macaque. Rostrodorsal aspect of left half. ×3. (Larsell, 1953a.)

178A and 181. Riley's lobulus 4B of the rhesus monkey and the posterior part of his lobulus 4 of *Cynocephalus* and *Cebus* correspond except for variations in the depth of the principal fissure (intraculminate fissure 2). The surface lamellae of lobule V in *M. rhesus* continue as two broad hemispheral lamellae that constitute the superficial part of lobule HV (fig. 179). Lamella Ve extends into the hemisphere as a broad leaflike fold in the anterior wall of the fissura prima, and lamella Vf reaches the floor of this fissure. The posterior wall of intraculminate fissure 2 also is foliated in the hemisphere as well as in the vermis. Lobule HV, accordingly, has a much larger cortical surface than its superficial folia would suggest.

The lobules of the anterior lobe of *M. rhesus* as interpreted above present a fairly uniform pattern in my material and in the published illustrations of this species; the principal variations involve lobules I and II. From species to species of the macaques, the photographs of Retzius show greater variations in these and other segments of the lobe. These variations are no doubt individual, in part, within a given species, but some probably reflect differences in the physical characteristics, briefly described above, between the several species.

It appears justifiable to identify the fissures and lobules of the anterior lobe of other species of *Macacus* on the basis of the developmental history of the lobe in *M. rhesus*. The pattern of four deep fissures and five lobules is evident in all cerebella of which adequate illustrations are available. An attempt to correlate differences in the size of lobules and depth of fissures, so far as these features are shown in median sagittal sections of the cerebella illustrated, with differences in relative size and presumptive functional significance of body parts, however, does not yield entirely concordant results. The individual lobules, if defined on the basis of the four deepest fissures in each species illustrated in figures 176 and 177A–C, vary so much both in relative size and, in some instances, in the lamellae included that they differ greatly not only from one species to another but also within the same species. In the outlines of the anterior lobe in median sagittal sections of two cerebella of *M. nemestrinus*, two of *M. maurus*, and two of *M. inuus*, illustrated in figures 182A–F, the lobules are very similar in both cerebella of *M. nemestrinus*, but in *M. maurus* and *M. inuus* they differ considerably within each species. In one specimen of *M. inuus* (fig. 182E) the lobules are almost identical with those of *M. erythraeus* (fig. 182B).

Lobule V has the most constant pattern of secondary subdivisions; lamellae Va to Vf as represented in *M. rhesus* can be easily identified in figures 183 (*M. speciosus*), 182C, D (*M. maurus*), and 182E (*M. inuus*). In a second specimen of *M. inuus*, however, lamella Va as interpreted in figure 182F is so large and intraculminate fissure 3 is so deep that the lamella resembles lobule IV of *M. rhesus* and several other species. Unless it is regarded as lamella Va, however, the remainder of lobule V is

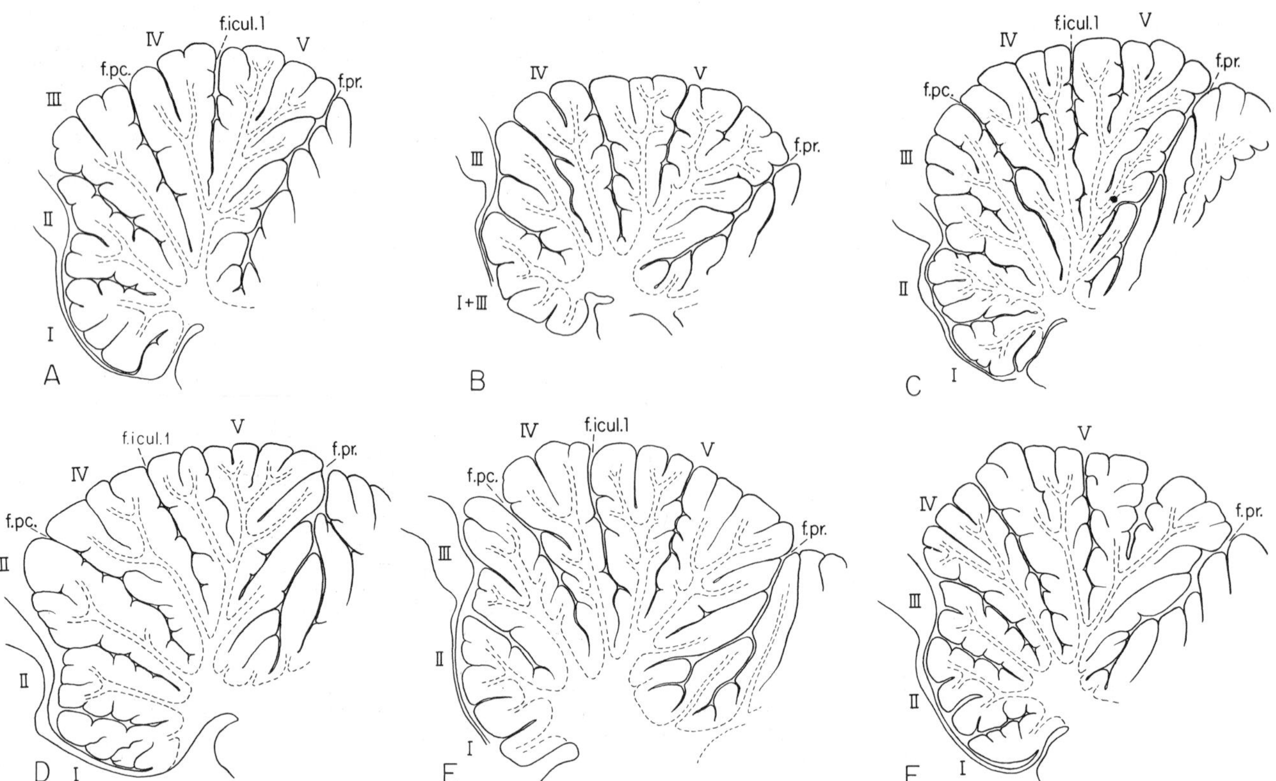

Figure 182. Midsagittal sections of anterior lobe of macaque cerebellum. A. *Macacus nemestrinus.* B. *Macacus erythroseus.* C, D. *Macacus maurus.* E, F. *Macacus inuus.*

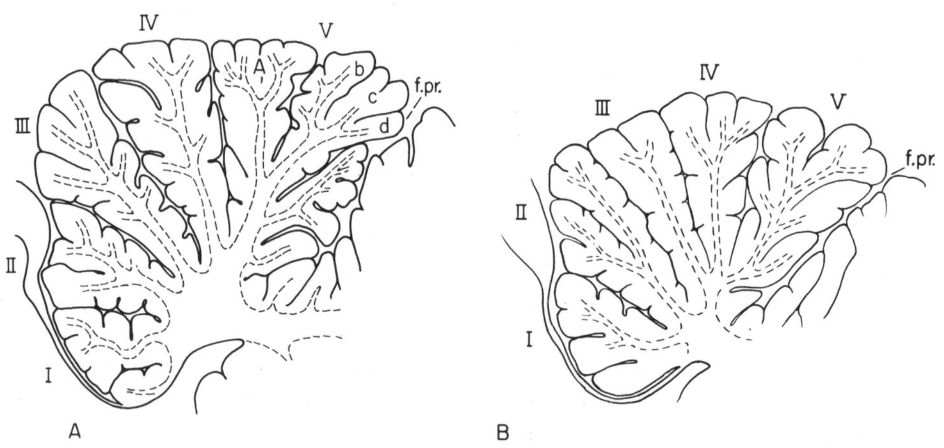

Figure 183. Midsagittal sections of anterior lobe of macaque cerebellum.
A. *Macacus speciosus.* B. *Macacus cynomolgus.*

atypical in this cerebellum; on the other hand, if so regarded, the most ventral subdivision of this specimen must be considered as combining lobules I and II. In the other cerebellum of *M. inuus* lobules I and II together comprise three subdivisions. Whether the intermediate one should be considered part of lobule I or of lobule II cannot be determined from the depths of the intervening fissures, although the three together correspond to the two lobules if lobules III, IV, and V were correctly interpreted.

On the basis of experimental evidence in *Ateles* (Chang and Ruch, 1949) of a connection between the lingula (lobules I and II, as I defined the lingula) and the caudal segments of the spinal cord, one might expect lobule I of the Barbary ape, the only tailless monkey, to be absent or greatly reduced. The relatively large area in sagittal section of these combined lobules in this species suggests that they may be functionally related to the perineum and that lobule I is differentiated in the tailed species.

The two species of stump-tailed monkeys illustrated, namely *M. speciosus* (fig. 183A) and *M. maurus* (fig. 182C, D), both distinctly show a differentiated but relatively small lobule I, while lobule II is comparable with that of other species in which lobules III, IV, and V are fairly typical. In *M. nemestrinus* and *M. cynomolgus* lobule I is relatively large, but in the latter species (fig. 183B) the remaining lobules of the anterior lobe do not readily fall into the typical pattern, at least as seen in the small number of cerebella actually studied.

Although five major subdivisions, separated by four deeper fissures, are apparent in all macaque cerebella the variations in size of the lobules and some of their lamellae are so great within a given species as well as between species that no strict somatotopical relationship of each seems probable unless the extent of the individual cortical areas involved also varies in individuals as well as between species. Lobules I and II vary in size more or less inversely with each other. Although lobule III is fairly constant in relative size, it appears to vary somewhat, again inversely, with the size of lobule II. Lobule IV is most prominent in species of larger body size, but varies inversely with lamella Va.

Because of the large size of the anterior lobe the fissura prima opens onto the dorsal cerebellar surface in *M. rhesus* and other species of macaques. It is the deepest of the cerebellar fissures and its walls are the most deeply folded. The lamellae that form these walls have the same pattern with respect to relative position and size as the lamellae in the walls of the fissura prima of subprimates. The vermal lobules of the posterior lobe are more uniform than those of the posterior lobe in the macaques.

Lobule VI of adult *M. rhesus* is narrow anteroposteriorly and its superficial lamellae usually are more or less elongated outward. On the basis of the fetal cerebella described above I found it necessary to modify my earlier (Larsell, 1953a) interpretations of these lamellae in the adult. Lamella VIa sometimes is combined with VIe and also may face the fissura prima instead of reaching the outer cerebellar surface. In other specimens VIa and VIe are distinct while VIb and VIc are separated only by a shallow furrow (fig. 176). Lamella VIc usually includes two folia, the superficial one and a more flattened fold facing the posterior superior fissure, but when lobule VI is very narrow both folia may face this fissure. A furrow in the upper anterior wall of the posterior superior fissure delimits VIc from the lower wall of the fissure, which may show one or two flattened folia. The superficial lamellae of the lobule, although in some cases apparently arbitrary as seen in median sagittal section, are borne out by their hemispheral continuations, described below, and by comparison with lobule VI of other species of monkeys as well as subprimates. Lamellae VId and VIf always occur as elongated folds in *M. rhesus*, with VId usually being the more prominent. In the large cerebellum illustrated in figure 177A lamellae VIa, VIb, and VIc are fairly large and a fold between VIa and VId corresponds to lamella VIe of subprimates. In other specimens VIe is very small, as is often the case in subprimates, or it may be combined with VIa, which it is always closely related to. Lamella VIb and VIc may be reduced to folia separated from each other by a shallow furrow; a similar furrow in the upper part of the anterior wall of the posterior superior fissure delimits VIc from the lower anterior surface of this fissure. In some cerebella lamella VIb is the caudal superficial fold of the lobule, while lamella VIc faces the posterior superior fissure. Sometimes one or two shallow grooves subdivide the lower anterior wall of this fissure into low folia (figs. 174A, 177A, 184B). The vermal segment of the posterior superior fissure varies in depth. Its posterior wall is formed by a lamella that often closely resembles the typical folium vermis of the human cerebellum (fig. 176) and, like the latter, may be attached to the medullary ray of lobule HVI instead of to the one leading to the superficial lamellae of sublobule VII, as is more common. In either case the lamella was regarded as lamella VIIAa. Sometimes a shallow groove occurs on its anterior surface, to which special reference is made in the description of lobule HVI.

Lobule VII does not change, except in size, from the pattern described in the later fetal stages. It includes two or three superficial sublamellae as well as three or four facing posteriorly in the wall of the compound prepyramidal-ansoparamedian fissure. The ansoparamedian fissure retains the relations described in the fetus and divides the lobule into sublobules VIIA and VIIB (figs. 176, 177). The latter is relatively smaller than in fetal stages because of the greater expansion of sublobule VIIA. The large medullary ray shared by lobules VI and VII is represented in carnivores, ungulates, and some other groups by a relatively much larger band of white substance that divides into large sheets to sublobules VIIA and VIIB and a smaller sheet to lobule VI. In the rhesus monkey the relatively much smaller primary ray bifurcates to lobule VI and sublobule VIIA, a smaller ray passes into sublobule VIIB from the level of bifurcation and below (fig. 176). These smaller vermal rays become reduced laterally and dip beneath the paravermian sulcus to the medullary sheet that extends into lobule HVIIB; their hemispheral continuations form the cores of folia that correspond to and frequently are continuous with those of sublobule VIIB. The ray to sublobule VIIA sometimes gives a branch to lamella VIc, as defined in the fetus, when a deep fissure occurs anterior of, rather than behind this lamella.

The most anterior of the superficial lamellae of sublobule VIIA, designated lamella VIIAa on the basis of its hemispheral relations and by reason of its form and position in most of the cerebella examined, corresponds to the folium vermis of the human cerebellum. The deep part of its medullary ray is continuous with a medially tapering band of white substance that connects crus Ia with the vermis. The furrow between it and lobule VI, in many instances, is a simple continuation of the posterior superior fissure. The furrow behind it, although its continuity with the hemispheral part of the intercrural fissure is obscured in the paravermian sulcus, may be regarded as the vermal segment of the intercrural fissure. In the large cerebellum illustrated in figures 176 and 178A, lamella VIIAa does not reach the cerebellar surface and the two fissures merge superficially but separately below the surface. Laterally the lamella, in this cerebellum, is superficially continuous with the caudalmost folium of lobule VI, but its medullary ray has a deep connection with the white substance of crus Ia. The deep furrow rostral of lamella VIIAa is directly continuous on either side with the posterior fissure of lobule HVI. A short caudally directed notch on either side of the lamella, however, appears to represent a partially interrupted connection with a compound fissure formed by the union of the hemispheral segments of the posterior superior and intercrural fissures (fig. 178A). On the basis of the relations of the hemispheral lobules to the vermis, described below, and the variations of the folium vermis in the human cerebellum, described by Ziehen (1899) and in a later section I came to regard the deep furrow rostral of lamella VIIAa of the large monkey cerebellum as the vermal segment of the posterior superior fissure. The photograph of Retzius of a median sagittal section of a *M. rhesus* cerebellum shows a much larger lamella corresponding to VIIAa and similar delimiting furrows. The hemispheral relations of the lamella and the furrows, however, are not shown in this series of photographs. In other specimens, lamella VIc, as interpreted from its hemispheral continuity, resembles lamella VIIAa in sagittal section and has a deep fissure anterior to it, while the furrow delimiting it posteriorly is relatively shallow. On the grounds of hemispheral relations it appears justifiable to consider the shallow furrow in such instances the posterior superior fissure and the smaller superficial fold behind it as lamella VIIAa.

The superficial sublamellae behind VIIAa and those on the anterior wall of the prepyramidal-ansoparamedian fissure correspond to the tuber vermis of the older terminology, but the homology of those below the entrance of the ansoparamedian fissure into this wall with sublobule VIIB should be recognized.

The reduced nature of sublobule VIIB was pointed out in the fetal stages of *M. rhesus*. The vermal segment of the ansoparamedian fissure is deeper in the adult; with some modifications resulting from the enlargement of lobule HVIIB, the vermal segment usually maintains its relations with the hemispheral segments of the fissure. In some cerebella that have a relatively shallow paravermian sulcus the continuity between folia of sublobule VIIB and those of HVIIB is only slightly obscured, but in others the folia themselves are interrupted in the depths of the narrow cleft of the paravermian sulcus. The medullary substance, however, is continuous with the large medullary ray shared by lobules VI and VII.

Lobule VIII is large in the adult *M. rhesus* and is divided by a relatively deep intrapyramidal sulcus into sublobules VIIIA and VIIIB (figs. 176, 177). Sublobule VIIIA is unusually large and the occasional displacement of part of the vermis away from the midline involves this sublobule and the adjacent part of sublobule VIIIB.

Lobule IX, the uvula, is separated from the pyramis by a deep fissura secunda. The lobule is narrow from side to side but has a large area in sagittal section (figs. 176, 177). The four superficial lamellae, IXa, IXb, IXc, and IXd, are larger in adult than in fetal stages but otherwise they are similar.

The six species of *Macacus* whose cerebella are shown in median sagittal sections in the photographs of Retzius present a very similar pattern of lobules and secondary folds in the posterior lobe. The greatest degree of variation is shown in lobules VI and VII. Lobule VIII is divided into two large sublobules in all; sublobule VIIIA is somewhat smaller in specimens (or species?) that have a relatively large lobule VII, or possibly sublobule VIIB. The figure of *M. rhesus*, already mentioned, in this series of photographs shows a pattern of the posterior lobe almost identical with what I found in this species.

HEMISPHERAL LOBULES OF POSTERIOR LOBE

Lobule HVI comprises four elongated superficial folia and the folia and lamellae of its surfaces facing the fissura prima and the posterior superior fissure. The pattern of the fissures separating the superficial folia differs in the two hemispheres of the individual cerebellum and usually varies more or less from specimen to specimen in both hemispheres. Oblique sagittal sections of the hemisphere, however, show that the lobule is divided into a pars anterior and a pars posterior; each includes two su-

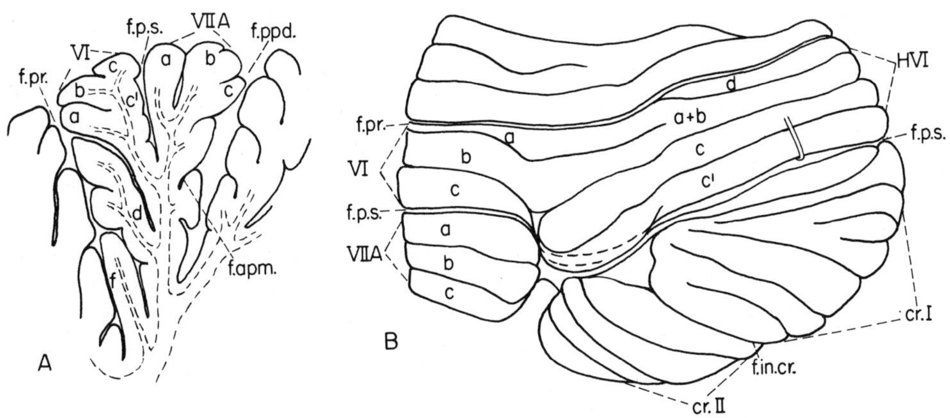

Figure 184. Cerebellum of *Macacus rhesus.* A. Midsagittal section of lobules VI and VII with adjacent parts of V and VIII. B. Dorsal view of corresponding parts of right hemisphere.

perficial folia and variable folds in the depths of the intervening fissures (figs. 184A–C). The pars anterior and pars posterior of the lobule in the two hemispheres are very similar and there is little variation between one lobule HVI and another. The intralobular fissure separating the two divisions is the deepest in the lobule.

The variations in the superficial folial pattern are due to differences in the connections of the individual folia with those of lobule VI. They involve submergence on one side of folia or parts of folia that may be superficial contralaterally. The pattern of two long superficial folia, however, is constant in both the pars anterior and the pars posterior of the right and left lobules. In the simplest arrangement of superficial folia the anterior elongated superficial folium of the pars anterior is continuous with vermal lamella VIa, while the second folium is continuous with lamella VIb. As illustrated in figure 178A (left side), a short hemispheral continuation of VIe may appear medially, rostral to VIa. The anterior folium of the pars posterior is continuous with VIc and the posterior one with the anterior wall of the vermal segment of the posterior superior fissure. The intralobular sulcus in this simple type of the lobule is a hemispheral continuation of declival sulcus 2 of the vermis. In variations of this pattern the rostral folium of the pars anterior may be continuous with VIe or, when that is small, with VId. The furrow between VIe and VIa may disappear laterally of the vermis; the hemispheral continuations of the two sublamellae may fuse into one superficial sublamella or sublamellae VIa and VIb may fuse laterally (fig. 184A); sometimes VIb becomes submerged laterally, with the furrow between it and VIa continuing into the anterior wall of the intralobular sulcus. When the rostral superficial folium of one side is continuous with vermal lamella VIa, the corresponding contralateral folium is continuous with VIa + e, VIe, or VId. In general the vermal connections of the remaining contralateral folia are advanced forward one folium. The picture, however, is greatly confused in many instances by the fact that some superficial fissures may dip into the walls of other fissures or may end blindly on the surface. The pars anterior is always related to VIa, VIb, VIe, and VId, while the pars posterior is related to VIc, the walls of the vermal segment of the posterior superior fissure, and in varying degree to lamella VIIAa (fig. 184A).

Lobule HVIIA, the ansiform lobule of Bolk, changes little, except in size, from this lobule in the later fetuses already described. The intercrural fissure is deeper and its walls have more foliation. About midway between the lateral hemispheral surface and the paravermian sulcus

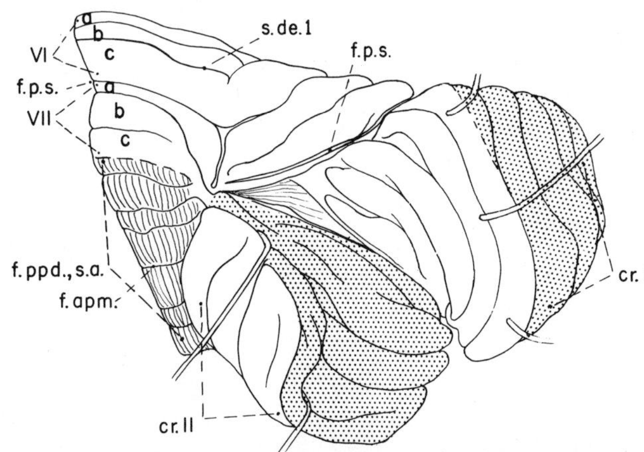

Figure 185. Dissection of macaque cerebellum showing walls of intercrural fissure spread apart, exposing the connection between crus I and sublobule VIIA. In this specimen the connection was a medullary sheet which was joined medially by the two posterior folia of HVI, interrupting the posterior superior fissure. ×3. (Larsell, 1953a.)

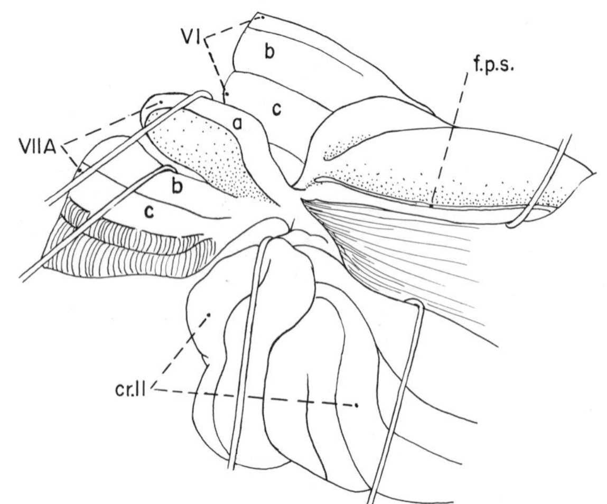

Figure 186. Cerebellum of macaque. Outline drawing, at higher magnification, of sublobule VIIA and its connections with crus I and crus II. ×6. (Larsell, 1953a.)

the intercrural fissure unites with the posterior superior fissure to form a compound fissure in the floor of which the medially tapering lamellae of lobule HVIIA and the medullary sheets connecting them with the vermis are hidden from surface view (figs. 178A, 185, and 186).

Crus I and crus II both are large and together they constitute the greater part of the hemisphere (figs. 178, 181, 187A). Crus I is divided into three groups of lamellae by two furrows: the more caudal one always opens onto the superficial cerebellar surface but varies in depth in different specimens; the rostral furrow, intracrural sulcus 1, is deeper and may extend to the border of the vermis. In the adult intracrural sulcus 1 may open onto the anterior superficial surface of crus I or onto the posterior wall of the posterior superior fissure. Penetrating deeply behind the compact group of small lamellae that consti-

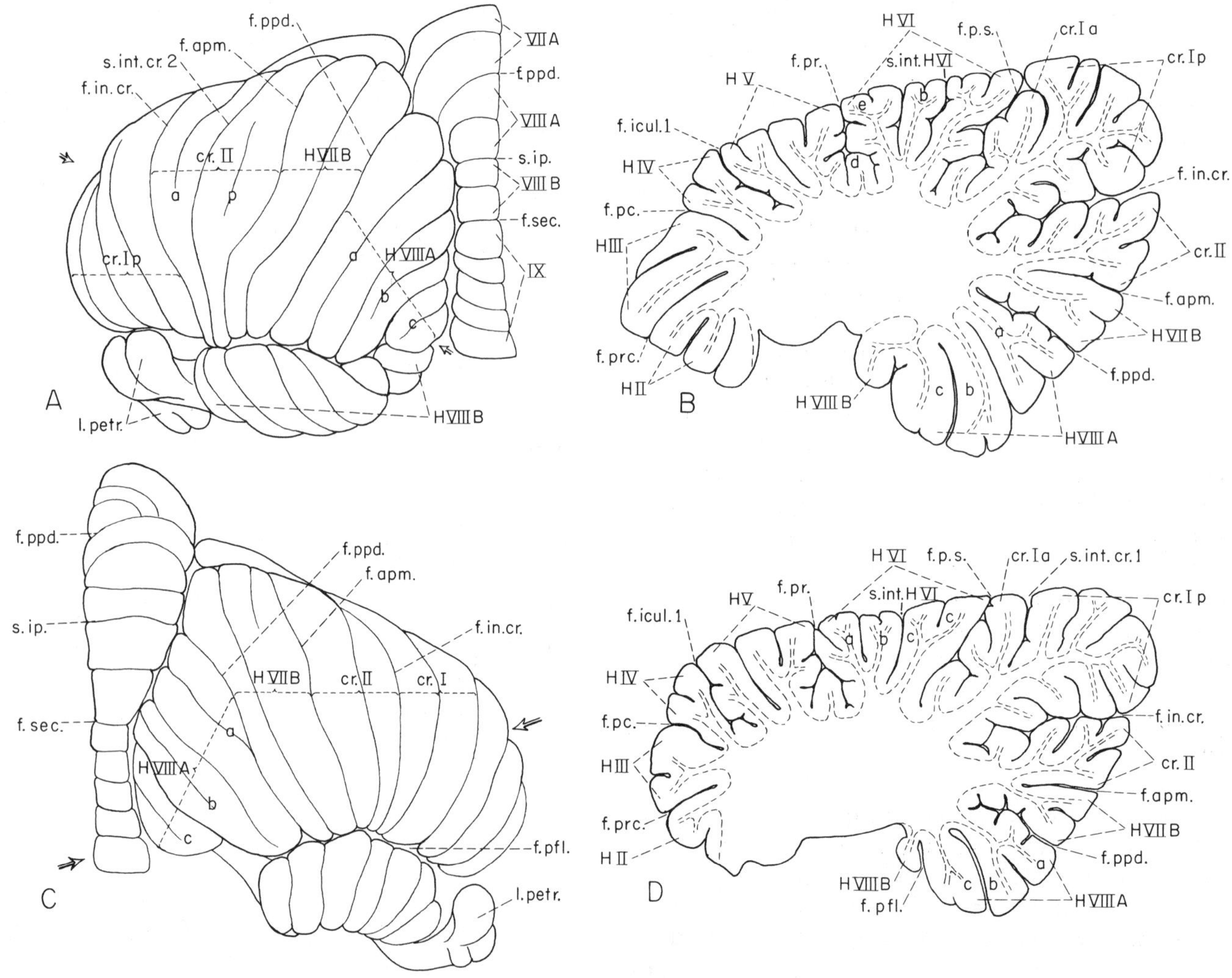

Figure 187. Cerebellum of *Macacus rhesus.* A. Posterior aspect of left half. B. Oblique section through left hemisphere. Arrows in A indicate plane of section. C. Posterior aspect of right half. D. Oblique section through right hemisphere. Arrows in C indicate plane of section.

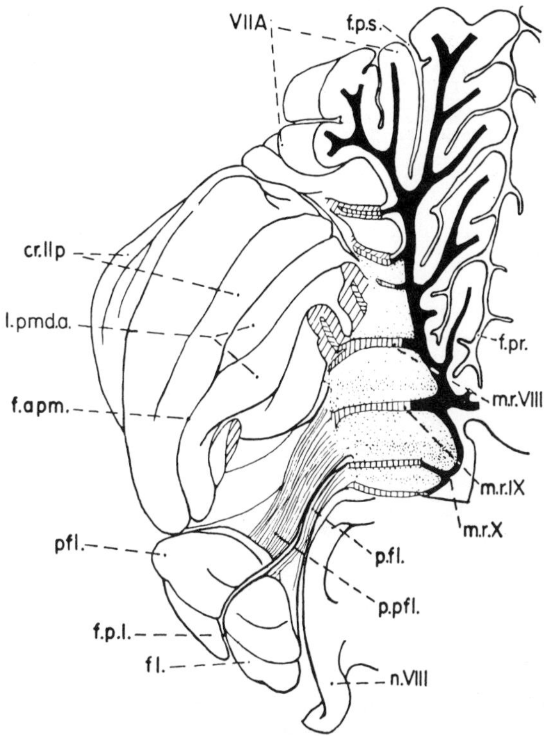

Figure 188. Cerebellum of macaque. Dissection showing pars anterior of paramedian lobule forming the lower part of anterior wall and the floor of prepyramidal fissure and continuous medially with the lower part of lobule VII, corresponding to sublobule VIIB and with the base of lobule VIII. ca. ×2.5. (Larsell, 1953a.)

tute crus Ia, intracrural sulcus 1 delimits this sublobule from the remainder of crus I. Crus Ia is exposed in subprimates. In the rhesus monkey it is exposed to a greater degree than in the human cerebellum described later on. There were an insufficient number of individual cerebella of other primates available to validate comparisons, but submergence of the sublobule, related to expansion of the hemispheral cortex as described in the fetal monkey, appears to be substantiated by its comparative relations in adult cerebella. As already stated, the lateral part of crus Ia appears to correspond to the middle portion of the cerebellar autonomic eye field of Hampson (1949) and Hampson, Harrison, and Woolsey (1952) in the monkey. It is continuous medially with lamella VIIAa, as already mentioned, by a medullary band of variable length. Crus Ip differs from this sublobule in the fetal monkey by its size and in connecting by a longer medullary band with the principal medullary ray of sublobule VIIA (fig. 185).

Crus II comprises two lamellae whose broad superficial surfaces are partially foliated. They represent crus IIa and crus IIp, respectively, and are separated by intracrural sulcus 2. Their medullary sheets converge medially and are continuous with the vermal ray leading to sublobule VIIA (fig. 186).

Lobule HVIIB retains the relations described in fetal stages, that is the ansoparamedian fissure separates lobule HVIIB from lobule HVIIA in the anterior wall of the prepyramidal fissure (fig. 176). Folia cross the floor of the hemispheral segment of the prepyramidal fissure from lobule HVIIB to the lower anterior surface of the base of the pyramis as in the fetus; the cleft of prepyramidal sulcus 1 extends farther laterally before merging with the prepyramidal fissure. The superficial surface of the lobule is divided into two folia that can be short or can extend almost to its full length.

Lobule HVIIIA is not changed, except in size, from the structure and relations described in fetal stages. Lamellae HVIIIAa, HVIIIAb, and HVIIIAc are well illustrated in figure 187. Lamella HVIIIAc is readily dissected away, exposing its attachment to the medullary sheet whose medial part continues to the sublobule VIIIB as the vermal attachment of the dorsal paraflocculus (fig. 188).

Lobule HVIIIB, the dorsal paraflocculus, begins as

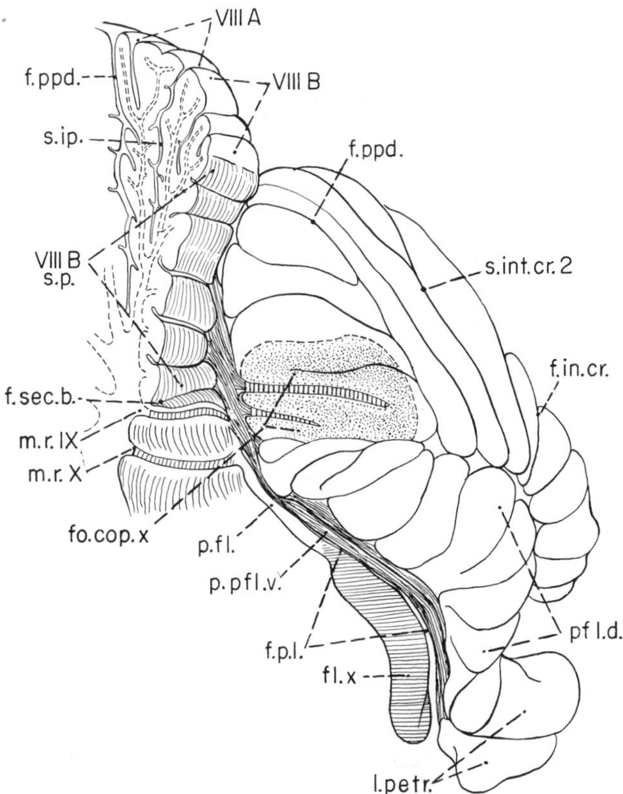

Figure 189. Cerebellum of macaque. Dissection of posterior portion of right half showing relations of medullary rays of copula to stalk of paraflocculus and of the latter to base of sublobule VIIIB. ×5. (Larsell, 1953a.)

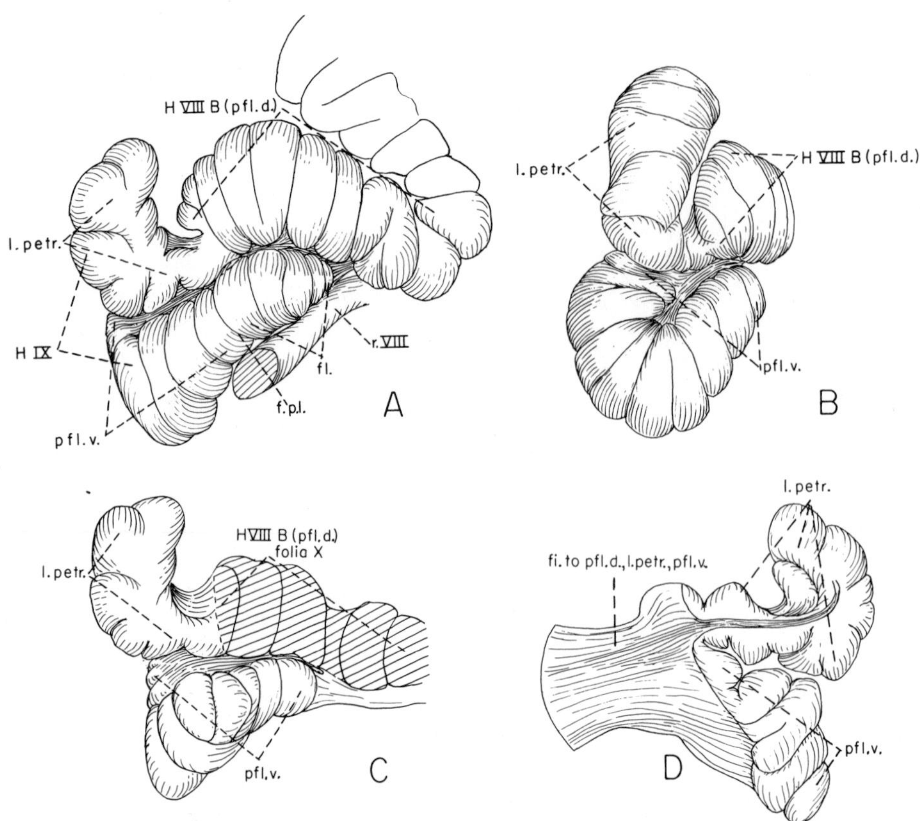

Figure 190. Paraflocculus and flocculus of *Macacus rhesus.* A. Posterior view. B. Anterior view. C. Dorsal view, after removal of paraflocculus dorsalis. D. Dissection showing the relations of lobulus petrosus and ventral paraflocculus to the parafloccular peduncle.

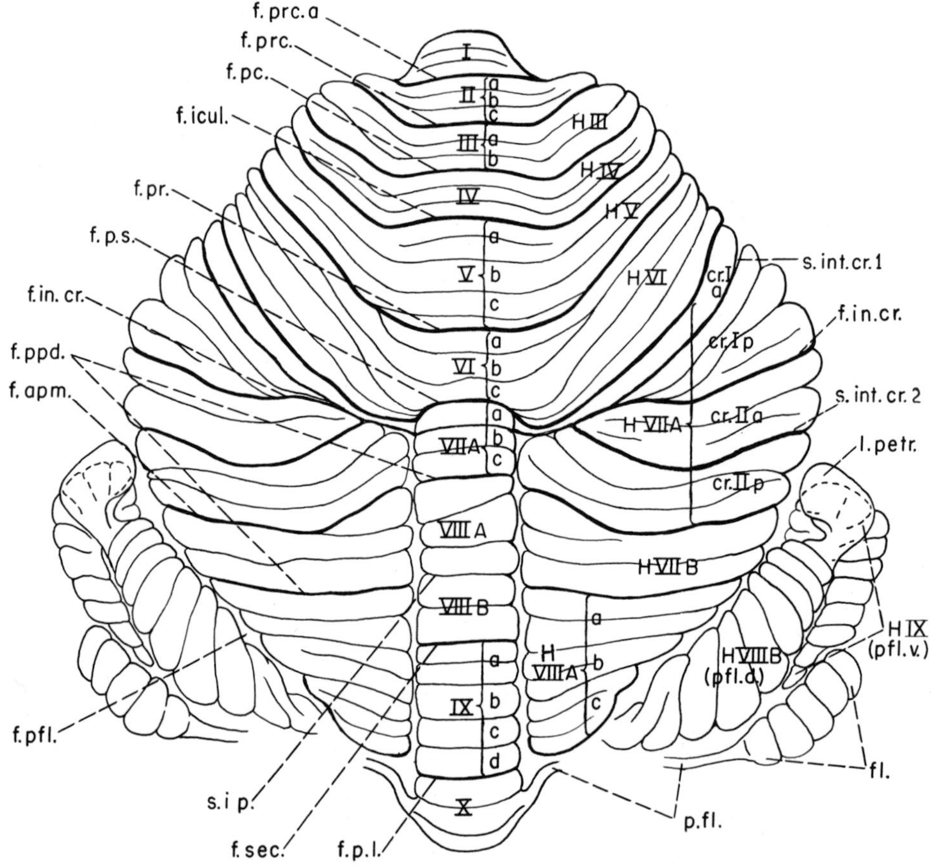

Figure 191. Diagram of the cerebellum of *M. rhesus.* The cortex is folded out in one plane.

several small folia on the parafloccular peduncle, distal to the separation of this peduncle from the medullary sheet of lobule HVIIIA (fig. 189), and continues as a series of folia that increase in size beneath the posterolateral part of the hemisphere and then diminish distally toward the lobulus petrosus (fig. 190). The concealed rostromedial surfaces of these folia form the posterolateral wall of the parafloccular fissure. This fissure continues medialward between the initial small folia of the dorsal paraflocculus and the overhanging lamella HVIIIAc; laterally the parafloccular fissure forms a cleft between the hemisphere and the rostrolateral part of the paraflocculus.

Lobule HIX, the ventral paraflocculus (fig. 190), is larger but is otherwise little changed from its late fetal features. The lobulus petrosus varies in size and form in individual cerebella of the adult monkey.

FLOCCULONODULAR LOBE

The flocculonodular lobe of the adult cerebellum differs from that of the fetus only in the size of the nodulus and flocculus. The floccular peduncle, that is the fibrous connection between nodulus and flocculus, is closely associated with the posterior border of the flattened sheet of fibers that lead to the dorsal and ventral paraflocculi, but a small groove, the posterolateral fissure, usually is visible along the peduncle (figs. 188, 190).

The diagram (fig. 191) shows the folial pattern of the cerebellum of the rhesus monkey and the relations between the vermal and hemispheral lobules.

BABOON

Cynocephalus sphinx or *papio* is one of the smaller baboons. The cerebellum is relatively wide. A prominent vermal ridge begins on the anterior surface and continues to the posterior surface; the posterior portion is separated from the hemispheres by a deep paravermian sulcus on either side. The hemispheres extend caudolaterally and cover the paraflocculus, with only the lobulus petrosus being visible in dorsal view (fig. 193).

CORPUS CEREBELLI

In median sagittal section (fig. 192) the corpus cerebelli has a nearly oval form and is divided into approximately equal anterior and posterior lobes. Lobules I and II form components of a large ventral projection which at first seems to constitute a unit. Study of the lateral relations of the lamellae and of the surface folia and fissures, however, reveals a furrow that reaches the cortical margin. Although this furrow is relatively shallow in sagittal section, it evidently represents precentral fissure *a*. A small lobule I, comprising folia Ia, Ib, and Ic, accordingly, is delimited from lobule II; folium Ic extends slightly toward the hemisphere. Lobule II has two surface lamellae and a small lobule HII is formed by extension onto the hemisphere.

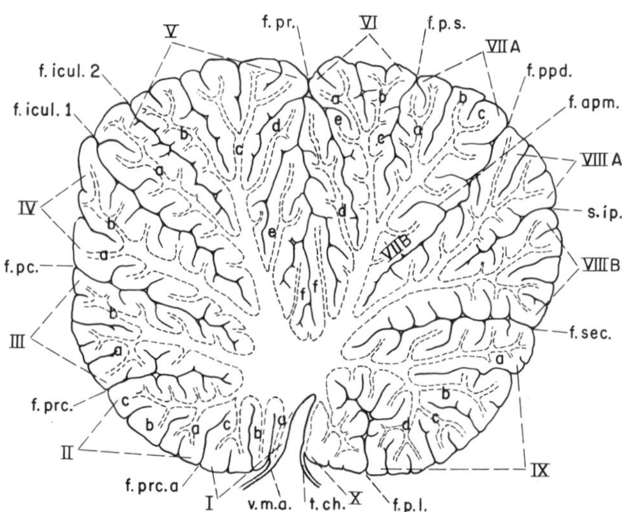

Figure 192. Cerebellum of baboon (*Cynocephalus sphinx*). Midsagittal section.

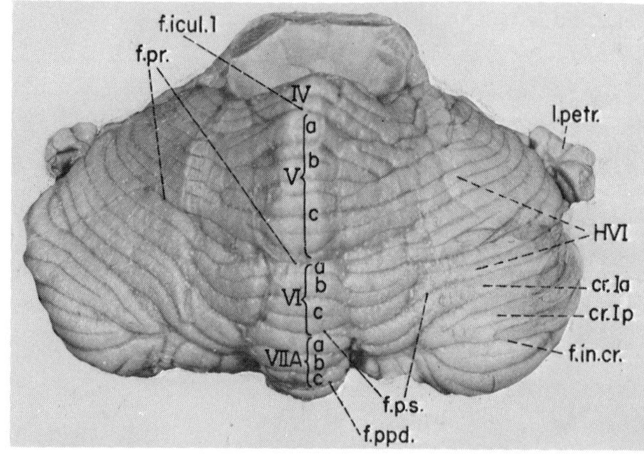

Figure 193. Cerebellum of baboon. Dorsal view.

To establish its identity, lobule III must be considered together with lobule HIII. In median sagittal section the lobule is elongated rostralward and divides into two large terminal lamellae. These continue into the hemisphere, forming the superficial part of lobule HIII, which is delimited from lobule HII by a lateral extension of the precentral fissure and from lobule HIV by the preculminate fissure; both fissures are deep and reach the cerebellar margin (fig. 193).

Lobules I, II, and III, as defined above, correspond to Bolk's lobuli 1, 2, and 3 of *C. sphinx* as illustrated in median sagittal section. Photographs of corresponding sections of two cerebella of the same species in the monograph of Retzius show some variations. In one specimen lobule I is relatively smaller but lobule II is larger and is divided by a relatively deep but simple furrow into two lamella that correspond, except in their greater size, to those of figure 192. Another cerebellum has a still smaller lobule I and a larger lobule II. Lobule III is relatively smaller in both than in my specimens. Retzius' figure of *C. babuin*, a larger species with a short tail, shows relatively small lobules I and II and a large lobule III. The fissures of the lower part of the anterior lobe are too indistinct for comparison with the photograph of *C. mormon*, the largest of the baboons, which also is characterized by a stump tail.

Lobule IV is large and intraculminate fissure 1 is deep, as also shown in Bolk's figure of a median sagittal section of *C. sphinx* and in Retzius' photograph of *C. babuin*. Retzius' figure of *C. sphinx* shows a large segment behind the corresponding lobule which perhaps should be considered a subdivision of lobule IV. In *C. babuin* a similar segment, although relatively much larger, corresponds to lamella Va of the rhesus monkey. Evidently this segment varies in the baboons as does lamella or sublobule VA in the macaques. The hemispheral relations of this segment are not shown in any of the photographs of Retzius, but in my baboon specimens the segment is continuous with the anterior superficial lamella of lobule HV. This is delimited from lobule HIV by a deep hemispheral segment of intraculminate fissure 1. Lobule HIV includes two superficial lamellae that widen before reaching the cerebellar margin (fig. 194).

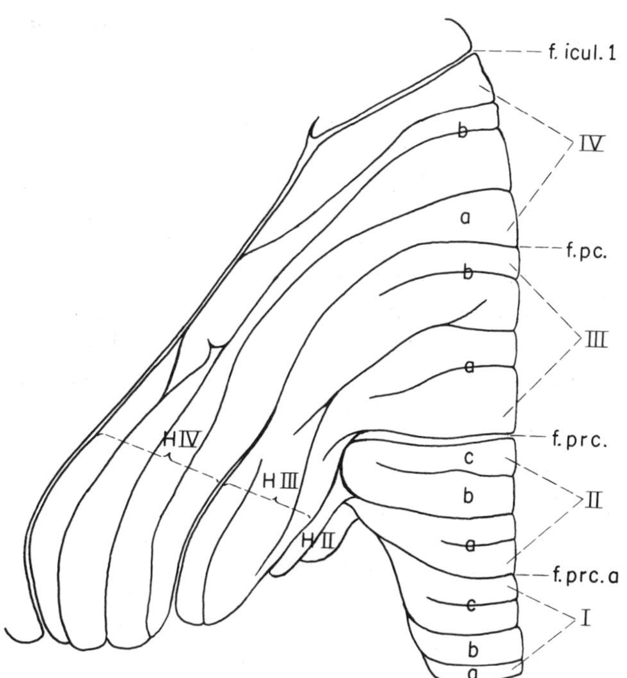

Figure 194. Cerebellum of baboon. Anteroventral view of right half of anterior lobe.

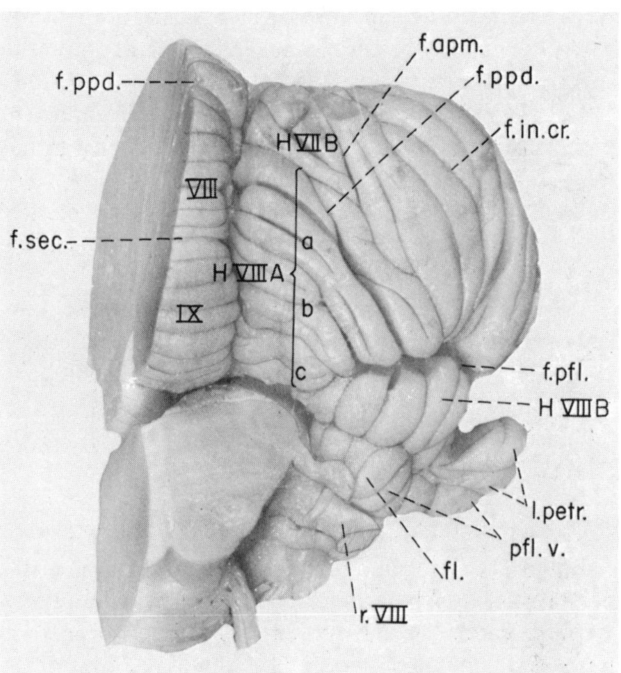

Figure 195. Cerebellum of baboon. Posterior view of right half.

Lobule V includes the large segment mentioned above, which is labeled VA in figures 192 and 193, since it may be regarded as a sublobule rather than a lamella. In addition superficial lamellae Vb and Vc, which seem greatly enlarged and foliated as compared with the rhesus monkey, and fissural lamellae Vd, Ve, and Vf are clearly shown. These all are recognizable in Retzius' figures of several species of baboons in typical form and relationships except that lamella Vc is divided into relatively larger secondary lamellae in *C. sphinx* than in the other species illustrated. Sublobule VA varies in size inversely with lobule IV in individual cerebella. Lobule HV comprises four elongated superficial folia and the folds in the appropriate walls of its limiting fissures. The superficial folia are continuous, in various combinations, with sublobule VA and lamellae Vb and Vc, but the posterior hemispheral fold is formed by emergence of Vd to the surface (fig. 193).

Lobule VI, as in the monkeys, is relatively small superficially. Deep lamellae VId and VIf are large and characteristic but lamellae VIa, VIb, and VIc are difficult to identify in sagittal sections (fig. 192). On the basis of their relations to the folia of lobule HVI the two folds that reach the cerebellar surface appear to represent lamellae VIa and VIb; lamella VIc is reduced and faces the upper part of the posterior superior fissure. The furrow between VIa and VIb corresponds to declival sulcus 1, but declival sulcus 2 has merged with the posterior superior fissure.

Lobule VII comprises a typical lamella VIIAa, two or three superficial folia or small lamellae, and four or five folds in the anterior wall of the ansoparamedian-prepyramidal fissure (fig. 192). The two imperfectly separated ventral folia of this wall represent a rudimentary sublobule VIIB, as their hemispheral relations show.

Lobules VIII and IX are typical as found in the monkeys and are separated by a deep fissura secunda (fig. 195). The pyramis is divided into large sublobules VIIIA and VIIIB. Lobule IX is broad in sagittal section but narrow from side to side. Surface lamellae IXa, IXb, IXc, and IXd are relatively large (fig. 192).

HEMISPHERAL LOBULES OF POSTERIOR LOBE

Lobule HVI forms a large quadrilateral area on the dorsorostral cerebellar surface that tapers laterally toward the cerebellar margin and divides into the pars anterior and the pars posterior. The vermal relations of the folia, which differ in the right and left lobules, are indicated in figures 193 and 195. The intralobular sulcus of both right and left ansiform lobules is continuous with the vermal segment of the posterior superior fissure. The pars posterior is continuous on one side with the anterior

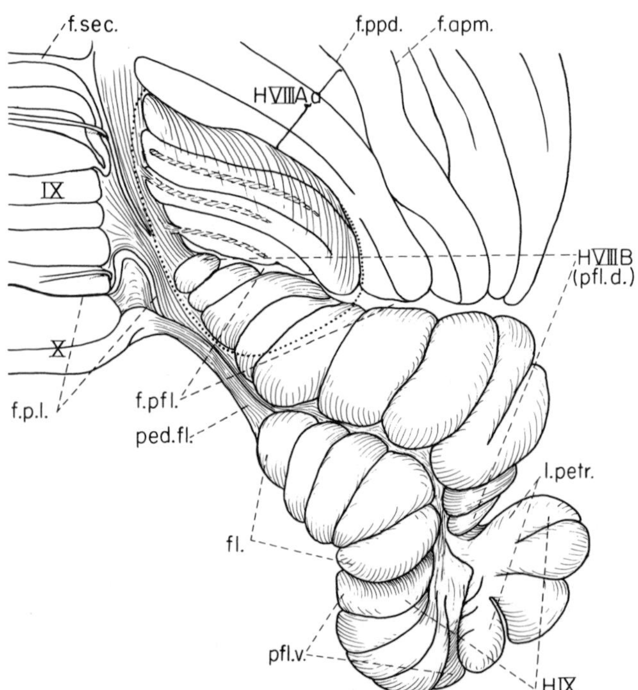

Figure 196. Cerebellum of baboon. Posteroventral view. Major part of paramedian lobule (dotted line) dissected away to expose floccular and parafloccular peduncles.

wall of the latter fissure, including the reduced folium VIc which forms the upper part of this wall; contralaterally it is continuous with the foliated posterior wall. The base of lamella VIIAa appears to have connections from both lobules but laterally the pars posterior is deeply divided from crus I in both hemispheres.

The hemispheral segment of the posterior superior and intercrural fissures converge medially to form a compound fissure before reaching the vermis. The floor of this furrow consists of medially tapering medullary bands that connect much of the expanded portion of the hemisphere with sublobule VIIA. The posterior wall is formed by the rostromedially directed ends of the lamellae of crus II. The posterior wall of the posterior superior fissure is formed by crus Ia. In the left hemisphere this sublobule emerges to the surface for a short distance laterally and again medially so that in these parts of its course intracrural sulcus 1 becomes distinct from the compound furrow which it forms elsewhere with the posterior superior fissure. The intercrural fissure is deep and there is considerable foliation in its walls. A shallower intracrural sulcus 2 divides crus II into crus IIa and crus IIp. The ansoparamedian fissure, as in *Macacus* and *Cercocebus*, emerges from its vermal position in the posterior surface of lobule VII to form the superficially visible hemispheral segment that separates lobule HVIIA from lobule HVIIB (fig. 195).

Lobule HVIIIA is delimited dorsolaterally by the hemispheral segment of the prepyramidal fissure. It comprises lamellae HVIIIAa, HVIIIAb, and HVIIIAc, as in the rhesus monkey, but these are much wider medially and the first two are relatively shorter, as seen superficially, than in the monkey (fig. 195). The paravermian sulcus into which they extend medially is deeper, thus adding to their length. Lamella HVIIIAa is continuous by constricted folia with the anterior surface of sublobule VIIIA. Lamella HVIIIAb is connected with the fibrous sheet that passes into sublobule VIIIA, and lamella HVIIIAc is attached to the lateral part of a band of fibers that divides before reaching the vermis; the lateral division passes into sublobule VIIIA and the medial division into sublobule VIIIB (fig. 196). Lamella HVIIIAc overhangs the proximal part of the peduncle of the paraflocculus and is separated from it by a medial continuation of the parafloccular fissure, as in the monkeys.

Lobule HVIIIB, the dorsal paraflocculus, comprises three or four small folia that are covered by lamella HVIIIAc, and a superficially visible series that at first successively increase in length and then shorten toward a constricted attachment of the lobulus petrosus (figs. 195, 196). The longer folia extend with a hollow beneath the ventrolateral margin of the hemisphere; they also expose

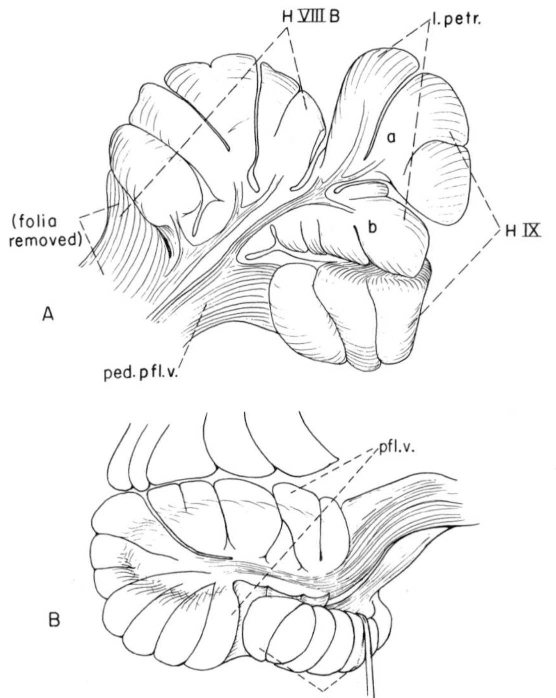

Figure 197. Cerebellum of baboon. A. Medial view of left paraflocculus after removal of flocculus. B. Dorsal aspect of ventral paraflocculus and flocculus after removal of lobulus petrosus and dorsal paraflocculus.

a considerable surface on the posterolateral wall of the parafloccular fissure.

Lobule HIX, the ventral paraflocculus, comprises a chain of folia that begins medial to the flocculus, which covers the initial three low folds, and then continues medially beneath the lobulus petrosus, arching dorsalward medial to the petrosus and the distal part of the dorsal paraflocculus. Including those hidden by the flocculus, there are fourteen or fifteen folia, with those at its medial end becoming reduced in size. The proximal folia are attached to a continuation of the ventral part of the parafloccular peduncle and the chain arches around the end of the stalk so formed (fig. 197). Distally the lobule is separated from the hemisphere and brachium pontis by a narrow space that represents the parafloccular fissure. A sheet of fibers, however, connects the white substance beneath the hidden medial part of the lobule with the medullary body of the hemisphere.

The lobulus petrosus is composed of several large lamellae which, as a group, are separated from the dorsal paraflocculus by a wide space (fig. 197A). The lobulus petrosus is attached to a fibrous band that branches from the parafloccular peduncle; as seen from the posterolateral aspect this band appears more closely related to the dorsal than to the ventral paraflocculus. In some of the photographs of this species in the Retzius monograph the petrosal lobule is larger than in figure 195; in others it is of about equal size.

FLOCCULONODULAR LOBE

Lobule X, the nodulus, is relatively small (fig. 192) and the vermian part of the posterolateral fissure is shallow. The fissure can be followed as a groove between the floccular and parafloccular peduncles while the flocculus comprises a chain of six foliá at the end of the floccular peduncle (figs. 196, 197).

MANGABEY

THE cerebellum of the mangabey (*Cercocebus* sp.) does not differ greatly from that of the rhesus monkey in external appearance. The contours and folial patterns of the hemispheres are very similar but the dorsal and anterior parts of the vermis form a somewhat more distinct ridge. The petrosal lobule is larger while the flocculus is somewhat narrower. In median sagittal section lobules I, II, and IV of *Cercocebus* are larger than those of the rhesus monkey but the other lobules are remarkably similar to those of most rhesus cerebella. The secondary lamellae of most of the lobules are somewhat more elongated, increasing the size of the lobules – this feature is probably related to the larger size of *Cercocebus*.

CORPUS CEREBELLI

The vermal part of the corpus cerebelli is divided into nearly equal anterior and posterior lobes, as seen in median sagittal section (fig. 198). The fissura prima opens on the dorsal cerebellar surface, but extends lateroventrally and rostrally in such a manner that the entire anterior lobe, including its hemispheral parts, is much smaller than the posterior lobe (fig. 199).

Lobule I has four large surface folia or sublamellae (fig. 200). Lamella Ia is large, as also shown in the illustrations of Bradley (1905) and Retzius (1906), depicting similar sections of the cerebellum of *C. fuliginosus* and *C. collaris*, respectively. Bradley's figure shows the remainder of the lobule, designated A_1, as being relatively larger than in my material, but the photograph of Retzius shows a smaller lobule in the corresponding position. Continuations of the folia into the hemisphere form a small lobule HI. Precentral fissure *a* is deep in the vermis, while laterally it reaches the cortical margin (fig. 200).

Lobule II is divided distally into elongated surface lamellae IIa and IIb, which continue into the hemisphere as a small lobule HII. The precentral fissure is deep and reaches the cortical margin (fig. 200A). It appears to correspond to Bradley's fissure *c* of *C. fuliginosus*. The cortical segment ventral of this fissure in Bradley's figure is similar in form and relative size to lobule II of figure 200; in the photograph of Retzius it is shorter but wider in sagittal section.

Lobule III also has two large surface lamellae, IIIa and IIIb, with lamella IIIb being the larger. The lobule is separated from lobule IV by the preculminate fissure that is slightly deeper than the precentral fissure. A rostrolaterally elongated lobule HIII reaches the anterior surface of the brachium pontis.

Lobule IV is separated from lobule V by intraculminate fissure 1, which is nearly as deep as the preculminate fissure. The lobule is divided into two large superficial lamellae, IVa and IVb, while lamellae IVb is composed of two sublamellae (fig. 198). The medullary ray can be regarded as arising from the central medullary body or from a branch common to lobules IV and V but it is much shorter in *Cercocebus* than in *M. rhesus*. Lobule HIV extends almost to the lateral margin of brachium pontis and terminates in a clublike expansion.

Lobule V has a prominent anterior subdivision and two smaller superficial lamellae. The anterior subdivision, which is composed of two surface lamellae and large folia on its fissural surfaces, is so large that it can properly be regarded as sublobule VA, which is delimited from the remainder of the lobule by a rather deep intraculminate fissure 2. The two surface folds behind this fissure are lamellae Vb and Vc. In the anterior wall of the fissura prima lamellae Vd, Ve, and Vf were readily identified (fig. 198). Lobule HV tapers rostrolaterally, reaching the lateral surface of the brachium pontis (fig. 199).

In the figure of Bradley mentioned above, the subdivision which I interpreted as lobule IV is attached to the

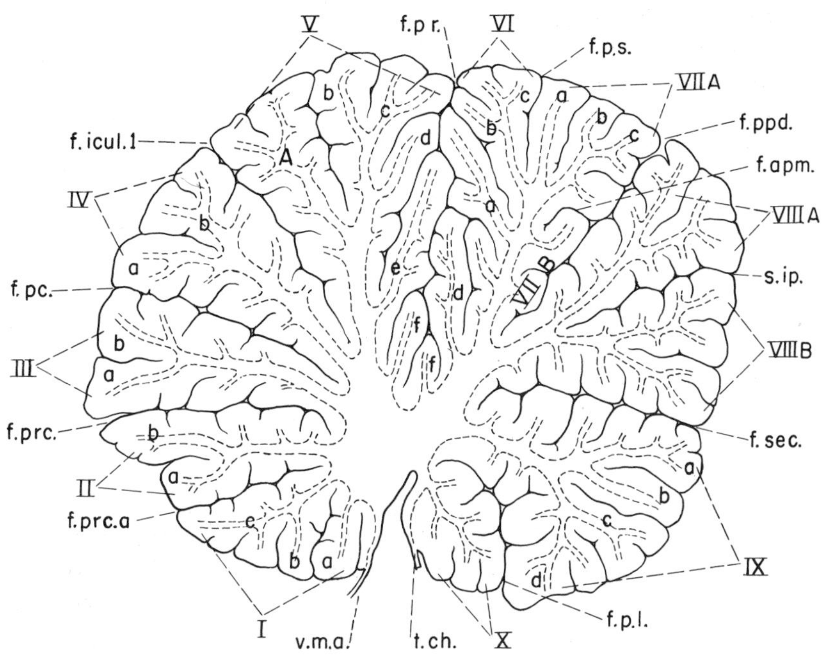

Figure 198. Cerebellum of mangabey (*Cercocebus* sp.). Midsagittal section.

medullary ray common to it and lobule V at a greater distance from the medullary body than in my specimen (fig. 198) and intraculminate fissure 1 is much shallower. Also sublobule VA, as designated in figure 198, is reduced to a lamella in Bradley's figure. According to my viewpoint, lobule V corresponds to the posterior part of lobe B of Bradley, which in his illustration is subdivided into a large anterior lamella and two smaller ones, with the three corresponding to my sublobule VA and lamellae Vb and Vc. In the photograph of Retzius the segment corresponding to lobule IV is very similar to this lobule as illustrated in figure 198. Its medullary ray, however, arises directly from the medullary body. Lamellae corresponding to Vd, Ve, and Vf are shown in the illustrations of both authors but are not designated. It is probable that the large size of lobule IV and sublobule VA of my specimen is a compensation for the relatively reduced lobules I, II, and III, as compared with these lobules in the figures cited.

Lobules VI and VII appear to constitute a single major division of the vermis in *Cercocebus* because the vermal segment of the posterior superior fissure is quite

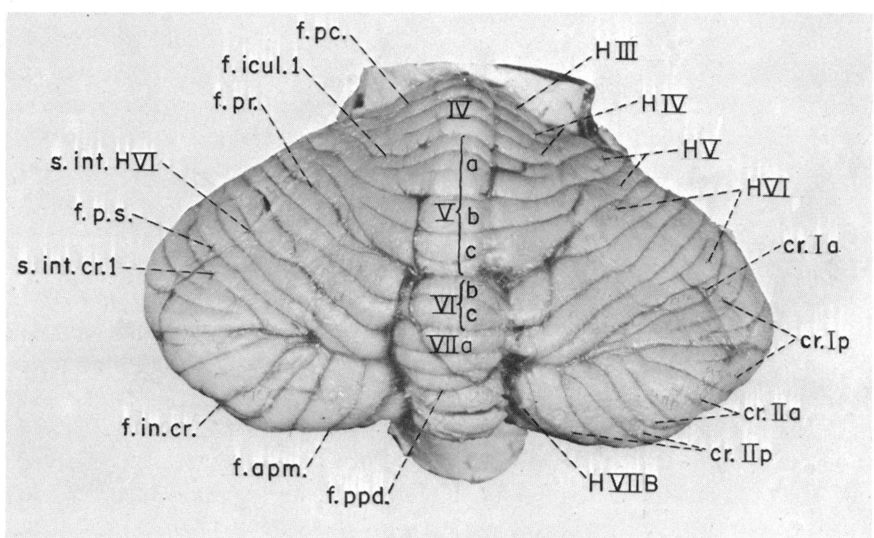

Figure 199. Cerebellum of mangabey. Dorsal view.

shallow and both lobules are small. The delimiting fissure, however, can be followed into the hemispheres where it forms a deep boundary between lobules HVI and HVIIA. The superficial folds of lobule VI are so small in median sagittal section that their identification, as indicated in figure 198, is far from certain but their existence appears to be supported by their hemispheral relations. Lamellae VId and VIf, however, are typical. In Retzius' photograph two elongated superficial lamellae are shown but there is no folding of either wall of the posterior superior fissure.

Lobule VII includes three surface lamellae and those of the anterior surface of the prepyramidal fissure. The superficial lamellae correspond to lamellae VIIAa, VIIAb, and VIIAc of other species and are continuous with medullary sheets leading to crus I and crus II of lobule HVIIA. The upper lamellae of the anterior wall of the prepyramidal fissure are continuous with crus II. The ansoparamedian fissure of one side of the hemisphere extends without interruption to the furrow so labeled in the anterior surface of the prepyramidal fissure (fig. 198); contralaterally it less certainly reaches the immediately dorsal deeper arched furrow. The large folium between these two fissures is continuous on one side with crus II, and on the other side, less clearly, with lobule HVIIB. The folia of the lower part of the anterior surface of the prepyramidal fissure are continuous with some of the medially converged folia of the posteromedial surface of lobule HVIIB, thus corresponding on a reduced scale to sublobule VIIB of *Macacus* and *Cynocephalus*. The medullary sheet leading to sublobules HVIIB and HVIIIA is continuous with the large medullary band which also gives rise to the rays leading to lobules VI, VII, and VIII.

Lobule VIII is divided into the usual sublobules VIIIA and VIIIB, which are separated by a deep intrapyramidal sulcus. The anterior surface of sublobule VIIIA is related to some of the medially converged folia of lobule HVIIIA but there is no distinct ala corresponding to the copula pyramidis of subprimates.

Lobule IX is compressed from side to side but is large in median sagittal section. Surface lamellae IXa, IXb, IXc, and IXd are well developed (fig. 198).

HEMISPHERAL LOBULES OF POSTERIOR LOBE

Lobule HVI is divided into pars anterior and pars posterior (fig. 199), which are typical and nearly identical in the right and left lobules, as seen in section. The intralobular furrow is confluent, on the left side, with the shallow declival sulcus 1 of the vermis. In the right lobule the furrow is directly confluent with the vermal segment of the posterior superior fissure, but a shallow groove on

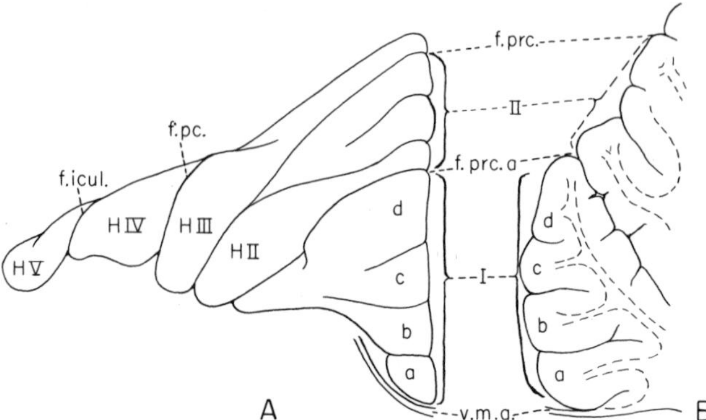

Figure 200. Cerebellum of mangabey. Lower segment of anterior lobe. A. Rostroventral view of right half. B. Midsagittal section. ×5.

the anterior wall of the latter fissure appears to represent its real continuation in the vermis. Since both pars anterior and pars posterior are broad lamellae in *Cercocebus*, and the connections with the vermis are constricted beneath the paravermian sulcus, a clearer picture of their individual relations to the subdivisions of lobule VI emerges by describing the continuity of each with the lobule rather than by considering them as hemispheral continuations of the smaller vermal folia and lamellae.

The two superficial folia of the pars anterior of the left lobule HVI merge before reaching the vermis but the large folium so formed is continuous with lamellae VIa and VIb. In the right lobule the rostral superficial folium of the pars anterior is continuous with lamella VId; the second one, which expands medially, is continuous with lamellae VIa, VIb, and VIc. The pars posterior on the left side has three superficial folia: the rostral one is continuous with lamella VIc; the two posterior folia are continuous with the deep part of lamella VIIAa and with both walls of the vermal segment of the posterior superior fissure. In the right lobule the pars posterior includes two principal folia; the posterior one is partially subdivided. The two folia are continuous with the deep part of lamella VIIAa and, by a connection beneath the posterior superior fissure, with the anterior wall of this fissure. Including the two partial folia of the right pars posterior, *Cercocebus* has five superficial folia on either side but their vermal connections differ on the two sides. Thus there is an additional superficial folium, as compared with *M. rhesus*, and the pars posterior is relatively much larger.

Lobule HVIIA is greatly expanded laterally but its continuity with the vermis is effected by medially tapering folia that give way to medullary bands in the floor of a compound furrow formed by the confluence of the posterior superior and intercrural fissures (fig. 199), as in

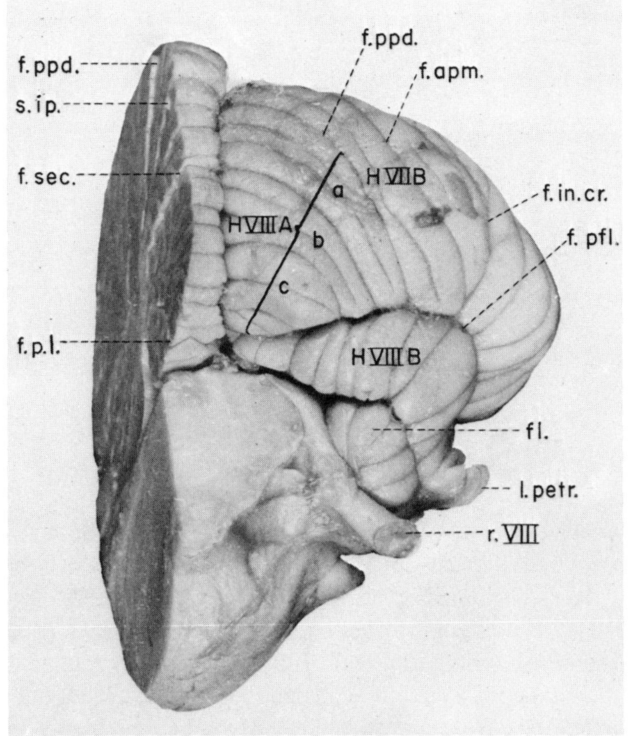

Figure 201. Cerebellum of mangabey. Posteroventral view of right half.

the baboon. The lobule is divided into the typical crus I and crus II, each of which is subdivided in turn into anterior and posterior parts. Crus Ia reaches the surface as a narrow folium but includes three deep folia, throughout most of its length, which constitute the posterior wall of the posterior superior fissure. Medially crus Ia is continuous with the deep and posterior portions of lamella VIIAa by a slender medullary band. Crus Ip expands laterally into many folia (fig. 199); medially it is continuous with the medullary substance of sublobule VIIA by a band of white substance which unites with the deeper portion of the band from crus Ia. Crus IIa and crus IIp converge into a broad medullary band that is connected with the large ray of the vermis leading to sublobules VIIA and VIIB. Two large folia forming the hidden posterior surface of crus IIp are continuous with the medially converged superficial folia.

Lobule HVIIB is so similar to this lobule in *Macacus* and *Cynocephalus*, both in vermal and hemispheral relations, that further description is unnecessary. The hemispheral segment of the ansoparamedian fissure dips into the posterior surface of lobule HVII, delimiting the two folia of crus II, mentioned above, from lobule HVIIB. The cleft between lobules HVIIA and HVIIB, on the one hand, and lobule HVIIIA, on the other hand, has the same relations as in the two species already described (fig. 201).

Lobule HVIIIA also is similar to the rhesus monkey and baboon in vermal relations and in its subdivision into lamellae HVIIIAa, HVIIIAb, and HVIIIAc. Lamella HVIIIAc is connected with the medullary ray of the superficial part of sublobule VIIIA by a fibrous band which merges with the one connecting sublobule VIIIB with the dorsal paraflocculus.

In *Cercocebus* lobule HVIIIB, the dorsal paraflocculus, as in the rhesus monkey, begins as small folia on a fibrous band that can be followed medially to sublobule VIIIB. The folia increase in size, as the series is followed laterally, and then diminish toward the petrosal lobule (fig. 201). The larger folia have a more extensive surface in the ventral wall of the parafloccular fissure than is true in *M. rhesus.*

Lobule HIX, the ventral paraflocculus, is larger than in the rhesus monkey but otherwise it is similar. Somewhat more so than in the rhesus monkey, this lobule appears to be a continuation of the flocculus but dissection shows hidden folia beneath the latter and a cleft between the two which is a continuation of the posterolateral fissure.

The lobulus petrosus was unsatisfactory for analysis in my material, since part of it had been torn off on both sides of the one mangabey cerebellum available. In the photographs of Retzius it is shown as a large lobule in several species of *Cercocebus*. The part of the lobule that remained in my material evidently corresponds to group *b* of the other monkeys and the baboon described.

FLOCCULONODULAR LOBE

Lobule X, the nodulus (fig. 198), is relatively small in sagittal section but is wide between the floccular peduncles. The flocculus, as in *M. rhesus*, conceals the proximal folia of the ventral paraflocculus and is relatively large (fig. 201). The floccular peduncle is short. The posterolateral fissure is distinct from the vermis to its confluence with a deep cleft between the ventral paraflocculus and the flocculus.

SPIDER MONKEY

THE cerebellum of the spider monkey (*Ateles ater*) is relatively narrow from side to side and high from the fastigium to the mouth of the fissura prima, which is on the dorsal surface. The anterior part of the dorsal surface slopes rapidly on either side of a ridgelike dorsorostral projection but the caudal part of the hemisphere is rounded laterally and posteriorly. The vermis is narrow and the paravermian sulcus is shallow except on the posterior surface, where it forms a deep cleft. A large petrosal lobule projects upward and laterally from the ventral paraflocculus, which it largely hides (fig. 203). The dorsal paraflocculus is closely apposed to the inferior lateral surface of the hemisphere.

CORPUS CEREBELLI

In surface view the anterior lobe is much smaller than the posterior lobe but in median sagittal section the anterior lobe has a considerably larger area. The fissura prima is unusually deep (fig. 202). The vermal lobules of the corpus cerebelli are elongated and the fissures between them are relatively deep. The lobules are similar in general to those of *Macacus rhesus* but are larger and more elongated; the pattern of the fissures corresponds to that in the 90-day-old *Macacus* embryo.

Lobule I in sagittal section shows three surface lamellae as in the macaques. In *Ateles*, however, the lobule has a much greater extension onto the ventrorostral surface of the hemisphere, forming a lobule HI which is larger in relation to the total size of the cerebellum than in any other species investigated. The hemispheral part represents chiefly a lateral continuation and expansion of folius Ic, as shown in figure 204. Precentral fissure *a*, separating lobules I and II and also extending between lobules HI and HII, reaches the lateral margin of the cortex.

Lobule II is relatively large and is composed of two elongated lamellae separated by a rather deep furrow which does not quite reach the cortical margin. Both extend onto the hemisphere as ovoid expansions, which together constitute a relatively prominent lobule HII (fig. 204). The precentral fissure, delimiting lobule II from lobule III, is deep and reaches the cerebellar margin.

Lobule III is greatly elongated in sagittal section, and extends rostrally beyond lobule II. It has three surface folia but the two small dorsal ones shown in figure 202 merge a short distance lateral of the midline and the lobule continues onto the hemisphere as two broad folia that reach the cerebellar margin and constitute lobule HIII (fig. 203A). The preculminate fissure is not much deeper than the precentral fissure but its dorsal wall is somewhat more foliated.

Lobule IV includes two large surface lamellae, six folia that form the dorsal wall of the preculminate fissure, and three folia in the rostral wall of intraculminate fissure

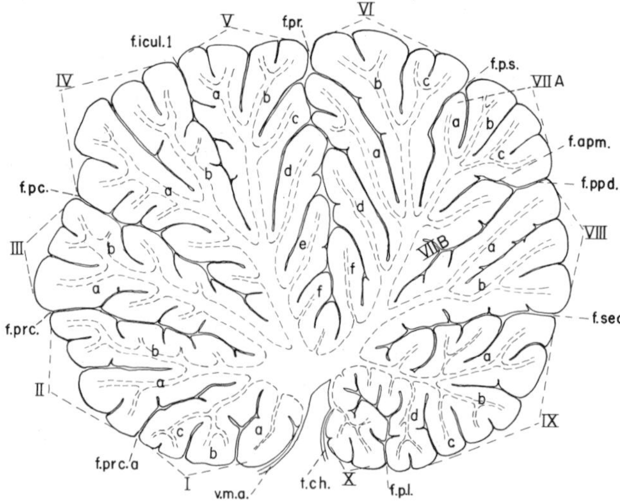

Figure 202. Cerebellum of spider monkey (*Ateles ater*). Midsagittal section. ×4.5.

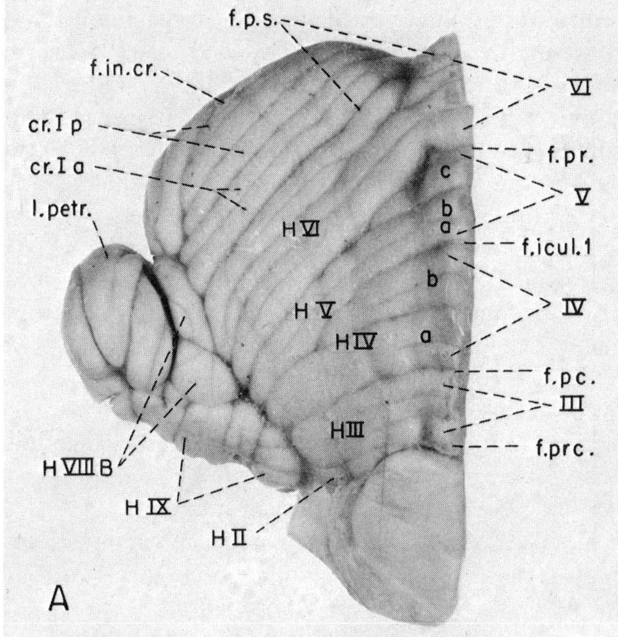

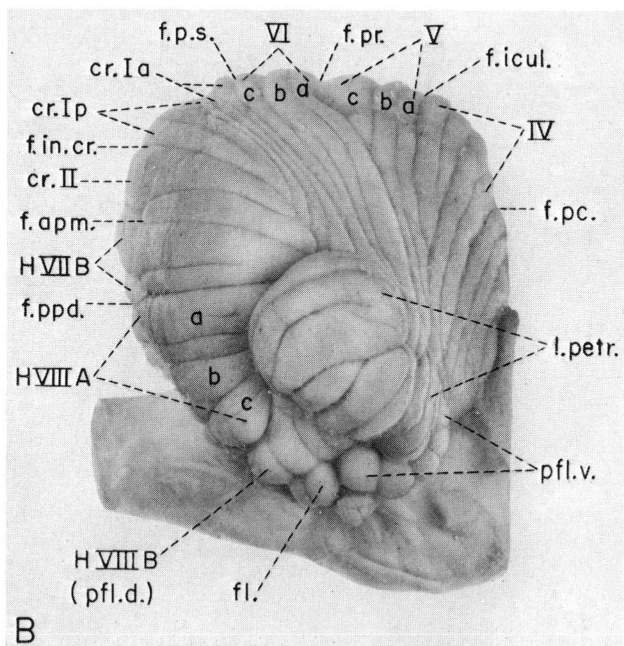

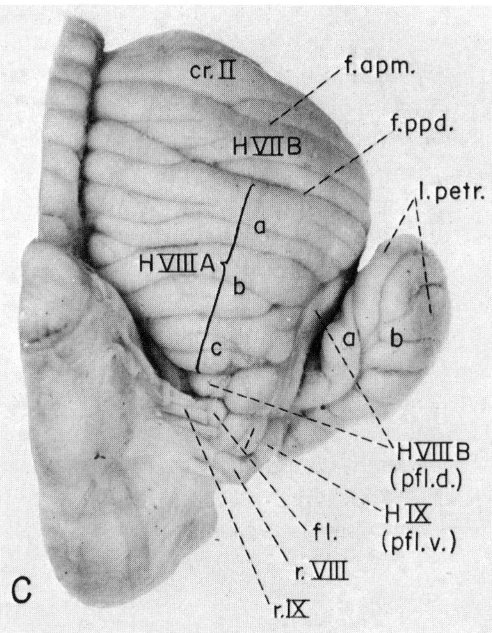

Figure 203. Cerebellum of spider monkey (*Ateles ater*). A. Anterior view of right half. B. Lateral view of right half. C. Posterior view of right half. Photographs, slightly retouched.

1. As in *Macacus*, intraculminate fissure 1 is shallower than the preculminate fissure but it reaches the cerebellar margin. The two superficial vermal lamellae continue into the hemisphere as lobule HIV, the more dorsal one sinks into the anterior wall of intraculminate fissure 1 (fig. 203A).

Lobule V is relatively narrow in the sagittal plane and has but four surface folia. If these are regarded as folia of lamellae Va and Vb, as indicated in figure 202, and the elongated folia forming the rostral wall of the fissura prima are regarded as folia Vc to Vf, as labeled, then the typical pattern of lobule V is present except that folia Vc and Vd both face this fissure. The superficial part of the lobule is unusually small as compared with other monkeys but the fissura prima is unusually deep. The two folia of lamella Va and the most dorsal folium of the caudal wall of intraculminate fissure 1 merge laterally into a single surface fold which continues to the cerebellar margin (fig. 203A). The superficial folia of lamella Vb merge laterally and the resulting single folium continue lateroventrally as a part of the upper rostral wall of the fissura prima. Folia Ve and Vf taper lateralwards for varying distances, forming the remainder of the rostral wall of the fissure. Lobule HV tapers rapidly lateroventrally into two elongated surface folia that merge before reaching the cerebellar margin (figs. 203A, B).

Lobule VI is relatively large in *Ateles* owing to the elongation of its lamellae and the depth of the fissura prima. Lamella VIa + e faces the fissura prima and lamellae VIb and VIc are both subfoliated. In an apparently immature spider monkey of undetermined species the same pattern is present but the cortex is less expanded and lamella VIa + e faces the mouth of the fissura prima as in the rhesus monkey. Lamella VId is similar in the two specimens and corresponds to this fold in other species of monkeys.

Lobule VII is small but the superficial folds behind the

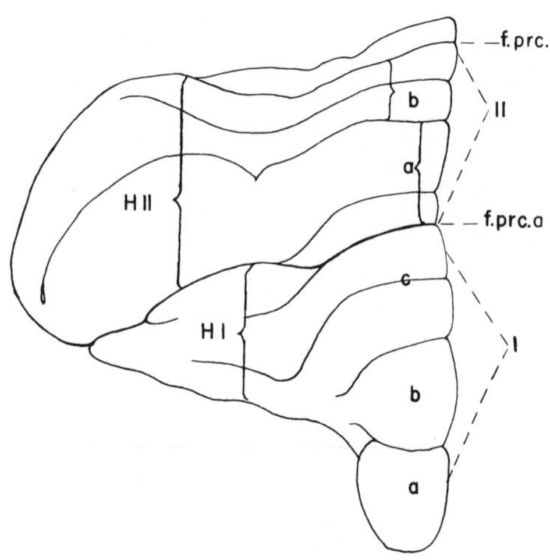

Figure 204. Cerebellum of spider monkey. Right half of lower segment of anterior lobe in rostroventral view. ×2.

posterior superior fissure (VIIAa, VIIAb, VIIAc, fig. 202) correspond in their hemispheral relations to the similarly designated folds of the rhesus and other monkeys described above. It therefore seems logical to regard these superficial folds as a small sublobule VIIA. The hemispheral relations of the two folds in the anterior wall of the prepyramidal fissure are obscured by the depth of the paravermian sulcus. The hemispheral segment of the ansoparamedian fissure, however, is continuous on one side with the vermal fissure so labeled in figure 202; on the opposite side the continuity appears to be with the more ventral and shallower fissure that is not labeled. The medullary ray of the larger lamella passes into lobule HVIIB. The two folds of the anterior wall of the prepyramidal fissure accordingly correspond to sublobule VIIB of other monkeys. The opening of the vermal segment of the ansoparamedian fissure into the compound furrow is nearer the cerebellar surface.

Lobule VIII is relatively small; sublobule VIIIA is reduced to an elongated lamella without superficial secondary folds and sublobule VIIIB is reduced to a lamella superficially divided into two folia. The lobule also is narrow from side to side. The medullary substance of its base expands laterally into a flattened band.

Lobule IX is large in median sagittal section and presents the four characteristic superficial lamellae, IXa, IXb, IXc, and IXd (fig. 202).

HEMISPHERAL LOBULES OF POSTERIOR LOBE

Lobule HVI is narrow and is delimited by deeper fissures than in other monkeys. The pars anterior and pars posterior are attached to the medullary body by a common medullary band (fig. 205). Superficially the lobule is divided into three lamellae, of which the anterior two constitute the pars anterior. The intralobular sulcus is deeply continuous on either side with the vermal segment of the posterior superior fissure. The two lamellae of the pars anterior are directly continuous with vermal lamellae VIa and VIb. A flattened folium in the anterior wall of the intralobular sulcus, in both right and left lobules of the larger cerebellum, is continuous with lamella VIc. In the smaller specimen a deep folium in the posterior wall of the fissure, on one side, crosses the fissural floor and emerges medially to continue with lamella VIc. Aside from such continuity with lamella VIc and evidence of fibrous connection with the deep part of the pars anterior, the pars posterior of both right and left lobules appears to be connected medially only with the deep part of lamella VIIAa and its anterior surface.

Lobule HVIIA is large and is divided into crus I and crus II, each of which is separately continuous with sublobule VIIA. Each also is subdivided into anterior and posterior parts as in other monkeys (figs. 203, 205). Crus Ia, however, emerges to the surface throughout its length (fig. 203A), medially it is continuous with lamella VIIAa and apparently also with VIIAb, by means of a fibrous band. Crus Ip has only three superficial lamellae medially but its posterior surface that faces the deep intercrural fissure is largely foliated.

Posterior of the intercrural fissure the hemisphere presents difficulties of analysis owing to the deep and narrow paravermian sulcus and the lack of recognizable continuity of vermal and hemispheral folia across the bottom of the sulcus. The ansoparamedian fissure, however, is deep and can be readily followed from the left hemisphere to the bottom of its vermal segment. On the right side the hemispheral segment of the fissure is entirely similar but its continuity with the vermal segment is less certain. It appears to end in the second furrow below the ansoparamedian fissure on the anterior wall of the

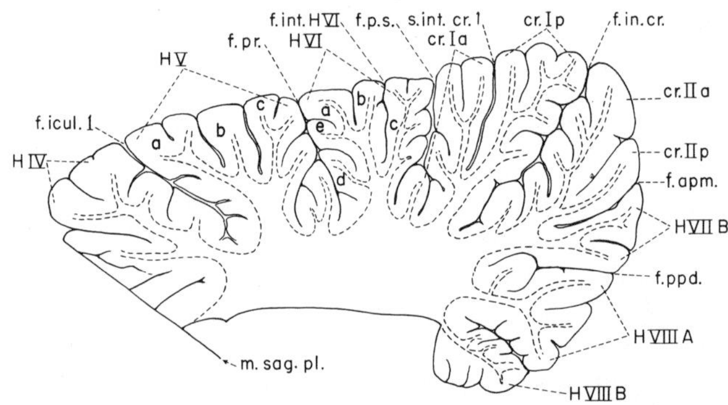

Figure 205. Cerebellum of spider monkey. Oblique, posterolateral to anteroventral section through right hemisphere.

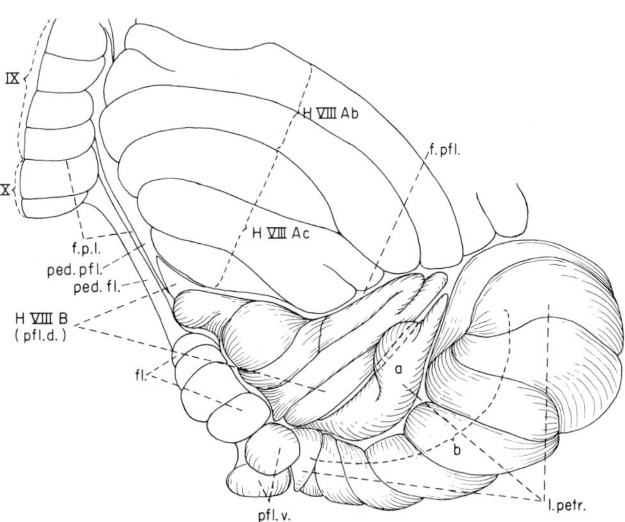

Figure 206. Cerebellum of *Ateles.* Posterolateral and ventral view of flocculus and paraflocculus.

prepyramidal fissure. Assuming that the developmental history of the ansoparamedian fissure of *Ateles* corresponds to that of the rhesus monkey, one concludes that the differences between the two sides probably represent failure of presumably separate vermal and hemispheral segments of the furrow to meet on one side, as in some cerebella of *Macacus.* The right hemispheral segment of the fissure in *Ateles* is continuous with the vermal segment (fig. 203C), and the vermal relations of crus II are entirely with the posterior part of sublobule VIIA. The surface lamella that is immediately ventral of the ansoparamedian fissure on both hemispheres and connected medially with sublobule VIIB must be recognized as lobule HVIIB.

Crus II of lobule HVIIA is composed of two broad lamellae, the dorsal one which is crus IIa and the ventral one which is crus IIp (figs. 203B, C). The furrow separating them corresponds to intracrural fissure 2 of the monkeys and baboon. Crus IIa is divided laterally into two large folds; the inferior one dips into intracrural sulcus 2 medially and forms part of the roof of this furrow. This fold appears to correspond to the second superficial lamella of crus IIa in the Old World monkeys and the baboon. Crus IIp is subdivided into narrower folia that dip into the roof of the ansoparamedian fissure.

Lobule HVIIB is broad medially, elongated laterally, and ends on the lateral surface of the hemisphere (figs. 203B, C). The limiting furrow behind the lobule is continuous medially with the deep part of the prepyramidal fissure of the vermis. It may be regarded therefore as the hemispheral segment of this fissure which, in *Ateles*, is not part of a compound furrow but is completely separated from the hemispheral segment of the ansoparamedian fissure.

Lobule HVIIIA comprises three lamellae that correspond to HVIIIAa, HVIIIAb, and HVIIIAc of the Old World monkeys and baboon (fig. 203C). Their medullary sheets are continuous with the ray of the base of lobule VIII which extends into the reduced sublobule VIIIA. Lamella HVIIIAc is relatively much larger than in the species just mentioned but its vermal connections are with a medullary sheet which divides medially into bands leading to the base of sublobules VIIIA and VIIIB. Distally the medial part of this sheet is elongated to form the peduncle of the dorsal paraflocculus (fig. 206).

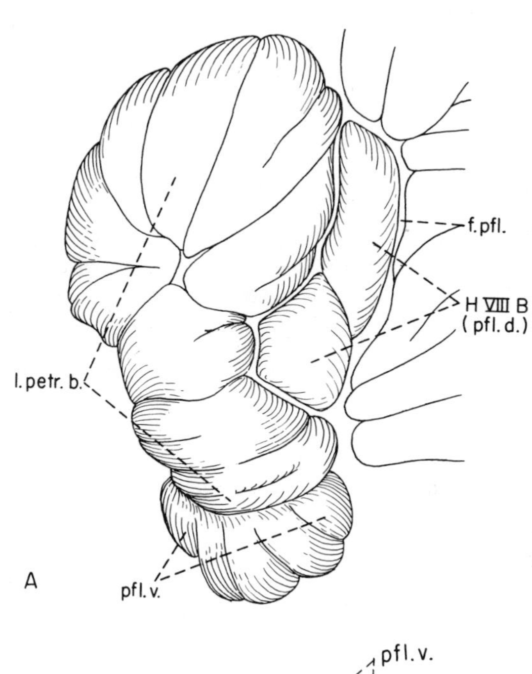

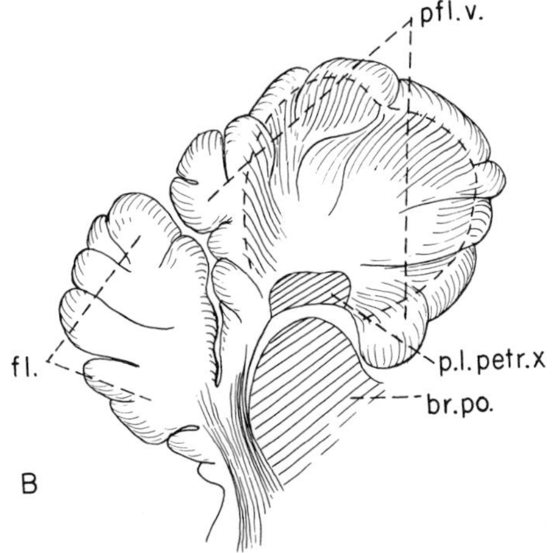

Figure 207. Cerebellum of *Ateles.* A. Anterior view of paraflocculus. B. Dorsal view of flocculus and ventral paraflocculus after removal of lobulus petrosus.

Lobule HVIIIB, the dorsal paraflocculus, in the smaller *Ateles* cerebellum is very similar in appearance to the dorsal paraflocculus of the Old World monkeys and baboon, as is also that of the larger specimen viewed ventrally (fig. 206). From the lateral aspect, after removal of the lobulus petrosus, however, it is clear that the folia are greatly elongated rostralward in the large cerebellum. Some continue between the lobulus petrosus and the hemisphere almost to the anterior cerebellar surface and form a narrow but dorsoventrally extensive rostral surface of the lobule (figs. 203A, 207A). Others continue as elongated folia onto the posterolateral surface of the parafloccular fissure which is greatly deepened in *Ateles* but is reduced to a narrow cleft by close apposition of lobule HVIIIB to the hemispheral surface. The lobule appears to receive a larger contingent of fibers from the brachium pontis than in the other monkeys and the baboon described above. Other fibers, upon dissection, appear to pass into the medullary body of the hemisphere. Presumably these are chiefly efferents from the parafloccular cortex.

Lobule HIX, the ventral paraflocculus, as in the rhesus and other monkeys, is composed of a series of folia that begin under cover of the flocculus and arch rostromedially and dorsally around the base of the petrosal lobule (fig. 203B). The folia surround the end of the parafloccular peduncle, forming the fringe of a concavo-convex plate in whose hollow the base of the petrosal lobule rests (fig. 207B). A thin sheet of fibers, separable from the brachium pontis, accompanies the latter into the medullary body of the hemisphere.

The lobulus petrosus comprises two principal divisions, both attached to the parafloccular peduncle. As shown in the photographs of Retzius, illustrating ventral views of the brain of several species of *Ateles*, the lobulus petrosus varies in size and degree of tilt dorsalward. In *Ateles ater* (fig. 203) it is relatively large and is strongly deflected upward and medially against the hemisphere. On dissection the lobulus petrosus appears to receive a considerable contingent of fibers from the brachium pontis.

FLOCCULONODULAR LOBE

The flocculus is superficially similar to that of other monkeys but upon dissection one sees that it is expanded terminally into a cluster of folia, at the end of the floccular peduncle, that has a somewhat rounded form (fig. 207B). The nodulus is small in my specimens; however, as illustrated by Riley in *Ateles ater* it is unusually large, relatively speaking, for a primate cerebellum. The floccular peduncle is short. The posterolateral fissure distinctly separates the flocculus and its peduncle from the parafloccular peduncle but the vermal part of the fissure is relatively shallow due to the small nodulus (fig. 206).

CAPUCHIN MONKEY

THE cerebellum of the capuchin monkey (*Cebus* sp.) has a high ridge anteriorly and dorsally from which a broad expanse of hemispheral surface slopes rapidly toward the ventrolateral cerebellar margin (fig. 209). A suggestion of a paravermian sulcus on the dorsal surface and a cleft on either side of the posterior part of the vermis mark the general boundary between hemispheres and vermis. The hemisphere is rounded laterally and posteriorly. The paraflocculus is nearly hidden beneath it posterolaterally but the lobulus petrosus is large and projects laterally, caudally, and slightly dorsalward (figs. 209–211).

CORPUS CEREBELLI

As in *Ateles* the anterior lobe has a much smaller superficial surface than the posterior lobe, but in median

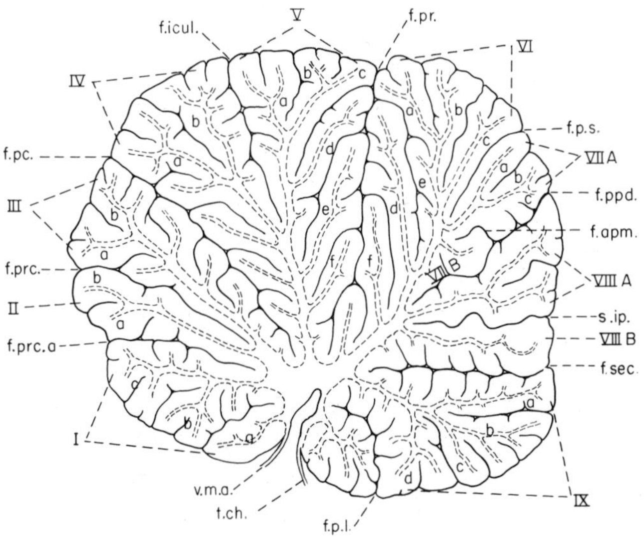

Figure 208. Cerebellum of capuchin monkey (*Cebus* sp.). Midsagittal section.

sagittal section (fig. 208) it is considerably larger. Lobule I is relatively large. The typical pattern of surface folds found in other monkeys is present in the form of definitely subfoliated lamellae rather than sublamellae and folia. Lamellae Ib and Ic extend to the hemisphere, forming lobule HI which is nearly as large, relatively speaking, as in *Ateles* (fig. 210).

Lobule II is narrow and elongated. It terminates as two surface sublamellae and extends to the hemisphere as a rostrolaterally elongated lobule HII. Precentral fissure *a* extends to the cortical margin, completely separating lobules I and HI from lobules II and HII. The photographs of Retzius include median sagittal sections of the cerebellum of *C. capucinus*, in which lobule II is shown as being shorter than in figure 210 but also thicker, so that it has approximately the same area as lobule I. The latter is smaller in these figures than in my specimens but the lamellar pattern of both lobules is similar to that illustrated in figure 210. In Bradley's (1905) figure of the cerebellum of *C. capucinus* the furrow that appears to correspond to precentral fissure *a* is shallow, which makes the two lobules appear as a single unit.

Lobule III is greatly elongated in the sagittal plane. It continues onto the hemisphere as an extended but narrow lobule HIII. The preculminate fissure, delimiting lobules III and HIII dorsally, is nearly as deep in the median plane as the fissura prima (fig. 208).

Lobule IV shares with lobule V a large medullary ray that extends one-third of the distance from the medullary body to the cerebellar surface before branching to the individual lobules (fig. 208). Intraculminate fissure 1, accordingly, is shallower than in most of the other monkeys described. Lobule IV has two large surface lamellae which continue onto the hemisphere as tapering folds that, together with the folia in the fissural walls, consti-

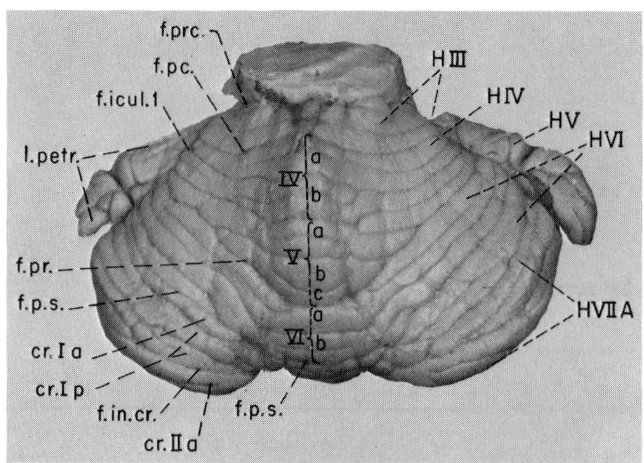

Figure 209. Cerebellum of capuchin monkey. Dorsal view.

tute lobule HIV (figs. 209, 210). In *C. capucinus*, as illustrated by Retzius, the two terminal lamellae of lobule IV are larger and intraculminate fissure 1 is deeper.

Lobule V shows the surface folds characteristically found in other species. Lamella Va is slightly larger than in *Ateles*, but Vb and Vc are small, with the posterior surface of the latter facing the mouth of the fissura prima. Lamellae Vd, Ve, and Vf are prominent in the anterior wall of this fissure. Lobule HV superficially includes only the hemispheral continuation of lamella Va except that medially, lamellae HVb and HVc converge on either side of the vermis and dip into the fissura prima of which the resulting lamella forms the dorsal part of the anterior wall of this fissure. Lamellae Vd, Ve, and Vf extend into the hemisphere as deeper but shorter folds of the anterior wall of the fissure. The folia in the posterior wall of intraculminate fissure 1 add to the cortical area of lobule HV but do not reach the surface.

Lobule VI is separated from lobule VII by a relatively shallow vermal segment of the posterior superior fissure in contrast with the deep fissures delimiting the other vermal lobules. This feature and the large medullary ray shared by the two lobules give the appearance of a single large lobule (fig. 208), as in the 90-day-old fetus of the rhesus monkey. When closely examined in comparison with other primates and with subprimates, and especially with reference to their relations to the hemispheral lobules, two distinct lobules are recognizable. Lobule VI includes three fairly large and elongated superficial lamellae, namely, VIa, VIb, and VIc and lamellae VId and VIf, which are also more elongated than in the Old World monkeys, while lamella VIe is represented by a folium. The elongation of lamellae VIa, VIb, and VIc makes declival sulci 1 and 2 more prominent than in the other monkeys that were examined.

Lobule VII is small but is divided into sublobules VIIA and VIIB, if one interprets the formation on the basis of the development of the corresponding segment in the rhesus embryo. The three lamellae reaching the cerebellar surface correspond to VIIAa, VIIAb, and VIIAc of other species. The ansoparamedian fissure from each hemisphere is continuous with the hooked furrow of the posterior surface of the lobule (fig. 208).

Lobule VIII is divided by a deep intrapyramidal sulcus into sublobule VIIIA, consisting of two lamellae, and sublobule VIIIB which is formed from a single much foliated lamellalike segment (fig. 208). In the photograph of Retzius mentioned before, the two sublobules are larger and the intrapyramidal sulcus is shallower.

Lobule IX is large and has considerable foliation. The fissura secunda is unusually deep, which results in a greatly lengthened fissural surface of the lobule (fig. 208). Four superficial lamellae, apparently corresponding to IXa, IXb, IXc, and IXd, are recognizable, but the pattern of their intervening fissures is not typical.

HEMISPHERAL LOBULES OF POSTERIOR LOBE

Lobule HVI, as in *Ateles*, is divided into a pars anterior with three superficial folia, and a pars posterior including two; the intralobular sulcus is deeper than in the

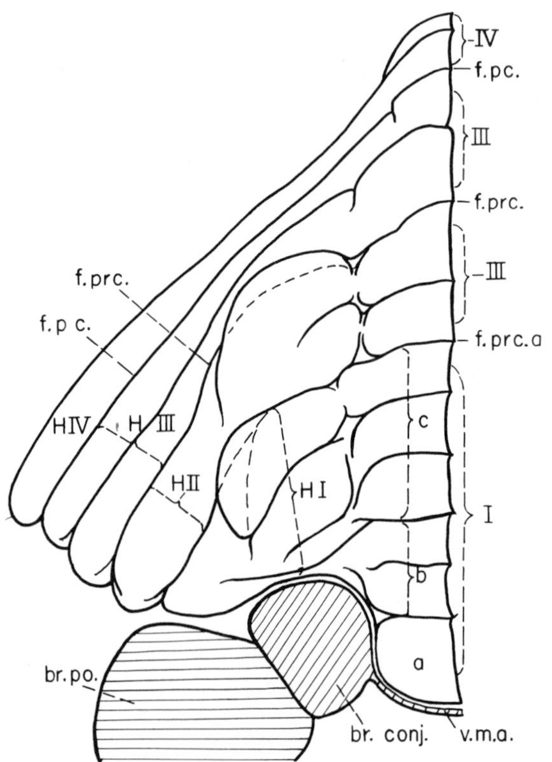

Figure 210. Cerebellum of capuchin monkey. Ventral view of right half of anterior lobe. ×5.

spider monkey so that the two parts are more distinct (fig. 212). This fissure of both sides is continuous with the posterior superior fissure of the vermis. The pars posterior superficially appears more closely related to lamella VIIAa than with VIc, but it has deep connections with the latter.

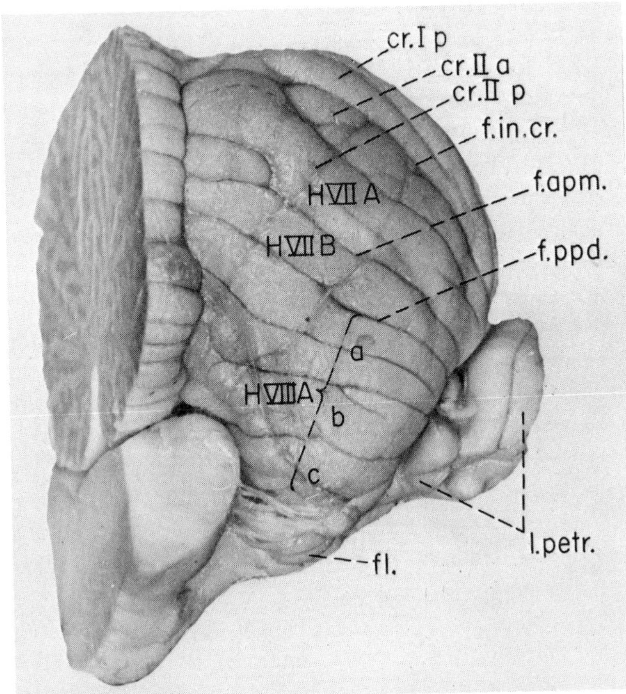

Figure 211. Cerebellum of capuchin monkey. Posteroventral view of right half.

Lobule HVIIA forms the posterior part of the dorsal surface and the upper part of the posterior surface of the hemisphere (fig. 211). The intercrural fissure is deep and its walls are considerably foliated (fig. 212). It opens externally near the posterior margin of the dorsal surface, running parallel with this margin. Crus I has but four principal superficial folds, with the folia in its deep related fissures accounting for the greater part of its cortical surface. The two anterior folds and their subjacent folia are separated from the posterior group by a deep furrow that opens onto the superficial surface and corresponds to intracrural sulcus 1. The lamella comprising two superficial folia anterior to this fissure constitutes crus Ia; it is continuous with the posterior and deep part of lamella VIIAa. The posterior group forms crus Ip and is continuous by a medullary band with the medullary ray of sublobule VIIA. Crus II is less deeply subdivided into crus IIa and crus IIp, and the latter tapers onto the lateral surface as a relatively small lamella (figs. 209, 211). Crus II is continuous medially with the caudal folia of sublobule VIIA and the medullary ray leading to them.

Lobule HVIIB is divided medially into two superficial sublamellae; the dorsal one dips into the inferior wall of the ansoparamedian fissure and continues lateralward as entirely submerged folia. Submerged folia of the superior wall of the prepyramidal fissure also add to the cortical surface of the lobule; some of these emerge to the surface and blend laterally with the superficial sublamella. The medullary sheet of the lobule is, in part, a continuation of the rays of sublobule VIIB and, in part, a branch of the common medullary ray leading to lobules VI and VII.

Lobule HVIIIA, as in other monkeys, comprises three lamellae (fig. 211). Lamella HVIIIAa is subdivided into two superficial folia throughout its length on the right side; in the left hemisphere the anterior folium disappears in the hemispheral segment of the prepyramidal fissure. Lamellae HVIIIAb and HVIIIAc include two and three superficial folia, respectively. Lamella HVIIIAc is relatively large and is crowded ventralward and laterally so that it extends onto the ventrolateral surface of the hemisphere. The connections of all three lamellae are similar to those of the corresponding lamellae in the other monkeys and the baboon.

Lobule HVIIIB, the dorsal paraflocculus, is similar to that of *Ateles* in both its resemblance to this lobule in other monkeys when seen from the ventrolateral angle and the elongation of its folia. As seen from the dorsolateral angle the more lateral folia extend dorsorostrally as long terminally expanded plates separated by relatively deep furrows, while the medial folia continue into the lateral wall of the narrow but deep parafloccular fissure. The result is an elongated lobule of considerable size which is closely pressed against the inferior part of the

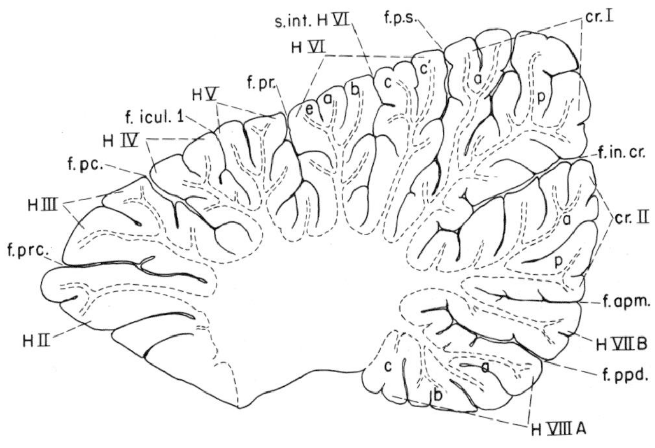

Figure 212. Cerebellum of capuchin monkey. Oblique section, posterolateral to anteromedial, through right hemisphere.

posterolateral surface of the hemisphere (fig. 213). As in *Ateles*, the dorsal paraflocculus of *Cebus* represents a transitional form between that of the Old World monkeys and the baboon, on the one hand, and the medial division of the biventral lobule of the chimpanzee and gorilla, described below.

Some of the dorsal parafloccular folia are more elongated in the baboon than in the Old World monkeys, and they also have a larger surface facing the parafloccular fissure. All are short, however, in comparison with *Cebus* and *Ateles*, and none in the baboon extend dorsolaterally and forward between the principal mass of the hemisphere and the petrosal lobule. Also the dorsal paraflocculus of the baboon and the Old World monkeys is more distinct from the hemisphere.

The ventral paraflocculus of *Cebus* (fig. 213) has the same general relationships as in *Ateles* but the terminal rosette lies medial of the laterally projecting lobulus petrosus, the base of which rests in a caplike depression of the ventral paraflocculus. This relation of the lobulus petrosus and the ventral paraflocculus (called paraflocculus by Bradley, 1903) is illustrated in figure 56 of Bradley.

The lobulus petrosus extends lateroposteriorly and dorsally as a thick stalk which ends in a rounded expansion (figs. 209, 211, 213). Surrounding most of the base of the expanded part is a rounded groove that evidently had been formed by the bony margin of the petrosal recess. The lobule comprises two series of folia separated by a deep fissure. The anterolateral series forms the anterior part of the stalk and most of the terminal expansion. The posteromedial series ends in a clublike process. When the flocculus and ventral paraflocculus were removed one could see the petrosal lobule attached to the parafloccular peduncle. The two series of folia apparently correspond to subdivisions *a* and *b*, respectively, of the rhesus

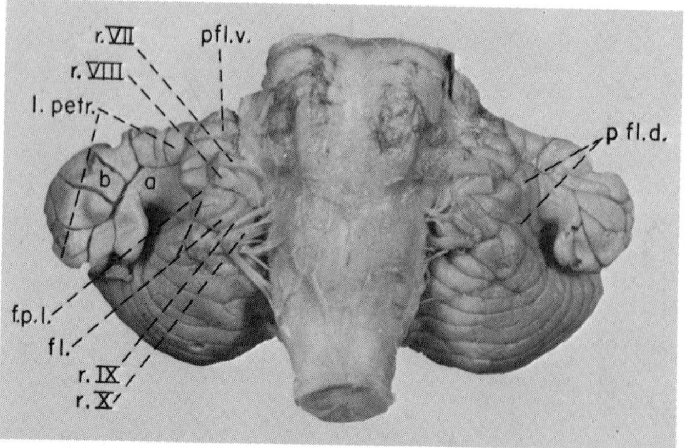

Figure 213. Cerebellum of capuchin monkey. Ventral view of cerebellum, medulla oblongata, and pons.

embryos but the relations of their attachments could not be determined.

A review of the petrosal lobule in the monkeys and baboon leaves questions about its relations to the dorsal and ventral paraflocculus, respectively. In the 90-day- and 115-day-old fetuses of *M. rhesus* its connections appear to be with the ventral parafloccular part of the parafloccular peduncle. Folia which I grouped as *a* of the adult cerebellum, however, appear to be more closely related to the dorsal paraflocculus and group *b* appears to be more closely related to the ventral paraflocculus in all the species studied. Scholten (1946) referred to the lobulus petrosus of *Cebus* as an appendage of the ventral paraflocculus but I was unable to wholly eliminate a relationship with the dorsal paraflocculus also in any of the adult cerebella studied.

Many earlier authors regarded the Nebenflocke of Henle in man as the homolog of the paraflocculus of animals, but the homology of the ventral paraflocculus with the tonsilla and the dorsal paraflocculus with part of the biventral lobule makes it necessary to seek another structure that corresponds to the Nebenflocke or accessory paraflocculus, as I designated it (Larsell, 1947) in the human fetus. The relations of the accessory paraflocculus to the tonsilla in the human embryo are more fully described later.

Jansen (1954, p. 57) regarded the accessory paraflocculus in the whale, elephant, and seal as being homologous with the human Nebenflocke. Whether the lobulus petrosus of monkeys and such subprimates as the rabbit and other species in which part of the paraflocculus complex has been similarly named also corresponds to the accessory paraflocculus or Nebenflocke remains an open question at present. Experimental studies are needed to establish the vermal and other connections of the lobulus petrosus and its relations to the dorsal and the ventral paraflocculus, respectively, more accurately than was possible by dissection. Should it prove to be connected with the ventral paraflocculus part of the peduncle and, through it, with the uvula, homology with the accessory paraflocculus would be favored. Although I was inclined to regard the lobulus petrosus of the monkeys and baboon as corresponding to the reduced accessory paraflocculus of the great apes and man, described later on, this homology is still not established beyond question. In addition to experimental studies on primates a comprehensive restudy of the lobulus petrosus of the rabbit and other subprimates is also needed.

FLOCCULONODULAR LOBE

Lobule X, the nodulus, is small in median sagittal section as illustrated in figure 208, as well as in the figures of

Cebus in the publications of Bradley and Retzius. In Riley's figure of a corresponding section of *C. capucinus* this lobule is usually large in comparison with other monkeys. The flocculus comprises a series of five or six folia and is directed rostrolaterally, abutting against lamella HVIIIAc posteriorly (fig. 213). A short floccular peduncle connects it with the nodulus and spreads out beneath the proximal floccular folia as a medullary layer of the lobule. The floccular and parafloccular peduncles are separated by a shallow groove which is continuous with the vermal segment of the posterolateral fissure. In the lateral direction, this is continuous with the parafloccular fissure, between the dorsal paraflocculus and lamella HVIIIAc.

CHIMPANZEE

THE anthropoid ape material available included one cerebellum from a young chimpanzee, one from an evidently mature chimpanzee, and one from a young gorilla. The cerebellum of both species is much more similar to the human than to any of the monkey cerebella described. The homologies of many of the fissures and lobules with those of subprimates and monkeys, however, could be established only by following their development in the fetus. Since fetal stages of the apes were unavailable it seemed safe to apply the results of developmental studies of the monkey cerebellum, already described, and the human cerebellum, described in a subsequent volume, to the interpretation of the lobules and fissures of the anthropoid apes. We will consider the chimpanzee cerebellum first for several reasons. First, the chimpanzee cerebellum more closely resembles the human cerebellum than it does that of the gorilla. Second, the photographs of Retzius (1906) and the figure of Flatau and Jacobsohn (1899), Bolk (1906), and Riley (1929) provide six median sagittal sections and various aspects of surface views of eight chimpanzee cerebella for comparison with my own specimens.

The cerebellum of the chimpanzee (*Pan pan*) is large and wide. Its hemispheres are prominent and rounded posteriorly; their dorsoanterior surface (fig. 214) presents a broad, slightly concave expanse that slopes forward and laterally and then turns ventromedially at the lateral margin to form the anterior part of the ventral cerebellar surface. This surface is separated from the posterior ventral surface (fig. 215) by a prominent cleft corresponding to the human transverse cerebellar fossa except that it is directed ventromedially instead of transversely from the rounded lateral surface of the hemisphere. The paravermian sulcus is deep and prominent posteriorly; in the larger cerebellum it continues forward on the dorsorostral surface almost to the fissura prima. The vermis lies below the surface contour of the hemispheres as a narrow sunken ridge, projecting beyond the hemispheral surface only anteriorly. Lobules resembling the human biventral lobule and the tonsilla were found in the medial part of the posteroventral surface (fig. 218). The flocculus is relatively large.

CORPUS CEREBELLI

The anterior lobe differs in the number and size of its subdivisions in my specimens and also in the illustrations of other authors. In the small cerebellum illustrated in figure 217 three deep fissures divide this lobe into four major segments. The adult cerebella represented in figure 216A, B show five and four major divisions, respectively, if the furrow labeled intraculminate fissure 1 in both may be regarded as homologous with that designated as such in figure 217. The interpretation of these segments in terms of the typical lobules of the anterior lobe is dependent upon establishing the preculminate fissure. As labeled, the fissure corresponds to the preculminate fissure of monkey and human fetuses. In the human fetus, in which the development of the vermal fissures and lobules has been followed in numerous stages, the preculminate fissure is the first to appear between the fissura prima and the anterior medullary velum; it divides the anterior lobe into dorsal and ventral segments, as in fetal subprimates. These segments do not undergo subdivision in the shrews and small bats, as already pointed out, and the preculminate fissure remains as the only one in the lobe. In man, as in all subprimates of which fetal material has been available, except the small bat *Corynorhinus*, the ventral segment differentiates into lobules I, II, and III; the dorsal one divides into lobules IV and V. As more fully described in a later section lobules I and II are subject to a great deal of variation in the human fetus but lobule III, the central lobule, is fairly constant

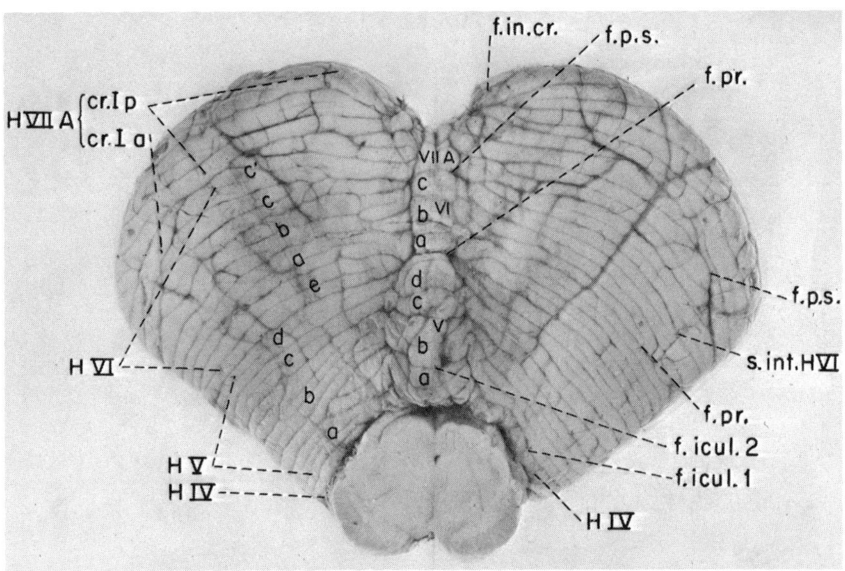

Figure 214. Cerebellum of chimpanzee (*Pan pan*). Large specimen. Dorsal view.

in size and pattern. The culmen, especially its anterior portion, also varies in pattern but intraculminate fissure 1 divides it into lobules IV and V. The preculminate fissure is recognizable from fetal stages to the adult as the boundary between vermal lobules III and IV and between the alae of the central lobule (lobule HIII) and the rostral part of the anterior quadrangular lobule (lobule HIV).

The fissure interpreted as the preculminate in the chimpanzee corresponds, with respect to position and relation to the culmen and the hemispheral lobules, to the furrow so designated in man, monkeys, and subprimates. Only two obvious segments, however, have their position ventral of the preculminate fissure in my specimens, in contrast with three in subanthropoids and sometimes in man (fig. 217). The more ventral of the two in the chimpanzee varies in size and form. In the small cerebellum (fig. 217) and in Riley's (1929) figure this segment is relatively large and its subdivisions all appear to be folia of one lobule. In my larger specimen (fig. 216A) and in two of the photographs of Retzius (1906, plate 51, fig. 6 and plate 51, fig. 7) it is smaller, whereas the folium covering the base of the anterior medullary velum is more elongated and also is separated from the other folia by a deeper furrow (fig. 216B). The figures of Retzius show the folium as being

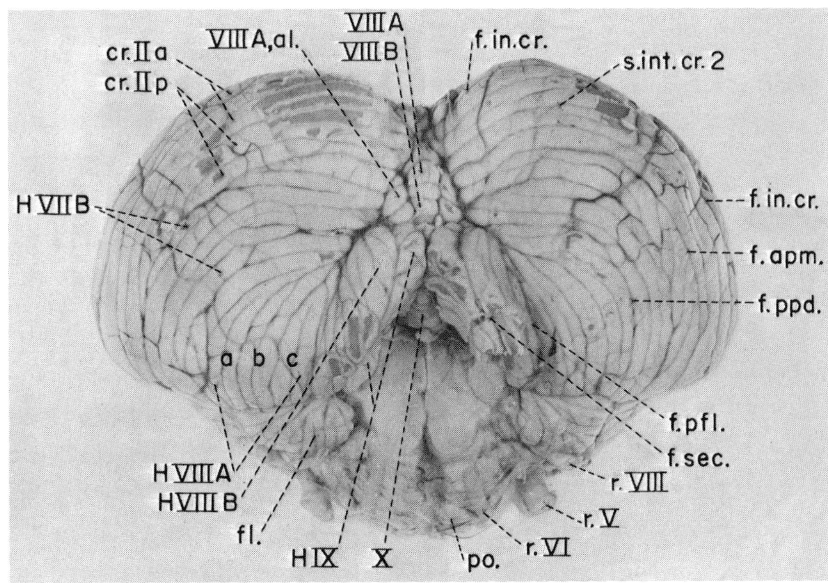

Figure 215. Cerebellum of chimpanzee. Large specimen. Ventral view.

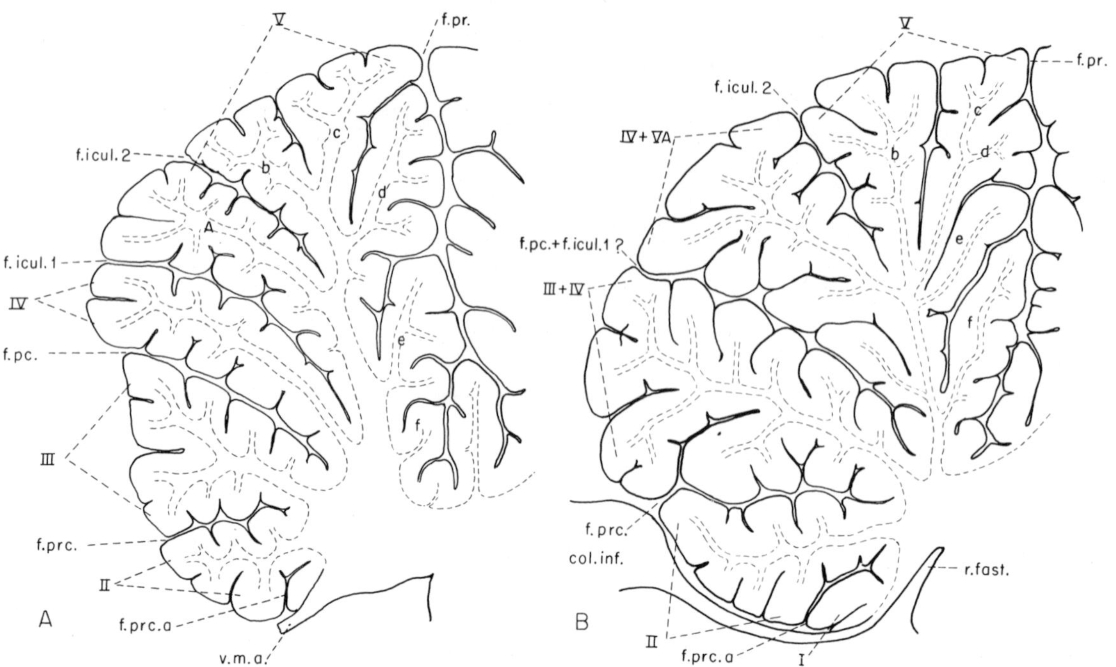

Figure 216. Cerebellum of chimpanzee. Midsagittal sections. A. Large specimen. ×4.5. B. Tracing from Retzius (1906, fig. 6, plate 3).

longer than in figure 216A, and the magnifying glass reveals several small folia so that it may be regarded as a lamella.

The adult human cerebellum has a similar but more elongated layer of cortex extending to the anterior medullary velum when the sublobulus centralis anterior of Ziehen is present, but it is much less extensive than the lingula as usually described. The sublobulus centralis anterior, as more fully pointed out in the description of the human cerebellum, is lobule II; the folia covering the medullary sheet which is continuous with the anterior medullary velum represent a rudimentary lobule I. In the illustrations mentioned above of six chimpanzee cerebella which have been compared, a segment corresponding to the sublobulus centralis anterior, i.e., lobule II, is present but in some cerebella the folia that represent lobule I are merged with it. The distinct units, when present, seem to be lobules I and II as in man, and the single larger segment of some cerebella seem to combine these two lobules. In none of the six illustrations nor in my specimens does lobule II become reduced to a series of folia covering a rostral extension of cerebellar medullary substance as frequently happens in man.

Lobule I, as interpreted in the chimpanzee, does not extend into the hemisphere in my specimens. The furrow, homologous with precentral fissure *a*, which separates it from lobule II reaches the anterior cortical margin at a short distance lateral of the midline. In the young specimen the first folium of the apparently combined lobules probably represents lobule I and the furrow immediately rostral of this folium is precentral fissure *a* (fig. 217). The remaining ventral folia converge laterally and extend onto the hemisphere as lobule HII, which is composed of two superficial folia on the right side (fig. 218) but with only one on the left. The adult specimen has only one hemispheral folium on each side, and this one is a continuation of the vermal folium most rostrally situated in lobule II.

Lobule III is elongated rostralward and divides into two superficial sublamellae in the small cerebellum (fig. 217). In the larger one and in the photographs of Retzius it is more massive and terminates as two large lamellae (fig. 216). The corresponding segment, designated lobulus 2 in Riley's (1929) figure, is similar. Lobule HIII is relatively large in both my specimens; the rostralmost folia extend to the lateral part of the anterior surface of the brachium pontis (fig. 218).

Lobule IV of the young cerebellum is an elongated segment divided into two large superficial lamellae. Its medullary ray is attached to a large branch from the central medullary body that also leads to lobule V (fig. 217). In two of the photographs of Retzius a more massive segment, corresponding to lobule IV, has a similar attachment and is likewise divided into large terminal lamellae. Intraculminate fissure 1 in these cerebella is shallower than the preculminate fissure. In my larger speci-

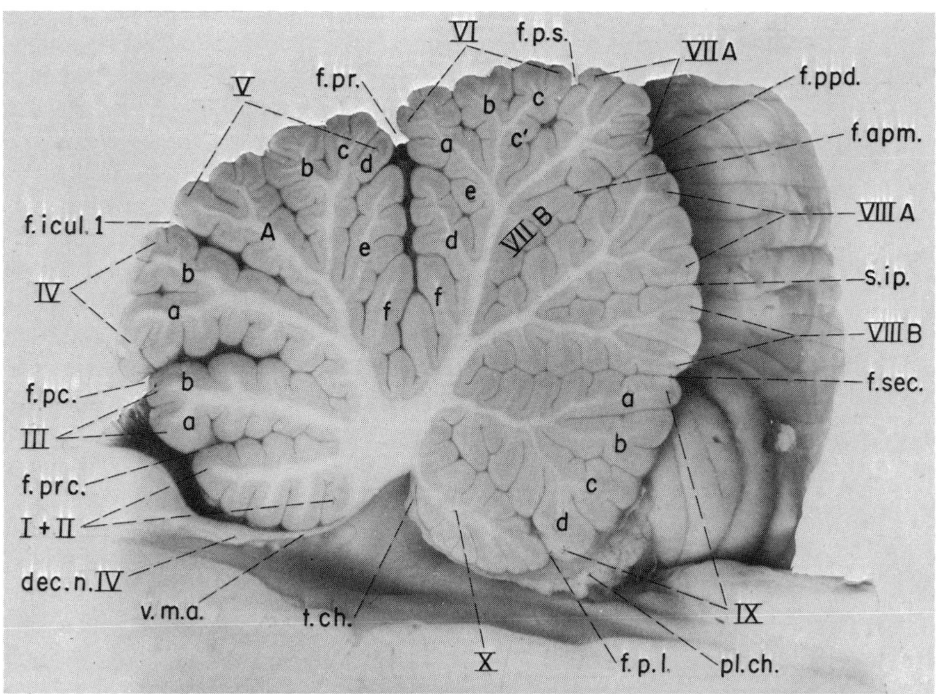

Figure 217. Cerebellum of small chimpanzee. Midsagittal section.

men, lobule IV is more slender in sagittal section and the terminal lamellae are relatively small. Its medullary ray may be regarded as branching directly from the medullary body which intraculminate fissure 1 almost reaches (fig. 216). The hemispheral continuation of this fissure was found on the upper rostroventral cerebellar surface, since expansion of the hemisphere evidently displaced it forward and downward from the dorsoanterior position which it occupies in the young cerebellum (fig. 218). The smaller size of lobule IV in the adult cerebellum appears to be compensated by a relatively large sublobule VA. Lobule HIV of the small cerebellum comprises the two anterior folia of the dorsorostral surface and a number on the rostral border and inferior surface of the anterior lobe (fig. 218). Intraculminate fissure 1, in contrast with the preculminate fissure, does not quite reach the cortical margin; a thin zone of cortex around its end connects lobules HIV and HV.

Lobule V varies considerably in the size of its subdivisions and the depth of its fissures. The pattern of the surface lamellae shown in the small cerebellum (fig. 217) is also represented in the larger one, as seen in the figures of Bolk and Riley and in one of the photographs of Retzius; in two of the photographs of Retzius the pattern of the surface lamellae is very different. In my specimens three lamellae, corresponding to lamellae Va, Vb, and Vc of subanthropoids, reach the surface but lamella Va is so large that it must be regarded as sublobule VA. In the large cerebellum (fig. 216) and in one of the photographs of Retzius, lamella Va is very large while in Bolk's figure the corresponding segment is relatively small. Lamellae Vb and Vc in my two specimens are similar to correspondingly situated folds in one of the photographs of Retzius and in Bolk's illustration; Riley's figure shows a much deeper fissure between the apparently homologous subdivisions than in the other figures mentioned or in my specimens. Lamellae Vd, Ve, and Vf, as illustrated in figures 216 and 217, conform with the general pattern in other primates except that Vd, if correctly interpreted, is small relative to the others in the young cerebellum and unusually large in the adult specimen. Two folds in Riley's figure correspond pretty closely to lamellae Vd and Ve of figure 216, and a more ventral one corresponds to Vf of figure 217 rather than to the small folium so labeled in figure 216. The corresponding parts of the photographs of Retzius are too indistinct for comparison and the figure of Bolk is too schematic. Lobule HV forms a broad surface area which, with lobule HIV obviously corresponds to the anterior quadrangular (anterior semilunar) lobule of man. It is separated, however, from lobule HIV by the deep hemispheral continuation of intraculminate fissure 1.

The anterior lobe as seen in median sagittal section of one of the cerebella illustrated by Retzius was reproduced in outline, magnified, and then carefully traced with the camera lucida, because it shows a striking varia-

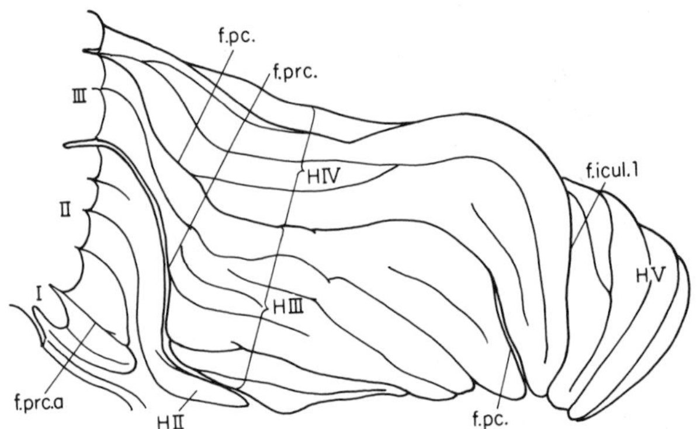

Figure 218. Cerebellum of small chimpanzee. Anteromedial view of left half of anterior lobe.

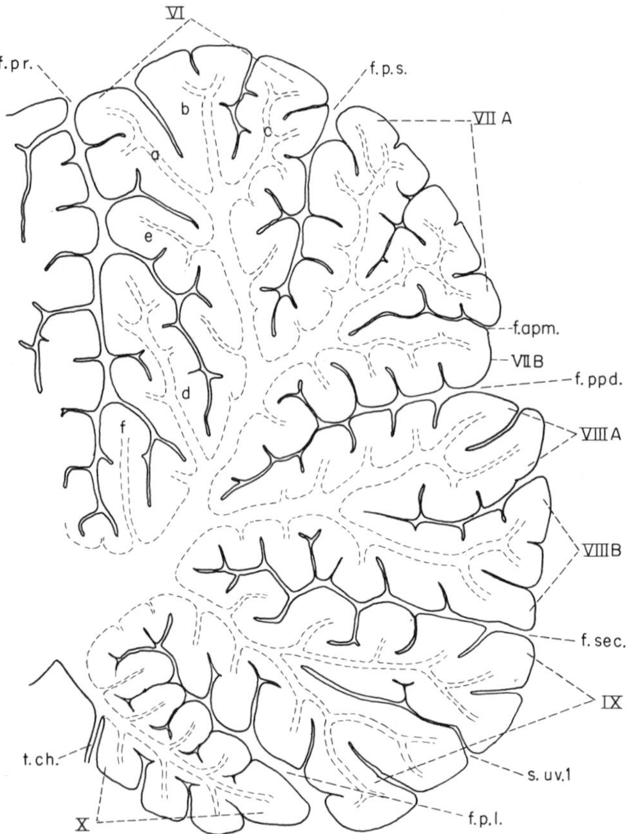

Figure 219. Cerebellum of large chimpanzee. Midsagittal section of posterior lobe.

tion from the apparently more common pattern described above (fig. 216B). In this cerebellum four large segments are shown, the most anterior of which can be subdivided into a small lobule I and a lobule II which is much larger than that in either of my specimens or in any other chimpanzee cerebellum illustrated in the literature. Lobule III, if the interpretation attempted in figure 216B is correct, is very large. Lobule IV appears to be combined in part with sublobule VA. Lamellae Vb, Vc, and those of the anterior wall of the fissura prima were interpreted as indicated in the figure because of their resemblance to the similarly situated folds in other specimens. The entire pattern of the anterior lobe of this cerebellum appears to have resulted from an unusual manner of initial folding of the cortex in the fetus. The large size of lobules II and III suggests that the former includes a portion of the cortex which usually becomes folded into the inferior part of lobule III and that the latter includes part of lobule IV as represented in other specimens. If part of lobule V is incorporated with lobule IV, as suggested above, the large size of the latter segment and the small size of the remainder of lobule V may have a plausible explanation.

In the posterior lobe, lobule VI is divided into distinct superficial lamellae VIa, VIb, and VIc and the characteristic lamellae VIe, VId, and VIf in the posterior wall of the fissura prima. Lamella VIe is a mere folium in the smaller cerebellum but in the large one it is a definite lamella, distinct from VIa (figs. 217, 219).

Lobule VII is divided into sublobules VIIA and VIIB. In the smaller cerebellum (fig. 217) the ansoparamedian fissure is situated as in the monkeys; in the larger one (fig. 219) the ansoparamedian fissure is represented by a deep furrow which opens on the cerebellar surface, with an elongated lamella intervening between it and the prepyramidal fissure. In one of the photographs of Retzius a similar deep fissure and an elongated lamella reaching the surface are pictured in the chimpanzee. The lamellae of sublobule VIIA are typical in the small cerebellum except that VIIAa is small. In the large specimen they form an atypical (as compared with the human cerebellum) combination of VIIAa, VIIAb, and VIIAc. In the photograph of Retzius, mentioned above, a lamella similar in general to the folium vermis (lamella VIIAa) of the human cerebellum occupies a corresponding position.

Sublobule VIIB, in the large cerebellum, includes the lamella which on one side separates the ansoparamedian fissure from the prepyramidalis; the contralateral ansoparamedian fissure ends more ventrally on the anterior surface of the prepyramidal fissure and overlaps the opposite fissure.

Lobule VIII is subdivided by a deep intrapyramidal sulcus into sublobules VIIIA and VIIIB. On either side of the lobule a group of short folia is separated from it by a sagittal cleft beneath which the folia are continuous with sublobule VIIIA, with the more anterior ones continuing onto its upper anterior surface. Apparently they are unrelated to sublobule VIIIB. These clusters of folia correspond to the alae of the pyramid, as designated by

Dejerine (1901), and the Nebenpyramiden of Henle (1871) in the human cerebellum. I have used the term copula pyramidis as was done for the homologous structure in other species described in this volume. These folia are shown in all of Retzius' photographs of the chimpanzee brain from appropriate angles but, as in man, they may not always be present as a distinct group.

Lobule IX (figs. 217, 219) is large in median sagittal section but is narrow from side to side. The fissura secunda and uvulonodular segment of the posterolateral fissure both are relatively deep. The lobule is divided into dorsal and ventral segments that are almost as large as the sublobules of lobule VIII by uvular sulcus 1 which is unusually deep in both my specimens and the photographs of Retzius. The dorsal segment is subdivided into two superficial lamellae which differ somewhat in the two specimens but appear to correspond to lamellae IXa and IXb. The ventral segment is subdivided into IXc and IXd.

HEMISPHERAL LOBULES OF POSTERIOR LOBE

Lobule HVI presents a broad superficial area very similar to the posterior quadrangular lobule of the human cerebellum. As in *M. rhesus* and other monkeys it comprises four superficial divisions which are expanded into definite lamellae and into the lamellae and folia facing its delimiting fissures. The lamellae are continuous with those of lobule VI in the pattern clearly shown in the smaller chimpanzee cerebellum (fig. 220), which also shows the division of the lobule into pars anterior and pars posterior (typically as compared with the monkeys).

The pars anterior of one side of both cerebella is continuous with vermal lamellae VIe, VIa, and VIb, as indicated in figures 214 and 222. Contralaterally the large anterior lamella of the larger cerebellum is continuous with lamella VIe only; the second and third lamellae, which are less deeply separated from each other, are continuous with lamellae VIa and VIb respectively. In the smaller cerebellum the secondary lamella of the pars anterior, which is continuous with VIe, emerges to the surface in the left hemisphere but is not deeply divided from what continues with vermal lamella VIa. The hemispheral continuation of lamella VId remains submerged in both cerebella.

The pars posterior of the smaller specimen is composed of two large lamellae. The anterior one is continuous, by deep folia from its rostral surface, with lamella VIc. The posterior lamella of the pars posterior is related medially principally with the deep part of sublobule VIIA and with the folia forming the surfaces of the vermal segment of the posterior superior fissure (fig. 220). Contralaterally, deep folia of the anterior lamella are continuous with the walls of the posterior superior fissure, and the posterior lamella is continuous with sublobule VIIA. The intralobular sulcus from the right hemisphere is confluent with declival sulcus 1; in the left hemisphere it appears superficially to be continuous with the posterior superior fissure but this results from the deep submergence into its floor of the folia of the anterior lamella of the pars posterior which are connected with lamella VIc. The left lobule HVI of the larger specimen conforms with the smaller cerebellum in its subdivisions and fissures (fig. 214). On the right side, however, although the pattern is almost identical as seen in section (fig. 222), the vermal relations of the three anterior lamellae appear to place them in the pars anterior, while the elongated fourth lamella seems to be the pars posterior. In general, beginning with the posterior lamella of the pars posterior, all the superficial lamellae of lobule HVI are advanced farther rostralward on one side than on the other with respect to their connections with the vermal lamellae. Dejerine (1901) described a similar pattern in the human cerebellum.

Lobule HVIIA corresponds to the combined superior and inferior semilunar lobules of man; the two lobules are separated by a deep furrow that is homologous with the horizontal fissure. The development of the subdivisions of the lobule and the horizontal fissure in the human fetus and the development of their homologs in the monkey and subprimates show that the superior and inferior semilunar lobules correspond to crus I and crus II, respectively, and the horizontal fissure corresponds to the intercrural fissure of subanthropoids. For convenience in further descriptions the terminology of comparative anatomy will be used.

Crus I is subdivided into two parts by a sulcus which appears at the surface medially and laterally on the right side of the small cerebellum but is hidden in the upper posterior wall of the posterior superior fissure on the left side. In the larger specimen the sulcus is hidden on both sides. This furrow, which corresponds to intracrural sulcus 1 of monkeys, delimits an elongated spindle-shaped lobule that is homologous with the deep lobule of the posterior superior fissure (lobule profond du sillon superieur de Vicq d'Azyr of Dejerine) in man, which I also found in the human cerebellum. This lobule also corresponds to crus Ia of subanthropoids. The posterior subdivision of crus I, which is relatively very large in the chimpanzee, corresponds to crus Ip.

The intercrural and ansoparamedian fissures, delimiting crus II, are deep and have a great deal of foliation in the walls. The intercrural or horizontal fissure is the deepest cleft in the hemisphere of the larger cerebellum.

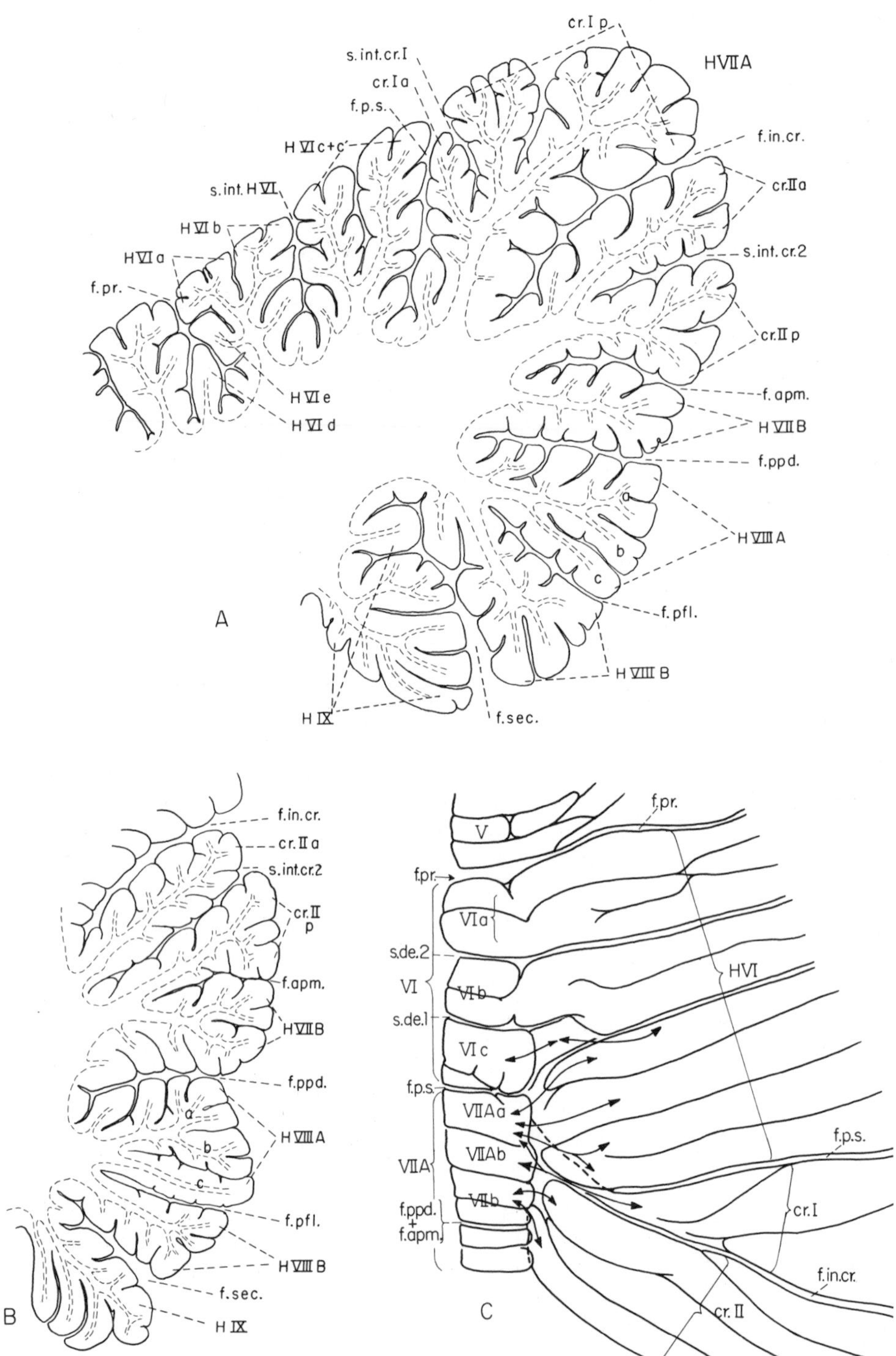

Figure 220. Cerebellum of small chimpanzee. A, B. Sagittal sections through right hemisphere (B more lateral). C. Dissection to show the relationship between vermal lobules VI and VIIA and the corresponding hemispheral lobules, HVI and crus I. ×6.

It arches from the vermis to the transverse cerebellar fossa in a wide arc on the upper posterior surface of the hemisphere and corresponds in every respect to the horizontal fissure of the human cerebellum. In the smaller specimen, with a less expanded hemisphere, the intercrural fissure is situated farther dorsally so that only its lateral part appears in posterior view of the hemisphere (fig. 218). It also is shallower than the ansoparamedian fissure, apparently because of incomplete dorsocaudal expansion of the hemisphere.

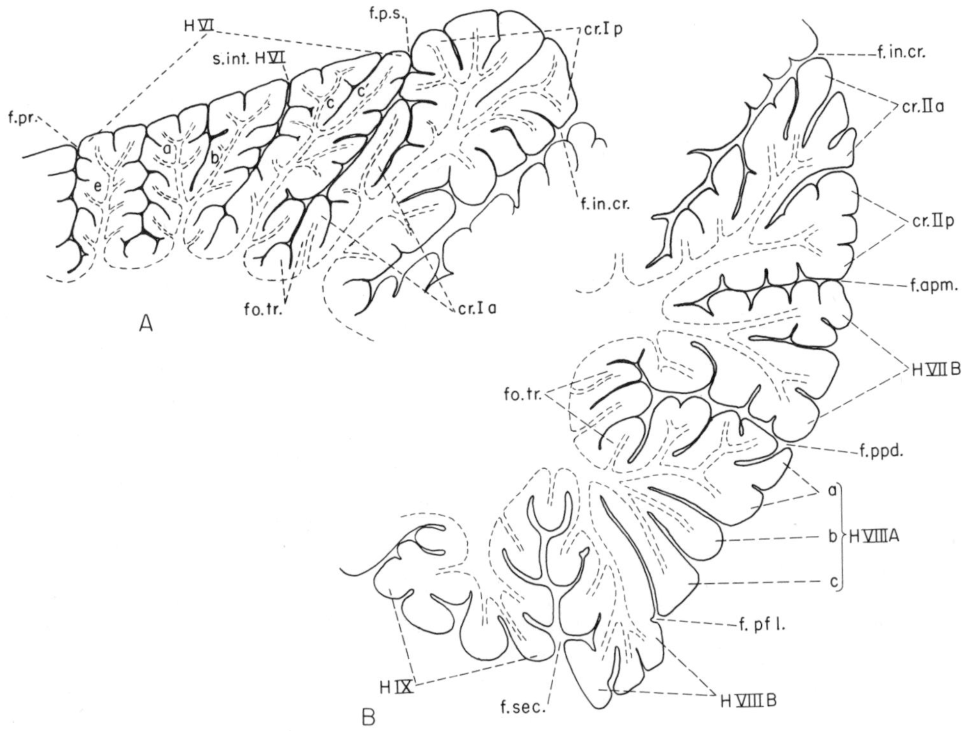

Figure 221. Cerebellum of large chimpanzee. Oblique sections through lobules HVI and HVII of right (A) and left (B) hemisphere.

The ansoparamedian fissure corresponds to the one so interpreted in the human cerebellum by Løyning and Jansen (1955) and to the posterior inferior fissure of conventional terminology. Dejerine (1901) referred to the ansoparamedian fissure in man as the "sillon inférieur de Vicq d'Azyr" (inferior groove of Vicq d'Azyr) and Schafer and Symington (1908) called it the sulcus postgracilis. In the chimpanzee the ansoparamedian fissure penetrates deeply between crus II and the remaining lobules of the posterior part of the hemisphere. The hemispheral and vermal segments of the fissure are directly continuous on both sides of the smaller specimen and on one side of the larger cerebellum. On the right side of the latter the vermal segment disappears in the depths of the paravermian sulcus which, on this side, intervenes between the elongated terminal lamella of sublobule VIIB and the hemisphere; the hemispheral segment of the fissure is confluent with a shallow furrow at the base of this lamella. In the 180-mm- and 200-mm C.R. length human fetuses (described in volume III) the ansoparamedian fissure continues from the left hemisphere across the vermis to the constricted zone between the vermis and the right hemisphere, but no definite confluence with the right hemispheral segment of this fissure is in evidence. The hemispheral and vermian segments of the fissure apparently fail to meet on this side of the vermis.

Crus II, situated between the intercrural and ansoparamedian fissures, is divided into sublobules crus IIa and crus IIp by a fissure which extends from the paravermian sulcus to the transverse cerebellar fossa. On one side of both specimens this fissure is visible on the posterior surface throughout its course, on the other side it disappears laterally into the ansoparamedian fissure but can be followed to the fossa. This furrow is intracrural sulcus 2. Crus IIa, which lies between it and the intercrural fissure, is a broad, much-curved lobule, which is subdivided into two large lamellae and medially is connected by a short medullary band to the similar band of white substance from crus I. The combined mass is continuous with the deep part of the medullary ray of sublobule VIIA (fig. 222). Laterally crus IIa reaches the transverse fossa and forms the greater part of its posterior wall in the larger cerebellum. Crus IIp, as seen superficially, is narrower. On one side it tapers lateralward and disappears into the ansoparamedian fissure but its folia form a thin plate in the lateral part of the roof of this fissure. It is not the same on the other side (right side of fig. 215); here crus IIp is visible superficially as far as the transverse fossa, with its lower lateral folia turning into the roof of the ansoparamedian fissure.

The hemispheral segment of the ansoparamedian fissure forms the dorsal boundary of two related lobules in one hemisphere and one lobule in the other (figs. 215,

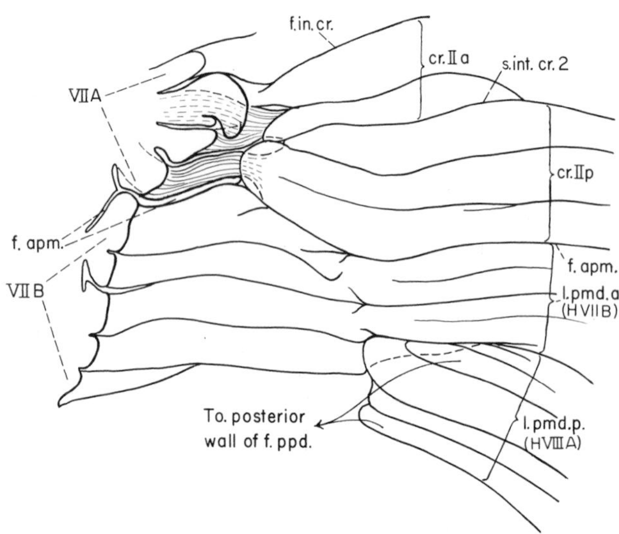

Figure 222. Cerebellum of small chimpanzee. Dissection to show the relations between the vermal sublobules VIIA and VIIB and the respective hemispheral lobules. ×6.

218) which arch from the posteromedial to the lateral inferior cerebellar surface. These lobules, on a reduced scale, resemble the lobulus gracilis of the human cerebellum as described by Dejerine (1901). The single unit, which is larger than either subdivision of the double lobule, corresponds to the single lobulus gracilis frequently found in man. In the large specimen this unit continues through many folia to sublobule VIIB but in the smaller one direct continuity with this sublobule is more limited (fig. 222), with most of the folia arching to the floors of its limiting fissures.

The vermal connections of both the dorsal and ventral sublobules of the double lobulus gracilis of the large specimen are with the folia below the elongated lamella and, across sublobule VIIB, with lamella VIIIAa. The ventral sublobule of the small cerebellum reaches the vermis by a single broad folium, which appears to be continuous contralaterally with lamella HVIIIAa. The remaining folia of the inferior surface of the ventral sublobule arch to the floor of the hemispheral segment of the prepyramidal fissure (fig. 222).

On the basis of its vermal connections and relations to the ansoparamedian and prepyramidal fissures, the lobulus gracilis of the chimpanzee appears to be homologous with lobule HVIIB of *Ateles* and *Cebus*.

Bolk (1906) included these lobules with his inferior semilunar lobule of the chimpanzee and favored the view of Flatau and Jacobsohn (1899) that the lobulus gracilis of this species is represented by segments corresponding to the lobulus biventer of man. Riley (1929), however, discriminated between crus II of the ansiform lobule and the "lobulus paramedianus" of the chimpanzee, and Løyning and Jansen (1955) homologized the lobulus gracilis of man with the paramedian lobule. Consideration of the remaining lobules of the hemisphere indicates that the lobulus gracilis of the chimpanzee (and of man) corresponds only to the anterior or dorsal part of the paramedian lobule of Bolk as represented in subanthropoids.

Medial of and parallel to the concavity of lobule HVIIB of the chimpanzee a smaller segment is situated whose vermal connections are chiefly with the anterior surface of sublobule VIIIA, although some of the deeper folia of its upper surface continue with the deeper folia of sublobule VIIB as already mentioned. This segment corresponds to lamella HVIIIa of monkeys and will be so designated for simplicity of terminology although it could well be considered a sublobule. The furrow separating it from lobule HVIIB is continuous with the prepyramidal fissure of the vermis as in *Ateles* and *Cebus*; this furrow, which appears to correspond to the sulcus prebiventeris of Ziehen (1934a) in man, was regarded as the paraflocular fissure by Løyning and Jansen (1955).

Medial of lamella HVIIIAa a group of folia that tapers strongly upward, medialward, and forward appears to be homologous with lamellae HVIIIAb and HVIIIAc of monkeys. On the left side of the large cerebellum this group is separated by a fairly deep furrow into medial and lateral divisions, each of which is composed of several folia; on the right side and in the smaller cerebellum

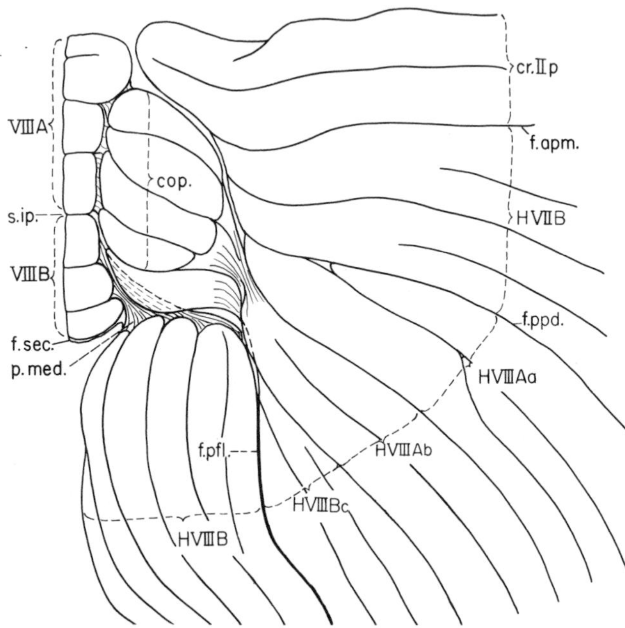

Figure 223. Cerebellum of small chimpanzee. Dissection showing relationship between the vermal lobule VIII, copula pyramis, and the hemispheral lobules. ×6.

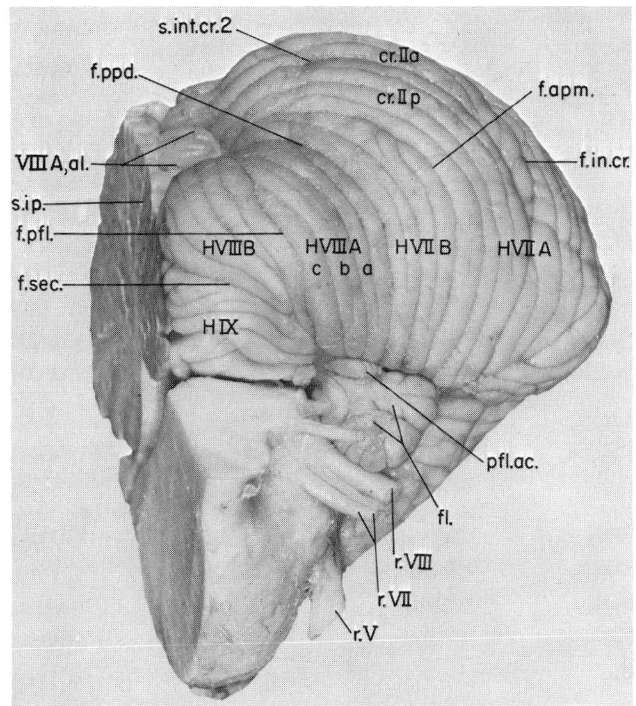

Figure 224. Cerebellum of small chimpanzee. Posteroventral view of right half.

such divisions are less obvious. The sublobule formed by these two lamellae is continuous with the copula pyramidis by a narrow collection of elongated folia (fig. 223). The three lamellae, HVIIIAa, HVIIIAb, and HVIIIAc, with little question, correspond to the lateral division or belly of the biventral lobule of man. Løyning and Jansen (1955) regarded the human biventral lobule, including the medial belly, as being homologous with the dorsal paraflocculus. In the chimpanzee, however, lobule HVIIIB corresponds to the medial belly of the biventral lobule and alone is homologous with the dorsal paraflocculus of monkeys. The furrow corresponding to the sulcus interbiventeris of Dejerine rather than the sulcus prebiventeris appears to be homologous with the parafloccular fissure of the monkeys.

Lobule HVIIIB (figs. 215, 218) is an almond-shaped structure which is connected with the base of sublobule VIIIB by a short peduncle that separates from the medially directed vermal attachments of lamellae HVIIIAb and HVIIIAc (fig. 223). This connection corresponds to that of the dorsal paraflocculus of monkeys. The folia are elongated as in *Ateles* and *Cebus* but are directed forward and downward, instead of forward and upward, owing to the increased size of the hemisphere. The lobule is not so flattened against the hemisphere as in these two species and is relatively larger. The lobule is separated from lobule HIX, the tonsilla, which lies medial of it, by a furrow that corresponds to the intraparafloccular fissure of Løyning and Jansen or to the sulcus inferior anterior of Ziehen (1934a) in man. Lobule HVIIIB corresponds to the medial belly of the biventral lobule of man which it resembles in general contour, position, and relations.

Wedged between the dorsal paraflocculus or medial divisions of the biventral lobule, on the one hand, and the medulla oblongata and uvula (lobule IX), on the other hand, is a lobule which bears little resemblance to the

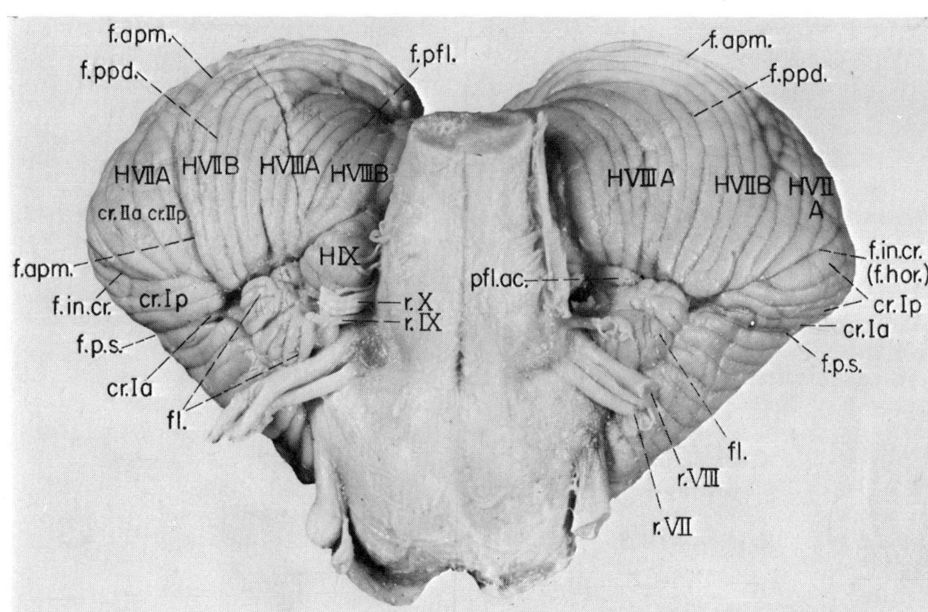

Figure 225. Cerebellum and brainstem of small chimpanzee. Ventral view.

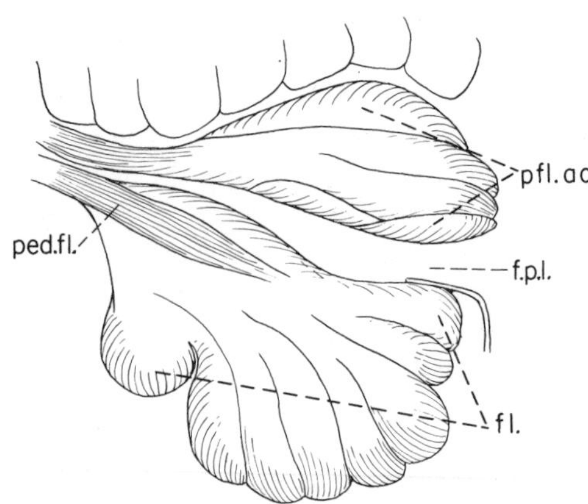

Figure 226. Cerebellum of large chimpanzee. Dissection showing the relations between flocculus and paraflocculus accessorius.

ventral paraflocculus of monkeys but corresponds to the tonsilla of man. Its vermal connections are with the base of lobule IX by means of a short, fibrous band. There is little continuity of cortex, however, from the uvula to the tonsilla; most of the folia of the uvula end on the lower part of its lateral surface and those of the tonsilla end on the short peduncle. The vermal part of the deep fissura secunda opens on either side into the paravermian sulcus which penetrates to the deeply situated peduncles of the tonsilla and the dorsal paraflocculus. No distinct continuity of the fissura secunda with the intraparafloccular fissure of Løyning and Jansen could be demonstrated in the chimpanzee material. In the human fetus, however, such continuity is clear so that it seems justifiable to regard the intraparafloccular fissure as the lateral segment of the fissura secunda. The connections of the tonsilla of the chimpanzee with lobule IX, and its development and lateral relations, as interpreted from the human fetus, make it clear that this lobule is homologous with the ventral paraflocculus of subanthropoids (figs. 215, 224, 225).

A small nodule composed of two reduced folia and situated between the ventral margin of the biventral lobule and the flocculus appears to correspond both to the Nebenflocke of Henle and to the accessory paraflocculus of Jansen. This nodule is attached to a medullary sheet extending from the peduncle of the tonsilla beneath the deep anterior surface of this lobule (figs. 225, 226). As noted below a similar lobule occurs in the gorilla. The accessory paraflocculus of Jansen in the whale, elephant, and seal and the apparently corresponding lobule of man, as shown in the human fetus, are related to the ventral paraflocculus. The lobulus petrosus of monkeys, which is very large in some species, also is related to the ventral paraflocculus but possibly may have connections with the dorsal parafloccular part of the parafloccular peduncle, as already mentioned. It does not seem probable, however, that so prominent a feature of the monkey cerebellum as the lobulus petrosus would entirely disappear in the great apes and it seems justifiable to regard the accessory paraflocculus of the chimpanzee and gorilla as being homologous with the lobulus petrosus of monkeys.

FLOCCULONODULAR LOBE

Lobule X, the nodulus, is relatively large and the vermal segment of the posterolateral fissure is deep (figs. 217, 219). The lobule is connected with the flocculus by a rather broad flattened peduncle which spreads distally into a rosettelike cluster of the floccular folia. The flocculus is relatively large (fig. 226) and extends farther laterálward than in man and the gorilla (figs. 215, 224). Together with the nodulus it constitutes a flocculonodular lobe which in proportion to the corpus cerebelli is somewhat larger than that in the human and, apparently, in the gorilla cerebellum.

GORILLA

THE cerebellum of a young gorilla (*Gorilla gorilla*) forms the basis of the description of the organ in this species. Comparisons have been made between the photographs in the monograph of Retzius (1906) of two adult specimens and the description and figures of an apparently adult cerebellum by Riley (1929). Superficially the specimen at hand mostly resembles that of the young chimpanzee already described. In median sagittal section, however, the vermis is higher and shorter and most of the fissures, except for the fissura prima, are shallower than their counterparts in the chimpanzee. Most of the vermal lobules are more massive in the gorilla.

CORPUS CEREBELLI

The ventralmost subdivision of the anterior lobe is small and at first sight it appears to correspond to lobule I of the subanthropoids. Comparison of the remaining lobules of the anterior lobe with those of other primates and man makes it clear that the vermal segment immediately above the ventral segment is lobule III, the central lobule. The first obvious segment then must represent either lobules I and II combined, or lobule II. Riley designated it lobulus 1, but his illustration shows a tongue of cortex extending onto the anterior medullary velum. Comparison with the variations of this region of the human cerebellum indicates that this layer of gray, shown as a flattened lamella in figures 227 and 228, represents lobule I, and the larger rostrally projecting segment immediately dorsal of it is lobule II. So interpreted lobule II is composed of three flattened folia on its surface and four larger folia dorsally. Only the most proximal folium of the dorsal surface extends onto the hemisphere as lobule HII; it is prolonged as a slender fold of cortex lying between the superior cerebellar peduncle and lobule HIII (fig. 229). Riley (1929) also illustrated a lateral extension of the anterior folium to the hemisphere. Retzius (1906) reproduced only one photograph of the cerebellum of the gorilla in median sagittal section. In this section the lobule, which I interpreted as corresponding to "lobule II" in my specimen and in Riley's figure, is reduced to an elongated series of folia resting on a rostrally directed sheet of medullary substance which is continuous with the anterior medullary velum. The folia correspond to the lingula as most frequently found in the human cerebellum.

Lobule III is large and compact (figs. 227, 228, 229). It has two large surface lamellae, IIIa and IIIb, which are similar to correspondingly placed lamellae of the typical central lobule of the human cerebellum. Lamella IIIb is the larger one in the gorilla, as is usually the case in man. The outline of the entire lobule in sagittal section is simi-

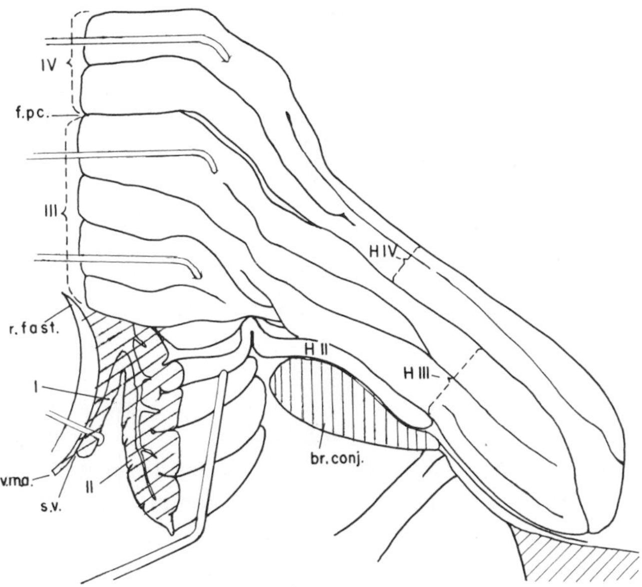

Figure 227. Cerebellum of *Gorilla gorilla.* Ventral view of left half of anterior lobe. Dissection. ×5.

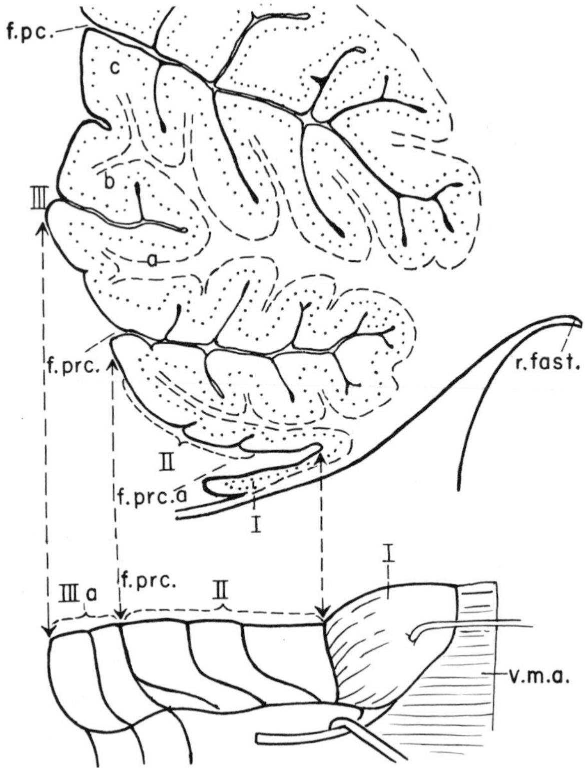

Figure 228. Cerebellum of *Gorilla gorilla.* Midsagittal section of lower segment of anterior lobe. ×7.

lar to that of the human central lobule, except that the lobule is relatively short in the gorilla. The large medullary ray leading to it is a direct branch of the medullary body. Lobule HIII comprises three folia which, as a group, form a winglike area similar to the ala of the central lobule in man. The preculminate fissure is deep and extends to the rostrolateral cortical margin. It is the most prominent fissure of the anterior lobe. The segment in the illustrations of Retzius and Riley that corresponds to lobule III is relatively smaller. Riley, who designated it lobule 2, described and illustrated a hemispheral extension similar to lobule HIII of figure 227.

Lobule IV is slightly longer than lobule III in the cerebellum illustrated in figure 229, but it has approximately the same area in sagittal section, and intraculminate fissure 1 is nearly as deep as the preculminate fissure (fig. 229). The corresponding segment in the figures of Retzius (fig. 230A) and Riley is relatively much larger. In all three cerebella its medullary ray branches from a thick stalk leading to that of lobule V. Riley designated the corresponding segment as lobulus 4A, omitting lobulus 3 in the gorilla because only two medullary rays leading to his lobuli 1 and 2 occur ventral of the large stalk that branches in the remainder of the anterior lobe. He subdivided this lobule into lobuli 4A and 4B. These two lobuli correspond to lobules IV and V, respectively, of figure 229. Lobule HIV is represented in the left hemisphere by a lamella on the anterior surface, which expands as it approaches the margin of the cerebellum, and by one on the dorsorostral cerebellar surface. In the right hemisphere both lamellae face the anterior surface.

Lobule V is relatively large in the gorilla; it is composed of three subdivisions that reach the superficial surface: one that faces this surface and the mouth of the fissura prima and three lamellae in the anterior wall of the fissura prima (fig. 229). If the subdivision immediately dorsal of lobule IV is regarded as lamella Va (or sublobule VA because it is larger and more deeply separated from the remainder of lobule V in the illustrations of Retzius and Riley), then the others correspond to lamellae Vb, Vc, Vd, Ve, and Vf of other species. All these lamellae are relatively large and Vd, reaching the dorsal surface, displaces those in front of it to a more rostral position than is usual with reference to the fissura prima. Lobule HV is represented by a large quadrangular area on the dorsorostral cerebellar surface (fig. 231). Together with lobule HIV it corresponds to the anterior quadrangular lobule of the chimpanzee and man.

Lobule VI is represented by one large and three small superficial lamellae, to which the typical lamellae VId and VIf in the posterior wall of the fissura prima must be added. In the Retzius photographs of the gorilla cerebellum the same pattern occurs but the lamella corresponding to the large superficial one of figure 229 is much smaller and faces the fissura prima (fig. 230B). In both cerebella this lamella appears to represent VIe. The three smaller folds behind it correspond to lamellae VIa, VIb, and VIc but they are smaller than in the chimpanzee and man. Their identity appears to be established in my specimen, however, by their relations to the lamellae and fissures of the hemispheres described below. The lamellae of the Retzius photograph that correspond to VId and VIf are reversed in relative size as compared with my specimen of the gorilla and with other primates as well as subprimates. The posterior superior fissure is much deeper in the Retzius photograph (fig. 230B) than in figure 229; Riley's figures of the gorilla cerebellum are too diagrammatic for detailed comparison but the lamella which I interpreted to be VIe is similar in size and position to my specimen. Lamellae VIa, VIb, and VIc are larger, and VId and VIf are similar to the folds so designated in figure 229.

Lobule VII is much smaller in my specimen than in the Retzius photograph, although the sagittal section in both instances was cut somewhat to one side of the median plane. Lamella VIIAa, as identified by its relation to crus Ia, is a mere folium in my specimen while in the

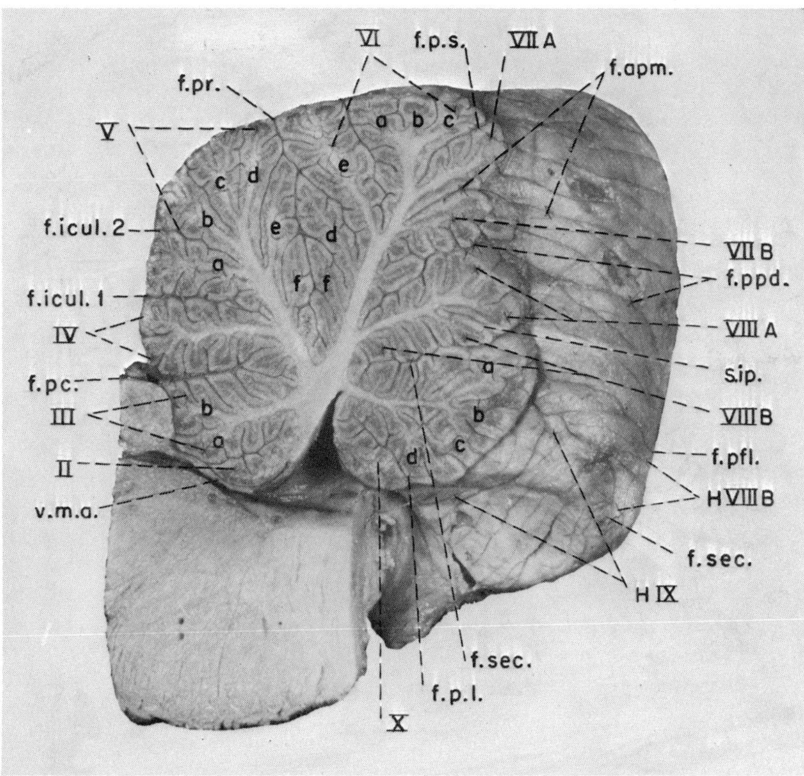

Figure 229. Cerebellum of *Gorilla gorilla.* Midsagittal section. Retouched photograph.

photograph of Retzius it forms a large and typical folium vermis (fig. 230B). The lobule is divided by the ansoparamedian fissure into dorsal and ventral subdivisions. The dorsal one, including lamella VIIAa, corresponds to sublobule VIIA; the ventral subdivision, facing the prepyramidal fissure, corresponds to sublobule VIIB (figs. 229, 230B). As in the chimpanzee and man sublobule VIIB is relatively large as compared with other primates.

Lobule VIII, the pyramis, is relatively small as compared with monkeys. Two superficial subdivisions, whose relations correspond to sublobules VIIIA and VIIIB, are separated by a shallow intrapyramidal sulcus. Sublobule VIIIA is continuous on either side with a small and almost hidden series of folia that correspond to the Nebenpyramiden of Henle of the human cerebellum and the copula folia of other mammals. On one side of lobule VIII the folia dip ventrally from the exposed surface of the pyramis and, after collecting into a somewhat constricted group, continue caudolaterally and expand in the lateral division of the biventral lobule (fig. 232A). On the other side the dorsalmost folium passes directly from the external surface of sublobule VIIIA to the lateral division of the biventral lobule. The deeper folia of this side arch caudolaterally from the lobular surface facing the outer portion of the prepyramidal fissure and continue into the lateral division of the biventral lobule. Sublobule VIIIB, which is reduced to a lamella superficially, includes the series of cortical folds facing the fissura secunda (fig. 229). These folds converge laterally to form a constricted zone, beyond which they expand onto the medial division of the biventral lobule. The group of folia connected with sublobule VIIIB is separated from that continuous with sublobule VIIIA by a wide lateral continuation of the intrapyramidal sulcus.

Lobule IX, the uvula, is roughly triangular in sagittal section (fig. 229); the apex of the triangle attaches to the central medullary body by a prominent medullary ray. From this apical region the lobule expands caudally and ventrally, which creates an extensive area in sagittal section. A deep cleft on either side separates the lobule from the tonsilla so that it forms a narrow, caudally projecting plate. A short fibrous peduncle connects the basal part of its medullary ray with the medullary substance of the tonsilla. The superficial surface is divided into four lamellae that appear to correspond to IXa, IXb, IXc, and IXd of other species.

HEMISPHERAL LOBULES OF POSTERIOR LOBE

Lobule HVI presents four superficial lamellae on either side. The most anterior one represents a direct hem-

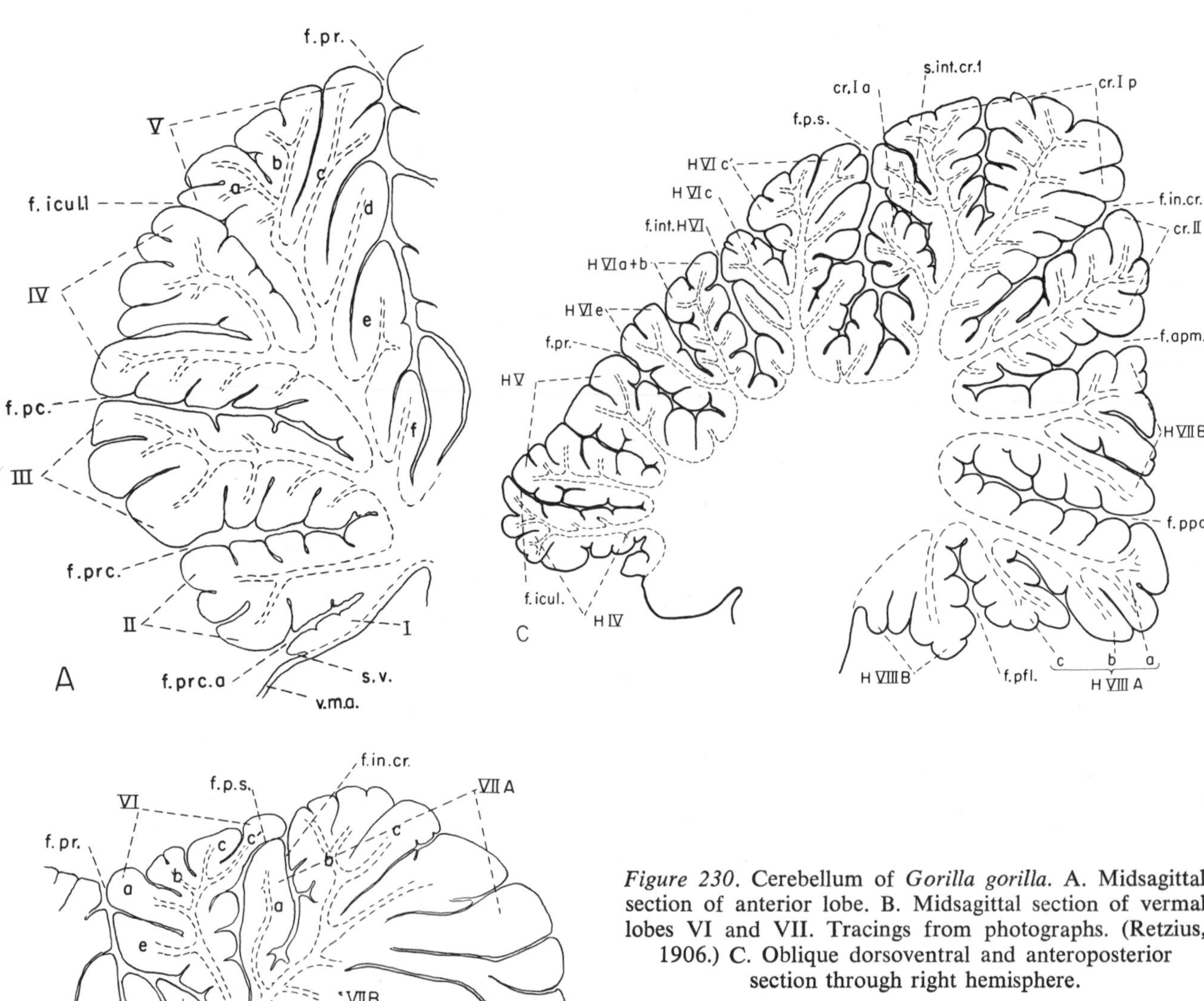

Figure 230. Cerebellum of *Gorilla gorilla.* A. Midsagittal section of anterior lobe. B. Midsagittal section of vermal lobes VI and VII. Tracings from photographs. (Retzius, 1906.) C. Oblique dorsoventral and anteroposterior section through right hemisphere.

ispheral continuation of the large lamella VIe of this specimen. The second lamella on both sides is continuous with vermal lamellae VIa and VIb. The depth and relations of the fissure behind the second lamella correspond to those of the intralobular fissure of the chimpanzee (except in the right lobule HVI of the larger cerebellum) and it was so interpreted in the gorilla. The anterior lamella of the posterior division is continuous with VIc of the vermis, and the posterior lamella, which is relatively large, is continuous with the posterior surface of the combined posterior superior and intercrural fissures and with sublobule VIIA.

Lobule HVIIA forms the caudal and lateral part of the hemisphere, extending from the vermis to the transverse fossa and from the posterior and lateral parts of the dorsal surface to the posterior and lateral inferior surfaces (figs. 231, 232). Lobule HVIIA is the largest lobule of the cerebellum. The posterior superior fissure, separating it from lobule HVI, penetrates obliquely downward and forward in the hemisphere instead of nearly vertically as in monkeys. This fissure forms a deep cleft which has heavily foliated walls. In the upper part of the posterior wall a deep fissure delimits a large, completely submerged sublobule, which is composed of many folia on both its posterior and anterior surfaces. This sublobule corresponds to crus Ia of the chimpanzee and in the

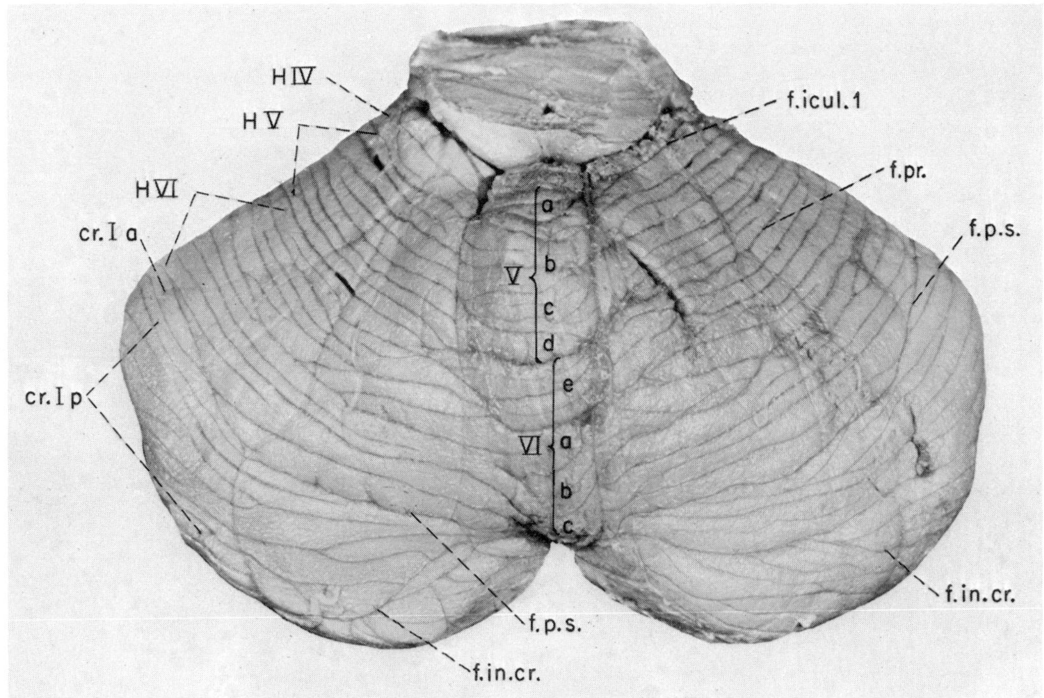

Figure 231. Cerebellum of *Gorilla gorilla.* Dorsal view. Retouched photograph.

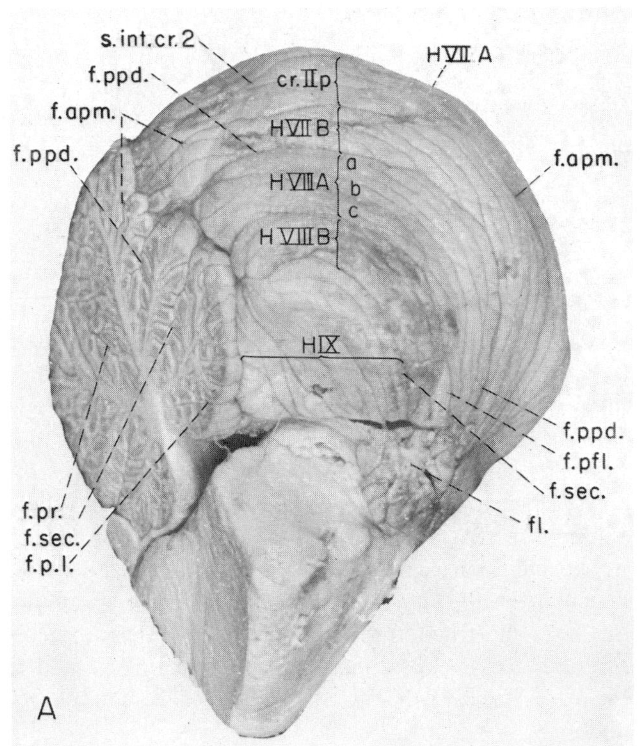

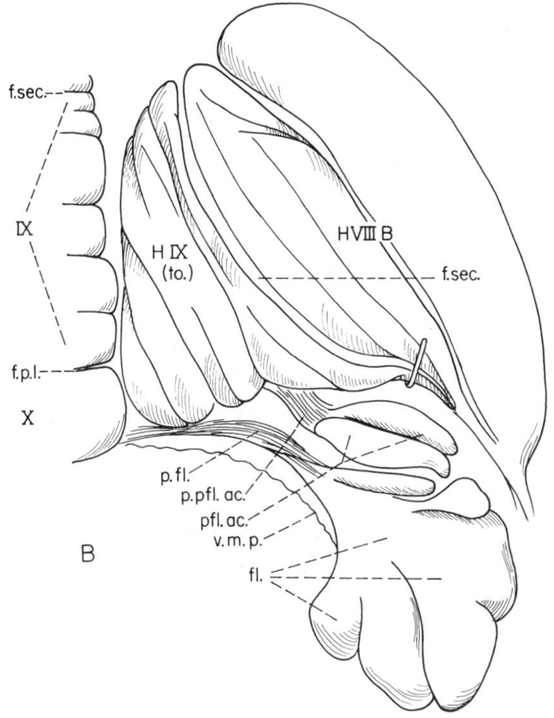

Figure 232. Cerebellum of *Gorilla gorilla.* A. Posteroventral view of right half. Retouched photograph. B. Posteroventral view of right tonsil, paraflocculus accessorius, and flocculus.

gorilla (fig. 231). The delimiting fissure was regarded as intracrural sulcus 1. The remainder of crus I is similar to crus Ip of the chimpanzee.

The intercrural fissure was found on the dorsal surface of the hemisphere; it has a course that is parallel with the

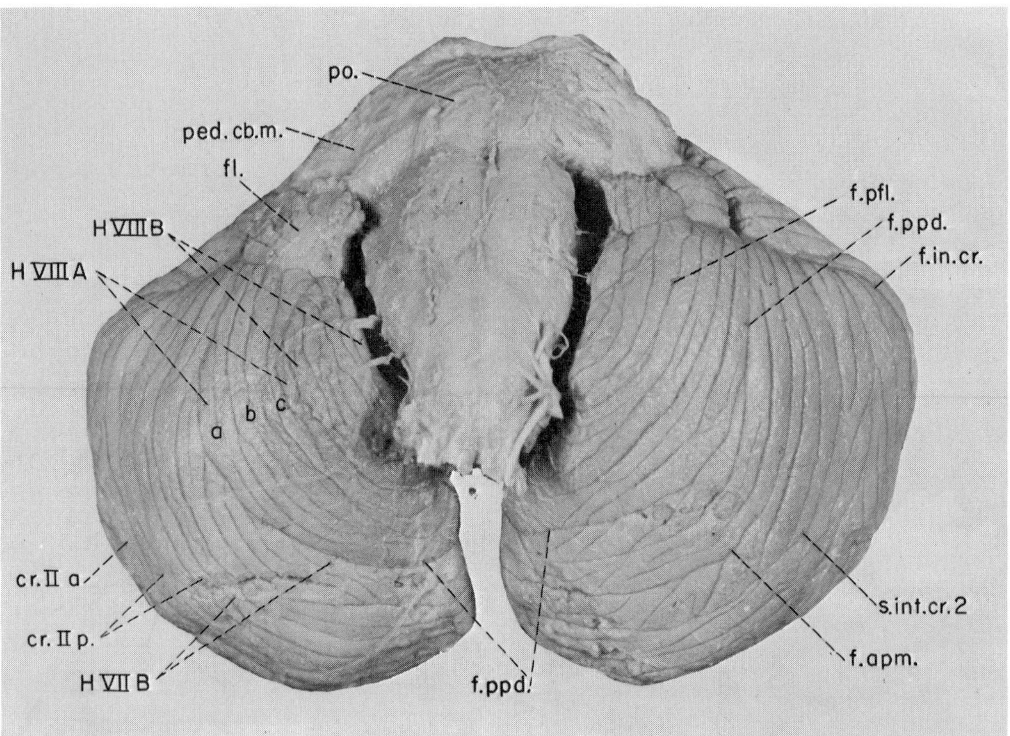

Figure 233. Cerebellum of *Gorilla gorilla.* Ventral view. Retouched photograph.

posterior border of the hemisphere and reaches the transverse fossa on the ventral surface. Crus II, which it separates from crus I, is considerably larger superficially than the latter division. It is divided by intracrural sulcus 2 into a wide crescent-shaped crus IIa which extends to the transverse fossa and a narrower sickle-shaped crus IIp which forms the upper wall of the ansoparamedian fissure. This fissure penetrates rostroventrally and is very deep, which greatly increases the cortical surface of crus IIp that forms its roof. It also is directly confluent, on both sides, with its vermal segment.

Both lobules HVIIB are directly continuous with sublobule VIIB; the paravermian sulcus is very shallow on either side of the latter (fig. 232). In the right hemisphere the lobule is subdivided into dorsal and ventral segments by a furrow that corresponds to the intragracile fissure of the chimpanzee. The dorsal segment tapers lateralward and disappears into the intragracile fissure. The ventral segment tapers medialward and continues, in the anterior wall of the prepyramidal fissure, to the outer posterior folia of sublobule VIIB. Lobule HVIIB of the left hemisphere comprises two lamellae that are continuous with the superficial folia of sublobule VIIB. Except for the relatively smaller size, superficially, of the dorsal and ventral divisions in the right hemisphere lobule HVIIB corresponds in all respects to the lobulus gracilis of the chimpanzee and man.

Lobule HVIIIA comprises three superficially narrow but deep lamellae that appear to correspond to HVIIIAa, HVIIIAb, and HVIIIAc of monkeys (figs. 232, 233). Lamella HVIIIAa is continuous on one side with the anterior surface of sublobule VIIIA. Contralaterally it appears to continue onto the inferior part of the anterior wall of the prepyramidal fissure, but this could not be established with certainty in the one cerebellum available. The two remaining lamellae of the lobule are continuous with the copula (ala) of the pyramis as in the chimpanzee.

Lobule HVIIIB is separated from lobule HVIIIA by a furrow which is less deep than those already named in the posterior part of the hemisphere. It penetrates, however, to the medullary body and medially is continuous with the intrapyramidal sulcus (fig. 229). This furrow corresponds to the interbiventral fissure that Løyning and Jansen (1955) noted in the human cerebellum and, as in the chimpanzee, I concluded that it was the parafloccular fissure (fig. 232). Lobule HVIIIB is continuous by a short peduncle with sublobule VIIIB and corresponds to the dorsal paraflocculus of monkeys and to the medial belly of the biventral lobule of the chimpanzee and man.

Situated between the biventral lobule and lobule IX is a triangular lobule (in surface view) whose base tapers laterally between the peduncle of the flocculus and the medial part of the biventral lobule (figs. 229, 232). Dissection reveals that it is attached by a short peduncle to the medullary body. It corresponds entirely to the tonsilla of the chimpanzee and man. The fissure between it and the biventral lobule (the intraparafloccular fissure of Løyning and Jansen in man) is deep and except for the interruption by the deep paravermian sulcus between the uvula and the tonsilla it appears to be a direct continuation of the fissura secunda. The tonsilla represents the greater part of the ventral paraflocculus and it together with the small accessory paraflocculus constitutes lobule HIX.

When the laterally extending part of the tonsilla is retracted or dissected away two small folia attached to the lateral part of the underside of the tonsilla are brought into view (fig. 232B). They have already been mentioned in connection with the similar lobule of the chimpanzee and, furthermore, their probable homology with the Nebenflocke or accessory paraflocculus of man and the lobulus petrosus of monkeys has previously been pointed out.

FLOCCULONODULAR LOBE

Lobule X, the nodulus, is relatively smaller than in the chimpanzee but comparison with the figures of other authors, already cited, shows considerable variation in size. The choroid tela is attached to its base near the fastigium (fig. 229). An arched peduncle attaches the flocculus to the nodulus in typical fashion. The flocculus comprises an expanded group of folia that is situated in a notch between the anterior and posterior ventral cerebellar surfaces (fig. 232). A narrow folium, attached to the floccular peduncle, lies above the main part of the flocculus and parallel with the folia of the accessory paraflocculus. It is quite distinct from the latter, however, and probably is part of the flocculus. The nodulus, the flocculus, and the peduncle connecting them constitute a typical flocculonodular lobe. The posterolateral fissure is deep in the vermis and for a short distance on either side. Along the floccular peduncle it appears to be represented by a shallow groove between this peduncle and a sheet of medullary substance which forms the floor of a tonsillar recess corresponding to the nidus avis of the human cerebellum.

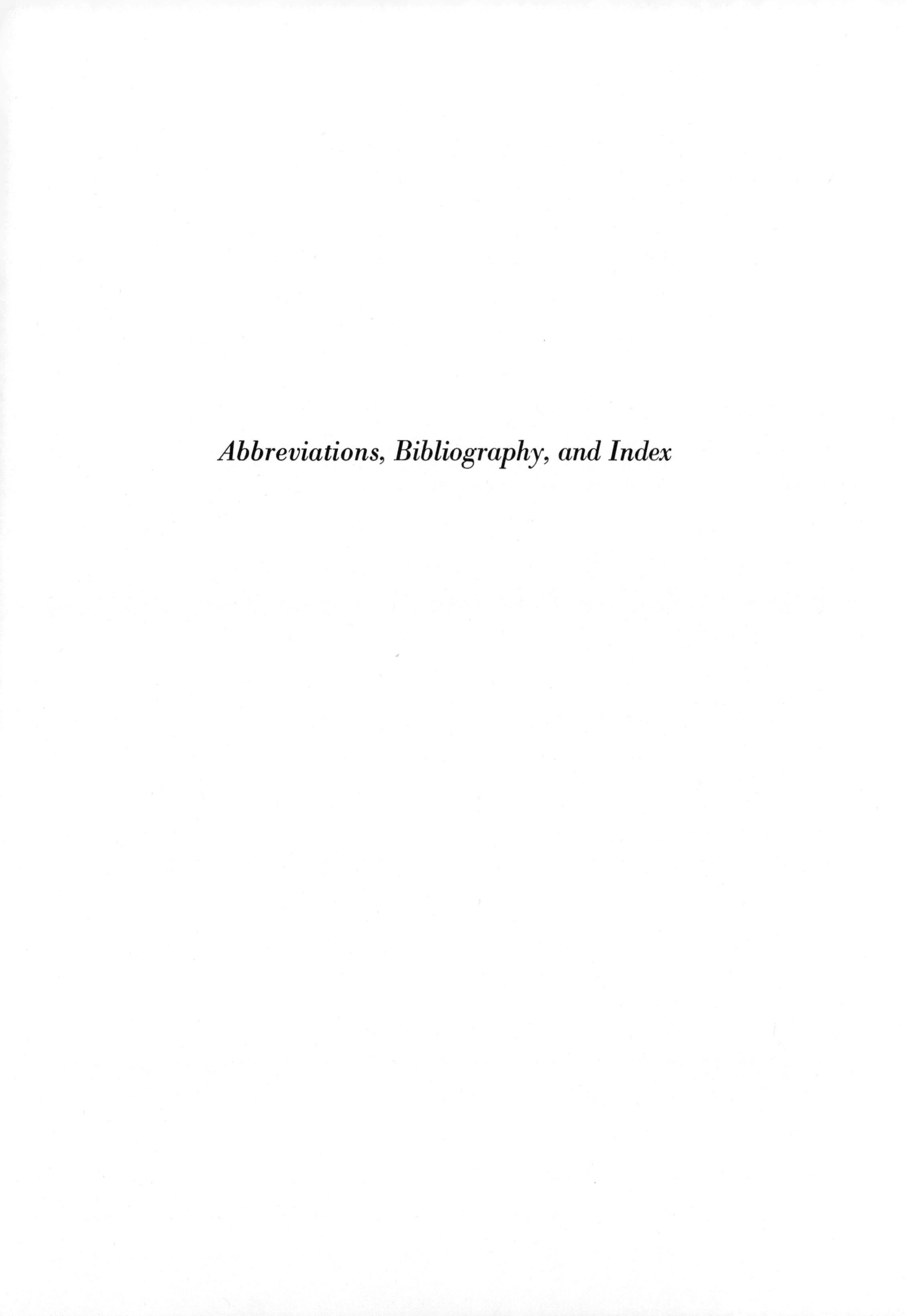

Abbreviations, Bibliography, and Index

ABBREVIATIONS USED IN THE FIGURES

I, vermian lobule I
II, vermian lobule II, the ventral lobule of lobulus centralis
III, vermian lobule III, the dorsal lobule of lobulus centralis
IV, vermian lobule IV, the ventral lobule of culmen
IVA, ventral sublobule of lobule IV
IVB, dorsal sublobule of lobule IV
V, vermian lobule V, the dorsal lobule of culmen
VA, sublobule A of lobule V
VI, vermian lobule VI, the declive
VID, sublobule D of lobule VI
VII, vermian lobule VII, the folium and tuber vermis lobule
VIIA, anterior sublobule of lobule VII
VIIAa,s.a., anterior surface of folium *a* of sublobule VIIA
VIIB, posterior sublobule of lobule VII, the posterior tuber vermis
VIIB,p., peduncle of sublobule VIIB
VIIB,ped., peduncle of sublobule VIIB
VIII, vermian lobule VIII, the pyramis
VIIIA, anterior sublobule of lobule VIII
VIIIA,al., ala of sublobule VIIIA
VIIIA, cop., copular part of sublobule VIIIA
VIIIB, posterior sublobule of lobule VIII
VIIIB,s.p., posterior surface of sublobule VIIIB
VIIIBx, lobule VIII removed
IX, vermian lobule IX, the uvula
IX,al., ala of lobule IX
IX,b., base of lobule IX
X, vermian lobule X, the nodulus

al.lam., lamina alaris
an.fl.nod., ansa flocculonodularis
aq.cer., cerebral aqueduct
aq.S., aqueduct of Sylvius
ar.med., medullary area

β, subnucleus *β* of medial accessory olive
b.a., area devoid of cortex
b.f.pr., bottom of fissura prima
b.R., furrowed band of Reil

ba.lam., lamina basalis
br.col.inf., brachium of inferior colliculus
br.conj., brachium conjunctivum
br.p., brachium pontis
br.po., brachium pontis
bu.po.ext., bulbopontine extension

c.cb., corpus cerebelli
c.po.b., corpus pontobulbare
c.r., restiform body
c.rest., restiform body
c.tr., trapezoid body
cb., cerebellum
cl., claustrum
co.V, intertrigeminal commissure
co.cb., cerebellar commissure
co.vest., vestibular commissure
col.inf., inferior colliculus
cop., copula pyramidis
cop.pyr., copula pyramidis
cop.s.a., anterior surface of copula
cop.x, copula, cut
cr.I, crus I
cr.Ia, anterior primary folium of crus I
cr.Ip, posterior folia of crus I
cr.II, crus II
cr.IIa, anterior folia of crus II
cr.IIp, posterior folia of crus II
cr.IIs.p., posterior surface of crus II
crb.hem., cerebral hemisphere
cul., culmen

d.c., dorsal cap
d.l., dorsal lamella of principal olive
D.l.h., dorsolateral "hump" region (of nucleus interpositus)
D.m.c., dorsomedial crest region (of nucleus interpositus)
d.m.c.c., dorsomedial cell column
de., declive
dec.n.IV, decussation of the trochlear nerve

f.apm., ansoparamedian fissure
f.apm.l., left ansoparamedian fissure
f.apm.r., right ansoparamedian fissure
f.apm. + in.cr., ansoparamedian and intercrural fissures
f.ax., fossa axillaris (of Ziehen)
f.de.1, declival sulcus 1
f.h., horizontal fissure
f.hor., horizontal fissure
f.i.pfl., intraparafloccular fissure
f.ib.x, fibrous band, cut
f.ic., intraculminate fissure
f.ic.1, 2, intracentral fissures 1, 2
f.icul.1, 2, 3, intraculminate fissures 1, 2, 3
f.in.cr., intercrural fissure
f.int.HVI, intralobular (HVI) fissure
f.p.l., posterolateral fissure
f.p.s., posterior superior fissure
f.p.s.,a.w., anterior wall of posterior superior fissure
f.p.s.,b., bottom of posterior superior fissure
f.pc., preculminate fissure
f.pfl., parafloccular fissure
f.ppd., prepyramidal fissure
f.ppd.,ant.w., anterior wall of prepyramidal fissure
f.ppd. + apm., prepyramidal and ansoparamedian fissures
f.ppd.b., bottom of prepyramidal fissure
f.ppd.,s.a., anterior surface of prepyramidal fissure
f.pr., fissura prima
f.pr.b., bottom of fissura prima
f.prc., precentral fissure
f.prc.a, precentral fissure a
f.sec., fissura secunda
f.sec.b., bottom of fissura secunda
f.unc., uncinate bundle of Russell
f.v., folium vermis
fasc.ang.L., angular bundle of Löwy
fasc.unc., uncinate bundle of Russell
fast.r., fastigial recess
fi.b.x., fibrous band, cut
fi. to pfl.d.,l.petr.,pfl.v., fibers to dorsal paraflocculus, lobulus petrosus, and ventral paraflocculus
fis.pr., fissura prima
fl., flocculus

fl.x, flocculus, cut
fo.cop.x, folia of copula, dissected away
fo.isth., fovea isthmi
fo.tr., transitional folia
fo.tr.pyr., transitional folia to pyramis
fo.v., folium vermis
folia x, folia, cut

g.z., germinal zone
gn.V, ganglion of V nerve
gn.VIII, ganglion of VIII nerve

HII–HX, hemispheral lobules II–X
HVIIA cr.I, cr.II, crus I and II of lobule HVIIA
HVIIB,f.s., fissural surface of lobule HVIIB
HVIIB,s.s., superficial surface of lobule HVIIB
HVIII,cop., copular part of lobule HVIII
HVIIIA,B, sublobules A, B of lobule HVIII
HVIIIA,d.f.s., deep fissural surface of lobule HVIIIA
HVIIIA,s.s., superficial surface of lobule HVIIIA
h.cb., cerebellar hemisphere
h.cer., cerebral hemisphere
hyp., hypothalamus

i.fppd., indication of prepyramidal fissure
isth., isthmus

L., left
l.ans., ansiform lobule
l.ant., anterior lobe of corpus cerebelli
l.apmd., ansoparamedian lobule
l.biv., lobulus biventer
l.c., central lobule
l.grac., lobulus gracilis
l.int.cal. of Z., intercallated lobule of Ziehen
l.m., medial lemniscus
l.pet., lobulus petrosus
l.petr., lobulus petrosus
l.petr.b., folia b of lobulus petrosus
l.pm.x, paramedian lobule, cut
l.pmd., paramedian lobule
l.pmd.a., pars anterior of paramedian lobule
l.pmd.a.x, pars anterior of paramedian lobule, cut
l.pmd.c., copular part of paramedian lobule
l.pmd.c.x, copular part of paramedian lobule, cut
l.pmd.cop., copular part of paramedian lobule
l.pmd.cop.x, copular part of paramedian lobule, cut
l.pmd.p., pars posterior of paramedian lobule
l.pmd.x, paramedian lobule, cut
l.quad.a., anterior quadrangular lobule
l.quad.p., posterior quadrangular lobule
l.quad.post., posterior quadrangular lobule
l.s.l.i., inferior semilunar lobule
l.s.l.s., superior semilunar lobule
l.sim., lobulus simplex
l.subm., submerged lobule of Dejerine
l.sub.mer., submerged lobule of Dejerine
la.term., lamina terminalis
ling., lingula
lm.med., medial lemniscus
lo.ant., anterior lobe of corpus cerebelli
lo.ant.s.d., dorsal segment of anterior lobe
lo.ant.s.v., ventral segment of anterior lobe
lo.fl.nod., flocculonodular lobe
lo.post., posterior lobe of corpus cerebelli
lu.opt.st., lumen of optic stalk

m., margin of cerebellar cortex
m.r.VIII, medullary ray of lobule VIII
m.r.IX, medullary ray of lobule IX
m.r.X, medullary ray of lobule X
m.sag.pl., midsagittal plane
med.obl., medulla oblongata
mes., mesencephalon
mes.Vc., mesencephalic V cells
myel., myelencephalon

n.IV, trochlear nerve
n.V, trigeminal nerve
n.VII, facial nerve
n.VIII, statoacoustic nerve
N.i., nucleus interpositus
N.l.l., lateral (dentate) nucleus, magnocellular part
N.l.s., lateral (dentate) nucleus, parvicellular part
N.m.dlp., medial (fastigial) nucleus, dorsolateral protuberance
N.m.m., medial (fastigial) nucleus, middle part
N.r., nucleus ruber
nid.av., nidus avis
nm., neuromeres
nod., nodulus
nuc.Vsup., superior V nucleus
nuc.co.cb., nucleus of cerebellar commissure
nuc.coch.d., dorsal cochlear nucleus
nuc.coch.v., ventral cochlear nucleus
nuc.dent., dentate nucleus
nuc.dorsolat.po., dorsolateral pontine nucleus
nuc.fast., fastigial nucleus
nuc.i.ant., nucleus interpositus anterior
nuc.i.post., nucleus interpositus posterior
nuc.ic., nucleus intercalatus
nuc.int., nucleus interpositus
nuc.lat., lateral (dentate) cerebellar nucleus
nuc.lat.dent., lateral (dentate) cerebellar nucleus
nuc.lat.po., lateral pontine nucleus
nuc.md.po., median pontine nucleus
nuc.med., medial (fastigial) nucleus
nuc.Vmes., mesencephalic V nucleus
nuc.mes.V, mesencephalic V nucleus
nuc.ol.ac.dors., dorsal accessory olive
nuc.ol.ac.med., medial accessory olive
nuc.ol.p.pr., principal olive
nuc.p.h., perihypoglossal nucleus
nuc.ped.po., peduncular pontine nucleus
nuc.pmd.po., paramedian pontine nucleus
nuc.ret.pmd., paramedian reticular nucleus
nuc.ret.po., reticular pontine tegmental nucleus (of Bechterew)
nuc.Ro., nucleus of Roller
nuc.v.sup., superior vestibular nucleus (Bechterew)
nuc.ventr.po., ventral pontine nucleus
nuc.vest.inf., inferior (descending) vestibular nucleus
nuc.vest.lat., lateral vestibular nucleus (Deiters)
nuc.vest.med., medial vestibular nucleus
nuc.vest.sup., superior vestibular nucleus (Bechterew)

ol.inf., inferior olive
ol.sup., superior olive
opt.ch., optic chiasm
os.lab., osseous labyrinth

p., pyramis
p.VIIA, peduncle of lobule VIIA
p.a.g., periaqueductal gray
p.cb., cerebellar peduncle
p.fl., floccular peduncle
p.h., perihypoglossal nuclei
p.i., pars intermedia of cerebellar cortex
p.l.petr.x, peduncle of lobulus petrosus, cut
p.med., medullary peduncle of HVIIIB
p.pfl., parafloccular peduncle
p.pfl.ac., peduncle of accessory paraflocculus
p.pfl.d., peduncle of dorsal paraflocculus
p.pfl.v., peduncle of ventral paraflocculus
p.pfl.x, parafloccular peduncle, cut
Pall., globus pallidus
ped., cerebral peduncle (and its continuation through pons)
ped.cb.i., inferior cerebellar peduncle
ped.cb.inf., inferior cerebellar peduncle
ped.cb.m., middle cerebellar peduncle
ped.cb.med., middle cerebellar peduncle
ped.cb.s., superior cerebellar peduncle
ped.cb.sup., superior cerebellar peduncle
ped.fl., floccular peduncle
ped.fl.sag., floccular peduncle of Burdach
ped.fl.x, floccular peduncle, cut
ped.pfl., parafloccular peduncle
ped.pfl.d., peduncle of dorsal paraflocculus
ped.pfl.v., peduncle of ventral paraflocculus
ped.to.med., peduncle of medial part of tonsilla
pfl., paraflocculus
pfl.ac., accessory paraflocculus
pfl.d., dorsal paraflocculus
pfl.d.fo.r., dorsal paraflocculus, folia removed
pfl.d.x, dorsal paraflocculus, cut
pfl.v., ventral paraflocculus
pfl.v.x, ventral paraflocculus, cut
pl.ch., choroid plexus
po., pons
Put., putamen
pyr., pyramis

R., right
r.IV, root of IV nerve
r.V, root of V nerve
r.Vm., motor root of V nerve
r.Vmes., mesencephalic root of V nerve
r.Vs., sensory root of V nerve
r.Vsp., spinal V nerve
r.VI, root of nerve VI
r.VII, root of VII nerve
r.VIII, root of statoacoustic nerve
r.VIIIa., acoustic root of statoacoustic nerve
r.VIIIc., cochlear root
r.VIIIv., vestibular root
r.IX, root of IX nerve
r.X, root of vagus nerve
r.XII, root of XII nerve
r.fast.v.4, fastigial recess of fourth ventricle
r.l., lateral recess of fourth ventricle
r.l.v.4, lateral recess of fourth ventricle
r.mes.V, mesencephalic root of V nerve
re.fast.v.4, fastigial recess of fourth ventricle
rec.fast.v.4, fastigial recess of fourth ventricle
rec.lat., lateral recess of fourth ventricle
rhomb., rhombencephalon

s.a., anterior surface
s.cop., copular sulcus
s.d., dorsal segment of anterior lobe
s.de.1, 2, 3, declival sulci 1, 2, 3
s.ic., intracentral sulcus
s.in.cr., intercrural sulcus
s.inf.post., posterior inferior sulcus
s.int.cr.1, 2, intracrural sulcus 1, 2
s.int.HVI, intralobular sulcus of HVI
s.int.HVIIIA, intralobular sulcus of HVIIIA
s.ip., intrapyramidal sulcus
s.ip.1, 2, intrapyramidal sulcus 1, 2
s.ip.b., bottom of intrapyramidal sulcus
s.ip.l., lateral part of intrapyramidal sulcus
s.l., sulcus limitans
S.L.P., small-celled part of nucleus lateralis (dentatus)
S.M.P., small-celled part of nucleus medialis (fastigii)
s.n., substantia nigra
s.p.VIa, b, c, d, sublobules a, b, c, d of lobule VI
s.pm., paramedian sulcus
s.ppd.1 b., bottom of prepyramidal sulcus 1
s.prebiv., prebiventral sulcus
s.t., sulcus taenia
s.ta., sulcus taenia
s.uv.1, 2, 3, uvular sulcus 1, 2, 3
s.v., ventral segment of anterior lobe
s.v.cb., sulcus ventralis cerebelli
s.v.m.a., sulcus of anterior medullary velum
str.gr., stratum granulosum, granular layer
str.gran., stratum granulosum, granular layer
str.mol., molecular layer

t.ch., tela choroidea
t.ch.x, tela choroidea, cut
t.v., tuber vermis
t.v.4, taenia of fourth ventricle
ta., taenia of fourth ventricle
ta.v.4, taenia of fourth ventricle
thal., thalamus
to., tonsilla
to.,p.l., lateral part of tonsilla
to.,p.m., medial part of tonsilla
tr.Vcb., trigemino-cerebellar tract of the V nerve
tr.sp.cb., spino-cerebellar tract
tr.sp.cb.d., dorsal spino-cerebellar tract
tr.sp.cb.v., ventral spino-cerebellar tract
tr.t.cb., tecto-cerebellar tract
tr.tec.cb., tecto-cerebellar tract
tr.trig.cb., trigemino-cerebellar tract
tu.ac., acoustic tubercle

uv., uvula
uv.f.1, uvular fissure 1

v.4, fourth ventricle
v.cb., cerebellar ventricle
v.i., inferior vestibular nucleus
v.l., lateral vestibular nucleus
v.l., ventral lamella of principal olive
v.l.o., ventrolateral outgrowth
v.m., medial vestibular nucleus
v.m.a., anterior medullary velum
v.m.p., posterior medullary velum
v.m.p.l., lower surface of posterior medullary velum
v.m.p.x, cut margin of posterior medullary velum
v.pfl., ventral paraflocculus
v.s., superior vestibular nucleus

BIBLIOGRAPHY

Abbie, A. A., 1934. The brain stem and cerebellum of Echidna. Phil. Trans. Roy. Soc. (Lond.) Ser. B, 224:1–74.

Aciron, E. E., 1950. Fissuración del cerebelo en la rata blanca (*Epimys norvegicus*). Arch. Anat. Antrop. (Lisboa), 27:215–261.

Addens, J. L., 1934. A critical review of the occurrence of crossing root-fibers in the facialis, vestibular, glossopharyngeal, and vagus nerves. Psychiat. Neurol. Bl. (Amst.), 38:274–291.

Adrian, E. D., 1943. Afferent areas in the cerebellum connected with the limbs. Brain, 66:289–315.

Ärnbäck-Christie-Linde, A., 1900. Zur Anatomie des Gehirnes niederer Säugetiere. Anat. Anz., 18:8–16.

Agduhr, E., 1919. Über die plurisegmentale Innervation der einzelnen quergestreiften Muskelfasern. Anat. Anz., 52:273–291.

Alexander, G., 1904. Entwickelung und Bau des inneren Gehörorganes von *Echidna aculeata*. In R. Semon, Zoologische Forschungsreisen in Australien und dem malayischen Archipel, Bd 3, T. 2, pp. 3–118. Fischer, Jena.

Alix, E., 1877. Sur le cerveau à l'état foetal. Bull. Soc. d'Anthrop. (Paris), Sér. 2., 12:216–225.

Allen, W. F., 1923. Origin and distribution of the tractus solitarius in the guinea-pig. J. Comp. Neurol., 35:171–204.

———, 1924. Distribution of the fibers originating from the different basal cerebellar nuclei. J. Comp. Neurol., 36:399–439.

Anderson, R. F., 1943. Cerebellar distribution of the dorsal and ventral spino-cerebellar tracts in the white rat. J. Comp. Neurol., 79:415–423.

Ariens Kappers, C. U., 1947. Anatomie comparée du système nerveux. De Erven F. Bohn, Haarlem; Masson et Cie., Paris.

———, G. C. Huber, and E. C. Crosby, 1936. The comparative anatomy of the nervous system of vertebrates, including man. Macmillan, New York.

Ashcroft, D. W., and C. S. Hallpike, 1934. The function of the saccule. J. Laryngol., 49:450–458.

Baffoni, G. M., 1954. La citomorfosi degli elementi di Purkinje del cervelletto. Ricerca Sci., 24:1641–1647.

Barker, D., 1948. The innervation of the muscle spindles. Quart. J. Micr. Sci., 89:143–186.

———, 1959. Some results of a quantitative histological investigation of stretch receptors in limb muscles of the cat. J. Physiol., 149:7–9.

———, and N. K. Chin, 1961. Efferent innervation of mammalian muscle-spindles. Nature (Lond.), 190:461–462.

Bartels, M., 1925. Über die Gegend des Deiters- und Bechterewskernes bei Vögeln. Z. Anat. Entwicklungsgeschichte, 77:726–784.

Beauregard, 1883. Recherches sur l'encéphale des Balaenides. J. Anat. (Paris). (Cited by Jansen, 1950.)

Beccari, N., 1931. Studi comparativi sopra i nuclei terminali del nervo acustico nei Pesci. Arch. Zool. Ital., 16:732–739.

Bender, L., 1932. Corticofugal and association fibers arising from the cortex of the vermis of the cerebellum. Arch. Neurol. Psychiat. (Chic.), 28:1–25.

Bergquist, H., and B. Källén, 1953. Studies on the topography of the migration areas in the vertebrate brain. Acta Anat. (Basel), 17:353–369.

———, 1954. Notes on the early histogenesis and morphogenesis of the central nervous system in vertebrates. J. Comp. Neurol., 100:627–659.

Bolk, L., 1902. Hauptzüge der vergleichenden Anatomie des Cerebellums der Säugetiere mit besonderer Berücksichtigung des menschlichen Kleinhirns. Monatsschr. Psychiat. Neurol., 12:432–467.

———, 1906. Das Cerebellum der Säugetiere. Eine vergleichende anatomische Untersuchung. De Erven F. Bohn, Haarlem; Gustav Fischer, Jena.

Boyd, I. A., 1956. The tenuissimus muscle of the cat. J. Physiol. (Lond.), 133:35–36.

———, 1958. The innervation of mammalian neuromuscular spindles. J. Physiol. (Lond.), 140:14–15.

———, 1959. Simple and compound mammalian muscle spindles. J. Physiol. (Lond.), 145:55–56.

———, and M. R. Davey, 1959. β-efferent fibres in nerves to mammalian skeletal muscle. J. Physiol. (Lond.), 149:28–29.

Bradley, O. C., 1903. On the development and homology of the mammalian cerebellar fissures. J. Anat. (Lond.), 37:112–130; 221–240.

———, 1904. The mammalian cerebellum; its lobes and fissures. J. Anat. (Lond.), 38:448–475.

———, 1905. The mammalian cerebellum; its lobes and fissures. Part II. The cerebellum in primates. J. Anat. (Lond.), 39:99–117.

Brodal, A., 1940a. Experimentelle Untersuchungen über die olivo-cerebellare Lokalisation. Z. Ges. Neurol. Psychiat., 169:1–153.

———, 1940b. The cerebellum of the rabbit. A topographical atlas of the folia as revealed in transverse sections. J. Comp. Neurol., 72:63–81.

———, 1941. Die Verbindungen des Nucleus cuneatus externus mit dem Kleinhirn beim Kaninchen und bei der Katze. Experimentelle Untersuchungen. Z. Ges. Neurol. Psychiat., 171:167–199.

———, 1954. Afferent cerebellar connections. In J. Jansen and A. Brodal, Aspects of cerebellar anatomy, pp. 82–188. Grundt Tanum, Oslo.

———, 1960. Fiber connections of the vestibular nuclei. In G. L. Rasmussen and W. F. Windle, Neural mechanisms of the auditory and vestibular systems, pp. 224–246. Thomas, Springfield, Ill.

———, and J. Jansen, 1946. The ponto-cerebellar projection in the rabbit and cat. Experimental investigations. J. Comp. Neurol., 84:31–118.

Brodal, A., and O. Pompeiano, 1957. The vestibular nuclei in the cat. J. Anat. (Lond.), 91:438–454.

———, 1958. The origin of ascending fibres of the medial longitudinal fasciculus from the vestibular nuclei. An experimental study in the cat. Acta Morphol. Neerl. Scand., 1:306–328.

Brodal, A., and A. Torvik, 1957. Über den Ursprung der sekundären vestibulo-cerebellaren Fasern bei der Katze. Eine experimentelle anatomische Studie. Arch. Psychiat. Nervenkrankh., 195:558–567.

Brodal, A., K. Kristiansen, and J. Jansen, 1950. Experimental demonstration of a pontine homologue in birds. J. Comp. Neurol., 92:23–69.

Brodal, A., O. Pompeiano, and F. Walberg, 1962. The vestibular nuclei and their connections, anatomy and functional correlations. 193 pp. Oliver and Boyd, Edinburgh and London.

Brunner, H., 1919. Die zentralen Kleinhirnkerne bei den Säugetieren. Arb. Neurol. Inst. Univ. Wien, 22:200–277.

Buchanan, A. R., 1937. The course of the secondary vestibular fibers in the cat. J. Comp. Neurol., 67:183–204.

Burlet, H. M. de, 1929. Zur vergleichenden Anatomie der Labyrinthinnervation. J. Comp. Neurol., 47:155–169.

Burt, W. H., and R. P. Grossenheider, 1952. A field guide to the mammals. Houghton Mifflin, Boston.

Cajal, See Ramon y Cajal

Callender, G. W., 1874. The formation and early growth of the brain of man. Brit. Med. J., 1:731–763; 795.

Camis, M., 1928. La fisiologia dell'apparato vestibolare. Zanichelli, Bologna. Trans. R. S. Creed (1930): The physiology of the vestibular apparatus. Clarendon Press, Oxford.

Carpenter, M. B., 1959. Lesions of the fastigial nuclei in the Rhesus monkey. Amer. J. Anat., 104:1–34.

———, 1960a. Fiber projections from the descending and lateral vestibular nuclei in the cat. Amer. J. Anat., 107:1–21.

———, 1960b. Experimental anatomical-physiological studies of the vestibular nerve and cerebellar connections. In G. L. Rasmussen and W. F. Windle, Neural mechanisms of the auditory and vestibular systems, pp. 297–323. Thomas, Springfield, Ill.

———, and G. R. Hanna, 1961. Fiber projections from the spinal trigeminal nucleus in the cat. J. Comp. Neurol., 117:117–131.

———, 1962. Effects of thalamic lesions upon cerebellar dyskinesia in the Rhesus monkey. J. Comp. Neurol., 119:127–147.

Carpenter, M. B., F. A. Alling, and D. S. Bard, 1960. Lesions of the descending vestibular nucleus in the cat. J. Comp. Neurol., 114:39–49.

Carpenter, M. B., D. S. Bard, and F. A. Alling, 1959. Anatomical connections between the fastigial nuclei, the labyrinth and the vestibular nuclei in the cat. J. Comp. Neurol., 111:1–25.

Carpenter, M. B., G. M. Brittin, and J. Pines, 1958. Isolated lesions of the fastigial nuclei in the cat. J. Comp. Neurol., 109:65–90.

Cattanao, A., 1888. Organes nerveux terminaux musculo-tendineux, leurs conditions normales et leur manière de se comporter après la section des racines nerveuses et des nerfs spinaux. Arch. Ital. Biol., 10:337–357.

Chambers, W. W., and J. M. Sprague, 1955a. Functional localization in the cerebellum. I. Organization in longitudinal cortico-nuclear zones and their contribution to the control of posture, both extrapyramidal and pyramidal. J. Comp. Neurol., 103:105–129.

———, 1955b. Functional localization in the cerebellum. II. Somatotopic organization in cortex and nuclei. Arch. Neurol. Psychiat. (Chic.), 74:653–680.

Chang, H.-T., and T. C. Ruch, 1949. The projection of the caudal segments of the spinal cord to the lingula in the spider monkey. J. Anat. (Lond.), 83:303–307.

Ciaccio, G. V., 1891. Sur les plaques nerveuses finales dans les tendons des vertébrés. Arch. Ital. Biol., 14:31–57.

Cilimbaris, P. A., 1910. Histologische Untersuchungen über die Muskelspindeln der Augenmuskeln. Arch. Mikr. Anat., 75:692–747.

Clark, S. L., 1926. Nissl granules of primary afferent neurones. J. Comp. Neurol., 41:423–451.

Clark, W. E. L., 1928. On the brain of the Macroscelididae (*Macroscelides* and *Elephantulus*). J. Anat. (Lond.), 62:245–275.

———, 1932. The brain of insectivora. Proc. Zool. Soc. (Lond.), 2:975–1013.

Cohen, D., W. W. Chambers, and J. M. Sprague, 1958. Experimental study of the efferent projections from the cerebellar nuclei to the brain stem of the cat. J. Comp. Neurol., 109:233–259.

Collier, J., and E. F. Buzzard, 1903. The degeneration resulting from lesions of the posterior nerve roots and from transverse lesions of the spinal cord in man. A study of twenty cases. Brain, 26:559–591.

Comolli, A., 1910. Per una nuova divisione del cerveletto dei mammiferi. Arch. Ital. Anat. Embriol., 9:247–273.

Cooper, S., 1953. Muscle spindles in the intrinsic muscles of the human tongue. J. Physiol. (Lond.), 122:193–202.

———, and P. M. Daniel, 1956. Human muscle spindles. J. Physiol. (Lond.), 133:1–3.

Corbin, K. B., 1940. Observations on the peripheral distribution of fibers arising in the mesencephalic nucleus of the fifth cranial nerve. J. Comp. Neurol., 73:153–177.

———, and F. Harrison, 1940. Function of mesencephalic root of fifth cranial nerve. J. Neurophysiol., 3:423–435.

Corbin, K. B., and J. C. Hinsey, 1935. Intramedullary course of the dorsal root fibers of each of the first four cervical nerves. J. Comp. Neurol., 63:119–126.

Craigie, E. H., 1928. Observations on the brain of the humming bird (*Chrysolampis mosquitus* Linn. and *Chlorostilbon caribaeus* Lawr.). J. Comp. Neurol., 45:377–481.

Cuajunco, F., 1927. Embryology of the neuromuscular spindles. Contrib. Embryol. Carnegie Inst., 19:45–72.

———, 1932. The plurisegmental innervation of neuromuscular spindles. J. Comp. Neurol., 54:205–235.

Dejerine, J., 1901. Anatomie des centres nerveux. 2 vols. Rueff, Paris.

Denny-Brown, D., 1932. Theoretical deductions from the physiology of the cerebral cortex. J. Neurol. Psychopathol., 13:52–67.

Diete-Spiff, K., and J. E. Pascoe, 1959. The spindle motor nerves to the gastrocnemius muscle of the rabbit. J. Physiol. (Lond.), 149:120–134.

Dillon, L. S., 1962. Comparative notes on the cerebellum of the monotremes. I. Contribution toward a phylogeny of the mammalian brain. J. Comp. Neurol., 118:343–353.

———, 1963. Comparative studies of the brain in the macropodidae. Contribution to the phylogeny of the mammalian brain. II. J. Comp. Neurol., 120:43–51.

Dogiel, A. S., 1902. Die Nervenendigungen im Bauchfell, in den Sehnen, den Muskelspindeln und dem Centrum tendinum des Diaphragmas beim Menschen und bei Säugethieren. Arch. Mikr. Anat., 59:1–31.

———, 1906. Die Endigungen der sensiblen Nerven in den Augenmuskeln und deren Sehnen beim Menschen und den Säugethieren. Arch. Mikr. Anat., 68:501–526.

Dohlman, G. F., 1960. Histochemical studies of vestibular mechanisms. In G. L. Rasmussen and W. F. Windle, Neural mechanisms of the auditory and vestibular systems, pp. 258–275. Thomas, Springfield, Ill.

———, J. Farkashidy, and F. Salonna, 1958. Centrifugal nerve-fibres to the sensory epithelium of the vestibular labyrinth. J. Laryngol., 72:984–991.

Donaldson, H. H., 1915. The rat. Mem. Wistar Inst. Anat. Biol., 6:1–278.

Dow, R. S., 1935. The relation of the paraflocculus to the movements of the eyes. Amer. J. Physiol., 113:296–298.

———, 1936. The fiber connections of the posterior parts of the cerebellum in the rat and cat. J. Comp. Neurol., 63:527–548.

———, 1938. Efferent connections of the flocculonodular lobe in *Macaca mulatta*. J. Comp. Neurol., 68:297–305.

———, 1939. Cerebellar action potentials in response to stimulation of various afferent connections. J. Neurophysiol., 2:543–555.

———, 1942a. Cerebellar action potentials in response to stimulation of the cerebral cortex in monkeys and cats. J. Neurophysiol., 5:121–136.

———, 1942b. The evolution and anatomy of the cerebellum. Biol. Rev., 17:179–220.

———, and R. Anderson, 1942. Cerebellar action potentials in response to stimulation of proprioceptors and exteroceptors in the rat. J. Neurophysiol., 5:363–372.

Dow, R. S., and G. Moruzzi, 1958. The physiology and pathology of the cerebellum. University of Minnesota Press, Minneapolis.

Edinger, L., 1910. Ueber die Einteilung des Cerebellums. Anat. Anz., 35:319–323.

Elftman, H., 1932. The evolution of the pelvic floor in primates. Amer. J. Anat., 51:307–346.

Elwyn, A., 1929. The structure and development of the proprioceptors. Assoc. Res. Nervous Disease Proc., 6:241–280.

Engström, H., 1958. On the double innervation of the sensory epithelia of the inner ear. Acta Oto-laryngol. (Stockh.), 49:109–118.

———, and J. Wersäll, 1958. The ultrastructural organization of the organ of Corti and of the vestibular sensory epithelia. Exptl. Cell Res. Suppl., 5:460–492.

Essick, C. R., 1907. The corpus ponto-bulbare — a hitherto undescribed nuclear mass in the human hind brain. Amer. J. Anat., 7:119–135.

———, 1912. The development of the nuclei pontis and the nucleus arcuatus in man. Amer. J. Anat., 13:25–54.

Fick, P. A. 1895. The central nervous system of Desmognathus Fusca. J. Morphol., 10:231–286.

Fischer, J. J., 1956. The labyrinth. Grune and Stratton, London.

Flatau, E., and L. Jacobsohn, 1899. Handbuch der Anatomie und vergleichenden Anatomie des Centralnervensystems der Säugetiere. Karger, Basel.

Foltz, F., and H. A. Matzke, 1960. An experimental study on the origin, course and termination of the cerebellifugal fibers in the opossum. J. Comp. Neurol., 114:107–125.

Forbes, H. O., 1894. A handbock of the primates. 2 vols. London.

Freiman, R., 1954. Untersuchungen über Zahl und Anordnung der Muskelspindeln in den Kaumuskeln des Menschen. Anat. Anz., 100:258–264.

Fuse, G., 1912. Die innere Abteilung des Kleinhirnstiels (Meynert, IAK) und der Deitersche Kern. Arb. Hirn-Anat. Inst. (Zürich), 6:29–267.

Gacek, R. R., 1960. Efferent component of the vestibular nerve. In G. L. Rasmussen and W. F. Windle, Neural mechanisms of the auditory and vestibular systems, pp. 267–284. Thomas, Springfield, Ill.

Galambos, R., 1956. Suppression of auditory nerve activity by stimulation of efferent fibers to cochlea. J. Neurophysiol., 19:424–437.

———, 1960. Studies of the auditory system with implanted electrodes. In G. L. Rasmussen and W. F. Windle, Neural mechanisms of the auditory and vestibular systems, pp. 137–151. Thomas, Springfield, Ill.

Ganser, S., 1882. Vergleichend-anatomische Studien über das Gehirn des Maulwurfs. Morphol. Jahrb., 7:591.

Gardner, E., 1944. The distribution and termination of nerves in the knee joint of the cat. J. Comp. Neurol., 80:11–32.

———, 1956. Nerves and nerve endings in joints and associated structures of monkey (*Macaca mulatta*). Anat. Record, 124:293.

Gehuchten, P. van, 1927. Recherches experimentales sur les terminaisons du nerf vestibulaire et sur les voies vestibulaires centrales. Rev. Oto-neuro-opthalmol., 5:777–791.

Gernandt, B. E., 1959. Vestibular mechanisms. In Handbook of physiology, Section I: Neurophysiology, Vol. I, pp. 549–564. American Physiological Society, Washington, D.C.

Golgi, C., 1880. Sui nervi dei tendini dell'uome e di altri vertebrati e di un nuovo organo nervoso terminale muscolo-tendineo. Opera Omnia, 1903, 1:171–198.

———, 1893. Sur l'origine du quatrième nervé cérébral et sur un point d'histophysiologie générale qui se rattache à cette question. Arch. Ital. Biol., 19:454.

Goodman, C. D., and J. T. Simpson, 1961. Functional localization in the cerebellum of the albino rat. Exptl. Neurol., 3:174–188.

Granit, R., 1955. Receptors and sensory perception. Yale University Press, New Haven, Conn.

———, O. Pompeiano, and B. Waltman, 1959. Fast supraspinal control of mammalian muscle spindles: extra- and intrafusal coactivation. J. Physiol. (Lond.), 147:385–398.

Gray, L. P., 1926. Some experimental evidence on the connections of the vestibular mechanism in the cat. J. Comp. Neurol., 41:319–364.

Greene, E. C., 1935. Anatomy of the rat. Hafner, New York.

Guldberg, G. A., 1885. Ueber das Centralnervensystem der Bartenwale. Christiania Vidensk.-Selsk. Forh., No. 4.

Häggqvist, G., 1960. A study of the histology and histochemistry of the muscle spindles. Z. Biol., 112:11–26.

Hagbarth, K.-E., and G. Wohlfart, 1952. The number of muscle-spindles in certain muscles in the cat in relation to the composition of the muscle nerves. Acta Anat., 15:85–104.

Hamberger, C. A., and H. Hydén, 1949. Transneuronal chemical changes in Deiters' nucleus. Acta Oto-laryngol. (Stockh.) Suppl., 75:82–113.

Hampson, J. L., 1949. Relationships between cat cerebral and cerebellar cortices. J. Neurophysiol., 12:37–50.

———, C. R. Harrison, and C. N. Woolsey, 1952. Cerebro-cerebellar projections and the somatotopic localization of motor function in the cerebellum. Res. Publ. Assoc. Nervous Mental Disease, 30:299–333.

Hardy, M., 1934. Observations on the innervation of the macula sacculi in man. Anat. Record, 59:403–418.

Harkmark, W., 1954. Cell migrations from the rhombic lip to the inferior olive, the nucleus raphe and the pons. A morphological and experimental investigation on chick embryos. J. Comp. Neurol., 100:115–209.

Hauglie-Hanssen, E., 1968. Intrinsic neuronal organization of the vestibular nuclear complex in the cat. A Golgi study. Ergeb. Anat. Entwicklungsgeschichte, 10, No. 5, pp. 1–105.

Hayashi, M., 1924. Einige wichtige Tatsachen aus der ontogenetischen Entwicklung des menschlichen Kleinhirns. Deut. Z. Nervenheilk., 81:74–82.

Held, H., 1892. Die Endigungsweise der sensiblen Nerven im Gehirn. Arch. Anat. Physiol., Anat. Abt., 33–39.

———, 1893. Beiträge zur feineren Anatomie des Kleinhirns und des Hirnstammes. Arch. Anat. Physiol., Anat. Abt., 435–446.

Henle, J., 1871. Handbuch der Nervenlehre des Menschen. In Handbuch der systematischen Anatomie des Menschen, Bd 3, Abt. 2. Vieweg, Braunschweig.

———, 1879. Handbuch der Nervenlehre des Menschen. In

Handbuch der systematischen Anatomie des Menschen, 2. Aufl. Vieweg, Braunschweig.

Herrick, C. J., 1891. Contributions to the morphology of the brain of bony fishes. I. Siluridæ. J. Comp. Neurol., 1:211–228.

Hines, M., 1925. The midbrain and thalamus of *Ornithorhynchus paradoxus*. Anat. Record, 29:361.

———, 1929. The brain of *Ornithorhynchus anatinus*. Phil. Trans. Roy. Soc. (Lond.) Ser. B., 217:155–287.

His, W., 1891. Die Entwicklung des menschlichen Rautenhirns vom Ende des ersten bis zum Beginn des dritten Monats. Abhandl. Math. Phys. Kl. Kön. Sächs. Ges. Wiss.. 17:1–74.

Hochstetter, F., 1929. Die Entwicklung des Mittel- und Rautenhirns. In Beiträge zur Entwicklungsgeschichte des menschlichen Gehirns, II, pp. 83–200. Deuticke, Wien and Leipzig.

Hohman, L. B., 1929. The efferent connections of the cerebellar cortex; investigations based upon experimental extirpations in the cat. Res. Publ. Assoc. Res. Nervous Mental Disease, 6:445–460.

Huber, G. C., and L. de Witt, 1900. A contribution on the nerve terminations in neuro-tendinous end-organs. J. Comp. Neurol., 10:159–208.

Hugosson, R., 1957. Morphologic and experimental studies on the development and significance of the rhombencephalic longitudinal cell columns. Ohlsson, Lund.

Huschke, E., 1854. Schädel, Hirn und Seele des Menschen und der Thiere. Mauke, Jena.

Hyde, J. B., 1957. A comparative study of certain trigeminal components in two soricid shrews, *Blarina brevicauda* and *Sorex cinereus*. J. Comp. Neurol., 107:339–351.

Ingvar, S., 1918. Zur Phylo- und Ontogenese des Kleinhirns. Folia Neuro-biol. (Lpz.), 11:205–495.

———, 1928. Studies in neurology. I. The phylogenetic continuity of the central nervous system. II. On cerebellar function. Bull. Johns Hopkins Hosp., 43:315–362.

Jacobsohn, L., 1909. Über die Kerne des menschlichen Hirnstammes. Abhandl. Preuss. Akad. Wiss., Phys.-Math. Kl., Anhang. Abhandl. I, 70 pp.

———, 1910. Struktur und Funktion der Nervenzellen. Neurol. Cbl., 29:1074.

Jakob, A., 1928. Das Kleinhirn. In von Möllendorff's Handbuch der mikroskopischen Anatomie des Menschen, Vol. 4, pp. 674–916. Springer, Berlin.

Jansen, J., 1950. The morphogenesis of the cetacean cerebellum. J. Comp. Neurol., 93:341–400.

———, 1953. Studies on the cetacean brain. The gross anatomy of the rhombencephalon of the fin whale (*Balaenoptera physalus*, L.). Hvalrådets Skrifter, No. 37, 1–35.

———, 1954. On the morphogenesis and morphology of the mammalian cerebellum. In J. Jansen and A. Brodal, Aspects of cerebellar anatomy, pp. 13–81. Grundt Tanum, Oslo.

Jansen, J., and A. Brodal, 1940. Experimental studies on the intrinsic fibers of the cerebellum. II. The cortico-nuclear projection. J. Comp. Neurol., 73:267–321.

———, 1942. Experimental studies on the intrinsic fibers of the cerebellum. The cortico-nuclear projection in the rabbit and the monkey (*Macacus rhesus*). Skrifter Norske Videnskaps-Akad. Oslo I. Mat. Naturv. Kl., No. 3, 1–50.

———, 1954. Aspects of cerebellar anatomy. Grundt Tanum, Oslo.

Jansen, J., and J. Jansen, Jr., 1955. On the efferent fibers of the cerebellar nuclei, in the cat. J. Comp. Neurol., 102:607–632.

Jansen, J., and J. K. S. Jansen, 1968. The nervous system of Cetacea. In H. Andersen, Biology of marine mammals, pp. 175–252. Academic Press, New York.

Jelgersma, G., 1934. Das Gehirn der Wassersäugetiere. Barth, Leipzig.

Johnson, F. H., 1954. Experimental study of spino-reticular connections in the cat. Anat. Record, 118:316.

Kaida, Y., 1929. Über den zentralen Verlauf des N. vestibularis und der Fasern aus dem Deiterschen Kerne. Fukuoka-Ikwadaigaku-Zasshi 22. (Quoted from Z. Ges. Neurol. Psychiat., 55:10, 1930.)

Kaplan, M., 1912–13. Die spinale Acusticus-Wurzel und die in ihr eingelagerten Zellsysteme. Nucleus Deiters. Nucleus Bechterew. Eine vergleichend-anatomische Studie. Arb. Neurol. Inst. Univ. Wien, 20:375–559.

Kellogg, W. N., 1959. Porpoise echolocation. Anat. Record, 134:592.

———, R. Kohler, and H. N. Morris, 1953. Porpoise sounds as sonar signals. Science, 117:239–243.

Klossowsky, B., 1933. Ueber eine bisher noch nicht beschriebene Zellgruppe im intramedullaren Teil der Wurzel des Nervus vestibularis beim Menschen und bei einigen Säugetieren (Nucleus intraradicularis nervi vestibularis). Arch. Psychiat. Nervenkrankh., 98:255–263.

Koelliker, A., 1879. Entwicklungsgeschichte des Menschen und der höheren Tiere. 2. Aufl., Leipzig.

———, 1891. Der feinere Bau des verlängerten Markes. Anat. Anz., 6:427–431.

Kohnstamm, O., 1910. Studien zur physiologischen Anatomie des Hirnstammes. III. J. Psychol. Neurol. (Lpz.), 17:33–57.

Kolmer, W., 1924. Mikroskopische Anatomie des nervösen Apparates des Ohres. In G. Alexander and O. Marburg, Handbuch der Neurologie des Ohres. Urban und Schwarzenberg, Berlin and Vienna.

Kooy, F. H., 1917. The inferior olive in vertebrates. Folia Neuro-biol. (Lpz.), 10:205–369.

Krause, W., 1884. Anatomie des Kaninchen. Engelmann, Leipzig.

Krishaber, M. K., 1865. Considérations sur le développement de l'encephale. Un. Méd. Paris Ser. 2, 27:586–588.

Künnemann, O., 1894. Ueber die Morphologie des Kleinhirns bei Säugetieren. (Dissertation), Erlangen.

Kuhne, W., 1863a. Ueber die Endigung der Nerven in den Muskeln. Virchows Arch. Pathol. Anat., 27:508–533.

———, 1863b. Die Muskelspindeln. Virchows Arch. Pathol. Anat., 28:528–538.

Kuithan, W., 1894. Die Entwicklung des Kleinhirns bei Säugetieren. Sitzungsberichte Ges. Morphol. Physiol., Munich.

———, 1895. Die Entwicklung des Kleinhirns bei Säugetieren. Münch. Med. Abhandl., 7:1–40.

Lam, R. L., and J. H. Ogura, 1952. An efferent representation of the larynx in the cerebellum. Laryngoscope (St. Louis), 62:486–495.

Lange, S. J. de, 1918. Le cervelet de l'Echidna. Festbundel Cornelis Winkler, pp. 466–471. van Rossen, Amsterdam.

Langelaan, J. W., 1919. On the development of the external form of the human cerebellum. Brain, 42:130–170.

Langworthy, O. R., 1932. A description of the central nervous system of the porpoise (*Tursiops truncatus*). J. Comp. Neurol., 54:437–499.

Larsell, O., 1934. Morphogenesis and evolution of the cerebellum. Arch. Neurol. Psychiat. (Chic.), 31:373–395.

———, 1935. The development and morphology of the cerebellum in the opossum. Part I. Early development. J. Comp. Neurol., 63:65–94.

———, 1936a. The development and morphology of the cerebellum in the opossum. Part II. Later development and adult. J. Comp. Neurol., 63:251–291.

———. 1936b. Cerebellum and corpus pontobulbare of the bat (*Myotis*). J. Comp. Neurol., 64:275–302.

———, 1937. The cerebellum: a review and interpretation. Arch. Neurol. Psychiat. (Chic.), 38:580–607.

———, 1947. The development of the cerebellum in man in relation to its comparative anatomy. J. Comp. Neurol., 87:85–130.

———, 1948. The development and subdivisions of the cerebellum of birds. J. Comp. Neurol., 89:123–189.

———, 1952. The morphogenesis and adult pattern of the lobules and fissures of the cerebellum of the white rat. J. Comp. Neurol., 97:281–356.

———, 1953a. The cerebellum of the cat and the monkey. J. Comp. Neurol., 99:135–199.

———, 1953b. The anterior lobe of the mammalian and the human cerebellum. Anat. Record, 115:341.

———, 1954. The development of the cerebellum of the pig. Anat. Record, 118:73–107.

———, 1967. The comparative anatomy and histology of the cerebellum from myxinoids through birds. (J. Jansen, ed.) University of Minnesota Press, Minneapolis.

———, and R. S. Dow, 1935. The development of the cerebellum in the bat (*Corynorhinus* Sp.) and certain other mammals. J. Comp. Neurol., 62:443–468.

Leidler, R., 1913. Experimentelle Untersuchungen über das Endigungsgebiet des Nervus vestibularis. Arb. Neurol. Inst. Univ. Wien, 20:256–330.

———, 1914. Experimentelle Untersuchungen über das Endigungsgebiet des Nervus vestibularis. Arb. Neurol. Inst. Univ. Wien, 21:151–212.

Leksell, L., 1945. The action potential and excitatory effects of the small ventral root fibers to skeletal muscle. Acta Physiol. Scand., 10, Suppl. 31.

Leuret, F., and P. Gratiolet, 1839–57. Anatomie comparée du système nerveux. J.-B. Baillière, Paris.

Lewandowsky, M., 1904. Untersuchungen über die Leitungsbahnen des Truncus cerebri und ihren Zusammenhang mit denen der Medulla spinalis und des Cortex cerebri. Neurobiol. Arb. II, Ser. 1, 63–147.

Liechtenhan, K., 1945. Über Gewicht und Volumen von Rinde und Mark im menschlichen Kleinhirn. Acta Anat., 1:177–190.

Loewe, L., 1880. Beiträge zur Anatomie und zur Entwicklungsgeschichte des Nervensystems der Säugethiere und des Menschen. Bd. I. Die Morphogenesis des Centralnervensystems. Denicke, Leipzig.

Löwenstein, O., 1936. The equilibrium function on the vertebrate labyrinth. Biol. Rev., 11:113–145.

———, and T. D. M. Roberts, 1949. The equilibrium function of the otolith organs of the thornback ray (*Raja clavata*). J. Physiol. (Lond.), 110:392–415.

———, 1951. The localization and analysis of the responses to vibration from the isolated elasmobranch labyrinth. A contribution to the problem of the evolution of hearing in vertebrates. J. Physiol. (Lond.), 114:471–489.

Löwy, R., 1916. Über die Faseranatomie und Physiologie der Formatio vermicularis cerebelli. Arb. Neurol. Inst. Univ. Wien, 21:359–382.

Løyning, Y., and J. Jansen, 1955. A note on the morphology of the human cerebellum. Acta Anat., 25:309–318.

Lorente de Nó, R., 1924. Études sur le cerveau postérieur. Trabajos Lab. Invest. Biol. Univ. Madrid, 22:51–65.

———, 1926. Études sur l'anatomie et la physiologie du labyrinthe de l'oreille et du VIIIe nerf. Deuxième partie. Quelques données au sujet de l'anatomie des organes sensoriels du labyrinthe. Trabajos Lab. Invest. Biol. Univ. Madrid, 24:53–153.

———, 1928. Die Labyrinthreflexe auf die Augenmuskeln nach einseitiger Labyrinthexstirpation nebst einer kurzen Angabe über den Nervenmechanismus der vestibulären Augenbewegungen. Urban und Schwarzenberg, Wien.

———, 1931. Ausgewählte Kapitel aus der vergleichenden Physiologie des Labyrinthes. Die Augenmuskelreflexe beim Kaninchen und ihre Grundlagen. Ergeb. Physiol., 32:73–342.

———, 1933. Anatomy of the eighth nerve. Laryngoscope (St. Louis), 43:1–38.

McCrady, E. Jr., 1938. The embryology of the opossum. Mem. Wistar Anat. Biol., No. 16.

McIntyre, A. K., 1953. Cortical projections of afferent impulses in muscle nerves. Proc. Univ. Otago. Med., 31:5–6.

McNally, W. J., and J. Tait, 1934. The function of the utricular macula of the frog. Acta Oto-laryngol. (Stockh.), 20:73–76.

MacNalty, A. S., and V. Horsley, 1909. On the cervical spino-bulbar and spino-cerebellar tracts and on the question of topographical representation in the cerebellum. Brain, 32:237–255.

Malacarne, M. V. G., 1776. Nuova esposizione della vera struttura del cerveletto umano. G. M. Briolo, Turin. (Cited by Ziehen, 1934a.)

———, 1780. Encefalotomia universale. Briolo, Turin.

Marburg, O., 1924. Die Anatomie des Kleinhirns. Deut. Z. Nervenheilk., 81:8–35.

Marchi, V., 1882. Ueber die Terminalorgane der Nerven (Golgi's Nervenkörperchen) in den Sehnen der Augenmuskeln. Arch. Ophthalmol., 28:203–212.

Meessen, H., and J. Olszewski, 1949. A cytoarchitectonic atlas of the rhombencephalon of the rabbit. Karger, Basel and New York.

Mehler, W. R., M. E. Feferman, and W. J. H. Nauta, 1960. Ascending axon degeneration following anterolateral chordotomy. An experimental study in the monkey. Brain, 83:718–750.

Merrillees, N. C. R., S. Sunderland, and W. Hayhow, 1950. Neuromuscular spindles in extraocular muscles in man. Anat. Record, 108:23–30.

Mihalkovics, V. von, 1877. Entwicklungsgeschichte des Gehirns. Engelmann, Leipzig.

Mott, F. W., 1895. Experimental enquiry upon the afferent tracts of the central nervous system of the monkey. Brain, 18:1–20.

Mountcastle, V. B., M. R. Covian, and C. R. Harrison, 1952. The central representation of some forms of deep sensibility. Res. Publ. Assoc. Nervous Mental Disease, 30:339–370.

Murie, J., 1874. Researches on the anatomy of Pinnipedia. Part III. Descriptive anatomy of the sea-lion (*Otaria jubata*). Trans. Zool. Soc. (Lond.), 8:501–582.

Nicholson, H., 1924. On the presence of ganglion cells in the third and sixth nerves of man. J. Comp. Neurol., 37:31–36.

Nulsen, F. E., S. P. M. Black, and C. G. Drake, 1948. Inhibition and facilitation of motor activity by the anterior cerebellum. Fed. Proc., 7:86–87.

Obenchain, J. B., 1925. The brains of the South American marsupials, *Caenolestes* and *Orolestes*. Publ. Field Mus. Nat. Hist., Zool. Ser., 14:175–232.

Ogawa, T., and S. Arifuku, 1948. On the acoustic system in the cetacean brain. Sci. Rep. Whales Res. Inst. Tokyo, 2:1–20.

Olszewski, J., and D. Baxter, 1954. Cytoarchitecture of the human brain stem. Karger, Basel and New York.

Onufrowicz, B., 1885. Experimenteller Beitrag zur Kenntniss des Ursprungs des Nervus acusticus des Kaninchens. Arch. Psychiat. Nervenkrankh., 16:711–742.

Oort, H., 1918. Über die Verästelung des Nervus octavus bei Säugetieren. (Modell des Utriculus und Sacculus des Kaninchens.) Anat. Anz., 51:272–280.

Osen, K. K., and J. Jansen, 1965. The cochlear nuclei in the common porpoise, *Phocaena phocaena*. J. Comp. Neurol., 125:223–257.

Osgood, W. H., 1925. A monographic study of the American marsupial *Caenolestes*. Pub. Field. Mus. Nat. Hist., Zool. Ser., 14:1–156.

Palmer, R. S., 1954. The mammal guide. Doubleday, New York.

Pascoe, J. E., 1958. Two types of efferent fibres to the muscle spindles of the rabbit. J. Physiol. (Lond.), 143:54–55.

Pearson, A. A., 1949a. The development and connections of the mesencephalic root of the trigeminal nerve in man. J. Comp. Neurol., 90:1–46.

———, 1949b. Further observations on the mesencephalic root of the trigeminal nerve. J. Comp. Neurol., 91:147–194.

Petroff, A. E., 1955. An experimental investigation of the origin of efferent fiber projections to the vestibular neuroepithelium. Anat. Record, 121:352–353.

Pilleri, G., 1963. Zur vergleichenden Morphologie und Rangordnung des Gehirnes von Weisswal, *Delphinapterus leucas Pallas* (Cetacea, Delphinapteridae). Rev. Suisse Zool., 70:569–586.

———, 1964. Morphologie des Gehirnes des Southern Right Whale *Eubalaena australis* Desmoulins 1822 (Cetacea, Mysticeti, Balaenidae). Acta Zool. (Stockh.), 46:245–272.

———, 1966. Morphologie des Gehirnes des Seiwals, *Balaenoptera borealis* Lesson (Cetacea, Mysticeti, Balaenopteridae). J. Hirnforsch., 8:221–267.

Poljak, S., 1926. Untersuchungen am Oktavussystem der Säugetiere und an den mit diesem koordinierten motorischen Apparaten des Hirnstammes. J. Psychol. Neurol. (Lpz.), 32:170–231.

———, 1927. Über die Nervenendigungen in den vestibulären Sinnesendstellen bei den Säugetieren. Z. Anat. Entwicklungsgeschichte, 84:131–144.

Pompeiano, O., and A. Brodal, 1957a. The origin of vestibulospinal fibres in the cat. An experimental-anatomical study, with comments on the descending medial longitudinal fasciculus. Arch. Ital. Biol., 95:166–195.

———, 1957b. Spino-vestibular fibers in the cat. An experimental study. J. Comp. Neurol., 108:353–381.

Pompeiano, O., and F. Walberg, 1957. Descending connections to the vestibular nuclei. An experimental study in the cat. J. Comp. Neurol., 108:465–503.

Porta, A., 1908. I muscoli caudali e anali nei generi Pavo e Meleagri. Zool. Anz., 33:116–120.

Portmann, M., and C. Portmann, 1952. Les fibres efférentes cochléaires. Bull. Acad. Nat. Méd., 136:225–226.

Powell, T. P., and W. M. Cowan, 1962. An experimental study of the projection of the cochlea. J. Anat. (Lond.), 96:269–284.

Pupilli, G. C., and G. P. von Berger, 1956. Le risposte della corteccia cerebellare a impulsi trasmessi per le vie ottiche. Arch. Sci. Biol. (Bologna), 40:541–601.

Putnam, I. K., 1928. The proportion of cerebellar to total brain weight in mammals. Proc. Koninkl. Ned. Akad. Wetenschap., 31:1–14.

Ralston, H. J., III, M. R. Miller, and M. Kasahara, 1960. Nerve endings in human fasciae, tendons, ligaments, periosteum, and joint synovial membrane. Anat. Record, 136:137–147.

Ramon y Cajal, S., 1896. Studium der Medulla oblongata, des Kleinhirns und des Ursprungs der Gehirnnerven. Barth, Leipzig.

———, 1908. Los ganglios centrales del cerebelo de las aves. Trabajos Lab. Invest. Biol. Univ. Madrid, 6:177–194.

———, 1909. Histologie du système nerveux de l'homme et des vertébrés. Vol. 1. Maloine, Paris.

———, 1911. Histologie du système nerveux de l'homme et des vertébrés. Vol. 2. Maloine, Paris.

Rasmussen, A. T., 1932. Secondary vestibular tracts in the cat. J. Comp. Neurol., 54:143–171.

———, 1933. Origin and course of the fasciculus uncinatus (Russell) in the cat, with observations on other fiber tracts arising from the cerebellar nuclei. J. Comp. Neurol., 57:165–197.

Rasmussen, G. L., 1946. The olivary peduncle and other fiber projections of the superior olivary complex. J. Comp. Neurol., 84:141–220.

———, 1953. Further observations of the efferent cochlear bundle. J. Comp. Neurol., 99:61–74.

———, 1960. Efferent fibers of the cochlear nerve and cochlear nucleus. In G. L. Rasmussen and W. F. Windle, Neural mechanisms of the auditory and vestibular systems, pp. 105–115. Thomas, Springfield, Ill.

———, and R. R. Gacek, 1958. Concerning the question of an efferent fiber component of the vestibular nerve of the cat. Anat. Record, 130:361–362.

Rasmussen, G. L., and W. F. Windle, 1960. Neural mechanisms of the auditory and vestibular systems. Thomas, Springfield, Ill.

Reil, J. G., 1807–08. Fragmente über die Bildung des kleinen Gehirns im Menschen. Arch. Physiol., 8:1–58.

Retzius, G., 1881–84. Das Gehörorgan der Wirbelthiere. 2 vols. Samson and Wallin, Stockholm.

———, 1906. Das Affenhirn. Fischer, Jena.

Reysenbach de Haan, F. W., 1958. Hearing in whales. Acta Oto-laryngol. (Stockh.) Suppl. 134.

———, 1960. Some aspects of mammalian hearing under water. Proc. Roy. Soc. (Lond.) Ser. B., 152:54–62.

Ries, F. A., and O. R. Langworthy, 1937. A study of the surface structure of the brain of the whale (*Balaenoptera physalus* and *Physeter catadon*). J. Comp. Neurol., 68:1–47.

Rijnberk, G. van, 1908. Das Lokalisationsproblem im Kleinhirn. Ergeb. Physiol., 7:653–698.

Riley, H. A., 1929. The mammalian cerebellum. A comparative study of the arbor vitae and folial pattern. Res. Publ. Assoc. Nervous Mental Disease, 6:37–192.

Rollett, A., 1876. Ueber einen Nervenplexus und Nervenendigungen in einer Sehne. Sitzungsberichte Akad. Wiss. Wien, Math.-Nat. Kl., 7:142. (Quoted from Ariens Kappers *et al.*, 1936.)

Romer, A. S., 1955. The vertebrate body. 2nd ed. Saunders, Philadelphia and London.

Rosenthal, F. C., 1831. Zur Anatomie der Seehunde. Nova Acta Acad. Caesar. Leopoldina, 15, Abt. 2, 313–348.

Ruffini, A., 1893. Sur la terminaison nerveuse dans les fuseaux musculaires et sur leur signification physiologique. Arch. Ital. Biol., 18:106–114.

———, 1897–98. On the minute anatomy of the neuromuscular spindles of the cat and on their physiological significance. J. Physiol. (Lond.), 23:190–208.

Russell, J. S. R., 1897. The origin and destination of certain afferent and efferent tracts in the medulla oblongata. Brain, 20:409–440.

Sabin, F. R., 1897. On the anatomical relations on the nuclei of reception of the cochlear and vestibular nerves. Bull. Johns Hopkins Hosp., 8:253–259.

Saetersdal, T. A. S., 1956. On the ontogenesis of the avian cerebellum. Part I. Studies on the formation of fissures. Univ. Bergen Årb. Nat.-Vit. R., No. 2, 1–15.

Sanders, E. B., 1929. A consideration of certain bulbar, midbrain, and cerebellar centers and fiber tracts in birds. J. Comp. Neurol., 49:155–222.

Schimert, J., (or Szentágothai-Schimert), 1938. Die Endigungsweise des Tractus vestibulo-spinalis. Z. Anat. Entwicklungeschichte, 108:761–767.

Scholten, J. M., 1946. De plaats van den paraflocculus in het geheel der cerebellaire correlaties. Noord-Hollandsche Uitgevers Maatschappij, Amsterdam.

Schwalbe, G. A., 1881. Lehrbuch der Neurologie. Eduard Besold, Erlangen.

Serres, A. E. R. A., 1824–27. Anatomie comparée du cerveau dans les quatre classes des animaux vertébrés. Gabon, Paris.

Sherrington, C. S., 1894. On the anatomical constitution of nerves of skeletal muscles; with remarks on recurrent fibres in the ventral spinal nerve root. J. Physiol. (Lond.), 17:211–258.

———, 1918. Observations on the sensual role of the proprioceptive nerve-supply of the extrinsic ocular muscles. Brain, 41:332–343.

Shute, C. C. D., 1951a. Nervous pathways in developing human labyrinth. J. Anat. (Lond.), 85:359–369.

———, 1951b. The anatomy of the eighth cranial nerve in man. Proc. Roy. Soc. Med., 44:1013–1018.

Sisson, S., and J. D. Grossman, 1953. The anatomy of domestic animals. Saunders, Philadelphia.

Smith, C. A., 1956. Microscopic structure of the utricle. Ann. Otol. Rhinol. Laryngol., 65:450–469.

———, and G. L. Rasmussen, 1963. Recent observations on the olivo-cochlear bundle. Ann. Otol. Rhinol. Laryngol., 72:489–506.

Smith, G. E., 1899. The brain in the Edentata. Trans. Linnean Soc. Lond., Sec. Ser., 7:277–394.

———, 1902. The primary subdivision of the mammalian cerebellum. J. Anat. (Lond.), 36:381–385.

———, 1903a. Notes on the morphology of the cerebellum. J. Anat. (Lond.), 37:329–332.

———, 1903b. Further observations of the natural mode of subdivision of the mammalian cerebellum. Anat. Anz., 23:368–384.

———, 1903c. On the morphology of the brain in the mammalia. The cerebellum. Trans. Linnean Soc. Lond., Sec. Ser., 8:425–432.

———, 1903d. The morphology of the human cerebellum. Rev. Neurol. Psychiat., 1:629–639.

Snider, R. S., 1943. A fifth cranial nerve projection to the cerebellum. Fed. Proc., 2:46.

———, and A. Stowell, 1942. Evidence of a representation of tactile sensibility in the cerebellum of the cat. Fed. Proc., 1:82–83.

———, 1944. Receiving areas of the tactile, auditory, and visual systems in the cerebellum. J. Neurophysiol., 7:331–358.

Steg, G., 1962. Efferent fibres of the rat tail muscles. Intern. Congr. Physiol. Sci., 12th, Leiden.

Stilling, B., 1864–67. Untersuchungen über den Bau des kleinen Gehirns des Menschen. 2 Bd. Krieger, Cassel.

———, 1878. Neue Untersuchungen über den Bau des kleinen Gehirns des Menschen. Untersuchungen über den Bau des Bergs und der vorderen Oberlappen. Theodor Fischer, Cassel.

Stokes, J. H., 1912. The acoustic complex and its relations in the brain of the opossum (*Didelphys virginiana*). Amer. J. Anat., 12:401–445.

Stowell, A., and R. S. Snider, 1942a. Projection of an auditory pathway to the cerebellum of the cat. Anat. Record, 82:491.

———, 1942b. Evidence of a representation of auditory sensibility in the cerebellum of the cat. Fed. Proc., 1:84.

Stroud, B. B., 1895. The mammalian cerebellum. J. Comp. Neurol., 5:71–118.

———, 1897. A preliminary account of the comparative anatomy of the cerebellum. Proc. Assoc. Amer. Anat.

Swan, J., 1835. Illustrations of the comparative anatomy of the nervous system. London.

Swett, J. E., and E. Eldred, 1960a. Distribution and numbers of stretch receptors in medial gastrocnemius and soleus muscles of the cat. Anat. Record, 137:453–460.

———, 1960b. Comparisons in structure of stretch receptors in medial gastrocnemius and soleus of the cat. Anat. Record, 137:461–473.

Szentágothai-Schimert, J., 1941. Die Bedeutung des Faserkalibers und der Markscheidendicke im Zentralnervensystem. Z. Anat. Entwicklungsgeschichte, 111:201–223.

———. See also Schimert

Tello, J. F., 1906. Terminaciones en los músculos estriados. Trabajos Lab. Invest. Biol. Univ. Madrid, 4:104–114.

———, 1909. Contribución al conocimiento del encéfalo de los teleósteos. Los núcleos bulbares. Trabajos Lab. Invest. Biol. Univ. Madrid, 7:1–29.

———, 1917. Genesis de las terminaciones nerviosas motrices y sensitivas. Trabajos Lab. Invest. Biol. Univ. Madrid, 15:101–199.

———, 1940. Histogenèse du cervelet et ses voies chez la souris blanche. Trabajos Inst. Cajal Invest. Biol., 32:1–72.

Thiele, F. H., and V. Horsley, 1901. A study of the degenerations observed in the central nervous system in a case of fracture dislocation of the spine. Brain, 24:519–531.

Thomas, D. H., R. P. Kaufman, J. M. Sprague, and W. W. Chambers, 1956. Experimental studies of the vermal cerebellar projections in the brain stem of the cat (fastigiobulbar tract). J. Anat. (Lond.), 90:371–384.

Tiedemann, F., 1816. Anatomie und Bildungsgeschichte des Gehirns im Foetus des Menschen.

———, 1821. Icones cerebri simiarum et quorundam mammalium rariorum. Mohr and Winter, Heidelberg.

———, 1837. Das Hirn des Negers mit dem des Europäers und Orang-Outangs verglichen. Winter, Heidelberg.

Torvik, A., 1956. Transneuronal changes in the inferior olive and pontine nuclei in kittens. J. Neuropath. Exptl. Neurol., 15:119–145.

Tozer, F. M., 1912. On the presence of ganglion cells in the roots of III, IV and VI cranial nerves. J. Physiol. (Lond.), 45:15–16.

Treviranus, G. R., 1822. Biologie, oder Philosophie der lebenden Natur, für Naturforscher und Aerzte. Bd 6. Göttingen.

Troughton, E. L., 1947. Furred animals of Australia. Scribner, New York.

Tsai, C., 1925. The optic tracts and centers of the opossum, *Didelphis virginiana*. J. Comp. Neurol., 39:173–216.

Versteegh, C., 1927. Ergebnisse partieller Labyrinthextirpation bei Kaninchen. Acta Oto-laryngol. (Stockh.), 11:393–408.

Vicq d'Azyr, F., 1786–90. Traite d'anatomie. Paris.

Voit, M., 1907. Zur Frage der Verästelung des Nervus acusticus bei den Säugetieren. Anat. Anz., 31:635–640.

Voris, H. C., and N. L. Hoerr, 1932. The hindbrain of the opossum, *Didelphis virginiana*. J. Comp. Neurol., 54:277–355.

Voss, H., 1937. Untersuchungen über Zahl, Anordnung und Lange der Muskelspindeln in den Lumbricalmuskeln des Menschen und einiger Tiere. Z. Mikr.-Anat. Forsch., 42:509–524.

Vraa-Jensen, G., 1956. On the correlation between the function and structure of nerve cells. Acta Psychiat. Scand., Suppl. 109:1–96.

Walberg, F., and J. Jansen, 1961. Cerebellar corticovestibular fibers in the cat. Exptl. Neurol., 3:32–52.

Walberg, F., D. Bowsher, and A. Brodal, 1958. The termination of primary vestibular fibers in the vestibular nuclei in the cat. An experimental study with silver methods. J. Comp. Neurol., 110:391–419.

Walberg, F., O. Pompeiano, A. Brodal, and J. Jansen, 1962. The fastigiovestibular projection in the cat. An experimental study with silver impregnation methods. J. Comp. Neurol., 118:49–75.

von Waldeyer, W., 1891. Das Gibbon-Hirn. Internationale Beiträge zur Wissenschaftlichen Medizin. 1:1–40 (Festschrift, R. Virchow), Hirschwald, Berlin.

Walker, L. B., 1958. Diameter spectrum of intrafusal fibers in muscle spindles of the dog. Anat. Record, 130:385.

Wallenberg, A., 1898. Die secundäre Acusticusbahn der Taube. Anat. Anz., 14:353–369.

Weinberg, E., 1928. The mesencephalic root of the fifth nerve. A comparative anatomical study. J. Comp. Neurol., 46:249–405.

Wenderowič, E., and B. Klossowsky, 1932. Über die efferenten Fasern im Bestande des Nervus vestibularis bei der Katze. Z. Anat. Entwicklungsgeschichte, 98:314–326.

Wenzel, J., and C. Wenzel, 1812. De penitiori structura cerebri hominis et brutorum. Apud Cottam, Tübingen.

Wersäll, J., 1954. The minute structure of the crista ampullaris in the guinea pig as revealed by the electron microscope. Acta Oto-laryngol. (Stockh.), 44:359–369.

———, 1956. Studies on the structure and innervation of the sensory epithelium of the cristae ampullares in the guinea pig.

A light and electron microscopic investigation. Acta Oto-laryngol. (Stockh.) Suppl., 126:1–85.
———, 1960. Electron micrographic studies of vestibular hair cell innervation. In G. L. Rasmussen and W. F. Windle, Neural mechanisms of the auditory and vestibular systems, pp. 247–257. Thomas, Springfield, Ill.
———, H. Engström, and S. Hjorth, 1954. Fine structure of the guinea-pig macula utriculi. A preliminary report. Acta Oto-laryngol. (Stockh.), Suppl. 116:298–303.
Weston, J. K., 1936. The reptilian vestibular and cerebellar gray with fiber connections. J. Comp. Neurol., 65:93–200.
———, 1938. Observations on the distribution of ganglion cells and fibers related to the saccule and the basal coil of the cochlea. Acta Neerl. Morphol., 1:136–150.
———, 1939. Notes on the comparative anatomy of the sensory areas of the vertebrate inner ear. J. Comp. Neurol., 70:355–394.
Whitlock, D. G., 1952. A neurohistological and neurophysiological study of afferent fiber tracts and receptive areas of the avian cerebellum. J. Comp. Neurol., 97:567–635.
Wilson, R. B., 1933. The anatomy of the brain of the whale (*Balaenoptera sulfurea*). J. Comp. Neurol., 58:419–480.
Winkler, C., 1907. The central course of the nervus octavus and its influence on motility. Verhandl. Koninkl. Ned. Akad. Wetenschap., Sect. II, 14:1–202.
———, and A. Potter, 1911. An anatomical guide to experimental researches on the rabbit's brain. Versluys, Amsterdam.
———, 1914. An anatomical guide to experimental researches on the cat's brain. Versluys, Amsterdam.
Wolter, J. R., 1955. Morphology of sensory nerve apparatus in striated muscle of human eye. Arch. Ophthalmol., 53:201–207.
Yee, J., and K. B. Corbin, 1939. The intramedullary course of the upper five, cervical, dorsal root fibers in the rabbit. J. Comp. Neurol., 70:297–314.
Ziehen, T., 1897. Das Centralnervensystem der Monotremen und Marsupialier. Teil I. Makroskopische Anat. Jena. Denkschr., 6:168–187.
———, 1899. Centralnervensystem. In Bardelebens Handbuch der Anatomie des Menschen. Bd 1, 1. Abt., pp. 1–576. Fischer, Jena.
———, 1901. Ueber die Furchen und Lappen des Kleinhirns bei Echidna. Maandschr. Psychiat. Neurol., 10:143–149.
———, 1903. Centralnervensystem. In Bardelebens Handbuch der Anatomie des Menschen. Bd 4, 1. Abt., pp. 403–501. Fischer, Jena.
———, 1934a. Mikroskopische Anatomie des Gehirns. In Bardelebens Handbuch der Anatomie des Menschen. Bd 4, 2. Abt., pp. 863–1546. Fischer, Jena.
———, 1934b. Beiträge zur vergleichenden Anatomie des Kleinhirns. Anat. Anz., 78:182–187.

INDEX